# OFFICE UROLOGY
## *THE CLINICIAN'S GUIDE*

---

Compliments
of
**sanofi~synthelabo**

Sanofi-Synthelabo Inc. New York, NY 10016

---

© Sanofi-Synthelabo Inc.
47-020089

# CURRENT CLINICAL UROLOGY

Eric A. Klein, SERIES EDITOR

***Prostate Cancer Screening*** edited by **Ian M. Thompson, Martin I. Resnick, and Eric A. Klein,** 2001

***Bladder Cancer:*** *Current Diagnosis and Treatment,* edited by **Michael J. Droller,** 2001

***Office Urology:*** *The Clinician's Guide,* edited by **Elroy D. Kursh and James C. Ulchaker,** 2001

***Voiding Dysfunction:*** *Diagnosis and Treatment,* edited by **Rodney A. Appell,** 2000

***Management of Prostate Cancer,*** edited by **Eric A. Klein,** 2000

# Office Urology

## *The Clinician's Guide*

*Edited by*

# Elroy D. Kursh, MD
*and*
# James C. Ulchaker, MD
*Cleveland Clinic Foundation, Cleveland, OH*

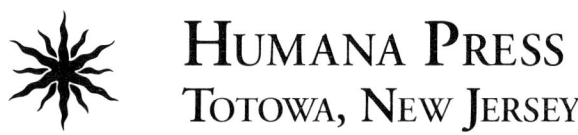

Humana Press
Totowa, New Jersey

© 2001 Humana Press Inc.
999 Riverview Drive, Suite 208
Totowa, New Jersey 07512

For additional copies, pricing for bulk purchases, and/or information about other Humana titles, contact Humana at the above address or at any of the following numbers: Tel: 973-256-1699; Fax: 973-256-8341; E-mail: humana@humanapr.com or visit our Website at http://humanapress.com

All rights reserved. No part of this book may be reproduced, stored in a retrieval system, or transmitted in any form or by any means, electronic, mechanical, photocopying, microfilming, recording, or otherwise without written permission from the Publisher.

All articles, comments, opinions, conclusions, or recommendations are those of the author(s), and do not necessarily reflect the views of the publisher.

Due diligence has been taken by the publishers, editors, and authors of this book to assure the accuracy of the information published and to describe generally accepted practices. The contributors herein have carefully checked to ensure that the drug selections and dosages set forth in this text are accurate and in accord with the standards accepted at the time of publication. Notwithstanding, as new research, changes in government regulations, and knowledge from clinical experience relating to drug therapy and drug reactions constantly occurs, the reader is advised to check the product information provided by the manufacturer of each drug for any change in dosages or for additional warnings and contraindications. This is of utmost importance when the recommended drug herein is a new or infrequently used drug. It is the responsibility of the treating physician to determine dosages and treatment strategies for individual patients. Further it is the responsibility of the health care provider to ascertain the Food and Drug Administration status of each drug or device used in their clinical practice. The publisher, editors, and authors are not responsible for errors or omissions or for any consequences from the application of the information presented in this book and make no warranty, express or implied, with respect to the contents in this publication.

This publication is printed on acid-free paper. ∞

ANSI Z39.48-1984 (American National Standards Institute)
Permanence of Paper for Printed Library Materials.

Cover design by Patricia F. Cleary.

Cover illustration:

**Photocopy Authorization Policy:**
Authorization to photocopy items for internal or personal use, or the internal or personal use of specific clients, is granted by Humana Press Inc., provided that the base fee of US $10.00 per copy, plus US $00.25 per page, is paid directly to the Copyright Clearance Center at 222 Rosewood Drive, Danvers, MA 01923. For those organizations that have been granted a photocopy license from the CCC, a separate system of payment has been arranged and is acceptable to Humana Press Inc. The fee code for users of the Transactional Reporting Service is: [0-89603-789-4/01 $10.00 + $00.25].

Printed in the United States of America. 10 9 8 7 6 5 4 3 2

Library of Congress Cataloging-in-Publication Data

Office urology: the clinician's guide/edited by Elroy D. Kursh and James C. Ulchaker.
    p.;cm.—(Current clinical urology)
  Includes bibliographical references and index.
  ISBN 0-89603-789-4 (alk. paper)
  1. Urinary organs—Diseases. 2. Urology. 3. Ambulatory medical care. I. Kursh, Elroy D. II. Ulchaker, James C. III. Series.
  [DNLM: 1. Urology. 2. Urologic Diseases—diagnosis. 3. Urologic Diseases—therapy. WJ 100 O32 2000]
  RC871.O36 2000
  616.6—dc21
                                                                                                00-033560

# Preface

Although urology is a surgical specialty, it has become apparent that changes in health care delivery and financing have led to an increasing volume of care being provided by urologists in their offices. A major part of the revenue of a urology practice depends on office production and efficient management. To have a successful practice, the productive, committed urologist must have a thorough understanding of the procedures and problems that need to be dealt with in the office. Moreover. the urologist must play an active role in the administration and business aspects of running the office. Surprisingly, very little has been written about the office practice of urology.

*Office Urology: The Clinician's Guide* presents a fresh, practical, and concise textbook covering the vital issues that the urologist must face on a daily basis in the office. The initial chapters of the textbook cover the critical aspects of managing the urologic office, such as principles of management, marketing the practice, proper billing and coding, advanced information systems, and important legal issues. The book is not intended to review in detail the academic aspects of the various pathologies pertaining to urology, which have been well covered in several other textbooks. Instead, the clinical chapters deal with practical issues, such as selecting appropriate treatment and counseling patients on the optimal therapy for the problems that the urologist frequently manages. The individual authors have demonstrated expertise in their fields. They provide practical information about their respective subjects, with references limited to only the most important sources. Individual chapters cover the diagnostic procedures or treatments that are specifically done, or are now being done more often, in the office, such as intravesical therapy for bladder cancer, minimally invasive treatment of benign prostatic obstruction, transrectal ultrasound and prostate biopsy, and office urodynamics. The chapter on practical dermatology for the urologist is very thorough and well-illustrated, making it an extremely handy reference. *Office Urology: The Clincian's Guide* includes other subjects that are not generally covered in urology textbooks, such as genital pain and managing incontinence in the geriatric patient. We believe there is no single comprehensive textbook in urology dealing with all of the topics covered in *Office Urology: The Clinician's Guide*, making it an invaluable addition to every urologist's library.

**This book is dedicated to the memory of Maxine Pollack, who bravely coauthored an invaluable chapter despite her grave illness.**

*Elroy D. Kursh,* MD
*James C. Ulchaker,* MD

*To our devoted familes,*
***Dee, Matt, Franci, Gabriella, Danielle***
*and*
***Elise, Eric, Stanley, Margaret, Margie***

# LIST OF COLOR PLATES

All color plates appear in Chapter 24, in an insert following p. 338.

**Plate 1, Fig. 1.**     Pearly penile papules.

**Plate 2, Fig. 3.**     Sclerosing lymphangitis.

**Plate 3, Fig. 4.**     Angiokeratomas of Fordyce.

**Plate 4, Fig. 5.**     Lichen sclerosis et atrophicus.

**Plate 5, Fig. 6.**     Chronic lichen sclerosis et atrophicus with foci of invasive SCC.

**Plate 6, Fig. 7.**     Balanoposthitis.

**Plate 7, Fig. 12.**     Lichen planus.

**Plate 8, Fig. 14.**     Zoon's balanitis.

**Plate 9, Fig. 16.**     Decorative tatoo of the glans.

**Plate 10, Fig. 28.**     Capillary hemangioma of glans in a child.

**Plate 11, Fig. 29.**     Capillary hemangioma of glans.

**Plate 12, Fig. 32.**     Erythroplasia of Queyrat. *In situ* SCC presenting as velvety red plaque on glans and periurethral skin.

**Plate 13, Fig. 33.**     Erythroplasia of Queyrat. *In situ* SCC of prepucial skin and glans presenting as chronically inflamed red plaque with verrucous foci.

**Plate 14, Fig. 34.**     Verrucous carcinoma.

**Plate 15, Fig. 35.**     Bowenoid papulosis.

**Plate 16, Fig. 36.**     Kaposi's sarcoma.

**Plate 17, Fig. 37.**     Extramammary Paget's disease.

**Plate 18, Fig. 38.**     Metastatic prostate carcinoma. Discrete and confluent pink papules and plaques.

**Plate 19, Fig. 39.**     Metastatic prostate carcinoma. Massive erythematous tumors and nodules.

**Plate 20, Fig. 40.**     Metastatic SCC of the lung to the scrotum.

# Contents

Preface ............................................................................................. v
List of Color Plates ........................................................................ vii
List of Contributors ...................................................................... xiii

## I  The Urologic Office ............................................................. 1

**1** Principles of Managing the Urologic Office .......................... 3
*Maxine Pollack and Jean Kouris*

**2** Marketing Your Urologic Practice Ethically, Effectively, and Economically ................................................................ 15
*Neil Baum*

**3** Proper Billing and Coding .................................................. 33
*Ray Painter*

**4** Advanced Information Systems in the Modern Physician's Office ................................................................................ 45
*Steve Gardilcic*

**5** Important Legal Issues in the Current Health-Care Environment ...................................................................... 55
*Alan E. Schabes and David M. Levine*

## II  Patient Evaluation ............................................................. 75

**6** Urologic History, Physical Examination, and Urinalysis ...... 77
*Mark R. Licht*

**7** Endoscopy and Instrumentation in the Office ..................... 89
*Steven H. Selman*

## III  Infections and Inflammation of the Genitourinary Tract ............................................ 103

**8** Evaluation and Management of Recurrent Urinary-Tract Infections ......................................................................... 105
*Howard B. Goldman*

**9** Prostatitis ........................................................................ 113
*J. Curtis Nickel*

**10** Sexually Transmitted Diseases ......................................... 121
*Jeannette M. Potts*

**11** The Diagnosis and Treatment of Interstitial Cystitis ......... 131
*Kenneth M. Peters and Ananias C. Diokno*

## IV The Renal Mass .................................................. 143

**12** Evaluation of the Renal Mass .................................................. 145
*Norm D. Smith and Steven C. Campbell*

**13** Selecting the Optimal Treatment for Localized Renal Tumors and Long-Term Follow-Up .................................................. 165
*Andrew C. Novick*

## V Bladder Tumors .................................................. 173

**14** Evaluation and Management of Low-Grade, Low-Stage Bladder Cancer .................................................. 175
*Michael J. Droller*

**15** Intravesical Therapy for Superficial Bladder Cancer: *A Practical Guide* .................................................. 185
*Michael O'Donnell*

**16** Selecting and Counseling Patients for Cystectomy or Cystoprostatectomy .................................................. 203
*James E. Montie and Robert Marcovich*

## VI Prostate—Benign .................................................. 213

**17** Evaluation of Lower Urinary-Tract Symptoms .................................................. 215
*Rasmus H. Krogh and Reginald C. Bruskewitz*

**18** Medical Management of Benign Prostatic Obstruction .................................................. 225
*Michael J. Barry and Claus Roehrborn*

**19** The Advent of Minimally Invasive Treatments for Benign Prostatic Obstruction .................................................. 237
*Christopher S. Ng, James C. Ulchaker, and Elroy D. Kursh*

## VII Prostate—Malignant .................................................. 253

**20** Evaluation of Prostate Cancer .................................................. 255
*Robert L. Grubb III and Gerald L. Andriole*

**21** Transrectal Ultrasound and Prostate Biopsy in the Office .................................................. 265
*Christopher A. Haas and Martin I. Resnick*

**22** Selecting and Counseling Patients on Appropriate Treatment of Prostate Cancer .................................................. 277
*Faiyaaz M. Jhaveri and Eric A. Klein*

**23** Prostate Cancer: *Endocrine Therapy* .................................................. 291
*Hamed A. Daw and David M. Peereboom*

## VIII Penile Disorders .................................................. 303

**24** Practical Dermatology for the Urologist .................................................. 305
*Scott Podnos and Allison T. Vidimos*

**25** Erectile Dysfunction .................................................. 343
*Drogo K. Montague and Milton M. Lakin*

| | | | |
|---|---|---|---|
| IX | | **The Scrotal Contents** | **353** |
| | 26 | Evaluation and Management of the Scrotal Mass and Acute Scrotum | 355 |
| | | Edward E. Cherullo and James C. Ulchaker | |
| | 27 | Genital Pain | 369 |
| | | Elroy D. Kursh | |
| | 28 | A Practical Approach to Male Infertility | 381 |
| | | James A. Daitch and Anthony J. Thomas, Jr. | |
| | 29 | Elective Sterilization | 395 |
| | | Roy A. Brandell and Marc Goldstein | |
| X | | **Voiding Dysfunction** | **405** |
| | 30 | Office Urodynamics | 407 |
| | | John P. Lavelle, Michael W. Phelan, Seamus Teahan, and Michael B. Chancellor | |
| | 31 | Assessment of the Incontinent Woman | 417 |
| | | Edward J. McGuire | |
| | 32 | Selection, Treatment, and Counseling for Women with Urinary Incontinence | 431 |
| | | Kathleen C. Kobashi and Gary E. Leach | |
| | 33 | Managing Incontinence in the Geriatric Patient | 453 |
| | | Patricia S. Goode and Kathryn L. Burgio | |
| XI | | **Other Problems** | **467** |
| | 34 | Evaluation and Differential Diagnosis of Hematuria | 469 |
| | | Dimitri Kuznetsov and Charles Brendler | |
| | 35 | Evaluation and Management of Recurrent Stone Disease | 483 |
| | | Stephen J. Savage and Stevan B. Streem | |
| | 36 | Common Pediatric Problems | 495 |
| | | Jonathan H. Ross and Robert Kay | |
| Index | | | 513 |

# Contributors

GERALD L. ANDRIOLE, MD • *Division of Urologic Surgery, Washington University School of Medicine, St. Louis, MO*
MICHAEL J. BARRY, MD • *Medical Practice Evaluation Center, Massachusetts General Hospital, Boston, MA*
NEIL BAUM, MD • *Department of Urology, Tulane Medical School and Louisiana State University, New Orleans, LA*
ROY A. BRANDELL, MD • *Urology Department, New York Presbyterian Hospital, New York, NY*
CHARLES BRENDLER, MD • *Section of Urology, University of Chicago, IL*
REGINALD C. BRUSKEWITZ, MD • *Division of Urology, Clinical Science Center, University of Wisconsin Hospitals, Madison, WI*
KATHERINE L. BURGIO, PHD • *Department of Medicine, University of Alabama, Birmingham, AL*
STEVEN C. CAMPBELL, MD, PHD • *Department of Urology, Northwestern University School of Medicine, Chicago, IL*
MICHAEL B. CHANCELLOR, MD • *Department of Urology, University of Pittsburgh School of Medicine, Pittsburgh, PA*
EDWARD E. CHERULLO, MD • *Department of Urology, The Cleveland Clinic Foundation, Cleveland, OH*
HAMED A. DAW • *Department of Hematology and Medical Oncology, The Cleveland Clinic Foundation, Cleveland, OH*
ANANIAS C. DIOKNO, MD • *Department of Urology, William Beaumont Hospital, Royal Oak, MI*
MICHAEL J. DROLLER, MD • *Department of Urology, Mt. Sinai School of Medicine, New York, NY*
STEVE GARDILCIC, MD • *Mansfield, OH*
HOWARD B. GOLDMAN, MD • *Department of Urology, University Hospitals of Cleveland, OH*
MARC GOLDSTEIN, MD • *Urology Department, New York Presbyterian Hospital, New York, NY*
PATRICIA S. GOODE, MD • *Department of Medicine, University of Alabama, Birmingham, AL*
ROBERT L. GRUBB, III, MD • *Division of Urologic Surgery, Washington University School of Medicine, St. Louis, MO*
CHRISTOPHER A. HASS, MD • *Department of Urology, Case Western Reserve School of Medicine, Cleveland, OH*
FAIYAAZ M. JHAVERI, MD • *Department of Urology, The Cleveland Clinic Foundation, Cleveland, OH*
ROBERT KAY, MD • *Section of Pediatric Urology, The Cleveland Clinic Foundation, Cleveland, OH*
ERIC A. KLEIN • *Department of Urology, The Cleveland Clinic Foundation, Cleveland, OH*
KATHLEEN C. KOBASHI, MD • *Tower Urology Institute for Continence, Los Angeles, CA*
RASMUS H. KROGH, MD • *Division of Urology, Clinical Science Center, University Wisconsin Hospitals, Madison, WI*
ELROY D. KURSH, MD • *Department of Urology, The Cleveland Clinic Foundation, Cleveland, OH*
DIMITRI KUZNETSOV, MD • *Section of Urology, Pritzken School of Medicine, University of Chicago, IL*
MILTON M. LAKIN • *The Cleveland Clinic Foundation, Cleveland, OH*

JOHN P. LAVELLE, MB • *Department of Urology, University of Pittsburgh School of Medicine, Pittsburgh, PA*
GARY E. LEACH, MD • *Tower Urology Institute for Continence, Los Angeles, CA*
DAVID M. LEVINE • *Benesch, Friedlander, Coplan, and Aronoff LLP, Cleveland, OH*
MARK R. LICHT, MD • *Boca Raton, FL*
ROBERT MARCOVICH, MD • *Department of Urologic Surgery, Section of Urology, Taubman Health Care Center, University of Michigan, Ann Arbor, MI*
EDWARD J. MCGUIRE, MD • *Section of Urology, Department of Surgery, The University of Michigan Medical Center, Ann Arbor, MI*
DROGO K. MONTAGUE • *Department of Urology, The Cleveland Clinic Foundation, Cleveland, OH*
JAMES E. MONTIE, MD • *Department of Urologic Surgery, Section of Urology, Taubman Health Care Center, University of Michigan, Ann Arbor, MI*
CHRISTOPHER S. NG, MD • *Department of Urology, The Cleveland Clinic Foundation, Cleveland, OH*
J. CURTIS NICKEL, MD • *Department of Urology, Queen's University, Kingston General Hospital, Kingston, ON, Canada*
ANDREW C. NOVICK, MD • *Department of Urology, The Cleveland Clinic Foundation, Cleveland, OH*
MICHAEL O'DONNELL, MD • *Division of Urology, Beth Israel Deaconess Medical Center, Boston, MA*
RAY PAINTER, MD • *Physicians Reimbursement Systems, Denver, CO*
DAVID M. PEEREBOOM • *Department of Hematology amnd Medical Oncology, The Cleveland Clinic Foundation, Cleveland, OH*
KENNETH M. PETERS, MD • *Department of Urology, William Beaumont Hospital, Royal Oak, MI*
MICHAEL W. PHELAN, MD • *Department of Urology, University of Pittsburgh School of Medicine, Pittsburgh, PA*
SCOTT PODNOS • *Department of Urology, The Cleveland Clinic Foundation, Cleveland, OH*
MAXINE POLLACK • *Pepper Pike, OH*[‡]
JEANNETTE M. POTTS, MD • *Department of Urology, The Cleveland Clinic Foundation, Cleveland, OH*
MARTIN I. RESNICK, MD • *Department of Urology, University Hospitals, Case Western Reserve School of Medicine, Cleveland, OH*
CLAUS ROEHRBORN, MD • *Department of Urology, University of Texas Southwestern Medical Center, Dallas, TX*
JONATHAN H. ROSS, MD • *Section of Pediatric Urology, The Cleveland Clinic Foundation, Cleveland, OH*
STEVEN J. SAVAGE, MD • *Department of Urology, The Cleveland Clinic Foundation, Cleveland, OH*
ALAN E. SCHABES • *Benesch, Friedlander, Coplan, and Aronoff LLP, Cleveland, OH*
STEVEN H. SELMAN, MD • *Department of Urology, Medical College of Ohio, Toledo, OH*
NORM D. SMITH, MD • *Department of Urology, Northwestern University School of Medicine, Chicago, IL*
STEVAN B. STREEM, MD • *Department of Urology, The Cleveland Clinic Foundation, Cleveland, OH*
SEAMUS TEHAN, MB • *Department of Urology, University of Pittsburgh School of Medicine, Pittsburgh, PA*
JAMES C. ULCHAKER, MD • *Department of Urology, The Cleveland Clinic Foundation, Cleveland, OH*
ALLISON T. VIDIMOS • *Department of Urology, The Cleveland Clinic Foundation, Cleveland, OH*

[‡]*Deceased*

# I THE UROLOGIC OFFICE

# 1 Principles of Managing the Urologic Office

*Maxine Pollack, MA†*
*and Jean Kouris, CPC*

**CONTENTS**

ORGANIZING YOUR PRACTICE
HIRE QUALITY STAFF
PROVIDE TRAINING AND GIVE FEEDBACK
BUILD A CULTURE OF PATIENT SATISFACTION
LEAD IN THE VISION
SELECTED READING

Running a medical practice today has become increasingly complex. Our work as consultants confirms what the research suggests: physicians expect their staff to be knowledgeable and well-trained, to possess excellent problem-solving skills, and to be able to function independently. Unfortunately, the staff does not always have the necessary tools or support from management to meet these expectations.

In this chapter our goal is to familiarize you with the main themes of a well-run practice:

- Organizing the practice;
- Hiring quality staff;
- Providing training and giving feedback;
- Building a culture of patient satisfaction; and
- Leading in the vision.

Most importantly, we hope to highlight the significant role you—the physician—play in the successful management of your practice.

We have provided you with sample job descriptions, an example of an organizational chart, interview questions, standards governing many aspects of the practice, and an outline of what a personnel policy and performance appraisal should contain.

This is just the beginning. We encourage you to explore additional resources that will expand on these topics and provide you with the tools that you and your staff need to accomplish what we recommend.

† Deceased.
From: *Current Clinical Urology: Office Urology: The Clinician's Guide*
Edited by: E. D. Kursh and J. C. Ulchaker © Humana Press Inc., Totowa, NJ

# ORGANIZING YOUR PRACTICE

## *Develop a Policy and Procedure Manual*

The first goal of the practice is to create a structure that will support the staff and give them a clear understanding of the practice's mission and purpose. This is accomplished through the development of policies and procedures.

Part of the process of developing policies and procedures is to be clear about who you are, what you do, and where you are going. Remember that your strongest competition is your own reputation—what people remember about your service. In order to excel, you must redefine your practice activities in terms of service to your patients.

The goals of a policy and procedure manual are:

- To reflect practice philosophy;
- To inform employees of regulations and expectations;
- To provide support for supervisors who must maintain operational standards;
- To minimize tension and confusion by providing consistent structure; and
- To define expectations and boundaries of the employment relationship.

Individuals need to know how their work contributes to the organization's goals. The policy and procedure manual will help to align practice activities, provide information about expectations, and help ensure that the goals of the practice are being met. Written policies help to provide consistency and structure, which the staff can rely on in their job functions.

### Factors to Consider When Developing Policies

A team approach to policy development results in better buy-in and commitment. When physicians, administrators, and staff work together, a variety of perspectives and needs are represented. Staff will be more invested in the success of the policies when their ideas are valued in policy development.

Staff meetings are a good vehicle for the development of policies and procedures. Be sure the policy manual includes a statement addressing how policies and procedures will be monitored and when they will be updated. Review the policies regularly to ensure that changing practice needs are addressed.

## *Developing Standards for Your Practice*

Standards provide a benchmark against which to measure the success of your practice policies. They help to determine whether the policies are being followed, and whether they are effective at accomplishing the practice goals.

Like policies, standards must be developed with input and cooperation from every member of the staff. Standards must be developed with one purpose in mind—meeting the needs and expectations of the patients. The following sections list suggested standards for various office procedures.

### Telephones

- All calls should be answered in three rings or fewer.
- The receptionist should identify the practice by name, and give his or her first name.
- No callers should be put on hold until they have been greeted properly, and asked whether they mind holding.

- Patients should not remain on hold for more than 30 seconds, except when the receptionist is on another call.
- Patients should wait no longer than two hours for a return call from the practice.
- There should be no complaints about lost or forgotten messages.
- There should be no more than two complaints per month about telephone procedures.

**Scheduling**

- No patient should wait more than seven days for an appointment.
- New patients should be seen within three days.
- There should be no more than two complaints per month about scheduling procedures.

**Patient Reception**

- All patients should be greeted by name within 30 seconds of their arrival.
- The reception area and lobby should be kept clean and neat at all times.

**Waiting Time**

- No patient should wait more than 15 minutes from the scheduled appointment time to see the doctor.
- If there is a change in the schedule, patients should be notified immediately upon arrival and given the option to reschedule or come back later in the day.
- There should be no patient complaints about waiting time.

## *Personnel Policies*

The personnel policy manual is the second important document to be developed. It will help staff understand their employment relationship with the practice and will provide support for supervisors. Every employee should be given a copy of this manual.

Personnel policies should address:

- **Philosophy, goals, and history of the practice:** This sets the tone for values and goals of the practice.
- **Employment policies:** Covers general issues, such as recruitment and hiring, orientation and training, and employee conduct.
- **Wage, salary, and bonus policy:** Defines full-time vs. part-time employment, work week, overtime policy, bonuses, profit-sharing and other incentives, and salary schedule and review procedures.
- **Time-off benefits:** Outlines the situations when employees may take time off: vacations, sick days, personal days, holidays, bereavement, leave of absence, family leave, disability, and jury duty. Also identifies which circumstances are paid and which are not paid. Develops a policy about carrying over unused benefits from one year to another. Reimbursement for continuing education should also be addressed here.
- **Health and related benefits:** Defines medical, dental, disability, and life insurance coverage for employees. Policy should also address pension and educational assistance plans.
- **Performance appraisals:** The policy defines how often and when appraisals will be conducted. We recommend annual appraisals in a one-to-one meeting format.
- **Termination and resignation:** Policies must be developed carefully, with legal guidance.

Personnel policies and procedures are affected by both federal and state laws which govern many aspects of the employer-employee relationship. All policies should be reviewed by your attorney.

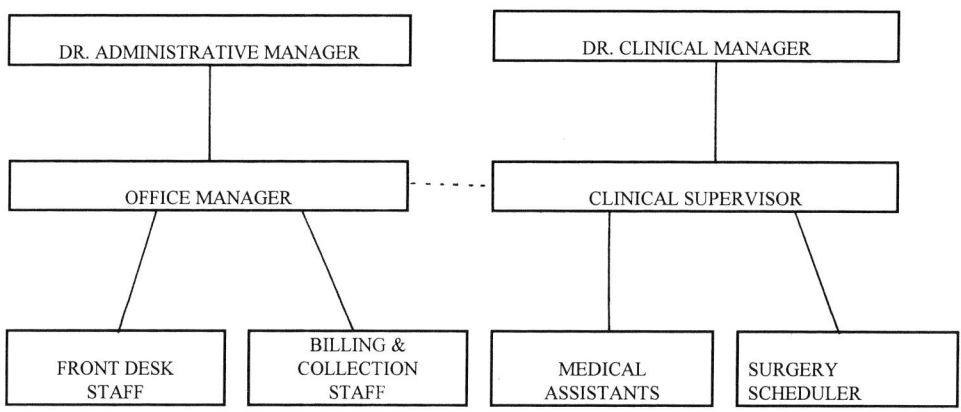

**Fig. 1.** Sample organizational chart.

## *Developing an Organizational Chart and Job Descriptions*

Once policies and procedures have been defined, the next step is to delineate each staff member's job responsibility and authority. The organizational chart (Fig. 1) defines levels of decision-making, responsibility, and accountability; promotes consistency of policy; discourages favoritism; minimizes inappropriate judgments; limits political infighting; and encourages two-way communication.

### Job Descriptions

An effective job description includes a written definition of the position with skills required, primary duties (performed daily), and secondary duties (performed occasionally). Include standards for each duty. For example, the duty is to answer the phone; the standard is to do so by the third ring. Clearly define reporting and authority boundaries.

**Sample Job Description**
**Position:** Receptionist
**Position Requires:**
1. High-school diploma
2. Medical office experience
3. Good communication skills
4. Basic computer and typing skills

| Primary Duties | Standards |
|---|---|
| 1. Answer telephones and direct calls | All calls will be answered by the third ring, in compliance with the telephone policy. |
| | All calls will be returned within two hours. |
| | A permanent log will be kept for all phone calls. |
| 2. Make appointments for patients. | Patients will be given the first available appointment, according to the scheduling policy |
| | All new patients will be given practice information as defined in the policy manual. |
| 3. Greet patients. | All patients will be greeted promptly, as defined in the policy manual. |
| | Patients will be notified of schedule delays by telephone when possible, or immediately upon arrival at the office. |

All billing and insurance information will be verified at each visit.

| Secondary Duties | Standards |
|---|---|
| 1. Type correspondence. | Completed promptly, as needed. |
| 2. Provide back-up support for other staff members. | Familiarity with basic job tasks in case of absence or illness. |
| 3. Perform other duties and tasks as may be assigned from time to time. | Willingness to be flexible and do extra work as needed. |

Reports to office manager. No supervisory responsibility.

## HIRE QUALITY STAFF

### *Recruiting and Interviewing*

Clearly the staff in a medical practice plays a critical role in carrying out its mission. Understanding the needs of the practice, based on job description is the first step in recruiting quality employees. Remember that skills can be taught, but attitude and personality cannot. A team player who needs additional training may be a far more valuable asset to your practice than one who has better training and skills but is less flexible.

Assessing the skills of a candidate can be difficult. The interviewer should focus on the needs of the practice, and should ask open-ended questions to elicit the most meaningful responses. When evaluating prior work experience, be specific, such as "Describe how you did. . ." or "Explain why it is important to. . ." It may also be helpful to interview prospective employees more than once to avoid an exaggerated focus on first impressions.

Give the candidate information about the practice without overwhelming her or him. Do not hide the negative aspects of the job.

#### Interview Questions

Federal discrimination laws affect the type of questions that can be asked during an interview. The following table gives examples of questions an interviewer may or may not ask:

| May ask. . . | May not ask. . . |
|---|---|
| 1. If hired, can you provide proof of age | What is your age? |
| 2. Nothing about race. | What is your race/color? |
| 3. Can you provide proof of employment eligibility? | What is your national origin or citizenship, or that of your spouse or parents? |
| 4. What language(s) do you speak and/or write fluently? | How did you learn a foreign language? |
| | Is it your native tongue? |
| | What is your religion? |
| | What is your sex? |
| | What is your marital status? |
| | Where/Does your spouse work? |

| | How many children do you have? |
| | Do you have plans to have children? |
| | What are your child-care arrangements? |
| 5. Are there any physical or mental impairments that would prevent you from performing the job duties as they have been described? | Do you have any handicaps? |
| 6. Have you ever been convicted a felony? What kind? How many times? | Have you ever been arrested? For what? How many times? |

| **Closed-end questions:** | **Open-ended questions:** |
|---|---|
| 1. Do you feel you are qualified for this position? | How have your past job experiences prepared you for a position like this? |
| | What are your strengths/weaknesses? |
| 2. Do you work well under pressure? | Under what kind of conditions do you do your best work? |
| 3. Do you consider yourself a leader? | In groups, do you naturally emerge as a leader? Describe such a situation. |
| 4. Are you ambitious? | How do you define success? |
| 5. Do you get along well with others? | Tell me about two significant interpersonal problems you have had on the job. |
| | Describe your best/worst boss. |
| 6. Are you a good decision maker? | Describe the methods you use to make decisions. |
| 7. Do you take criticism well? | Describe some situations in which you have been criticized. How did you respond, and why? |
| 8. Are you satisfied with your current state of professional development? | What would you like to be doing one year from now? Five years from now? |
| 9. Are you interested in this job? | Why are you interested in this job? |
| 10. May I contact your references? | What do you think your references will tell me when I call to inquire about your past employment? |

Be sure to verify references of all potential employees. Objective information is sometimes difficult to obtain, as previous employers may be concerned about legal repercussions. Have interviewees sign a release of information form to mail to former employers. It is also important to verify that potential employees have not been excluded from participation in federally funded patient care for noncompliant activities in the past.

## PROVIDE TRAINING AND GIVE FEEDBACK

### *Orientation and Training*

Too often in medical practices, sufficient time is not set aside for proper orientation and training. This is a great disservice to the practice, as the front line is the bottom line. Management knows 7%–9% of what is going on and middle-management knows 30%–40%. Those in the front line know 100%, and they are your most important resource.

If you spend time helping the staff to understand the practice goals, and provide the tools and techniques required to succeed at those goals, you will make major strides toward a successful practice.

Employee training can take several forms. Staff may be trained by others in the practice who have expertise in a particular area, or may be sent to workshops offered by local resources, such as insurers or hospitals. These focused training sessions are invaluable tools for keeping your staff up to date with changing requirements.

Training should be an ongoing part of the practice, and not limited to new employees. Keeping the skills of the staff current is the only way to ensure that you are meeting the changing needs of patients, payers, and the practice. The payoffs of a well-thought-out training program include increased staff loyalty, better individual and organizational performance, increased job satisfaction, and less staff turnover.

### *Supervision and Performance Appraisals*

Supervision requires monitoring the employee's performance as it relates to the goals of the practice. Effective supervision provides valuable feedback to the employee about job expectations, accomplishments, and needed improvements. The supervisor uses the performance appraisal as a tool to provide feedback to the employee about his or her ability to meet practice objectives.

The performance appraisal may take a number of formats, ranging from subjective essays to weighted checklists based on objective standards. A simple objective format is the employee job description with its corresponding standards. Adding a second segment focusing on general behavioral expectations completes a simple but highly effective appraisal format. The following is a list of standards for evaluating general behavior and conduct:

- Exhibits respect for self, others, and the practice.
- Communicates a general feeling of goodwill.
- Conveys a supportive, positive attitude toward patients.
- Works in cooperation with other staff so work is done efficiently with minimal friction.
- Is willing to accept supervisor's direction.
- Accepts assigned work tasks.
- Demonstrates good judgement.
- Completes tasks in the time allotted.
- Maintains patient confidentiality.

A core element of the evaluation process is asking the employee to use the form for self-appraisal one week prior to the scheduled meeting. This will better ensure that the meeting becomes an interactive discussion about successes, meeting or exceeding practice expectations, and any needed improvements.

Hold the meeting in a confidential setting free of interruptions, and create an atmosphere that welcomes open discussion. The most positive outcome of this session is that it becomes a learning tool, helping the employee and supervisor to develop a plan for future improvement and growth. The plan should include *any and all* necessary support and resources from the practice to ensure that the employee can be successful.

Be sure to evaluate employee challenges fully and objectively. Research has shown that 85% of employee difficulties are a result of some inefficiency or inequity in the system, and only 15% are under the employee's direct control. Be creative and flexible in solving problems. For example, solutions may be as simple as a later start time to accommodate the arrival of a babysitter, or as complex as redefining an employee's job responsibilities.

## *Discipline and Termination*

Employees who are unable to succeed despite all attempts, or continue to have disciplinary problems, require dismissal. Although termination of employment is not a pleasant task, it is essential to overall staff morale. A poor performer puts a drain on everyone's attitude and work and gives the message that management ignores problems.

It is essential to document employee behavior, management's attempts at intervention, and lack of progress in the personnel file. Well-documented behavior leading up to dismissal will help avoid unemployment liability and protect against lawsuits.

Recommendations for a dismissal meeting are:

- Hold the meeting in a private place.
- Limit discussion to a maximum of 10 minutes.
- Request signatures from all parties involved.
- Explain the procedure for collecting the final paycheck and compensation for any earned benefits.
- Explain COBRA policies.
- Allow the employee to express opinions and emotions without prolonging the meeting.
- Accompany the employee to his or her desk, request keys, and escort him or her out of the office.

## BUILD A CULTURE OF PATIENT SATISFACTION

Changes in societal expectations have required a fundamental shift from the physician and the medical practice to the *people* the practice serves. Physicians have traditionally relied on their clinical expertise to keep patients coming back, but today's medical practice must also meet or exceed the expectations of its patients. This means that performance that encourages patient satisfaction and retention is the responsibility of everyone in the practice.

Research has shown that patients want:

- Access—to be seen within two weeks.
- Short waiting time—not longer than 20 minutes.
- A friendly and helpful environment.
- Attentive and responsive providers.
- To walk out with a treatment plan, written instructions or information.
- Test results in a timely manner.
- Simple billing procedures and up-front identification of out-of-pocket costs.
- Clear, easy-to-understand information about practice procedures.

Patients expect high-quality medical care, but are generally unable to determine what that is. What they do know is how they were treated during the medical encounter. This perception directly affects how a patient rates the quality of care. In other words, a negative experience with any aspect of the practice may influence the patient's perception of the quality of care. *From a patient's perspective, being treated as an individual is often more important than getting well.*

The payoff is large when patients feel that their needs are taken into consideration. Satisfied patients are loyal, are compliant with treatment, and pay their bills on time. Compliance improves the chances for a successful course of treatment, which further increases patient satisfaction and retention. Patient referrals increase. Malpractice claims decrease. Staff morale increases with personal and professional fulfillment, which decreases turnover. Creating a culture that promotes patient satisfaction is an absolute win-win situation for any practice.

Clear communication with patients is a core element of patient satisfaction. Patients who know what to expect feel a greater sense of control. Their attitudes are generally more positive, and they are more trusting of the physician/patient relationship.

### *Does the Patient Come First?*

The message a practice gives to patients begins with the first encounter and is carried on through every aspect of the practice—from the office design to the way the staff greets the patients and how follow-up care is provided.

Does the environment adequately represent your practice? The environment should be comfortable and welcoming, and contribute to good patient flow. Privacy and confidentiality are two areas where many practices fall short. Walking through the practice as if you were a patient and holding a staff meeting in your waiting room are two ways to evaluate your office from the patient's perspective.

Do patients routinely feel that they are intruding on a busy day at the practice? Do the practice hours and schedule fit patient needs, such as evening and Saturday hours? Are patients put on hold indefinitely? Are calls returned only at staff convenience? Does the patient feel valued?

A simple but impactful first encounter would include sending a Welcome Package to every new patient, which would include a personal welcoming letter; a practice brochure containing the physician's name, photo, and biographical information; an appointment card identifying the date, time, and physician for the appointment; a map and parking instructions; and registration and medical history forms.

Developing a policy to meet the needs of the new patient will help the patient feel appreciated before the first visit, and there are many significant payoffs for the practice as well. The patient feels commited to the practice and is less likely to no-show, and unnecessary calls into the practice are reduced because you have provided the patient with all necessary information.

Experience has shown that developing policies that take the needs of the patient into consideration increases practice efficiency and reduces office stress, again yielding many payoffs for both the patient and the practice.

### *Telephone*

The telephone is often the first contact patients have with your practice, so make sure it is a positive one. Poor access is one of the largest sources of patient complaints. Sufficient staffing to answer the phones is critical; more phone lines simply increase hold times if staff are not available to answer.

A telephone receptionist can make or break the relationship with the patient, even before the first appointment. Therefore, it is imperative to develop telephone policies and provide staff with sufficient training. The receptionist must be knowledgeable about many aspects of the practice, and anticipate patient's questions.

The scheduling staff is the next point of contact with the patient. A good triage policy is important in helping the scheduling staff to feel comfortable with making important decisions for appropriate scheduling. This requires good communication among the clinical and front-desk staff with direction from the physicians.

There is often a "split" between front-desk and clinical staff, and such poor communication among staff members will negatively affect patient care and satisfaction. Development of policies such as a triage policy, with the input of all staff members, will go a long way toward developing a team among the staff.

### *Schedule*

The schedule organizes the work of the practice. It is the goal of the schedule to allow for maximum productivity while meeting the needs of the patients. This is best accomplished by creating a customized schedule that is reflective of individual physician practice patterns. The physician's attitude is the single most influential factor in the success of the schedule, and reflects the physician's priorities in patient care. Because the schedule has such a significant impact on patient satisfaction, the physician must respect the integrity of the schedule, and take care not to sabotage the efforts of the staff.

### *Patient Follow-Up*

Finally, spending some time to develop a good follow-up policy will reap many rewards. Patients appreciate written information about their condition and treatment plan. They need information about when to schedule follow-up care, and under what circumstances they should call before their scheduled appointment. It is important to provide a system of easy access for patients to receive test results and other information about their care. A recall system should be developed to monitor and schedule ongoing care.

## LEAD IN THE VISION

Most physicians have no training as managers. However, today's need for a well-run, efficient practice requires strong leadership. It is the strong leader who will create the vision for the staff, and will make sure that the values, culture, and goals of the practice are aligned. Once the staff buys into the vision, they can be motivated to take responsibility for carrying forth that mission. Leadership, therefore, is about building a culture that empowers people to take more responsibility by giving them the skills and freedom to make decisions. This requires a high level of trust and confidence between management and staff. So how do you do this?

One effective technique is to hold a half-day (or longer) staff retreat, where awareness is built, people are able to put forth their vision of the practice, and hear the vision of everybody else. This exercise, especially if facilitated by a professional, is a powerful tool to define who you are, what your practice is about, and have a powerful staff buy-in. It opens the lines of communication among everybody, from doctors to technicians, crosses boundaries, and can create a real team with a strong commitment toward the success of the practice.

Openness and communication among staff are the most important results of such a retreat, and can be maintained through staff meetings—a core management tool. As an outgrowth of the retreat, identify the highest priority problem areas in the practice, ask staff to volunteer to work on committees to address each problem, and give each committee responsibility to report back to the entire staff at a future staff meeting.

Time management is always a problem in a medical practice. Yet committed staff who feel empowered to make a difference will drop much of their resistance to doing this "extra" work. Sometimes an entire staff meeting will be taken up by a single issue that is being evaluated, and sometimes a simple report is sufficient. Allow the staff to set the agenda for the staff meetings.

As the physician leader, you must be an integral part of this process. Turning this over to your office manager will indicate to the staff that your commitment is not as full as you expect theirs to be. In order to effect change there must be strong sponsorship from you—the leader of the practice.

Physicians often fail to recognize their employees' contributions to the practice. Remember, your staff is your most important resource, and they are willing to work exceptionally hard under difficult conditions. Recognition fulfills a basic human need to be noticed and valued. Praise your staff when appropriate, and be sure to recognize their contributions.

Get to know your staff. Offer opportunities for growth in employment, pay adequately to attract and maintain the best employees, and use incentives to reward employees individually or as a group. Most importantly, be involved.

## SELECTED READING

Pollack M, Kouris J (1999) *Smart Practices: Success in Changing Environment.* Chicago: American Medical Association.

# 2 Marketing Your Urologic Practice Ethically, Effectively, and Economically

*Neil Baum,* MD

**CONTENTS**

ATTRACTING NEW PATIENTS TO YOUR PRACTICE
MARKETING TO YOUR EXISTING PATIENTS
IMPROVING PRACTICE EFFICIENCY
MARKETING THROUGH REFERRING PHYSICIANS
DOES MARKETING WORK?
SELECTED READING

Urologists often feel uncomfortable with the concept of marketing their practices. After all, doesn't that place them in the crass world of slick newspaper ads and snappy radio and TV commercials? In a word—no!

Whether you realize it or not, you have been marketing your practice since you first opened your doors. When you put your name in the Yellow Pages under the heading "Physicians and Surgeons," you are marketing your practice. When you write a timely referral letter to a primary-care physician, you are marketing to your colleagues.

Simply put, marketing is making the public and your peers aware of your services and your areas of interest and expertise in a professional and ethical manner. In this chapter, I will present many ideas on how to market your urology practice ethically and economically.

The purpose of this chapter is to provide the tools to attract patients to your practice, and to effectively and efficiently manage them from the moment they make a call for an appointment until they exit the practice, when they can share their positive experience with you and your practice.

I will provide you with turnkey materials that will make it easy for your patients and the public to learn about your areas of interest and expertise. These materials and methods can easily be implemented into your practice with your existing staff and with minimal expense. The marketing techniques outlined here are tested and ethical, and will not offend your colleagues.

From: *Current Clinical Urology: Office Urology: The Clinician's Guide*
Edited by: E. D. Kursh and J. C. Ulchaker © Humana Press Inc., Totowa, NJ

This chapter is intended to accomplish the following goals and objectives:

1. Attract new patients to your practice.
2. Increase the awareness of all your services to patients already in the practice.
3. Improve the efficiency of your practice.
4. Offer practical ideas to assist with marketing to your referring physicians and other nonmedical referral sources.
5. Offer suggestions to increase your practice's communication with managed-care plans.
6. Provide you with techniques to measure the effectiveness of your marketing plan.

What are the benefits of marketing and promoting your practice? By implementing a marketing strategy into your practice, you will ensure that nearly every patient will have a positive experience with your practice. When a patient leaves your practice feeling satisfied with their expectations exceeded, they may not return as a loyal patient. They will tell others about their experience with you and your practice, thus generating new patients to your practice. Marketing also allows you to sculpt or carve out exactly the type of practice that you would like to have and enjoy. For example, marketing allows you to focus on diseases and symptoms that will bring the patient directly to your practice without the necessity of seeing a primary-care physician and waiting for physicians to refer patients to you. Examples in a urology practice include impotence, infertility, and incontinence—the three "I's." Even in this era of managed care, where patients need to ask for permission from the gatekeeper in order to see a urologist, we can market and promote our practice directly to managed-care plans.

## ATTRACTING NEW PATIENTS TO YOUR PRACTICE

The key to attracting new patients to your practice is to become visible in the community in a positive manner. Very few of us—unless we practice in a community with no other urologists—will have the luxury of simply hanging out our shingle and waiting for the patients to knock down the door to get in. Most of us will have to create a very definite, planned strategy to let the public know who we are, where we practice, and what our areas of interest and expertise are. It is the latter—educating the public about our areas of uniqueness—that will enable us to quickly build a practice. Of course, in this era of managed care, we will have to be cost-effective, demonstrate excellent outcomes, and provide outstanding service. But first we have to motivate the patients to call the office for an appointment. There is no shortcut to accomplishing this goal or objective. The techniques are simple: We have to become public speakers and to write for local magazines and newspapers.

### *Writing Articles for Lay Publications*

How many patients or referrals did you receive when you had an article published in *The New England Journal of Medicine* or *The Journal of the American Medical Association*? Your answer, like mine, is most likely zero. Most of us enjoy seeing our name and our articles in peer-reviewed journals, but we might question whether the hundreds of hours of research, writing, and editing of a manuscript for publication is a good return on our time investment. On the other hand, writing an article for a local lay publication takes only a few hours, and the results—new patients that enter our practices—can be significant and almost immediate. For example, the article written on urinary incontinence that appeared in a senior citizens' bulletin resulted in nearly 20 new patients, 15 diagnostic evaluations, and 3 surgeries. One of the spin-offs was that five family members became patients, and seven additional patients were generated from the word-of-mouth promotion of the original 20 patients. Perhaps these statistics will whet your appetite to consider writing articles for lay magazines.

An article written by you—or about you and your practice—that appears in the lay press will increase your visibility, your credibility, and ultimately your profitability. The public grants you the label "expert" when you have something published—they are more likely to believe what you say and do if you have published it first.

**Selecting a Topic**

There is no shortage of topics in your urology practice that can be created into an article for publication in a local magazine or newspaper. If you can provide interesting information, useful advice, a human-interest story, or best of all, a celebrity who will share his or her experience, you can be assured that some publication in your community will be interested in your article.

Do some research before you select your topic. Listen to and watch the news, and note which medical stories receive national attention. Look at national women's magazines, such as *Cosmopolitan*, *Mademoiselle*, *Ladies Home Journal*, and *Self*, or *American Health* and *Men's Health*. You will find that your local print media is interested in having local experts comment on these articles or provide a local angle to a national story.

### *You Have to Pitch in Order to Publish*

The key to being published is to write a pitch or query letter to the health editor of the local paper or magazine. This is a short letter that describes the subject of your article, indicates the angle you will take, and includes some information about yourself. This query letter is the equivalent of a sales pitch.

Address the query letter to the appropriate editor. If you do not know the editor, call the newspaper and ask for the name and address of the health and science editor of the paper or magazine. Do not send it to main editor of the publication, as he/she will most likely pass it to an assistant or division editor, and your letter may not end up on the desk or in the hands of the best person to accept your article.

Most health and science editors receive dozens and sometimes hundreds of letters every day. Your query letter should be written to make a positive first impression on the editor. The letter should be a condensed version of your proposed article, with a beginning (lead), a middle, and an end. Try to find a "hook" or unique beginning to attract the editor's attention. Begin with an eye-opening statistic, such as the number of people in the community affected with the medical condition you want to describe. The next paragraph could describe the benefits of the article to the readers, and finally, conclude with your qualifications to write the article. The letter should also contain information on how the editor can reach you. Above all, limit your letter to one page. A longer letter will not impress anyone, and it probably won't even get read.

Once you have sent the query letter, you must be prepared to track it. Unless you have a news-breaking story, such as a cure for cancer or a new pill to treat impotence, a follow-up call is a necessary part of the getting-published game. In many cases your query letter will not be looked at for weeks, so you will want to find out whether the editor received the letter and had an opportunity to read it. You might consider including a self-addressed, stamped envelope with the query letter to make it easier for the editor to reply. If, when you call the editor, he or she is "still thinking about it," offer to provide additional information. Make the call short, and don't be discouraged by the abruptness of editors. Most editors are under deadline pressure, and the stress of the job is comparable to an air traffic controller or a urologist with an office full of patients trying to manage a postoperative patient in retention and a patient with a kidney stone in the emergency room. If the editor does call back, make an effort to return the call promptly. If you plan to market and promote your practice to the media, you need to inform your staff that the media should be given the same priority as an emergency-room call or a call from a referring physician. Take the call immediately or return it as soon as possible.

One caveat on query letters. Do not send out more than one query letter at a time. You do not want to be embarrassed when two editors agree to publish your article and you have to turn one of them down. This will guarantee a closed door for future articles or stories with that editor. Remember the old adage: "you won't catch one rabbit if you are trying to chase two" applies to sending out multiple query letters.

Don't forget that there are more places to publish your article or story than the local newspaper. For example, if you are targeting men with erectile dysfunction, offer to write articles for the local branch of the AARP, and even local women's groups—i.e., Junior League, church groups, service organizations, and health clubs that have newsletters. There are also many city and regional magazines that will accept articles on medical topics.

### *Writing an Article That Gets Read*

Now that the editor has agreed to publish your article, how do you write an article that will be read and will generate patients for your practice? There are several approaches you can take to accomplish this task. First, ask the editor about the length of the article. Most magazine articles are 800–1000 words. This works out to be 3 typewritten pages of double-spaced type. A newspaper article is usually a little shorter: 300–500 words.

Of course, the easiest and most expensive method is to have someone write the article for you. This easy way out is not necessary or advisable unless you have a very tight deadline to meet. One of the best ways to start writing articles for lay publications is to tape-record a conversation with a patient. You will find that what you say to one patient, and the frequently asked questions that the patient asks you, can easily be translated to the written word and will work for hundreds and hopefully thousands of readers. Usually the 3- to 5-minute discussion that you have with a patient will supply you with ample material for an article in most newspapers and magazines.

One resource for editing your article is the hospital marketing and public relations departments. They can help you write the article and can assist with the placement was well. Most hospital public relations and marketing departments know the health and science editors, and can give you the guidelines for an acceptable article.

Another resource for editing and writing is the local colleges, universities, and high-school English teachers. Professors and A-students will provide editing assistance at a very reasonable fee.

### *Getting More Mileage from Your Masterpiece*

One advantage of print media is that you can get additional marketing mileage from your articles long after they have been published. For example, the articles can be framed and hung in your reception area or examination rooms. You will find that patients are much more interested in reading articles you have written than looking at your diplomas and medical memberships on the wall. You can also make copies of the articles and send them as a bill stuffer.

Take copies of your articles to one of the copy companies (Quick Copy or Kinko's) and have a few of them laminated. The cost is minimal, and laminated articles can be placed in your reception area and examination rooms. This allows patients to read the articles while waiting for the doctor and ensures a long shelf-life for your articles. It is unlikely that anyone will remove a large laminated article from your office.

I suggest that you have the original articles placed in a bound book in the reception area. Offer to provide copies to any patient who requests them. And finally, send copies of your articles to local radio and TV stations and suggest that you be interviewed for a story on the subject. The advantage of print material is its long shelf-life compared to radio and TV appearances, which only reach those who happen to be listening or watching. Finally, consider sending copies of your articles to your referring physicians along with your referral letters and also send copies of your articles to the managed-care plans that you belong to. This lets your referring doctors and the managed-care plans know that you are well-recognized for a certain area of expertise in your community.

In most instances, the first lay article you do will be the hardest to write and take the longest time to get published. But like any skill, the more you practice, the easier it gets.

### *Getting Your Point Across—Creating Powerful Presentations Through Public Speaking*

It has been said that the human brain starts working the moment you are born and never stops until you stand up to speak in public. But that doesn't have to be the natural reaction to public speaking. There is no better way to ethically escalate your reputation than through the medium of public speaking. Unfortunately, our medical training does not provide us with the skills necessary to become good public speakers. According to the *People's Almanac Presents the Book of Lists*, "most people fear speaking before a group more than sickness and even death!" The reason that people would rather die than speak in public is that they have not had the proper training, and they are out of their comfort zone when they get up in front of a group of strangers. However, like any other skill, public speaking can be learned and with practice we can become competent, proficient, and adept at getting up in front of others and getting our point across.

Whenever possible, try to use props as well as slides. Consider using a balloon and a clothespin as an analogy to the bladder and the sphincter to demonstrate the normal physiology of the lower urinary tract. For a talk on vasectomy, you can use a rubber band and apply the hemoclips to the rubber band and then cut between the clips to demonstrate the procedure. If you are discussing the principles of lithotripsy, consider showing a large kidney stone and then a vial of the sand-like particles to demonstrate how a large stone can be reduced and passed through the urinary tract without conventional surgery.

First, you will need an audience. Where do you look? Today's public is very interested in health topics and wellness. Social, civic, and professional associations frequently offer speakers and presentations on programs that accompany their regular membership meetings. Some of the most common organizations are the League of Women Voters, the local PTA, American Association of Retired Persons, church groups, and the Junior League. Your local chamber of commerce and your hospital marketing and public relations department can furnish you with a more complete list for your community.

In contacting most civic, social, and professional organizations, there are protocols to follow. If you would like to get a speaking engagement at a group or organization, call and find out the name of the program chairperson. Inform the organization of your topic or area of expertise and let them know that you are available for a speaking engagement. Many programs are scheduled 6–12 months in advance, so take this into consideration when you contact an organization.

Before you contact the organization, decide on several presentation topics. Then send a letter to the program chairperson offering to address a topic that would be of interest to their organization. This letter is very similar to the query letter you used for a written article to an editor for a magazine or newspaper. Notice that each letter mentions: 1) your qualifications to talk on the subject, 2) the length of your talk, 3) the content of the presentation, and 4) and the intention to follow up to the chairperson with a telephone call in a few weeks. In your letter, discuss the potential benefits of your topic to the group or audience. Not only will this get the attention of the program chairperson, but it will also form the basis of your presentation. Try to picture yourself as a member of the audience. Each member of the audience will be listening to Station WIIFM or "What's In It For Me!" When you can answer that question, you will have captured the attention of the meeting planner, and ultimately of your audience. The letter should also include your curriculum vitae, any articles that you have authored on the subject, the names of other organizations for which you have spoken, or any other materials that emphasize your expertise on the subject. Make a follow-up phone call 2-3 weeks after you send your introductory letter.

**Know Your Audience**

The more you know about your audience, the better you can tailor your presentation to their needs, and the more likely it is that some members of the audience will become your patients. Before preparing your speech, ask the program chairperson for background information about your audience. It is important to know the purpose of the organization, how many people are expected to attend, how much the audience already knows about the topic, who the previous speakers were and their topics, the age range of the audience and their educational background, and possible areas of challenge or resistance if your topic is controversial. For example, a talk on sexual dysfunction would be prepared differently for women at a Junior League meeting than for a mixed audience of men and women at a civic organization or a senior citizens' group of only men.

The best way to learn about your audience and the goals and objectives of the meeting planner is to send a survey to the meeting planner. This is particularly important if you are being paid to make the presentation, since you want to be sure that you truly understand the needs and desires of the audience. For example, if you are speaking on behalf of a pharmaceutical company, give the meeting planner (often the pharmaceutical representative) the survey and ask him or her to complete the survey and return it to you or to call you on the phone and answer the questions. By using this survey you avoid embarrassing yourself or the pharmaceutical representative if you review the questions in the survey before your presentation. You will also find that the meeting planners really appreciate this courtesy.

**Preparing Your Speech**

"Tell the audience what you are going to tell them, then tell them, and finally tell them what you told them," is the old adage about public speaking. It still holds true. All successful presentations have a circular structure (i.e., the end comes back to reinforce the beginning).

Begin your preparation by focusing on what action you want the audience to take as a result of listening to your speech. This goal or objective should be stated in the introduction and should also be stated emphatically at the conclusion. If, for example, you are talking to a group of middle-aged women, your objective might be "that women over 50 years of age frequently experience urinary incontinence and most of them can be cured of this embarrassing problem." Try to paint a word picture by referring to the fact that the number of men and women suffering from urinary incontinence in this community will be more than the capacity of the Superdome—a well-known landmark in my community. You might end your presentation by saying, "Some of you here in the audience may be suffering needlessly from urinary incontinence. Call your physician or your urologist and get an examination so that you can be dry for the rest of your life!" Another example is a talk on prostate cancer. Your goal or objective is to have all men over the age of 50 obtain a DRE and a PSA test. I suggest you begin with an eye-opening statistic or an anecdotal story about someone famous who has prostate cancer and the importance of early detection. You should end your presentation with the same call to action. Remember, what the audience hears in the first 30-60 seconds and the last few seconds of your presentation is what they take home from your presentation.

Essentially, your point of view in a presentation should be fired like a rifle hitting the center of the target. A speech without a single point of view ends up like a shotgun that scatters buckshot everywhere but on the target. However, a crystal-clear point of view strikes the one point that you want them to leave with at the end of your presentation. When you can accomplish this, you are indeed an effective public speaker.

Once you have the beginning and the conclusion, you can fill in the middle for a memorable speech that will motivate your audience to take positive action. In the middle portion of your speech, present 2-3 main points using illustrations, examples, stories, case histories, or visual aids whenever possible. When talking about urinary incontinence, use a balloon to illustrate the bladder. Your fingers compressing the neck of the balloon will serve as the urinary sphincter. When you release your fingers from the neck of the balloon it will make a sound that produces a predictable giggle or laughter from the audience. Then remark, "When it is a balloon leaking air, that's funny. But when it is your bladder losing urine, it's no laughing matter." This visual aid clearly explains the functional anatomy of the bladder and the urethra better than any slide from Gray's anatomy or a Frank Netter drawing from the Ciba-Geigy textbooks.

If you are comfortable talking to patients in a direct manner, then you can be a successful public speaker. The best speeches are those that are prepared well in advance. Giving a speech is not a situation in which you can "wing it." You cannot take a carousel of slides that you use for a presentation to physicians at grand rounds and use the same material for a lay audience. Giving the same speech that you used with your colleagues for a lay audience will result in a boring and confusing presentation, and you cannot expect members of the audience to leave the presentation and call your office for an appointment. Your fellow physicians may tolerate and even expect a talk punctuated by technical charts, graphs, anatomic drawings, photos of surgical specimens, and medical jargon. Lay audiences expect straightforward explanations of complicated subjects, direct information, and suggestions for improving their health and well-being. Good presentations are crisp, clear, and concise. In today's fast-paced world of sound bites, the audience expects clarity and simplicity.

If you support each main point with a variety of materials, anecdotes, or visuals, you keep your audience focused on your main goal or objective. If possible, include a personal story about yourself, a friend, or a family member. This adds the all-important ingredient—the human touch.

Another suggestion is to mention any celebrities or historical figures who have suffered from the medical condition you are describing. For example, when discussing complications of urinary incontinence, tell the story of Ben Franklin, who had bladder calculus that caused intermittent urinary retention. Franklin was able to relieve his urinary retention by standing on his head and allowing the bladder calculus to fall away from the bladder opening. "So," tell your audience, "Ben Franklin had to do handstands to solve his problem. You can get a helping hand for yours from your physician." If a well-known public figure has come forward to admit that they suffer or are afflicted with the disease or condition, then you might want to include that in your presentation. Examples are Senator Bob Dole and General Norman Schwarzkopf, who have prostate cancer and have been proponents of PSA testing and annual digital rectal exams for all men over the age of 50. Another is June Alyson, who is a spokesperson for urinary incontinence, or Lance Armstrong, the winner of the 1999 Tour de France cycling race, and a survivor of metastatic testicular cancer.

In this era of managed care, there is no better way to become attractive to the potential patients in the plan than to contact the employer or the company's nurse and offer to provide a 15–20 minute "brown bag" presentation on topics of health and wellness for their luncheon meetings. If you know your audience well and select your topic carefully, you can be sure that there will be several people in the audience who suffer from the condition or disease, or that they will have a friend or family member who needs your services. By being proactive with the employers, you demonstrate your emphasis on wellness and helping to keep their employees productive and gainfully employed.

## MARKETING TO YOUR EXISTING PATIENTS

### *Educating Existing Patients About Your Areas of Interest and Expertise*

Of course it is important to attract new patients to your practice, but don't forget the ones you already have. When I was in practice only a very short period of time, I operated on a lady with kidney stones. Six months later she came back with an incision on her abdomen, which she told me was from a bladder suspension performed by her gynecologist. When I asked her why she went to the gynecologist, she told me that she wasn't aware that I treated patients for incontinence. At that time, I made the decision to ensure that all of my existing patients were informed of the services my practice offered and my areas of urologic interest.

### *Softening the Bite of the Bill—and Educating Your Patients, Too*

By including information and educational materials in your monthly statements, you have an inexpensive method to provide your existing patients with information and news about your practice. You can include notices to your patients about new programs, support groups you are conducting, talks you have given or will be giving, or articles that you have written. The bill stuffer is also an excellent opportunity to distribute your office newsletter.

Many practices now have computerized billing that creates a statement ready for mailing in a special envelope that makes it difficult to insert other printed material. Most of the current software programs will allow you to customize a message on the statement. When I wanted to tell my existing patients that I was trained to do the laparoscopic bladder suspension, I included this on my monthly statements. Several of my existing patients called, asked for additional information, and even made appointments to discuss it further.

One other benefit of bill stuffers is that patients are more likely to open a bill that they know will provide useful information than just a reminder that they owe you money. Find topics that are related to your practice, wellness, nutrition, humor, and seasonal events. For example, in September of each year, we mention Prostate Cancer Awareness Month and provide the locations where the patients can receive a free PSA test and a rectal exam. We do a similar bill stuffer for urinary incontinence and erectile dysfunction.

### *Provide Value-Added Services to Your Existing Patients*

Patient advocacy groups provide useful information and support for your patients with certain medical conditions and diagnoses. Most metropolitan communities have one or several of the groups that meet on a regular basis. Most communities have an Ostomy Society, a diabetes support group, prostate cancer groups (Us Too), and interstitial cystitis groups. You provide value-added care for your patients when you can direct them to these groups for ongoing support.

Patients are often unable to pay for their medications. There is a government organization that provides free drugs to older Americans. This organization provides hundreds of prescription medications for indigent senior citizens. They can be contacted at (202) 224-5364, and they will provide you with a list and forms for your patient to complete. Also, many of your pharmaceutical representatives can provide discounted or free medication for the medically indigent.

### *Extra! Extra! Read All About It!*

In the last 10 years we have seen a real boom in health and medical information designed for public consumption. More than ever before, patients want to learn about health and fitness and the prevention, diagnosis, and treatment of medical problems. At the same time, patients often complain that their physicians do not communicate effectively. One of the most frequent reasons patients leave a practice is the doctor's failure to communicate. The average physician interrupts a patient discussing their present illness after 16 seconds! Patients and the public are very interested in receiving as much information as possible from their health-care providers. A newsletter will provide this information and will help to improve communication with your existing patients.

Writing a quarterly newsletter can be a formidable undertaking. I suggest that the easiest way to create a practice newsletter is to use one of the newsletter services. Many of your specialty organizations have template newsletters that allow you to use material and then modify it for your practice. Usually, the first and last page can be customized for your practice. The *Health Exchange* (Medical Group Management Association, 104 Inverness Terrace East, Inglewood, CO 80112, (303) 799-1111) can provide you with samples and all of the materials you will need to create your own newsletter.

Another possibility for creating a newsletter is to do it yourself. You can often find information at your annual conventions or in their publications that can be easily modified to become a newsletter for your patients. The only caveat is that it is necessary to "translate" the medical vocabulary into layman's language.

Most physicians who have tried newsletters indicate that they will only use them for a year or two and then quit. The reason most of them give for abandoning newsletters is an inadequate return on their investment. Like any marketing tool, it is necessary to track the results. The newsletter can contain a reply card or a special telephone number, which is the same method used in conjunction with a Yellow Pages ad. You may want to devise a code or system for distinguishing between new patients attracted to the practice and existing or established patients who have returned for new procedures or evaluations. Each time a reply card is returned or the special phone number is called, have your staff enter this information into your computer. By using this tracking method, you can determine the number of patients who enter your practice as a result of the newsletter. You can calculate the income derived as a result of the newsletter. This simple procedure allows you to accurately measure the return on investment of your newsletter. Now if you make a decision to discontinue the newsletter, you will be making an objective decision.

As with most marketing efforts, the results of a newsletter are not immediate. Don't become discouraged after you produce one or two issues. It does require persistence, reinforcement, and repetition.

**Other Uses of the Newsletter**

I suggest that you include a copy of your newsletter as part of your "welcome to the practice" package to new patients. I also send a copy to managed-care plans when I apply for inclusion in their panel. Copies of the newsletter are also included as part of the handout material when I speak to lay audiences. The newsletter is far more effective than giving out your business cards.

### *Networking—The Contact Sport of the 90s*

All of us have patients who have had successful results after we recommend a treatment or perform a surgical procedure. You can use these success stories to help new patients who are undecided about a treatment, procedure, or operation.

A patient network is similar to a support group, although it is not as formal. The medical profession has ethically used patients to discuss their experiences with other patients. For example, the ostomy support group has patients who have had ostomies impart their experience with those patients who are about to have the procedure or who have recently had the procedure. New or potential patients who attend these meetings have a better acceptance of their ostomy and have demonstrated a better adjustment to their new lifestyle. Patients develop confidence and security when they hear firsthand from someone who has "been there."

You will find that patients who have a medical condition or disease and have been helped are frequently willing to discuss their positive experiences with others who suffer from similar conditions. By connecting people with similar problems, you accomplish several goals:

- You help the patients considering the procedures to allay their fears and to arrive at a decision with confidence.
- You allow the patients who have completed treatment to give something back.
- You allow the patients who have completed treatment to help you with your marketing.

An example of how a patient network markets your practice to your existing patients is to allow a patient considering a procedure or treatment to call another patient who has undergone a similar procedure. For instance, if a woman is considering a surgical procedure to correct her incontinence, arrange for the patient to speak with another woman who has already had the surgery (and has had a good result).

Another spin-off from using this networking method is that patients who have benefited from the telephone conversation will volunteer to talk to new patients. They will usually say that they suffered from the medical problem for such a long period of time, and that talking to a fellow sufferer helped them to make the decision to have the surgery or the procedure. As a result of the benefit of using the networking system, they are happy to volunteer to talk to any prospective patients. You can be sure that once you start using this system you will never have a shortage of telephone numbers to recommend to new patients.

## IMPROVING PRACTICE EFFICIENCY

There is probably no area that will achieve as much attention in the near future as that of improving the efficiency of your practice. In the past we were able to see low volumes of patients with the luxury of enjoying high-profit margins. Today and tomorrow it will be the reverse—we will be seeing high volumes of patients with low profit margins. As a result, in order to see more patients in the same amount of time, it will be necessary to make our practices more efficient.

### *Do-It-Yourself Videos*

One of the best ways of improving the efficiency of your practice is to use videos of you and your colleagues to explain subjects and topics to your patients.

We are living in an electronic age. Most homes have videocassette recorders (VCRs) and most Americans are familiar and comfortable viewing videos. Using office videos is an effective method of educating your patients. Creating a video is easy and inexpensive, and can serve as a great marketing tool.

While one patient is viewing a videotape of an operation, a procedure, or a medical problem, you can be seeing other patients. An effective video can act as a surrogate assistant, addressing and answering the most frequently asked questions about a particular procedure or treatment. Because a video uses visuals, you can provide patients with a better understanding of such subjects such as anatomy, physiology, and complex technology.

Videos serve as medical-legal documentation that you have explained a procedure and its potential complications. To make the medical-legal protection stronger, have your patients sign the chart or add a sentence to the consent form that indicates that the video has been seen.

A video serves as a nice "giveaway" to your patients and their families or their friends. You can loan a videotape to a patient so that a friend or family member who suffers from the condition or problem has an opportunity to learn about the evaluation and treatment of the problem. If that friend does not have a physician who treats that condition, he or she is very likely to call your office for an appointment.

Subjects for videotapes include procedures or problems that you explain several times each day, and operations or procedures that you do frequently. Examples are: management of BPH, evaluation of urinary incontinence, vasectomy, interpretation of the PSA test, and treatment options for localized prostate cancer.

To create your own video, begin with a script or story. This is simply a narration that accompanies the visuals on the video. You can begin by recording a discussion with a patient on the topic you are considering for a video. Next, have the discussion transcribed and use it as a guide or an outline to prepare the video script. You can also review videos that are created by the medical manufacturing companies and pharmaceutical companies. For most topics you should avoid substituting a commercial video by the medical manufacturing or pharmaceutical company for a personalized, customized video of you and your story. Commercial videos are biased to their products or equipment and do not tell your story or point of view. Also, a video of you makes your patient feel that you are giving him or her a personalized message.

In most cases the video contains: a definition of the procedure or test; a description of how the procedure or test is performed; a detailed description of the necessary preparation; what the patient can expect after the procedure is performed; and the complications and their relative frequency. If your video is for a surgical procedure, it is important to include alternatives to the surgical procedure.

You can make notes on $8 \times 10$ cards, which can be used in place of a teleprompter. The only equipment necessary is a home video camera and a tripod. Most hospital audiovisual departments own this equipment and will frequently loan it to you or provide you with assistance in creating the video.

Finally, you need to edit your tape. You can easily edit your video with two videocassette recorders (VCRs). Keep the edited length between 7 and 10 minutes. Videos should not be longer than 15 minutes. Longer videos will not hold the interest of the patient and will also tie up your examination room or viewing area.

Offer the patient a written summary of each video after they have seen the tape. Always return to the room after they have seen the video to answer any questions the patient has. If you want to be sure that your patient understood the video, you can give them a short test on the material. This test should be included in the patient's chart in case it is needed for medical-legal purposes.

If you have or want to develop an incontinence practice, you will find that videos are a very effective method of giving the patients information, which significantly improves the efficiency of your practice. By using do-it-yourself videos you may find that you can see 15–20% more patients in the same time period.

## Color-Coded Prescription Pads

Most urologists use 20–25 drugs 95% of the time. We often have several dozen preprinted prescription pads in our examination rooms, and we fumble around the drawer to find the correct pad or take the time to write an individual prescription. You can avoid the "treasure hunt" for the correct prescription pad by having preprinted pads that categorize the drugs you frequently use. For example, the antibiotics you use can all be on one color-coded pad, drugs for incontinence on another color, and miscellaneous drugs on a third pad. When you write a prescription, just circle the appropriate drug, add the number that you wish to dispense, and circle the directions. The blank pad that you use for analgesics and other Class III drugs can be carried in your lab coat. You can save 15–30 seconds each time you write a prescription by using this system. If you see 30–40 patients a day and write 2–3 prescriptions for each patient, that's a savings of 25–50 minutes a day just by using this system. That translates to more than two hours a week and 80 hours a year. At $150 per hour (the value of physician time), that equates to nearly a $10,000 savings for an idea that is practically free. The take-home message is that managing care now means managing minutes!

Ask your pharmaceutical representative to make these pads for you. Offer to place their drug at the top of your list. One other advantage of the color-coded prescription pad is that you won't get any calls from the pharmacist that he or she can't read your writing!

## Educational Materials

Today our patients are much more medically sophisticated and more interested in their health and well-being than ever before. We can easily fill this need or desire of our patients by providing them with educational materials on their urologic problems. This educational material will also reduce the number of questions that you receive from your patients.

You will also reduce calls and questions from your patients by providing them with information on the drugs your prescribe for them. In addition to giving them the prescription, give the patient information on the purpose of the drug, common side effects, dosing instructions, common drug interactions, and when to take the medication, i.e., with or without meals. This information is available from *The Pill Book* or *The PDR Family Guide to Prescription Drugs*, and can be either photocopied or placed in a word-processor and then printed on your stationery. Much of this educational information, printed material, consents, pre- and post-operative forms and drug information is also available on software programs.

You can assist your patient with educational materials even before their first visit to your office. If the receptionist who makes the appointment for the patient asks about the nature of their visit to your office, she can send the patient a "welcome to the practice" package. In addition to a welcome letter, a practice brochure, a map of the location of the office, and a recent newsletter, include an article on incontinence and what is expected at the time of their first visit. Since most new patients are asked to provide a urine specimen, you can reduce the number of patients that void prior to their appointment by informing them in the letter that they will be asked to give a specimen and that they should consume extra fluid prior to coming to the office. This one sentence included in the "welcome to the practice" letter can help you maintain your schedule.

## *Calling Key Patients At Home*

Probably no better method exists to improve the efficiency and marketing of your practice than calling your key patients at home. Your key patients are: those who were recently discharged from the hospital; patients who had outpatient procedures or surgery; patients with significant medical problems; and patients who are going to be admitted early in the morning for surgery (AM admits).

Your nurse can contact the key patients and can usually answer most of the questions and triage her list down to one or two patients who you should contact. If your nurse tells a patient that you are going to call, give the patient an estimated time when you will call so that the patient is home and does not use the phone.

One of the benefits of calling your key patients is the wonderful response you will receive. Few things you do will be as appreciated as much as your calls to patients at home. You can almost hear the patient saying, "I can't believe my doctor is taking the time to call me at home." By calling your patients, you can anticipate problems that may require an office visit before the next scheduled appointment or admission to the hospital if they are not doing as well as expected.

Finally, when you call your patients at home, you reduce the number of calls you receive from them. If patients know that you are going to be calling, they are less likely to interrupt you with their calls. Thus, if you spend just 5–10 minutes a day calling your patients, you will ultimately have more time with your family and friends. There is no better way to develop a reputation as a caring, compassionate physician than to call your patients at home.

## MARKETING THROUGH REFERRING PHYSICIANS

In the past, the traditional methods of obtaining physician referrals usually involved trial and error. Perhaps you went to school with another physician and later he or she referred patients to you. Or you joined a group practice and got the overflow. Doing an excellent job with every patient gradually generated a word-of-mouth method that resulted in more physician referrals. Thus, slowly—usually in 2 or 3 years—a physician could build a reputation in the community. These methods worked in the past because there were enough primary-care doctors, patients, and referrals to go around. Although the traditional system will work, there are effective and economically practical methods of streamlining the development of physician referrals.

When referring physicians are surveyed about why they make referrals, they list prompt reporting first . . . way ahead of writing articles, teaching, and gifts and entertaining! You must always keep your referring physicians informed about their patients' progress.

When you see a patient by referral, follow this cardinal rule: Never allow the patient to arrive back in the referring physician's office before your report does. Nothing is more embarrassing to the referring physician than to be in the dark about what is going on with the patient. If a patient calls her ob-gyn doctor to talk about estrogen replacement therapy and medication to treat her incontinence, and that doctor has not received your report, you not only look bad in the eyes of the ob-gyn doctor, but the efficiency of your practice grinds to a halt. Now your staff has to retrieve the patient's chart, and then you are interrupted to answer any questions that the ob-gyn doctor may have.

The usual communication between a specialist and the referring doctor is 7–10 days after his or her patient is seen. During that hiatus, the patient will often be seen before the letter is sent to the referring doctor. One technique for handling this is to use the "lazy person's referral letter." The reason for this name is that it requires no dictating and absolutely guarantees that 100% of the time the letter arrives before the patient visits the referring doctor.

The three most important aspects of your referral letter are *the diagnosis, the medications prescribed, and the treatment plan*. These ingredients are referred to as the "buzz" words. These words are circled in the progress notes of the chart. For instance: a woman is seen with a problem of mild to moderate stress incontinence and you recommend a trial of alpha-adrenergic agonists and Kegel exercises; you plan to see her back in the office and check on her progress in 2 months. These key words are circled in the chart. At the end of the day, the nurse goes through the chart after the patient's visit and looks for the key words you have circled. She calls up our boilerplate referral letter on the computer screen, which has blanks to be completed. The nurse types in the appropriate referring physician's name, the diagnosis, and so on. The letter is printed and mailed that day or faxed directly to the physician's office the same afternoon that the patient is seen.

This type of referral letter delivers the essentials to the referring physician immediately. Whenever a referring physician gets a 2–3-page dictated report, he or she looks for the diagnosis, recommended treatment plan, and the follow-up. The referring doctor simply doesn't have time to read a long report.

Now if the patient calls with any questions, the physician can answer them without having to contact you or your office for clarification. Furthermore, the letter can usually be generated without any dictating at all. For those who must dictate the traditional 2- or 3-page referral letter, you might consider underlining or using boldface print for the essential information, including your impression, the medications, and your recommendations. A survey of referring physicians indicates that most of them prefer a timely computerized referral letter over a delayed 3-pager. Some specialists are concerned that referring physicians are upset when they receive a computerized, impersonal form letter. Surveys of referring physicians indicate physicians will value timely information more than a delayed personal letter.

If you do not have a computer, you can still employ the lazy person's referral letter. You can use photocopies of a typed letter with blanks in it. Simply fill in the blanks and send this to your referring physicians. When referring physicians are surveyed about these brief reports, they all indicate that they appreciate a timely report that highlights the three most important ingredients—ie, the diagnosis, the medications, and the treatment plan.

Unfortunately, many of us depend on our operative notes to inform referring doctors what tests and procedures have been done on their patients. Often these operative notes will not arrive for 10–14 days. In order to keep the referring doctor informed, consider using the "Stat Operative Note." By writing in the procedure, findings and recommendations, you can keep the referring doctor up-to-date on the status of his or her patient.

Niche marketing makes it possible to generate intraspecialty referrals or referrals from colleagues within your specialty. For example, if you provide a service or procedure that is not done by your colleagues you can inform them that you do the procedure and would be happy to work with them in the care of their patient. This concept of "their" patient is very important in generating intraspecialty referrals. If the patient is sent to you, make sure the patient is returned to the referring urologist.

Here's an example that might apply to your incontinence practice. If you have training and expertise in brachytherapy and no one else in your community is doing this procedure, you can offer this service for a colleague's patient. Perhaps the best way to get started working with your colleagues is to send them articles on the subject, especially if you have written articles that have been published in medical journals. You can also offer to do the surgery at the hospital of your colleague and allow your colleague to admit the patient. Your colleague can assist you with the surgery and participate in the postoperative care of the patient. The advantages to your colleague are that he continues to maintain control of the patient, participates in the surgery, and collects an admitting and discharge fee as well as any surgical assistant fee.

The keys to keeping the referral pipeline open from other physicians are communication and education. It is important to let the referring doctor know that incontinence is an area of interest or expertise that you enjoy. Some urologists may not enjoy treating incontinent patients, and you do not want to be placed in that category. Although many men and women have urinary incontinence, few primary-care doctors will ask their patients about their voiding habits. You can improve this situation by sending referring physicians articles on incontinence.

For example, if a patient has mild incontinence and you suggest that the patient take an alpha-adrenergic agonist, most primary-care doctors will not be aware of the urologic application of this medication. A tactful way to do this is to include with your referral letter an article that describes the use alpha-adrenergic agonists. It is unlikely that a referring physician will read the entire article or even the abstract. But you can significantly increase the likelihood that the information will be received by underlining the one or two sentences that are pertinent to the patient. Then place a Post-it™ on the article that will direct the referring doctors to the essential information.

Another method of keeping the primary-care doctors informed is to send a do-it-yourself newsletter about the latest developments in urology. If you attend the AUA you will have more than enough information for a short, 1-page newsletter that educates your referring physicians about the latest developments in urology.

## *Nontraditional Referrals*

We have the opportunity to communicate with other health-care professionals who could be sources of referrals. For example, nurses and hospital employees are frequently asked who they should see for various medical problems. Giving talks to the nurses both at your hospital and in the community can serve as an excellent method of letting these professionals know about your area of interest in the management of incontinent patients.

Pharmacists are another group from whom patients frequently seek advice. It's important to become an ally of the pharmacists in your community. Pharmaceutical representatives and medical manufacturing representatives are also a resource for generating good public relations and serve as referral sources for your practice. If pharmaceutical representatives see that you have an interest in incontinence, they will recommend your practice to other physicians, friends, and colleagues. If you want to endear yourself to the drug representatives and other salespeople who call on your practice, see them in a timely fashion. That's their hot button, and they really appreciate it if you don't ignore them or keep them waiting.

One way to improve the efficiency of the time you spend with pharmaceutical representatives is to request an agenda letter. This letter asks them to inform you what they want to talk about and how long they anticipate the visit will last. You can then decide if you want to see the representative on that subject, and can indicate that you accept the time frame of the representative. This method significantly focuses the representative's visit and reduces the amount of time you will spend with them to obtain information on their products.

## INCREASING COMMUNICATION WITH MANAGED-CARE PLANS

These days, we must ask permission or obtain authorization for nearly every procedure or operation. All of us have experienced the disaster that occurs when we fail to obtain the appropriate permissions, which may result in the managed-care plan not paying for the procedure. We can facilitate this process by using preprinted forms for our most common procedures.

We can streamline our communications with managed-care plans and gatekeepers by using fax sheets that clearly indicate the purpose of our referral and what action we would like taken. For example, if you plan to operate on a patient who is in a managed-care plan and need a clearance for surgery, you can complete the fax form by indicating the surgery, the date, and the request for a written document that clears the patient for surgery. This can be sent to the referring doctor to avoid a possible communication gap or failure for the gatekeeper to understand your request.

## DOES MARKETING WORK?

The answer is yes—but not immediately. You can't expect that after a talk to a lay audience the phone will start ringing off the hook with dozens of patients calling for appointments. The results of marketing are like creating a fine wine. It takes time for the marketing fermentation process to work. You will be amazed that months and even years after you appear on TV or write an article for a local publication, patients will decide to make contact with you and your office. Remember, it takes patience to attract patients!

Long delays in seeing results are not the norm for marketing to patients already in your practice. These results can occur almost immediately. Using the wine analogy, it's like uncorking the bottle and enjoying it right now. For example, I make it a point to ask every female patient about the ability of her husband/partner/significant other to engage in sexual intimacy and whether he has had a PSA test for prostate cancer. (Of course, I avoid this question when talking to a nun or a 90-year-old woman!) About 10% of the time, I find a woman who indicates that her husband is impotent, and I provide her with information on impotence for her husband to read and suggest he contact me if he is interested in solving this problem. About 30% of the time I ask about the PSA test, I identify men who have not had the test and have not established a relationship with a urologist. Providing educational material on prostate cancer to the woman will motivate her partner to make an appointment, and frequently she will actually make the appointment on his behalf.

This same approach applies to male patients. I ask all men about their partner's sexual performance, contraception, and incontinence. Occasionally this questioning will result in a vasectomy or a consultation for incontinence. Remember—the advice from the Good Book says "Ask and you shall receive." This certainly applies to marketing to the patients already in your practice.

Finally, not every one of these ideas is going to work for you, and I do not suggest you try them all. I do recommend that you find one or two that fit your personality and your style, and then try to implement an idea or two into your practice. I can promise you that you won't be sorry. Besides—it's ethical, exciting, and yes, for the most part, it is fun.

## SELECTED READING

Chfinick LD (1992) *The Pill Book.* New York: Bantam Books.
Sifton DW (1993) *The PDR Family Guide to Prescription Drugs.* Montvale, NJ: Medical Economics Data.
Wallechinsky D, et al. (1977) *The Book of Lists.* New York: William Morrow.

# 3 Proper Billing and Coding

*Ray Painter, MD*

**CONTENTS**

EXECUTIVE SUMMARY
THE CODING SYSTEM
E/M CODING
THIRD-PARTY PAYER
FRAUD AND ABUSE

## EXECUTIVE SUMMARY

The mere statement that the practice of medicine is changing is a gross understatement. HMOs, new technologies, government involvement, fraud, computerization of payments, and so forth have significantly changed the way urologists practice.

Realms of published rules and regulations fill shelves with mandated changes. One change that is ringing out loud and clear throughout the health care system is the mandate to incorporate good business principles into the practice of medicine. However, it is crucial for the urologist to keep the business of medicine in the proper perspective! Good patient care must continue to be *first and foremost* in your minds as you set up your business practices. Patients' needs, desires, and satisfaction cannot be ignored.

The payment system for physicians' services is somewhat complex. However, if broken down into its basic elements—the coding system, payment methodology, and payer-specific rules and interpretation—the mystery begins to diminish and gradually becomes comprehensible.

The specificity of the rules and the fine line between not getting paid and being fraudulent in your billing requires that:

1. The physician has a working knowledge of not only E/M coding but procedural and diagnostic International Classification of Diseases-Version 9-Clinical Modification (ICD-9) coding.
2. Each practice have expert coding/billing personnel.
3. Each office have access to the necessary current and updated extra materials (*see* Chart 1)
4. The protocol or methodology used in capturing coding and billing is detailed, precise, and strictly adhered to. (*see* Chart 2)
5. Billing is customized to the rules and regulations of the payer being billed.
6. The office is committed to a fully integrated compliance plan.

From: *Current Clinical Urology: Office Urology: The Clinician's Guide*
Edited by: E. D. Kursh and J. C. Ulchaker © Humana Press Inc., Totowa, NJ

---
Chart 1
Materials
---

1. Current Procedural Terminology (CPT)[a] updated annually.
2. International Classification of Diseases-Version 9-Clinical Modification (ICD-9-CM)[a] updated annually.
3. Health Care Financing Administration Common Procedure Coding System (HCPCS)[a] updated annually.
4. For Medicare:
   a. Quarterly updates on the Correct Coding Initiative (CCI).
   b. Quarterly updates on the ICD-9 mandates.
   c. Yearly updates of the Medicare rules and regulations.[a]
   d. Monthly bulletins from your carrier(s).
5. For private payers, your current contract containing detailed payment methodology rules and regulations.
6. Each office should establish a relationship with an outside consultant and/or hotlines to answer specific coding questions, to be alerted to specific changes and interpretation of rules, and to assist with office compliance, external audits, and so forth.
7. Computerized billing and electronic submission are a must. To be effective in collection, you must compile data reports that can only be achieved through computerization.

---
[a]Electronic subscriptions exist that combine all of these products into one source (e.g., Flash Code™ Expert Edition) that has an excellent search engine and quarterly updates.

---
Chart 2
Billing Methodology
---

1. Capture and identify all services using a verification process.
2. E/M coding and documentation (*see* Chart 3).
3. Determine specific diagnostic code for each service.
4. Determine chargeable services using payer-specific rules.
5. Use customized forms for accurate communication of the identified service codes with specific diagnostic codes.
6. Input flawless electronic data.
7. Check all codes prior to submission for payer-specific rules and fraud-free billing.

---

Each time a physician provides a service to a patient, someone owes the physician or their employer something. In this chapter, we will discuss the business principles and functions that should be incorporated in the everyday urology practice relating to the ethical and legal payment for services provided. Accurate, nonfraudulent efficient, and effective reporting of services—and collecting payment for these services—are our goals.

Strict adherence to the above business principles will increase your income (an estimate for many offices is as much as 10%–20%) and at the same time assure that your practice remains fraud-free.

## THE CODING SYSTEM

Physicians have to be very precise in identifying the code that accurately describes the service provided, as well as a diagnosis that conveys and verifies the specific reason for the medical necessity of the service. They must also be knowledgeable about the payment rules and the variations specific to the payer being billed, and correctly apply them in order to receive payment.

## E/M CODING

To charge for your E/M services, four separate decisions must be made:

1. Which category?
2. Which level?
3. Is there a global issue?
4. What is the diagnosis (ICD-9-CM), and the reason the service was provided?

### *Category*

Picking the correct category is easy. Patients are either new to the practice (patients who have not been seen or treated by that physician or partner of the same specialty for three years) or established; outpatient or inpatient. Consults are the wild cards in the deck and will be discussed in detail. Rules for documentation differ by category and at times by patient status. For example, inpatient consult requires the same documentation as an outpatient consult, but pays more, and if charging by time, requires more time.

Established patient work and required documentation is significantly less than that required for the same level of new patient code. For example, an established patient with a new problem requiring a work-up and drug therapy in which you have a complete history and *NO PHYSICAL,* would be at least a Level 4. A *new* patient would require a complete physical examination to charge a Level 4 code.

### Consults

Consults are the most misunderstood, underutilized (by physicians), and abused (by payers) set of codes in the Current Procedural Terminology (CPT) book. This section is intended to unravel the mystery of outpatient, inpatient, follow-up, and confirmatory consults.

**Outpatient Consults.** The outpatient consult code can be used regardless of whether the patient is new or established and whether they are seen in the office, in the emergency department, or other outpatient setting, if the visit satisfies the two sets of rules:

1. CPT specifies three criteria that must be met for the visit to be considered a consult:
   a. The patient must be referred by a physician;
   b. The evaluation performed during the visit must be documented; and
   c. The patient information must be conveyed back to the referring physician.
2. Medicare has added the requirement that a patient must be sent for your evaluation (as opposed to being referred for treatment). The 1999 CPT specifically states on page 15, second paragraph, under Consultations, that "A physician consultant may initiate treatment and/or therapeutic services." Medicare concurs with this policy. For private payers, the Medicare rule regarding evaluation versus treatment may or may not be required. Some payers may follow CPT only; others may not pay for a consult code at all. However, the three CPT criteria should be met in charging for any consult.

**Chart 3**
**E/M Coding Methodology**

---
1. Coding by physician.
2. Develop a "working knowledge."
3. Use history and physical examination intake forms.
4. Use quick-reference materials.
---

If these two sets of rules are met, the visit is considered to be a consult, even if:

1. The patient is an established patient;
2. The visit is in the global period of a different procedure;
3. You begin treatment;
4. You perform a diagnostic procedure;
5. You schedule a patient for a therapeutic surgery; or
6. The patient is in the ER or other outpatient setting.

**Exception:** Medicare has specifically stated that it is not a consult if an emergency-room physician refers the patient to the doctor's office.

Remember, it is "how" the patient was sent to you that counts—not how the patient left your office. You may start treatment, perform a cystoscopy, or remove a stone and still qualify for a consult if you meet the criteria as outlined.

**Inpatient Consult.** The inpatient consult is less controversial. The first time you evaluate the patient who has been admitted by another physician it should be charged as a consult, even if you—the consulting physician—assume responsibility for management of a portion or all of the patient's conditions.

**Follow-Up Consult.** The follow-up consult is an inpatient code and cannot be used in the outpatient setting. The follow-up consult may only be used under two conditions: 1) to complete the initial inpatient consult; or 2) if the consulting physician signed off the case and is requested by the attending physician to reevaluate the patient during the same hospitalization period. **Note:** Subsequent hospital visits should be used in all other circumstances.

**Confirmatory Consult.** Confirmatory consult may be performed at the request of the patient or third-party payer. The reason for the consult could be for a second opinion or possibly for appropriateness of care. The patient could be an inpatient or outpatient.

## *Level*

Documentation of all the work provided may be unnecessary for good patient care, and certainly picking the correct code is complex, but the process is not difficult or time-consuming if you set up and adhere to a strict methodology. (*see* Chart 3—E/M Methodology)

We recommend that you use the 1997 documentation guidelines because the Health Care Financing Administration (HCFA) has proposed new guidelines to be enacted in 2000 that will modify and somewhat simplify the 1997 guidelines. (Physicians are currently being audited by the federal government using either the 1995 or the 1997 guidelines.)

## Chart 4
## Established Patient

|  | Level 1 | Level 2 | Level 3 | Level 4 | Level 5 |
|---|---|---|---|---|---|
| Office/Outpatient | 99211 | 99212 | 99213 | 99214 | 99215 |

### ■ KEY COMPONENTS
MUST SATISFY TWO OF THE THREE KEY COMPONENTS

**History** — Content of Services

| | | | | | |
|---|---|---|---|---|---|
| History of Present Illness | Chief | 1 - 3 | 1 - 3 | 4+ * | 4+ * |
| Review of Systems | | | Pertinent | 2 - 9 | 10+ |
| PFSH -- Family and Social | | | | 1 | 2 - 3 |

*An extended can also be reached by documenting at least three (3) chronic or inactive conditions

**Physical**

| | System/Element | System/Element | System/Element | System/Element | System/Element |
|---|---|---|---|---|---|
| Single Organ System | None-Min | 1+/1-5 | 1+/6-11 | 1+/12+ (1+/9+ for eye & psych) | shaded/all unshaded/1 |
| Multi-System -- General | | 1+/1-5 | 1+/6-11 | 2+/12+ | 9+/ x 2 each |

**Medical Decision Making**
MUST SATISFY TWO OF THE THREE KEY COMPONENTS

| | | | | | |
|---|---|---|---|---|---|
| Number of Diagnoses | | Minimum | Limited | Multiple | Extensive |
| Amount of Data | | Minimum | Lim - Mult | Moderate | Extensive |
| Amount of Risk | | Minimum | Low | Moderate | High |

### ■ CONTRIBUTORY COMPONENTS

**Time**
BECOMES KEY COMPONENT AND OVERRIDES OTHER COMPONENTS IF OVER 50% OF SERVICE IS COUNSELING OR COORDINATING

| | | | | | |
|---|---|---|---|---|---|
| Time | | 5 | 10 | 15 | 25 | 40 |

**Problem**
PROBLEM MUST JUSTIFY TREATMENT

| | | | | | |
|---|---|---|---|---|---|
| Risk of Morbidity | | | Low-Mod | Mod-High | Mod-High |
| Risk of Mortality | | | Zero-Mod | Mod-High | Mod-High |

Don't try to memorize! Simply develop a working knowledge, and then use a quick-reference card or summary chart (*see* "Established Patient Minimum Work Chart" developed by PRS Chart 4) that tells you exactly what numbers you have to achieve in each of the categories, as outlined in the documentation guidelines. With a little study, you can take a look at a quick-reference chart and easily determine the proper level of code. When you have satisfied everything in a single level (history, physical, and medical decision-making), you have performed, documented, and should code that level.

### History

**New Patient.** You can simplify the process by collecting your history on a form that satisfies the Documentation Guidelines complete historical requirement, to be filled out by the patient and/or your office personnel before you see the patient. If the form is completed and used as part of your documentation in the chart, and you acknowledge its use by writing on it and signing it, you will automatically know that your history is at the fifth level.

**Established Patient.** For the established patient you have two choices. 1) If you have a complete history on your first visit you can simply review the complete history,

## Chart 5
This is an excerpt from a Physician's GU physical exam form created by PRS...

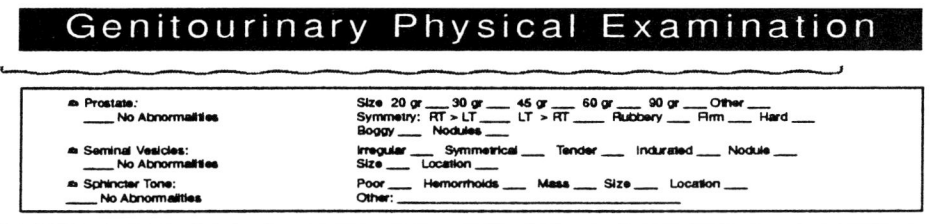

document the date, and update the ROS and PMS. Of course, you have to document the present illness. With that accomplished, you now have a fifth-level history. 2) Satisfy the specific requirements for each level of code referred to in the minimal work chart (*see* Chart 2). The requirements are much simpler for an established patient. Look at Level 3. The only requirements for history are that you have one element in the history of present illness and at least one in the review of systems.

### Physical Examination

**New patient.** Simplify by using a form! A checklist will make it easy to document all physical observations and examinations that you have provided for the patient. Counting the number of "bullets" or examination elements on an organized form is not only easy, but also more accurate and *will assist you in documenting higher levels* with less work. Most physicians currently observe and/or examine many elements they do not get credit for because of inadequate documentation. On a form, you can check "normal" for anything observed or examined that is a bullet—ie, well-developed, well-nourished. THIS COUNTS! You might want to take a look at one of the forms available to you and modify it to fit your practice needs. (*see* Chart 5, Excerpt from GU Physical Exam form.) There are three bullets recognized for a rectal exam. Many physicians document only findings of the prostate, missing two other bullets.

**Established Patient.** Since established inpatient documentation only requires two of the three key components, we do not need a physical examination (*see* Established Patient, Chart 4, Key Component "Must Satisfy 2 of the 3 Key Components.") Therefore, I do not recommend a form for follow-up examinations. Simply document what you do. No physical or only one bullet will not lower your code; you do not have to count it! However, if you performed a complete examination for hospitalization, and so forth, then use your history and physical examination forms and leave out medical decision-making in deciding which level to code.

### Medical Decision-Making

For this 2–3 step process you will need a quick-reference to the documentation guidelines or any number of sources for quick-reference materials. For medical decision-making you only need to use two of the three elements. Your medical decision-making level is the lowest level from the two elements you choose to use. First you have to determine the level of diagnoses, from minimum to extensive. To make this decision you must refer back to the documentation guidelines or use the quick-reference material,

## Chart 6
### Key Component for Medical Decision Making: Number of Problems/Diagnoses[a]

| Subelements | Content of service | Documentation required | Pocketcard says |
|---|---|---|---|
| Number of problems addressed during encounter | Minimum | 1 self-limiting problem | Minimum |
|  | Limited | 2 self-limiting problems or 1 established worsening | Limited |
| Type of problem addressed—new, established, self-limiting | Multiple | 1 new problem, no work-up required or 1 self-limiting + established problem worsening | Multiple |
| Problem worsening or improving | Extensive | 1 new problem, required additional work-up or 1 new problem no work-up + 1 self-limiting problem | Extensive |
| Additional work-up, no additional work-up | | | |

such as the wall chart developed by PRS. (*see* Chart 5). If this is a new problem requiring additional workup—then the diagnosis level is extensive. **Note:** for an established diagnosis you only have two choices, self-limiting or worsening. Any disease processes that are unresolved should be considered worsening. Data is merely a numbers game. Refer to the documentation guidelines or quick-reference to determine level. For risk the decision is quite simple; refer to the risk chart found in the documentation guidelines or other quick-reference materials and take the highest level from any of the three columns.

### Time vs. Components

The physician has a choice of using the components previously described or using time as a delimiter for the level of service. Specific rules must be used in each encounter. This process is quite detailed and is a "numbers game." If over 50% of the E/M encounter is spent counseling the patient, the use of time becomes an option. To use time, the physician must document the time spent. All physician, face-to-face E/M time—including history and physical—should be included. If you use time, you do not have to meet the requirements for the documentation for history, physical, and medical decision-making. However, you must document the content of the counseling session.

The physician who spends the few hours needed to develop a working knowledge of the coding system, assembles an expert team, purchases the needed educational and reference materials, and then organizes the process can be successful at the coding game.

### *E/M Global*

E/M services performed within the global period of a procedure will not be paid. However, if the service performed is unrelated to the procedure or is separate from the globe, then a modifier is applied and the service should be paid. Three modifiers are available to remove E/M services from a global:

1. Modifier –25 indicates that the service is separate from the global and is "significant." Can only be used on the day of a procedure.
2. Modifier –57 indicates that the decision to do the procedure was made during that E/M encounter.
3. Modifier –24 is used in the postoperative period to indicate that the service was unrelated to the procedure.

*An E/M service must satisfy the definition of the modifier if you are to use the modifier.* You must also know the specific payer rules. For example, if you decide to do a procedure, specific rules exist regarding whether you will be paid on the evaluation and management encounter. Using Modifier –57, the CPT rules differ from Medicare rules. If you are billing Medicare or a private payer who uses Medicare rules, follow these rules. Otherwise you should bill according to CPT rules.

## CPT

Use Modifier –57 on any E/M service in which you make the decision to do a procedure. If your E/M service is not within the global of the procedure, then you are not required to use the modifier to be paid.

## Medicare

Use Modifier –57 on E/M service in which you make the decision to provide a 90-d global procedure, if that E/M service falls on the day before or the day of the procedure (for Medicare the globe for a 90-d global procedure actually starts the day before the procedure). Do not use Modifier –57 for 0- or 10-d global procedures.

Medicare has determined that it will not pay for an E/M service on the same day as a diagnostic or minor procedure with Modifier –57 attached. **Note:** the E/M service would have to qualify for a –25 modifier to be paid.

For example, let us consider a patient who is seen for hematuria, and evaluated with the history, physical, and medical decision-making. A decision is made to proceed with the cystoscopy that day. Under Medicare, charge the E/M service with Modifier –25. This is justified because you have provided a significant E/M service that is separate from the procedure. Do not use modifier –57. **Note:** for CPT, and therefore for a private payer, both the –25 and the –57 modifier are technically correct to use. You have provided a "significant and separate E/M service" on the day of a procedure, and at the same time you "made the decision" to do the procedure. Use the modifier that works for the payer being billed. Diagnosis plays a significant role.

If there is a separate diagnosis for the E/M encounter, use it. However, all services that qualify for payment should be paid, even if you use the same diagnosis for both the E/M and the procedure. Unfortunately, some payers—including some Medicare carriers—do not honor this rule. Appeal any denials!

## ICD-9 Coding

The diagnosis code should be specific for each procedure or service provided. **Do not** use rule-outs or maybes; use symptoms if a definitive diagnosis is not available. Also, the ICD-9 code must be at its highest level of specificity—5th digit, if available.

## *Procedural Coding*

In Procedural Coding, the first step is to identify the code(s) (specificity). Following identification, payment rules should be applied to determine whether any of these services should not be charged because they are bundled or global or—if everything should be charged—how should they be charged? Do you need a modifier in order to evoke payment? Payment methodologies differ from payer to payer. To be successful, you should have a good working knowledge of the Medicare rules and regulations and compare other payer rules to identify the exceptions or determine how they differ from Medicare.

### Specificity

Procedural coding requires that every service a physician provides be reported using one or more 5-digit codes. Unfortunately, the CPT procedural coding system does not keep up with current technology, and physicians frequently find themselves providing services for which there are no specific CPT codes. In these circumstances, first check to see if Medicare has established HCPCS code locally or nationally. A temporary code may have been instituted by RVP (Relative Values for Physicians) and accepted by private payers. At times the physician can pick a very similar procedure and use the proper modifiers to accurately convey what service(s) were provided to the patient.

### Global

The term "global" must be understood conceptually. The idea is to combine the payments for all of the work related to a given procedure into one payment. This may include preoperative care, the procedure(s), and postoperative care. All E/M services and under certain circumstances, other procedures are assumed to be included in the global period. However, there are many exceptions to the global payment rules. These exceptions are conveyed by the use of the proper modifier, which notifies the third-party payers that payment is deserved for that particular service or procedure in addition to the procedural fee that triggered the global period.

Modifiers are defined and scrutinized in three levels of payment methodology. First, their specific uses are defined in the CPT. Second, the payment aspects of the modifiers—to pay or not to pay, circumstances under which they will pay, and at times percent of increase or decrease in payment—are defined in the payment methodologies as defined by Medicare and other Relative Value Systems (e.g., RVP) published by St. Anthony's. Third, the payer-specific rules regarding coverage or other payment issues are addressed.

### Bundling

By definition, bundling is the inclusion of one or more procedures that are an integral part of another procedure in payment for the more complex procedure. Bundling is the process of paying for each complete procedure instead of paying for all of the component parts of a procedure. The idea is to prevent the payment for "overlapping" procedures. The concept of bundling is valid and has merit. Physicians should be paid only once for providing a service. An excellent example would be a patient who has a cystoscopy and then a transurethral resection of a bladder tumor (TURBT). (Under that circumstance, the cystoscopy is an integral part of the TURBT and therefore should not be charged separately.)

Before billing, you must check for bundles each time more than one procedure is performed on the same day. Medicare has set up a complete bundling "edit," which is called the Correct Coding Initiative (CCI). Many bundles are correct; however, some codes are bundled to become an integral part of a procedure in certain circumstances and not in others. In addition, codes are bundled that are seldom, if ever, an integral part of the procedure into which they are bundled.

In April 1997, Medicare designated all codes in the bundle as either: 1) Unable to remove the procedure from the bundle with a modifier; or 2) Can be removed with a modifier. Does this mean that whenever you perform a procedure with this designation you should automatically use a modifier to remove it? No. It means that you can remove it if circumstances exist that satisfy the use of the modifier. A new modifier was added to the CPT in January 1997—Modifier 59. It is used to specifically remove codes from the bundle edit. However, its use must be satisfied by the circumstance surrounding the procedure. For example, if you do a cystoscopy at one patient encounter, such as in the office in the morning, and then excise a large bladder tumor (TURBT) in the afternoon at the hospital, the proper coding would be to charge for the TUR large bladder tumor and the cystoscopy using Modifier −59 and place of service as office. **Note:** LT/RT, 58,78,79 modifiers will also remove codes from the bundle if their use is appropriate.

In order to be paid properly for all services rendered, you must know your bundles, which are subject to change four times a year. A number of sources exist for this information, including the National Technical Information Services (NTIS), a for-profit publishing arm of the federal government, and The SourceBook, AccuSource™, or Flash Code™ Expert Edition (electronic versions of the SourceBook that are updated by PRS quarterly.) Follow this General Rule in the Private Section as well as in determining when to use a modifier to unbundle for Medicare. "If one procedure is an integral part of another procedure, do not charge for the included procedure. However, if the procedure is unrelated, performed at a different encounter, different part of the body, or for a different disease process, charge for both procedures and if they are bundled in the CCI, use the appropriate modifier to remove it from the bundle."

## THIRD-PARTY PAYER

The specifics of payment policies are revealed in the interpretation by the third-party payers. Knowing the variation in payment methodology of the different payers is critical to proper reimbursement. Frequently, a contract will state that the payer uses the "modified" St. Anthony/McGraw-Hill relative value schedule or a "modified" RBRVS (Medicare) schedule. This language is a euphemism for "Watch out! Changes have been made." An insurance company will often pick and choose between the specific rules of both value schedules to save themselves money in different payment situations. Some of the key elements to watch for are profiled below.

**Relative Values and Conversion Factor.** A third-party payer will frequently modify the relative values in a contract. They may lower the relative values for the top 10–20 procedures provided by the physician in the contract. This allows them to pay an excellent conversion factor, yet keep the payments lower than the physician anticipates. Payment equals relative value × conversion factor. High conversion and low relative value = lower payment, just as common relative value and low conversion factor = low payment.

**Consults.** Specific rules for consults are laid out in CPT and interpreted by Medicare. However, many insurance companies have decided that they will not pay for consults, or will pay for consults only under certain circumstances.

**Procedural Coding.** Payers have considerable variances on a given procedure regarding coverage for diagnosis and/or treatment (For example, erectile dysfunction).

**Modifiers.** Some insurance companies use all modifiers, some pick and choose, and others do not recognize modifiers at all.

**Bundling.** Currently, Medicare has the most comprehensive published bundling edits. Many private third-party payers also bundle procedures and services. Some may use Medicare's system, others have determined their own bundles, and many have no bundling edits in their payment system.

**Supplies.** Similarly, some payers pay for supplies in the physician's office (many use HCPCS codes for supplies, others do not), some pay selectively, and others pay for none. Medicare has "bundled" most supplies into the professional services.

**Multiple Procedural Reductions.** Medicare and St. Anthony/McGraw-Hill both suggest a payment of 100% for the highest or most complicated procedure and 50% for the additional procedures performed. Some payers pay on multiple procedures at the rate of 100% for the first, 50% for the second, 25% for the third, 10% for the fourth, and 5% for the fifth.

## FRAUD AND ABUSE

According to the Annual Office of the Inspector General (OIG) Report, in 1996, Medicare fraud was estimated to be about $23 billion; in 1997, this dropped to $20 billion; and in 1998, to $12.6 billion. In 1998, $3.7 billion of this was attributed to physicians. A total of $750 million was the result of poor or no documentation, $1.5 billion was from incorrect coding, and $394 million was because of lack of medical necessity—the only category that has increased since 1997.

The three categories for Medicare fraud and abuse are criminal, civil, and administrative. Fortunately, most wrongful billing cases are categorized as civil. Despite the anxicty surrounding fraud and abuse issues, most physicians will not have to go to prison for infringements of Medicare law. That punishment is reserved for criminal offenses by the very few who willfully and knowingly defraud the government. Proof "beyond reasonable doubt" is the standard required for conviction under criminal law.

For civil and administrative fraud and abuse, *ignorance of the law is no excuse.* Physicians utilizing the Medicare system are expected to *know the rules and regulations.* The law specifically states that if the physician "knew" or "should have known" when referencing defendants' knowledge of the law. Guilt is determined by "the preponderance of the evidence," as opposed to criminal law requirements for "beyond reasonable doubt."

In essence, if you code incorrectly, you are guilty. However, your "intent" and the magnitude of the offense determine your punishment.

The two basic levels of civil penalties for fraud and abuse with which the average practicing physician needs to be concerned are:

1. Recoupment or repayment of monies for which a physician has wrongfully billed; or
2. Repayment of three times the amount a physician has wrongfully billed, with a minimum of a $5000 fine per line item up to a maximum of $10,000 per line item.

Return of money erroneously collected is the general penalty for physicians if their intent to observe the Medicare laws is deemed genuine and the mistakes appear to be inadvertent. However, if errors are of a magnitude reflecting "reckless disregard" of the laws, the weighty civil money penalties mentioned above can be assigned.

Recently, June Gibbs Brown, Inspector General of the Department of Health and Human Services, stated in an open letter to physicians that providers could reduce fear of exorbitant fines by instituting in-office "compliance plans." HCFA has published the following seven elements that should be addressed in a compliance plan:

1. A clear commitment to compliance (mission, goals, and so forth).
2. Appointment of a trustworthy compliance officer with a high level of responsibility.
3. Effective training and education programs.
4. Auditing and monitoring (internal and external).
5. Communications.
6. Internal investigation and enforcement.
7. Response to identified offenses and application of corrective action initiatives (punitive actions, repayment, and so forth).

Physicians demonstrating a good-faith effort to comply with the rules (including a working compliance plan) should not have to worry about enormous fines. If they make a billing mistake, or even a series of coding errors, they will probably only have to repay the amounts improperly requested from Medicare. Consider your compliance plan your insurance plan against fraud.

# 4   Advanced Information Systems in the Modern Physician's Office

*Steve Gardilcic, MD*

**CONTENTS**

   COMPETING IN A PRICE COMPETITIVE ENVIRONMENT
   INFORMATION SYSTEMS FOR THE FUTURE
   BENEFITS OF ADVANCED INFORMATION SYSTEMS
   IMPLEMENTING THE NEW TECHNOLOGY:
      ASSURING A SUCCESSFUL TRANSITION

---

The delivery of health care has undergone dramatic changes in the last decade. The invention of managed care has had a profound impact on the practice of urology. Managed care, as well as advancement in technology, has decreased the need for urologists' services, resulting in a price-competitive environment. Our reimbursement is based on contracts; therefore, the business aspect of our practice is becoming more important. We are asked to deliver high-quality care at a lower cost. Capitation places even higher demands on those who accept this type of reimbursement. The capitated payment system works to the payer's advantage, guaranteeing a certain rate of profits while shifting the risk to providers. Having the precise knowledge of the cost of services provided—as well as the probability that those services will be needed—is the key to success. We are required to keep meticulous medical records and to comply with coding and reimbursement rules that often vary from payer to payer. New confidentiality regulations regarding medical records will require that we keep accurate logs about access to documents. Because of the time and effort needed to keep up with regulations and requirements, the practice of medicine in today's society is demanding for physicians and their staff. Managed care and government regulations have significantly increased the amount of paperwork we deal with, thus increasing the cost of running our practices.

It can be expected that reimbursement for our services will continue to decline as long as even a few physicians are willing to accept lower rates. Prices will stabilize at the point when competitors accepting contracts below their costs are driven out of the market.

Radical changes in the delivery of health care dictate radical changes within our practices. In the past, with generous reimbursement, the business aspect of the practice

From: *Current Clinical Urology: Office Urology: The Clinician's Guide*
Edited by: E. D. Kursh and J. C. Ulchaker © Humana Press Inc., Totowa, NJ

could be grossly neglected. Inefficiencies could be tolerated and the practice would still be successful. In the future, the delivery of high-quality care will, as before, remain a key element in the practice's success. Only those who have mastered the business aspect will enjoy long-term prosperity. To do this, *you must improve efficiency and productivity and make intelligent business decisions.*

## COMPETING IN A PRICE-COMPETITIVE ENVIRONMENT

The key elements needed for success have been determined by analyzing data from other industries that have gone through the stages of a price-competitive environment. As a rule, successful competitors have been able to prosper—not by selling more goods and services, but primarily by lowering their overhead costs. The reason for their success is a vital principle we must all adopt. Every dollar recovered from overhead will contribute 100% to your profits. For example, if you have an overhead ratio of 50%, each additional dollar in revenue generated will contribute 50% to your profits. Simply stated, lowering overhead expenses will contribute more to your practice's overall financial performance than providing additional services.

It is crucial to understand the difference between fixed and variable costs within your practice. Fixed costs, such as rent for your office space and malpractice insurance premiums, remain the same regardless of the number of patients you see in your office. Variable costs, such as staff salaries, will be higher if you see more patients. An increase in patients, therefore, will not contribute more to the overall financial performance of your practice if it leads to a significant increase in your overhead expense. The airline industry is a good example of this principle. Tickets are offered at a large discount just prior to the flight departure. This illustrates good business sense. The airplane amortization, fuel, and crew salaries are already paid off. Every additional ticket sold, even at a deep discount, will contribute 100% to the profit. In today's health-care environment, the decision to accept or not accept additional managed-care contracts requires careful financial analysis. This includes keeping an eye on the level of reimbursement. You must consider your fixed and variable costs as well as expected profit margins. More often than not, managed-care contracts are signed without a full understanding of the financial impact on the practice. Often, these contracts are signed without a realization that they are below the costs of providing services. In the past, with generous reimbursement, one or two nonperforming contracts would affect the practice performance but not necessarily lead to its demise. Within a price-competitive environment, a few nonperforming contracts could—and very well may—lead to the failure of the practice.

There is little you can do to lower your fixed costs. It is possible to renegotiate a better lease agreement for office space or join malpractice insurance purchasing groups to lower this expense. However, looking at the overall picture, the savings are minimal. You must do more than this to gain control of your variable expenses. One major item to consider is the salary and benefits for your staff. Lowering your staff compensation is the wrong strategy, and results in the loss of competent employees. To succeed in a price-competitive environment, you need to have a highly qualified and motivated staff. The solution is complex, yet simple. *You must increase staff productivity.* If this is carried out with careful planning and thought, you will be able to handle higher patient loads with the same amount of staff or the same patient load with fewer staff. This can only be accomplished with a full understanding of the basic efficiency concept. Any business activity resulting in a finished product or service is called a business process. Everything we do to provide care to patients can be defined as the sum of individual processes, and every process has its cost.

The process and associated costs can be clearly defined and analyzed. For example, your patient calls the office and would like to know his most recent PSA results. What should be a simple task turns into total chaos. The receptionist usually places the patient on hold and searches for the chart. If the chart is in its proper place, she looks for the results and finds they are not yet posted. Therefore, she informs the patient that she will have to call him back when the results are received. At this point, the task is passed to the nurse, and by the time the patient receives his results, two or three days have passed. The simple inquiry took a great deal of time, and incurred associated costs. In this particular case, we calculate the time the staff spent chasing the chart, filing the report, and contacting the patient. A simple question, in a paper environment, is thus very costly because staff wastes valuable time on the proverbial "paper chase." With electronic medical records, this same question would have taken a few seconds to answer. The reason for this is quite simple. If your office has fully computerized medical records, you have the capability of an interface to the local laboratory and therefore, you receive the results electronically. With an analysis of the difference in process, you can clearly understand the savings. When a patient calls, results are more likely to be posted in the electronic chart. With such a system, the results are transmitted electronically as soon as they are completed. The need to wait on mail and spend time placing this report in the patient's chart becomes obsolete. The receptionist simply locates the patient's chart with a few keystrokes and the chart and test results are immediately accessed. There is no need to involve anyone else in the process as long as the lab report is normal and no other medical action is needed. The cost for completing the same process under the worst-case scenario might be a few dollars vs—under the best-case scenario—a few cents. Electronic medical records also have a feature that enables you to notify the patient of his recent laboratory results with automatic customized letters. With the use of this feature, the call could have been completely avoided, thus saving time.

*If properly implemented, information technology will make your staff more productive, leading to an overall improvement of practice performance.*

## INFORMATION SYSTEMS FOR THE FUTURE

In order to succeed in a price-competitive environment, you must lower your overhead expenses, maintain or improve quality, and collect clinical and business data intelligently to make the right practice-management decisions. You can only accomplish this by properly implementing information technology. Document templates save a significant amount of time and money on transcription costs. This is only one example of how information systems can improve productivity. You can also enter clinical protocols in the electronic chart that will remind you of processes and steps in your clinical decision making. This will improve quality and efficiency. Clinical and business information is searchable and can be used to create customized reports about clinical outcomes as well as the cost of care. This will provide you valuable information needed for negotiating managed-care contracts and successful practice management.

The information system of the future will go far beyond the practice-management billing systems most practices are familiar with. The end point is a paperless medical office where all clinical and business information is received, stored, and transmitted into an electronic form.

The move toward a paperless environment started around 1996 with the availability of the first generation of electronic medical records for physician offices. *This is the key component of the entire system.* Currently, fewer than 1% of physicians around the country are using an information system more advanced than just a practice management, or billing, system. Only 1% of this small number has systems with a completely electronic clinical component. Even rarer are the offices that have computerized all business aspects of their practices.

Information systems for the futuristic physician's office are network-based. This means that the information can be accessed and shared at any time on the network. As a rule, the front office, back office, every patient examination room, and occasionally the waiting room, have computers that are connected to one network. The entire system should have the ability to connect to the Internet as well as access to dial-up connections. With these features the system can be accessed from satellite offices as well as the physician's home. Your information system should be capable of providing you with the costs of care. It should also have the ability to submit claims and receive payments electronically and verify patient enrollment and eligibility online. The proper information system should be capable of retrieving up-to-date information regarding your financial performance under various managed-care contracts. Your medical records should also be completely electronic. The system should communicate to other healthcare entities electronically through e-mail and network-based fax.

Every information system has two components. These components consist of hardware, including PCs, monitors, modems, and printers, and software, consisting of computer applications specifically designed to accomplish certain tasks.

The type of hardware, as well as the overall design of the computer network, will be dictated by the type of software applications you use as well as your clinical and business workflows. For example, if you are moving from room to room to see patients, you will need to have computers in every room. If the patients are coming to you and are consistently seen in the same room you may only need one computer.

## *Operating System*

Several types of software are used in the modern physician's office. These are the computer applications that run your network. The two major operating systems on the market are the Unix-based systems we may be familiar with from our old billing systems, and the newer Windows NT-based operating systems. Unix-based operating systems are highly proprietary, whereas Windows NT operating systems are built based on common standards. The software applications are designed specifically for each system. You should avoid having more than one operating system on your network; this situation will increase the maintenance cost. Almost all of the current electronic medical records programs are designed for Windows NT operating systems. I recommend that you base your entire network on this system, as it will serve your practice-management system, electronic medical records, and other applications.

## Practice Management—Billing

The practice-management systems of the past were based on one-way communication. The charges were entered and submitted to insurance companies, checks were received, and payments were posted. The newer practice-management systems are, as a rule, based on the Windows NT operating system. They receive payments electronically and post them automatically into the patient's account. This system saves a significant amount of time and also allows for online verification of the patient's insurance eligibility—an increasingly important factor as patients change insurance plans frequently and each insurance plan has a specific set of rules and requirements for providers. A good practice-management system should have built-in, sophisticated reporting capabilities. It is important that the system uses an open relational database and that the vendor is willing to provide you with the database scheme so you can customize and create your own reports as needed.

## Electronic Medical Records

*Electronic medical records are the key element in the success of a paperless physician's office.* Electronic medical records (EMR) is a sophisticated software application that allows for the creation and maintenance of complete paperless records. This application has a number of important features, such as the ability to verify that patient-encounter documentation meets specific coding requirements.

## Imaging Software

If you want your practice to be completely paperless, imaging software is a critical application. Much of the information we receive is on paper. These documents can be converted into electronic form. Examples of this include—but are not limited to—EKGs, such studies as urodynamics, and ultrasound images. These documents are scanned and then stored as electronic images with a reference within the electronic medical record. This application is also important because it allows you to scan existing patient medical records while moving from paper to the paperless environment. The same application can be used for converting other business information into electronic form, such as explanation of benefits, purchase orders, receipts, and other documents that are essential to keep.

## Network-Based Fax

Network-based faxing is another critical element of the entire system. If someone requests information from your electronic records, there is no need to print out the information. Your computer automatically transmits this. Incoming faxes can be viewed on the screen and forwarded to anyone in the office.

## E-Mail

E-mail is software that can be used for electronic communication as well as moving electronic documents within or outside the office. If medical records are sent outside via e-mail through the Internet, you must ensure that this software has the capability of encrypting for obvious privacy and patient confidentiality issues. If the computers on your network are multimedia-enabled, you can use voice-enabled e-mail within or outside the office via the Internet. This completely eliminates typing e-mail messages.

## *Electronic Time Clock*

The electronic time clock allows employees to clock in and out on their computers electronically. The advantages of this software include the data it provides to run payroll and its ability to provide reports about staff hours worked for each particular job capacity.

## *Accounting Software*

With the proper configuration of categories and subcategories offered by accounting software, you will be able to closely monitor your practice overhead. Modern accounting software will do this in astounding and sophisticated ways. Files sent to your accountant to be reviewed or modified can subsequently be automatically uploaded on your system in the office.

## BENEFITS OF ADVANCED INFORMATION SYSTEMS

### *Cost: Saving Time and Money*

It is very difficult for someone who has never worked in a truly paperless environment to appreciate the many benefits. The best way to gain a full understanding of this is to examine the most common processes as they occur and describe the resulting benefits. A properly implemented system provides access to information—whether clinical or business—in seconds instead of minutes or hours. This advantage is noted and appreciated by patients and referring physicians. The system allows for multiple access to information, thus improving efficiency. For example, a nurse who is scheduling surgery and an insurance person who is obtaining the precertification can access the information at the same time.

The cost of a paperless system vs. the cost of a paper system is another factor that must be considered. The cost of creating electronic patient records consists of the time needed to input the patient information. Once it is entered, it can be accessed in a matter of seconds at any location within the network. The cost of creating paper-based records is estimated to be approximately $10.00 per chart. The cost of processing the charts for patient visits—including pulling the chart, routing information, dictation, and filing the chart—is approximately $3.00 per visit.

### *Improved Accuracy of Records*

It is much easier for a physician to assess patients based on information in the electronic record as opposed to the paper chart. All notes within the chart are legible, categorized in groups, and offer selective viewing if desired. At the click of one button, you can view a flowsheet of PSA levels from the last year, with the capability to switch to a graphic form. It becomes nearly impossible for the physician to miss information. Reports, labs, and notes entered into the system by staff members are forwarded to the physician for review and electronic signature.

Electronic medical records also allow you to electronically respond and communicate with your staff via messages in any particular order as they relate to patient care. These particular electronic messages are called flags, and can be easily attached to the patient's chart. Each flag is stamped with the time and date, allowing you to selectively view what tasks have been forwarded to each staff member and check on completion status. If you notice that a particular staff member is have a difficult time keeping up with assigned tasks, you can electronically reroute them to others. This process replaces the commonly used "sticky notes" which so often get lost. The worry of "misplaced charts" also becomes a thing of the past.

Appointment scheduling is another feature worth mentioning. The appointment scheduler is capable of integrating and keeping track of all resources needed for appointments. For example, special directives—such as ultrasound equipment needed as well as availability of a specific staff member—are scheduled accordingly, eliminating conflict. At this point, optimal utilization of time and resources reaches its peak. Appointments can also be linked to certain electronic notes as appropriate with certain procedures. For example, let's say you have scheduled a cystoscopy appointment. The electronic chart will, at the time of the patient's arrival, automatically create a template in the patient's record accordingly.

The electronic chart has the capability of creating "structured notes." This means that during your patient assessment and examination, you can enter all the findings automatically without typing. The system will then automatically check the note for proper coding. If the documentation does not meet the requirement of the CPT code you select, you will be warned and the system will identify the portion of examination with the missing component. You can subsequently choose a different CPT code that will meet the requirements, or add to the examination if needed. Electronic records also allow for use of templates (text containing discussion with patients, handouts, and consents) that can be incorporated into the patient's chart as needed. If properly used, templates allow for a reduction of about 80% in transcription costs. The specific letter templates used for patient correspondence, referring physicians, and insurance companies, are especially valuable. Based on design, information from the patient's database, such as diagnosis, previous and current medications, and allergies, can be pulled automatically into a letter. This reduces a significant amount of transcription and adds quality to the accuracy of records.

Using a drop-down list, you can associate a particular diagnosis with particular visits. The physician codes the visits in terms of right diagnosis at the time of the patient's visit. This automatic check of the appropriate documentation for CPT coding eliminates potential coding errors. Prescriptions and handouts about potential side effects can be printed automatically. Prescriptions can be sent directly to the pharmacy, via network-based fax, right from the patient's room, or can be given to the patient to take. Also, every new medication is checked for side effects and cross-reactivity with all previously entered medications. If there is a potential problem with a combination, the system will display articles discussing this. Medication refills take seconds, with no need to search for patient charts. Allergies are entered into the electronic chart, making it impossible to write prescriptions in error. You can also enter any special directives the patient has given.

This system will also create order forms electronically, with appropriate insurance billing information, for different tests and procedures. The elimination of handwriting saves an enormous amount of time. Orders are checked for appropriate diagnosis and precertification requirements as defined by insurance carriers. If a precertification letter is required it can be created automatically.

### *Advanced Reporting Capabilities*

Electronic medical records offer sophisticated reporting capabilities. It takes seconds to identify all the patients who have been prescribed a certain medication, or had certain types of procedures. Any documents you are interested in researching can be displayed in seconds. This information can be further processed in order to calculate the total cost of care per specific condition or patient population as well as outcomes. Specific questionnaires can be sent automatically to groups of patients who meet certain clinical criteria.

Clinical protocols can be entered into the system and displayed on the screen while the physician is seeing the patient, and compliance and variation from protocols can be assessed.

In my practice, we have used all of the applications described here since the beginning of 1996. We have developed a completely paperless environment for patient records as well as business records. Our system is highly customized, with hundreds of documents, templates, handouts, protocols, and letters specifically designed for our specialty. We are also using specialty-specific workflows, and taking full advantage of this technology. Based on our benchmark analysis, we have shown that the creation of a completely paperless environment has resulted in an increased staff productivity of about 33% above the national average. I have also experienced increased patient satisfaction while using the system. Considering the fact that I am a solo practitioner with a highly motivated staff to embrace this technology, these results represent what can be accomplished under ideal circumstances.

## IMPLEMENTING THE NEW TECHNOLOGY: ASSURING A SUCCESSFUL TRANSITION

Based on my experience, I am confident that electronic medical records and paperless information systems are the wave of the future. Ten years from now it will be nearly impossible to practice without conversion. The transition from paper to a paperless office is an enormous task. Do not be disillusioned by electronic medical record vendors who tell you implementing their system will result in significant savings. Our experience is that electronic medical records *alone* will *not* produce a savings, but will incur additional expenses. As long as you need *any* paper records to be pulled for patient visits, savings will not be realized. You will notice a significant savings by acquiring imaging software and scanning paper records on active patients into the system. Reengineering of processes is critical to improve efficiency.

The first step, before deciding to implement an information system, is to perform a benchmark analysis. Spreadsheets that allow you to analyze the current efficiency of your practice by comparing your practice with national averages can be obtained by contacting the author by e-mail or telephone. The results will reveal your current standing and the potential savings associated with the implementation of advanced information technology.

Next, you will need to reach a consensus about the acquisition and implementation of the system. If you decide to implement electronic medical records, it is *crucial* that *all* physicians within the group are united in the decision to proceed with the project. Unlike the practice-management billing system, electronic medical records have a tremendous impact on the way physicians work. If there is dissension among the physicians regarding the project, *you are assured failure* with the implementation of the system.

Finally, in the implementation of the advanced information technology and reengineering of your practice, enlist the help of qualified consultants. Choosing components for your systems that are unreliable could have devastating effects. For example, if you cannot find a patient's record, you have to realize that you will not see that particular patient on this day. If your electronic medical records are not working, you will not see any patients at all. In evaluating which system to purchase and before making a final decision about a particular system, your consultant should provide you with a cost-benefit and return-on-investment analysis based on the data from your practice. As a rule, the paperless information system will pay for itself within two years. Moving from paper to a paperless environment is an enormous task. We recommend a gradual approach.

The first step is to develop a computer network. If you have one of the old Unix-based practice-management systems, you may want to convert to the modern Windows NT-based system. When your staff feels comfortable with this application, move to the next one. Next, you should consider adding internal/external e-mail and network-based fax software before implementing electronic medical records and document-imaging software. This is a major step that will affect not only the physicians, but the entire staff, and staff assessment is crucial. You should ask the following questions. How computer literate are they? Are they enthusiastic about technology? What will change in their job description? What kind of retraining is needed? These steps need to be planned well in advance.

The conversion from paper to electronic records must be carefully planned. All charts on active patients for two or three months in advance must be scanned into the system, and the remaining ones will be scanned as they are seen. The number will gradually decrease over the next couple of months. *Do not run a paper and paperless system at the same time*—it will lead to duplication of work and major confusion.

The move from paper to a paperless office is a very demanding process. People are normally resistant to change and only comply willingly if they see a clear benefit. For the physician, the benefit is to have a successful practice in the future. The staff will find their benefits in the ability to perform their jobs better and more easily with the elimination of dreaded tasks, such as hunting for information.

*Get an expert's advice.* You will be making a significant investment in your practice and should avoid repeating errors that others have made in implementing this technology.

Sound advice prior to proceeding with this major task will pay off later with a technology that works. In seeking this advice, you can avoid many disappointments along the way. Any additional information on this subject can be had by contacting the author at 419-756-4999, or by e-mailing your inquiry to doctor@urologycare.com

# 5  Important Legal Issues in the Current Health-Care Environment

*Alan E. Schabes*[1] *and David M. Levine*[2]

**CONTENTS**

    INTRODUCTION
    CRITICAL ISSUES
    CONCLUSION

## INTRODUCTION

This chapter addresses several of the more significant legal issues that arise in the physician office-practice setting. It cannot be disputed that the practice of medicine is a heavily regulated business—both at the state and Federal levels. Practical considerations preclude a discussion of the laws of any particular state; however, they have been addressed generically.

This chapter addresses two broad topics: A) the medical practice as a legal entity; and B) health care regulatory compliance, including: 1) the Federal antikickback statute, 2) the Federal physician "self-referral" statute, 3) compliance programs, and 4) voluntary disclosure of noncompliance to the government.

## CRITICAL ISSUES

### *The Medical Practice as a Legal Entity*

Previously, physicians could not practice medicine under a separate legal entity. It was feared that the existence of an entity would somehow corrupt the practice of a learned profession. This "corporate practice of medicine" doctrine has been significantly eroded, and today physicians are permitted to practice medicine under an array of legal structures. Although it is not required that a physician practice medicine under some form of legal entity, it is uncommon for a physician to operate as a "sole proprietorship" (i.e., a business conducted by a single individual in his[3] individual capacity, without the benefit of a separate legal entity).

The drawbacks of a sole proprietorship are significant—notably, the business owner is personally responsible for all liabilities of the business, and as an employer is also

From: *Current Clinical Urology: Office Urology: The Clinician's Guide*
Edited by: E. D. Kursh and J. C. Ulchaker © Humana Press Inc., Totowa, NJ

liable for the acts or omissions of his employees. Further, the sole proprietorship, by definition, is a business that is "owned" by only one person. Therefore, the addition of another owner necessitates the adoption of a new business structure, often with significant legal ramifications.

The principal benefit to conducting a business as a sole proprietorship is that there is no separate taxable legal entity—profits are taxed at the individual's tax rate and losses pass directly to the individual. As explained below, the principal benefit of a sole proprietorship can be realized, and the drawbacks can be avoided, through the appropriate selection and operation of a separate legal entity. The two most common choices are: 1) the professional corporation, and 2) the limited liability company (LLC).[4]

**Professional Corporation**

**In General.** There are two principle benefits of practicing as a professional corporation.

First, a professional corporation is easy to form. The filing of articles of incorporation with the state Secretary of State is commonly all that is required to "create" the entity. Other documents commonly used in conducting and governing corporate business (e.g., Code of Regulations, buy-sell agreements, directors and shareholders corporate resolutions, and so forth) are relatively straightforward. In many ways, the professional corporation is the simplest type of entity to manage.

Second, the professional corporation features *limited* liability for its owners (i.e., shareholders). Thus, shareholders of a professional corporation are not responsible for the corporation's liabilities. Of course, the physician shareholder risks losing his investment in the corporation in the event of insolvency.

In every instance, each physician remains personally liable for his own professional negligence—a fact that cannot be avoided through the selection of any type of legal entity form. One shareholder, however, is not liable for the professional liability of another shareholder or an employee (whereas partners of a partnership are jointly and severally liable not only for the partnership's liabilities, but also for the professional liability of each partner and that of the partnership employees).

The principal drawbacks of the corporate form arise in the tax area. First, the existence of a professional corporation can result in "double taxation" (at the level of the business entity, and again at the level of shareholder when the earnings are paid out as dividends or as liquidation proceeds), unless the corporation is an "S" corporation (discussed below). During operations, this double tax may be mitigated, to some degree, by payment of salaries (deductible to the corporation as a business expense) thereby "zeroing out" corporate income, and in turn, taxes. One potential pitfall is that amounts paid out in excess of "reasonable compensation" are not entitled to a deduction and, upon audit, will be reclassified as a nondeductible dividend.

Further, upon a sale of the business, double taxation may be mitigated to a limited degree, by structuring part of the purchase price as compensation for consulting services, non-compete agreements, and so forth, that will pass outside of the corporate entity directly to the shareholders. Otherwise, an asset sale will generate taxable income to the corporation, then another tax as the corporation liquidates and distributes proceeds to its shareholders. A purchaser will usually favor an asset sale, in order to increase the tax basis in the assets. A seller typically favors a stock sale, so that he may avoid some of the incidence of double taxation.

**S Corporations.** The Internal Revenue Code permits a corporation to make an election to be treated as an S Corporation (as opposed to a C Corporation). The principal benefit of this alternative is that there is only one level of tax (i.e., no tax at the entity level, absent unusual factors). Shareholders simply report income on their personal returns. There is also no concern related to the loss of a deduction for unreasonable compensation, discussed above.

The shareholders of an S Corporation, generally, must be individuals, and nonresident aliens may not be shareholders. Certain kinds of trusts and estates may be S Corporation shareholders. In addition, there may be only one class of stock, which for the medical practice is not typically a significant issue.

With regard to fringe benefits, S Corporations may provide their employees who are 2% shareholders with tax-free fringe benefits such as medical insurance only in partial amounts, which are 45% for 1998, 60% for 1999 through 2001, and will rise to 100% in 2003. By contrast, the C Corporation may provide tax-free fringe benefits that are generally fully deductible to the C Corporation without limitation.

## Limited Liability Company ("LLC")

The LLC is a relatively recent phenomenon—particularly in the practice of medicine. An LLC only requires the filing of Articles of Organization with the state Secretary of State. An "Operating Agreement" entered into by the LLC "Members" (the owners) dictates the internal governance. The Operating Agreement is similar in length and scope to a limited partnership agreement, and therefore is somewhat more involved than a "boilerplate" corporate Code of Regulations.

Limited liability for owners under state law, and "pass through" tax treatment (like a partnership or S Corporation), are the significant features of an LLC. Members who are active in the business pay tax on their entire K-1 pass through of income. Fringe benefits for employee owners are the same as for S Corporations.

In contrast to S Corporations, there are no restrictions on the types of persons and entities who may own interests. LLC's may, furthermore, have multiple classes of interests, which confer a degree of economic flexibility that does not exist with the S Corporation. In the absence of a personal guarantee, all debt of an LLC is treated as "nonrecourse" and is therefore allocated proportionately to all members for tax basis purposes. Under some state laws, an LLC may have as few as one member, although under Federal law, a single-member LLC is treated as a sole proprietorship for tax purposes, notwithstanding the protection it provides under state law.

## The Decision

As noted previously, it is rare for physicians to practice medicine as a sole proprietorship, and the authors do not recommend this option. As between the professional corporation and the LLC, most physicians currently opt for a professional corporation (also sometimes known as a "professional association"). Physicians, however, are electing to use LLCs with increasing frequency. The decision to elect S Corporation status is best made with the direct input of the corporation's accountant/tax adviser, since the issues turn largely on tax and employee benefits implications.

## *Health-Care Regulatory Compliance*

### Background

"Health-care regulatory compliance" is a catch-all phrase that covers issues arising under the Federal and state laws and regulations governing the activities of a particular provider-type. With respect to the practice of medicine, state licensure statutes and regulations impose significant regulatory requirements on physicians. Although the state "Medical Practice Acts" contain common features (e.g., prohibit "fee-splitting" or "grossly unprofessional or dishonest conduct"), the variations in statutory language and judicial interpretations on a state-by-state basis prohibit any type of generalization. Thus, although extremely important, state licensure laws and regulations are beyond the scope of this chapter.

Given the ever-increasing role of the Federal government in financing health-care delivery under the various Federal health-care programs (notably Medicare, Medicaid, and Tricare [formerly CHAMPUS]), and the increasing vigilance of the Federal "fraud fighters," this chapter will focus on four Federal regulatory issues affecting physicians—the Federal Anti-Kickback Statute, the Federal Physician "Self-Referral" Statute (aka, the Stark Law), the "Compliance Program," and the "Voluntary Disclosure" program.

### The Federal Anti-Kickback Statute

**The Statute.** Since 1972, the Medicare and Medicaid anti-kickback law (the "Federal Anti-Kickback Law") has provided for criminal and civil penalties for individuals or entities that offer, pay, solicit, or receive remuneration for referrals or for purchasing, leasing, ordering, arranging for or recommending goods or services for which payment is available, in whole or in part, under Medicare, Medicaid, or any other government health-care program.

The Federal Anti-Kickback Law (42 U.S.C. § 1320a-7b(b)) states:

1. Whoever knowingly and willfully solicits or receives any remuneration (including any kickback, bribe, or rebate) directly or indirectly, overtly or covertly, in cash or in kind—
    a. in return for referring an individual to a person for the furnishing of any item or service for which payment may be made in whole or in part under a Federal health-care program, or
    b. in return for purchasing, leasing, ordering, or arranging for or recommending purchasing, leasing or ordering any good, facility, service or item for which payment may be made in whole or in part under a Federal health care program,
   shall be guilty of a felony, and upon conviction, shall be fined not more than $25,000 or imprisoned for not more than 5 years, or both.
2. Whoever knowingly and willfully offers or pays any remuneration (including any kickback, bribe, or rebate) directly or indirectly, overtly or covertly, in case or in kind to any person to induce such person—
    a. to refer an individual to a person for the furnishing or arranging for the furnishing of any item or service for which payment may be made in whole or in part under a Federal health care program, or
    b. to purchase, lease, order, or arrange for or recommend purchasing, leasing or ordering any good, facility, service or item for which payment may be made in whole or in part under a Federal health care program,
   shall be guilty of a felony, and upon conviction, shall be fined not more than $25,000 or imprisoned for not more than 5 years, or both.

Violation of the Federal Anti-Kickback Law can result in severe criminal penalties (fines and imprisonment), as well as civil monetary penalties and exclusion from the Federal health-care programs. Further, conviction of a felony is typically grounds for severe sanctions under state physician licensure laws.

**The Safe Harbor Regulations.** In 1987, Congress directed the Office of the Inspector General (OIG) to promulgate regulations specifying those payment practices that would not be subject to sanctions under the Federal Anti-Kickback Law. If an arrangement falls within one of the safe harbors, the participants are assured that they will not be prosecuted. To fall within a safe harbor, *all* criteria for that safe harbor must be met. Failure to achieve safe harbor protection *does not* necessarily mean that the relationship violates the Federal Anti-Kickback Law, but it does mean that the arrangement is in a "zone of uncertainty" and, therefore, subject to possible scrutiny. The government must only show that at least one purpose of the remuneration was to induce referrals or the purchasing, etc, of goods and services reimbursable by a Federal health-care program.

A brief summary of the safe harbors is provided below.

1. *Investment Interests.* There is a safe harbor for investment interests in large public corporations. There is also a safe harbor for private investment interests, which protects investment interests that are held by either active or passive investors so long as several criteria are met, including the "40%" rules. No more than 40% of the value of the investment interests of each class of investments can be held in any fiscal year by investors who are in a position to make or influence referrals to, furnish items or services to, or otherwise generate business for the entity. In addition, no more than 40% of the entity's gross revenue in any fiscal year may come from referrals related to the furnishing of health care items or services or business otherwise generated from investors. Also, the terms on which the investment is offered to a passive investor, if any, who is in a position to make or influence referrals to, furnish items or services to, or otherwise generate business for the entity, can be no different than the terms offered to other (nonreferring) passive investors.
2. *Personal Service Contracts and Management Contracts.* Payments made by a principal to an agent (any person other than a bona fide employee of the principal) as compensation for the services of the agent are protected. The agreement must be in writing and have a term of not less than one year. The aggregate compensation paid over the term of the agreement must be set in advance, must be consistent with fair market value in an arms-length transaction, and must not be determined in a manner that takes into account the volume or value of any referrals or business otherwise generated between the parties. Further, the aggregate services contracted for must not exceed those that are reasonably necessary to accomplish the commercially reasonable business purpose of the services.
3. *Lease Agreements.* This safe harbor is applicable to payments for the rental or lease of equipment and office space. Similar to the personal services/management contract safe harbor, a lease must be in writing, for a term of not less than one year, and the rental charge must be set in advance, consistent with fair market value in an arms-length transaction and not be determined in a manner that takes into account the volume or value of any referrals or business otherwise generated between parties. Further, the aggregate equipment rental must not exceed that which is reasonably necessary to accomplish the commercially reasonable business purpose of the rental.
4. *Employees.* A safe harbor is available for payments made by an employer to an employee under a bona fide employment relationship, for rendering services for which payment is available under the governmental payment programs.

5. *Sale of Practice.* This safe harbor protects the sale of a physician's practice to another physician where the sale is completed within one year after the first agreement to sell the practice, and the selling physician will not be in a position to make or influence referrals to the purchaser after one year from the date of the first agreement pertaining to the sale.
6. *Warranties.* A safe harbor is available for a warranty that either 1) meets the Federal Trade Commission's definition of a warranty or 2) is a manufacturer's or supplier's agreement to replace another manufacturer's or supplier's defective item. The buyer must report any price reduction as a result of the warranty on the cost report or claim for payment and (upon the request of the Department of Health and Human Services or a state agency) must provide specified information. The manufacturer or supplier also must 1) inform the buyer of its obligation to report any price reductions, and 2) either report the price reduction on the invoice or, if not known at the time of the purchase, report the existence of a warranty and report the price reduction when its value is determined.
7. *Discounts.* This safe harbor protects reductions in price for goods or services based on an arms-length transaction and may include rebate checks, redeemable coupons, and credits subject to specified conditions. Discounts do not include cash payments, agreements to buy another good or service, price reductions not applicable to Medicare or Medicaid programs, routine reduction of a beneficiary's coinsurance or deductible warranties, or services provided in accordance with a personal or management services contract. Reporting obligations, similar to those for warranties, also apply.
8. *Referral Services.* Payments made to a referral service are protected, so long as the service does not exclude an otherwise qualified individual or entity, payment is assessed equally against all participants, and is based on the referral service's costs of operation and not the volume or value of referrals or business generated for which payment may be made under a Federal health care program.
9. *Group Purchasing Organizations ("GPO").* Payments by a vendor to a GPO are protected if the GPO has a written agreement with members of its group stating either that (a) vendors from which the members may purchase goods or services will pay a fee to the GPO of 3% or less of the purchase price; or (b) if the fee is not fixed at 3% or less, the agreement must specify the maximum amount the GPO will be paid by each vendor. Additionally, when the entity receiving the good or service from the vendor is a health care provider, the GPO must disclose in writing to the entity at least annually (and to the Department of Health and Human Services upon request) the amount received from each vendor.
10. *Waivers of Hospital Coinsurance and Deductibles.* If coinsurance or deductible amounts are owed to a hospital for inpatient hospital services for which Medicare or a State health care program pays under the prospective payment system, the hospital's waiver of such amounts is protected if the hospital does not later claim the amount as a bad debt, the waiver is offered to all Medicare beneficiaries without regard to length of stay or DRG, and the hospital's waiver is not made as part of a price reduction agreement between the hospital and a third-party payor. Routine waiver of coinsurance and deductibles by other providers/suppliers is illegal.
11. *Managed Care.* Complex safe harbors exist for managed care plans that are Medicare- or Medicaid-contract plans.
12. *Practitioner Recruitment.* Remuneration paid to a practitioner to locate or relocate to a Health Professionals Shortage Area is protected if nine standards are satisfied.
13. *Obstetrical Malpractice Insurance Subsidiaries.* Malpractice insurance subsidiaries

paid by a hospital or other entity are protected if the practitioner is serving a Health Professionals Shortage Area or a Medically Underserved Area.
14. *Investments in Group Practices.* This safe harbor protects returns on investments in a physician's own group practice, if the group practice meets the physician self-referral (Stark) law definition of a group practice. The safe harbor also protects returns on investment in solo practices where the practice is conducted through the sole practitioner's professional corporation or other separate legal entity. The safe harbor does not protect investments by group practices or members of group practices in ancillary services joint ventures, although such joint ventures may qualify for protection under other safe harbors.
15. *Cooperative Hospital Organizations.* Remuneration paid between a 501(c)(3) hospital and an affiliated cooperative hospital service organization is protected.
16. *Ambulatory Surgical Centers ("ASCs").* This safe harbor protects the return on certain investment interests in four categories of freestanding Medicare-certified ASCs: surgeon-owned ASCs; single-specialty ASCs (e.g., all gastroenterologists); multispecialty ASCs (e.g., a mix of surgeons and gastroenterologists); and hospital/physician-owned ASCs. In general, to be protected, physician investors must be physicians for whom the ASC is an extension of their office practice pursuant to conditions set forth in the safe harbor. Hospital investors must not be in a position to make or influence referrals. Certain investors who are not existing or potential referral sources are permitted. The ASC safe harbor does not apply to other physician-owned clinical joint ventures, such as cardiac catherization labs, end-stage renal dialysis facilities, or radiation oncology facilities.
17. *Specialty Referral Arrangements Between Providers.* This safe harbor protects certain arrangements where an individual or entity agrees to refer a patient to another individual or entity for specialty services in return for an agreement to refer the patient back at a certain time or under certain circumstances. For example, a primary care physician and a specialist to whom the primary care physician has made a referral may agree that, when the referred patient reaches a particular stage of recovery, the primary care physician should resume treatment of the patient.

**Fraud Alerts.** The OIG has issued several fraud alerts that identify suspect arrangements. Those most pertinent to physicians are summarized below.

1. *Joint Ventures.* A 1989 fraud alert listed the following features of questionable joint ventures between health-care providers:
   a. Investors are chosen because they are in a position to refer.
   b. Physicians who are expected to make a large number of referrals are offered a greater investment opportunity.
   c. The joint venture keeps track of referrals and disseminates such information to investors.
   d. Investors may be required to divest their ownership interests if they cease to practice in the service area.
   e. The joint venture is merely an investment "shell" that provides few services itself, but rather contracts with actual service providers.
   f. Physician investors are permitted to borrow the capital contribution from the venture and repay it through deductions from profit distributions.
   g. Investors are paid extraordinary returns in comparison with the business risk involved.
2. *Hospital-Based Physicians.* In a 1991 report, the OIG examined potential violations of the Federal Anti-Kickback Law in the financial arrangements between hospitals and hospital-based physicians. Suspect arrangements typically involve remuneration paid by the physician to induce the hospital to contract with the physician.

3. *Hospital Incentives.* A May 1992 fraud alert listed hospital incentive arrangements considered questionable by the OIG. Examples included:
   a. Payment of any sort of incentive each time a physician refers a patient to the hospital.
   b. Free or significantly discounted office space or equipment (in facilities usually located close to the hospital).
   c. Provision of free or significantly discounted billing, nursing, or other support services.
   d. Free training for a physician's office staff in such areas as management techniques, coding, and laboratory techniques.
   e. Income guarantees.
   f. Low interest or interest-free loans, or loans that may be forgiven if a physician refers patients to the hospital.
   g. Payment for services (which may include consultations at the hospital) which require few, if any, substantive duties by the physician, or payment for services in excess of the fair market value of the services rendered.
4. *Clinical Laboratory Services.* An October 1994 fraud alert identified suspect practices that involved remuneration paid by clinical laboratories to physicians and others in a position to refer patients/business to the lab. These laboratory practices included the provision of free phlebotomy services to physicians, free testing for physicians and their families, free disposal of biohazards, free computers and fax machines, and furnishing goods and services at below fair market value.
5. *Home Health Services.* In June 1995, the OIG issued a fraud alert regarding the home health-care industry. Examples of abusive practices included:
   a. Payment of a fee to a physician for each claim of care certified as medically necessary by the physician on behalf of the home health agency.
   b. Disguising referral fees as salaries by paying physicians for services not rendered, or in excess of fair market value for services rendered.
   c. Offering free services to beneficiaries, including transportation and meals, if they switch home health-care providers.
   d. Providing hospitals, at no cost or below fair market value, with discharge planners, home-care coordinators, or home-care liaisons in order to induce referrals.
   e. Providing other free services, such as 24-hour nursing coverage to retirement homes or adult congregate living facilities in return for home health referrals.
6. *Rental of Space in Physician Offices by Persons/Entities to Which Physicians Refer.* In February, 2000, the OIG issued a special fraud alert regarding leases between suppliers and physicians where the physician-landlords refer patients to the suppliers. The OIG is concerned about rental arrangements that may actually be disguised kickbacks to physician-landlords to induce referrals to the suppliers. The OIG identified the following lease arrangements as being suspect:
   a. Leases between physicians and comprehensive outpatient rehabilitation facilities that provide therapy services in the physician-office;
   b. Leases between physicians and mobile diagnostic testing companies that perform tests in the physician-office; and
   c. Leases between physicians and suppliers of durable medical equipment, prosthetics, orthotics and supplies, where the supplier sets up a "consignment closet" in the physician-office.

**Advisory Opinions.** Federal law now requires the OIG to issue advisory opinions to providers concerning the application of the Federal Anti-Kickback Law to a particular transaction or arrangement. In general, a requestor may ask the OIG to opine as to: 1) what constitutes illegal remuneration; 2) whether an arrangement or proposed arrangement fits within a statutory exception or safe harbor; and 3) whether an activity constitutes grounds for penalties under the Federal Anti-Kickback Law, civil monetary law, or exclusion statutes. The OIG may not give an opinion concerning: 1) the fair market value of goods, services, or property; or 2) whether a person constitutes a bona fide employee.

From the inception of the OIG advisory opinion process in 1997 through March 2000, the OIG has issued 40 advisory opinions. Notably, a favorable opinion insulates the participants in the subject arrangement from liability, but is binding only on the parties to the opinion. Health-care providers and their counsel should consider an OIG opinion to be an expression of the government's position concerning the propriety of a particular arrangement, which although clearly not binding on a court, could be given significant weight. As a practical matter, the vast majority of prosecutions under the Federal Anti-Kickback Law are resolved through negotiation (short of a judicial determination), since the stakes are so high for the health-care provider.

OIG advisory opinions, fraud alerts, safe harbor regulations, and even common sense should be used to guide health-care providers in structuring financial relationships that involve the furnishing of goods and services covered by the Federal health-care programs. Given the severe consequences of violating the Federal Anti-Kickback Law, experienced health-care counsel should evaluate all such arrangements.

## The Federal Physician "Self-Referral" Statute

**The Legislative History.** Section 1877 of the Social Security Act ("Limitation on Certain Physician Referrals"), also known as the "Stark" law, generally provides that a physician may not make a referral to an entity for "designated health services," and the entity may not present a claim under Medicare, if the physician (or the physician's immediate family member) has a "financial relationship" with the entity. This statute also applies to a significant extent in the context of referrals for Medicaid services.

Congress enacted the Stark law out of concern that many physicians were benefitting financially from the practice of referring patients to other providers with whom they (or their immediate family members) had financial relationships (through an ownership or investment interest, or a compensation arrangement). As with the Federal Anti-Kickback Law, Congress sought to insulate the practice of medicine from the corrupting influence of a referring physician's economic self-interest.

The original ban on physician "self-referrals" (Stark I) took effect in 1992, and covered only referrals to clinical laboratories for Medicare-covered services. In general, Stark I prohibited a physician who had a financial relationship with an entity (or a physician with an immediate family member who had a financial relationship with such an entity) from making a referral for clinical laboratory services for which Medicare would pay. Stark I also prohibited the entity from billing the Medicare program, an individual, a third-party payer, or another entity for an item or service furnished as a result of a prohibited referral. Finally, Stark I required a refund of any amount collected from an individual as the result of a prohibited billing.

In 1994, Congress greatly broadened the ban on physician self-referrals, and extended Section 1877 to cover ten additional "designated health services," beginning with referrals after December 31, 1994 (Stark II). On January 9, 1998, the long-awaited Stark II regulations were published as proposed rules. As of March 2000, the regulations have not been adopted as a final rule.

**The Statute and Regulations.** Section 1877(a) of the Social Security Act (42 U.S.C. § 1395nn) comprises the statutory ban on physician self-referrals. It states:

1. IN GENERAL.—Except as provided in subsection b), if a *physician* (or an *immediate family member* of such physician) has a *financial relationship* with an *entity* specified in paragraph 2), then—
   A. the physician may not make a *referral* to the entity for the furnishing of *designated health services* for which payment otherwise may be made under this title, and
   B. the entity may not present or cause to be presented a claim under this title or bill to any individual, third-party payer, or other entity for designated health services furnished pursuant to a referral prohibited under subparagraph A). (Emphasis added.)
   Several important terms are defined in Section 1877 or elsewhere in the Social Security Act and the Stark regulations.

- *Physician*—"Physician" means a 1) doctor of medicine or osteopathy, 2) doctor of dental surgery or dental medicine, 3) doctor of podiatric medicine, 4) doctor of optometry, or 5) chiropractor.
- *Immediate family member*—"Immediate family member" means "husband or wife; natural or adoptive parent, child, or sibling; stepparent, stepchild, stepbrother or stepsister; father-in-law, mother-in-law, son-in-law, daughter-in-law, brother-in-law, or sister-in-law; grandparent or grandchild; and spouse of a grandparent or grandchild."
- *Financial relationship*—"Financial relationship" means either an "ownership or investment interest" in an entity, or a "compensation arrangement" with the entity.
  42 C.F.R. § 411.351 expands the current definition to provide that a "financial relationship" means "a direct or indirect ownership or investment interest (including an option or nonvested interest) in any entity that exists through equity, debt, or other means and includes any indirect ownership or investment interest no matter how many levels removed from a direct interest (for example, a financial relationship in an entity furnishing designated health services exists if the individual holds an ownership or investment interest in any entity that furnishes designated health services), or a compensation arrangement with an entity."
- *Ownership or investment interest*—"[A]n ownership or investment interest ... may be through equity, debt, or other means and includes an interest in an entity that holds an ownership or investment interest in any entity providing the designated health service."
- *Compensation arrangement*—"Compensation arrangement" means "any arrangement involving any remuneration between a physician (or an immediate family member of such physician) and an entity. . . ."
  42 C.F.R. § 411.351 would define a "compensation arrangement" as "any arrangement involving remuneration, direct or indirect, between a physician (or a member of the physician's immediate family) and an entity."
- *Remuneration*—"Remuneration" includes "any remuneration, directly or indirectly, overtly or covertly, in cash or in kind." *See also* 42 C.F.R. § 411.351, which indicates that remuneration means "any payment, discount, forgiveness of debt, or other benefit." Section 1877(h)(1)(C) identifies certain types of remuneration that will not give rise to a "compensation arrangement." Remuneration does not include 1) forgiveness of amounts for inaccurate tests or procedures, mistakenly performed tests, or correction of minor billing errors; 2) the provision of items, devices, or supplies used solely to collect, transport, process, or store specimens, or to order or communicate test results; and 3) certain fee-for-service payments made to a physician by an insurer or self-insured plan.

- *Entity*—"Entity" means "a sole proprietorship, trust, corporation, partnership, foundation, not-for-profit corporation, or unincorporated association."
  42 C.F.R. § 411.351 defines an "entity" as "a physician's sole practice or a practice of multiple physicians that provides for the furnishing of designated health services, or any other sole proprietorship, trust, corporation, partnership, foundation, not-for-profit corporation, or unincorporated association."
- *Referral* and *referring physician*—"Referral" and "referring physician" mean:
  a. *Physicians' services*—Except as provided in subparagraph (C) (pertaining to referrals by pathologists, radiologists, and radiation oncologists), in the case of an item or service for which payment may be made under part B (of the Medicare program), the request by a physician for a consultation with another physician (and any test or procedure ordered by, or to be performed by (or under the supervision of) that other physician), constitutes a "referral" by a "referring physician."
  b. *Other items*—Except as provided in subparagraph (C), the request or establishment of a plan of care by a physician that includes the provision of the designated health service constitutes a "referral" by a "referring physician."
  
  The definition of referral is likely to be expanded to include "certifying or recertifying of the need for any designated health service, for which payment may be made under Medicare Part B" or a comparable service under Medicaid.
- *Designated health services*—"Designated health services" are: clinical laboratory services; physical therapy; occupational therapy; radiology services (including MRI, CAT scans, and ultrasound); radiation therapy, services, and supplies; durable medical equipment and supplies; parenteral and enteral nutrients, equipment, and supplies; prosthetics, orthotics, and prosthetic devices; home health services and supplies; outpatient prescription drugs; and inpatient and outpatient hospital services.

**Statutory Exceptions and Regulations (as proposed under Stark II).** The statutory ban on physician self-referrals is subject to a number of exceptions.

*Ownership and Compensation Arrangement Exceptions*

Physician Services. Section 1877(b)(1) excludes from the ban on self-referrals "physician services" that fall within the definition of a designated health service "provided personally by (or under the personal supervision of) another physician in the same group practice as the referring physician." This (seldom applicable) exception typically arises in connection with any "designated health services" that may be billed under Medicare as physician services, such as some pathology services.

In-Office Ancillary Services. Section 1877(b)(2) concerns designated health services furnished by a physician in his or her office, and is one of the most important statutory exceptions. All designated health services, except for certain durable medical equipment and nutrients, can be furnished under this exception, provided each element of the exception is satisfied. Section 1877(b)(2) applies (in the case of services other than durable medical equipment [excluding infusion pumps] and parenteral and enteral nutrients, equipment and supplies)

(A) either that are furnished:
  (i) Personally by the physician, personally by a physician who is a member of the same group practice as the referring physician, or personally by individuals who are directly supervised by the physician or by another physician in the group practice, and
  (ii) (I) In a building in which the referring physician (or another physician who is a

member of the same group practice) furnishes physician services unrelated to the furnishing of designated health services, or

(II) In the case of a physician who is a member of a group practice, in another building which is used by the group practice:

  (i) For the provision of some or all of the group's clinical laboratory services, or

  (ii) For the centralized provision of the group's designated health services (other than clinical laboratory services), unless the Secretary determines other terms and conditions under which the provision of such services does not present a risk of program or patient abuse,

(B) that are billed by the physician performing or supervising the services, by a group practice of which such physician is a member under a billing number assigned to the group practice, or by an entity that is wholly owned by such physician or such group practice.

Please note that all of the requirements of Section 1877(b)(2)(A)(i) and (ii) and (B) must be met.

Of central importance to this exception is the statutory definition of a "group practice." Section 1877(h)(4)(A) states:

*The term "group practice" means a group of 2 or more physicians legally organized as a partnership, professional corporation, foundation, not-for-profit corporation, faculty practice plan, or similar association:*

i. in which each physician who is a member of the group provides substantially the full range of services which the physician routinely provides, including medical care, consultation, diagnosis, or treatment, through the joint use of shared office space, facilities, equipment and personnel,

ii. for which substantially all of the services of the physicians who are members of the group are provided through the group and are billed under a billing number assigned to the group and amounts so received are treated as receipts of the group,

iii. in which the overhead expenses of and the income from the practice are distributed in accordance with methods previously determined,

iv. in which no physician who is a member of the group directly or indirectly receives compensation based on the volume or value of referrals by the physician, and

v. in which members of the group personally conduct no less than 75 percent of the physician-patient encounters of the group practice.

The proposed Stark II regulations address many of the important details of how Section 1877(b)(2) will be applied:

1. *Proposed Group Practice Definition*: The Stark II regulations, as proposed, would amend the definition of a group practice to include a group that may include an individual physician incorporated as a professional corporation. However, the definition still appears to exclude practices in which one physician holds 100% of the ownership interests but employs additional physicians. Accordingly, a single-owner practice should evaluate whether it needs to change its ownership structure to ensure compliance with the Stark statute. This is an issue that the Congress, with input from the Health Care Financing Administration (HCFA), may address in the future.

2. *Proposed Definition of a "Member"*: Under the Stark II regulations, the proposed definition of a "member" of a group practice would exclude independent contractors, and would define members as including owner and employee physicians only. Accordingly, an independent contractor could not "directly supervise" a group practice's in-

office ancillary services. Furthermore, an independent contractor could not refer to a group practice with which he has a compensation arrangement, unless an exception applies (for "personal services" or for "fair market value compensation" under the proposed Stark II regulations). Finally, the services of independent contractors could not be counted for purposes of determining whether 75% of all physician-patient encounters occur between group members and patients.

3. *The "Full Range of Services" and "Substantially All" Standards*: The "full range of services" and "substantially all" standards would be modified by the proposed Stark II rules. Specifically, the proposed definition of "patient care services" would include "any of a physician's tasks that address the medical needs of specific patients or patients in general, or that benefit the practice." This would mean that a physician's administrative or management duties would be counted toward determining whether the "full range of services" and "substantially all" standards have been met.

4. *Methods for Distributing Group Costs and Revenues*: Under the proposed rules, HCFA would require that the methods for distribution of costs and revenues must be established prior to the time in which the group earned the revenues or incurred the costs. With respect to the allocation of overhead expenses, HCFA reveals that the key question is whether the group practice is actually a unified business, with "centralized decision-making, pooling of expenses and revenues, and (has) a distribution system that is not based on each satellite office operating as if it were a separate enterprise."

5. *Compensation to Group Members*: HCFA has identified several compensation methodologies that are unrelated to referrals and would satisfy the applicable standard, including compensation based on "an even split, a physician's investment in the group, the number of hours a physician in general devotes to the group, or the difficulty of a physician's work."

6. *"Direct Supervision"*: The requirement that the services be provided either personally by the physician "or personally by individuals who are directly supervised by the physician or by another physician in the group practice" raises the issue of what constitutes "direct supervision." The proposed regulations largely retain the current restrictive definition (which incorporates the "in the office" and "readily available" supervision standards under the Medicare "incident to" provisions), but would permit the physician to take a lunch break. Regardless, the physician still must be physically present (except for lunch) in the office suite. Further, "after hours" testing (when the physician is not physically present) is not permitted.

Prepaid Health Plans. This exception applies to provider-payor integration activities, where a physician owns a qualifying health plan (e.g., HMO). This exception also permits the qualifying health plan to furnish designated health services either directly or through a subsidiary.

Other Permissible Exceptions. Congress authorized HCFA to create, by regulation, exceptions that "do not pose a risk of program or patient abuse." See 42 C.F.R. § 411.355(d) (relating to certain services furnished in an ambulatory surgical center, end-stage renal disease facility or hospice), because these services are paid for as part of a composite rate that cannot vary in response to utilization.

*Ownership or Investment Interest Only Exceptions*

Publicly Traded Securities and Mutual Funds. This exception carved out physician ownership of publicly traded securities and mutual funds, provided the company or mutual fund is sufficiently large, and the securities were purchased by the physician on terms generally available to the public.

Ownership of Hospitals in Puerto Rico, Ownership of Rural Providers, and Hospital Ownership. These exceptions are relatively straightforward, and there are no significant Stark II amendments proposed.

*Compensation Arrangement Only Exceptions*

Office and Equipment Rental. These exceptions are similar, and generally protect arrangements where:

1. the lease is in writing and signed by the parties;
2. the space or equipment does not exceed what is reasonable and necessary for legitimate business purposes and is used exclusively by the lessee when being used by the lessee;
3. the lease provides for a term of at least one year;
4. the rental charges over the lease term are set in advance, consistent with fair market value, and are not determined in any manner that takes into account the volume or value of any referrals or business generated between the parties; and
5. the lease would be commercially reasonable even if no referrals were made between the parties.

The term "fair market value" means the value in an arms-length transaction consistent with the general market value, and, with respect to rentals or leases, the value of rental property for general commercial purposes (not taking into account its intended use) and, in the case of a lease of space, not adjusted to reflect the additional value that the prospective lessee or lessor would attribute to the proximity or convenience to the lessor where the lessor is a potential source of patient referrals to the lessee.

The preamble to the Stark II regulations addresses the following additional details concerning leases:

- A lease that can be terminated "with good cause" can still satisfy the one-year term requirement, as long as the parties do not enter into a new arrangement within the originally established one-year time period. This seems to imply that a "without cause" termination right will not satisfy the one-year term requirement. This is an issue that HCFA may address in the future.
- Lease renewals must be for at least one year (i.e., month-to-month renewals will not satisfy the one-year term requirement).
- Subleases are not permitted (since the space or equipment must be used *exclusively* by the lessee).
- Capital leases will not qualify under the exception, since they are treated effectively as ownership of the property (and therefore, payment would not be "for use" of the equipment or space).
- Payments by a lessee to a physician lessor on a "per event" basis are permitted, provided the physician lessor does not also receive a "per event" payment for any patients referred to the lessee for the designated services the lessor is providing. This situation would arise, for example, where a physician (lessor) owns an MRI unit that is leased to and used by a hospital (lessee) (and the hospital pays rent on a "per click" basis), and the hospital pays the physician to interpret the studies. A "per read" payment to the physician would not meet the equipment rental exception.

Bona Fide Employment Relationships. This exception generally protects arrangements between employers and physicians (or their immediate family members) who have a bona fide employment relationship, determined under the common law/IRS test, where: 1) the employment is for the furnishing of identifiable services (not simply health-care services); 2) the amount of the compensation paid must be consistent with the fair market value of the services and not be determined in a manner that takes into account the volume or value of any referrals by the referring physician; and 3) the compensation is provided pursuant to an agreement that would be commercially reasonable even if no referrals were made to the employer.

The Stark II regulations, as proposed, would require that the compensation also not take into account other business generated between the parties. Further, productivity bonuses based on services personally performed by the physician (or an immediate family member) would be permitted, as long as the bonus "is not directly related to the volume or value of a physician's *own* referrals." An employee's bonus, however, could take into account nondesignated health services, noncovered services, as well as designated health services referred by another physician.

It bears noting that there are significant differences between the bona fide employee exception and the group practice exception, although at a glance they appear very similar. In short, bona fide employees who are not part of a group practice face greater compensation restrictions than physicians in a group practice.

Personal Service Arrangements. This exception protects compensation arrangements between a physician (or immediate family member) and an entity in which the physician is an independent contractor (not an employee) of the entity. The exception is satisfied where:

1. There is a written agreement, signed by the parties, specifying the services covered;
2. The arrangement covers all the services to be provided;
3. The aggregate services contracted for do not exceed those that are reasonable and necessary for the legitimate business purpose of the arrangement;
4. The term of the agreement is at least one year;
5. The compensation to be paid over the term is set in advance, does not exceed the fair market value, and except in the case of a physician incentive plan, is not determined in any manner that takes into account the volume or value of any referrals or business generated between the parties; and
6. The services to be performed do not involve the counseling or promotion of a business arrangement or activity that violates any State or Federal law.

The proposed Stark II regulations would slightly loosen the requirement that the arrangement cover all of the services to be furnished by the physician or family member, by permitting multiple agreements, as long as each agreement incorporates the others by reference. The proposed rule would also permit a physician or immediate family member to furnish personal services through employees they have hired for the purpose of performing the services.

The "physician incentive plan" (exception within the exception) generally applies where the physician is at substantial economic risk (through a withhold, capitation, bonus arrangement or otherwise), and the "compensation arrangement between an entity and a physician or physician group may directly or indirectly have the effect of reducing or limiting services provided with respect to individuals enrolled in the entity." The proposed Stark II rules would amend this exception by referencing and incorporating the physician incentive plan regulations that were published March 27, 1996 at 60 Fed. Reg. 13430 (1996).

Remuneration Unrelated to the Provision of Designated Health Services. This exception covers situations in which a hospital pays a physician for services that are unrelated to the furnishing of designated health services (e.g., for administrative duties, quality assurance, utilization review).

Physician Recruitment. This exception applies when a hospital pays remuneration to a physician to induce the physician to relocate to the geographic area to become a member of the hospital medical staff if:

1. The arrangement is set forth in writing and signed by both parties;
2. The physician is not required to refer patients to the hospital;
3. The amount of the remuneration is not determined in a manner that takes into account (directly or indirectly) the volume or value of any referrals by the referring physician; and
4. The physician is not precluded from establishing staff privileges at another hospital or referring business to another entity.

The proposed Stark II regulations would require that the compensation also not take into account the other business generated between the parties. Although the physician recruitment exception would not apply when the physician does not relocate to the geographic area, the newly proposed exception for "fair market value compensation" (discussed below) could apply.

Isolated Transactions. This exception applies to isolated transactions (like a one-time sale of property or a physician practice), if: 1) the amount of the remuneration paid is consistent with fair market value and not determined in a manner that takes into account the volume or value of any referrals by the referring physician; and 2) the remuneration is provided pursuant to an agreement that would be commercially reasonable even if no referrals were made.

The proposed Stark II regulations would require that the compensation also not take into account other business generated between the parties.

Certain Group Practice Arrangements with a Hospital. This exception applies when a physician group furnishes designated health services that are billed by the hospital. Other requirements are essentially the same as those for the personal services exception, and in addition, "substantially all of the services furnished to patients are furnished by the group under the arrangement."

The proposed Stark II regulations would replace the "substantially all" language with the 75% standard also found in the definition of a group practice. This standard requires that 75% of the patient-care services furnished by group members be furnished through the group. This provision recognizes that some degree of "moonlighting" may occur.

Payment by a Physician for Items and Services. Payments made by a physician to an entity as compensation for clinical laboratory services—or for other items or services if the items or services are furnished at a price that is consistent with fair market value—are exempt.

The proposed Stark II regulations would amend the fair market value standard to require that payments exempted thereunder are not specifically exempted by another exception. The proposed regulations also indicate that the reference to "services" includes any type of service, and not just Medicare-covered services.

Discounts. This proposed exception would exempt discounts to physicians, where the discounts are passed on, in-full, or to the patient or payer. Thus, a physician mark-up would not meet the exception, since the discount would not be passed on in-full.

De Minimis Compensation. This proposed exception would exempt compensation, in the form of items or services (but not cash or cash equivalents), that does not exceed a value of $50.00 per gift and an annual aggregate of $300.00, if: 1) the entity providing the remuneration makes it available to all similarly situated persons (regardless of whether they refer to the entity); and 2) the remuneration is not determined in a manner that takes into account the volume or value of any referrals by the referring physician.

Fair Market Value Compensation. This proposed exception contains most of the elements from the "personal services" exception, but also provides that the arrangement must meet a safe harbor under the Federal anti-kickback statute (42 U.S.C. § 1320-7b) in order to be exempt. The elements are:

1. The arrangement must be set forth in a written agreement, signed by the parties, which covers only identifiable items or services, all of which are specified in the agreement, and the agreement must cover all the services to be provided (or must contain a cross-reference to any other agreements for items or services between the parties);
2. The agreement specifies the time frame covered, which may be for any time period and may contain a termination clause, provided the parties enter into one arrangement for such items or services during the course of a year, and an arrangement made for less than a year may be renewed if the terms and compensation do not change;
3. The compensation must be specified, consistent with fair market value, and not be determined in a manner that takes into account the volume or value of referrals, payment for referrals for medical services that are not covered under Medicare or Medicaid, or any other business generated between the parties;
4. The arrangement must involve a transaction that is commercially reasonable and furthers the legitimate business purposes of the parties; and
5. The arrangement meets a safe harbor under the anti-kickback statute.

**Reporting Requirements.** In general, Section 1877(f) requires that entities providing Medicare-covered services must report to the Secretary information about their ownership, investment, and compensation arrangements. However, HCFA has not published the forms necessary to make the contemplated report. Thus, there is currently no reporting obligation.

**Advisory Opinions.** HCFA—pursuant to the Balanced Budget Act of 1997, and regulations promulgated thereunder—has established procedures for the furnishing of advisory opinions concerning the Stark statute. As of May 1, 1999, only two such opinions had been issued.

**Penalties and Sanctions.** The implications of noncompliance with the Stark statute are serious, and include:

1. denial of payment;
2. refund of monies collected;
3. a civil money penalty up to $15,000 for each bill or claim submitted that a person knows or has reason to know is for a service for which payment should not be made; and
4. a civil money penalty up to $100,000 for each arrangement or scheme that the physician or entity knows or should have known has a principal purpose of assuring referrals that, if made directly, would be unlawful (a "circumvention" scheme).

Exclusion from the Medicare and Medicaid programs is also possible. There is presently no criminal sanction under the Stark statute itself, although as discussed below, the retention of Federal health-care program funds received improperly is a basis for criminal sanctions.

**Practical Considerations**

- Any agreement or relationship between a physician and a possible recipient of a referral must be scrutinized carefully to ensure compliance with the Federal Stark statute.
- Many states have a physician "self-referral" of some kind. Most are patterned after the Federal statute, but some apply regardless of whether the subject health-care services are paid for under a governmental program.
- Any agreement or relationship that must be scrutinized in light of Stark must also be reviewed for compliance with the Federal Anti-Kickback Law (and analogous state statutes).
- Physicians in a medical practice must ensure that all financial relationships have been disclosed to the practice, so that impermissible referrals are avoided.

**The Compliance Program**

When asked why he robbed banks, Willie Sutton is reported to have said, "Because that's where the money is." For the same reasons, the Federal and state governments have devoted unprecedented resources to fighting fraud, waste, and abuse in the health-care industry. The implications of this increased governmental scrutiny are clear. Recognizing that the Federal government can detect only a small fraction of health-care fraud and waste, Congress, through the enactment of the Federal Sentencing Guidelines, set up incentives for health-care providers to regulate and police themselves. Compliance Programs and "Voluntary Disclosure" are two of the government's vehicles for engineering a "culture of compliance."

**Compliance Programs.** Under the Federal Sentencing Guidelines, the existence of an "effective program to prevent and detect violations of the law" must be taken into account in the Federal sentencing process. The plan must be appropriately designed, implemented, and enforced. The goal is to detect and prevent criminal activity. However, the entity's failure to detect or prevent a violation does not *per se* mean that the plan was not "effective."

A physician practice should establish a formal Compliance Program, the key elements of which should be:

- *Standards and Procedures*—embodied in policy and procedure manuals and corporate directives.
- *Oversight Responsibilities*—must be assigned specifically to high-level and trustworthy individuals within the organization, whose responsibility it is to monitor compliance.
- *Education and Training*—compliance standards and procedures must be adequately communicated to all persons acting on behalf of the organization (employees and other agents).
- *Monitoring and Auditing*—prospective monitoring of compliance, and retrospective audits of the organization's activities, must be conducted and documented.
- *Enforcement and Discipline*—standards and procedures must be enforced consistently; corrective action must be taken in the event of noncompliance, and for an individual's failure to detect and prevent noncompliance.
- *Response and Prevention*—the organization must respond swiftly and decisively when noncompliance is discovered; additional steps to prevent future noncompliance should be undertaken.

The design and implementation of an effective Compliance Program requires time and a commitment of resources. First, the organization's governing body should adopt a resolution authorizing the development of a Compliance Plan. Second, tailor a "sample" or "model" to fit the organization's activities—a "one size fits all" approach is not recommended. Third, a "legal audit" should be performed to identify all statutes and regulations applicable to the business. Fourth, key personnel should play an active role in identifying the areas of the business that could give rise to noncompliance (e.g., billing/claims submission, contracting with referral sources or recipients of referrals) (the "hot areas"). Fifth, a thorough review of the organization's documents pertaining to the "hot areas" should be conducted under the direction of legal counsel and with the involvement of accounting and other professionals where appropriate. Sixth, counsel should deliver a report to the governing body, which identifies any areas of noncompliance (or potential noncompliance), and recommend changes in the organization's standards and procedures. Finally, corrective action must be taken to avoid future noncompliance.

If drafted and conducted appropriately, a Compliance Program can detect and prevent violations of law that could result in severe criminal and civil sanctions.

**Voluntary Disclosure to the Government**

Another serious issue facing physician practices arises when the practice receives governmental reimbursement that the organization knows it is not entitled to based on an overbilling, upcoding, error, and so forth. Withholding such funds, combined with the requisite intent, is a Federal crime. If it is discovered that governmental reimbursement has been received improperly, disclosure is warranted. However, the practice should avoid making a disclosure without first conducting a reasonable investigation of the facts and circumstances surrounding the overpayment.

The *advantages* of voluntary disclosure are:

- The organization can control the manner and timing of the disclosure.
- Voluntary disclosure may permit the matter to be resolved privately, and will enhance the organization's credibility in the government's eyes.
- The government gives credit for disclosure in a penalty determination.
- The disclosure may even avoid program exclusion or criminal conviction.

The *disadvantages* of voluntary disclosure are:

- The government may have been unaware of the noncompliance without the voluntary disclosure.
- The government might initiate a wider investigation of the organization's activities.

Overall, the advantages of disclosure typically outweigh the disadvantages. What is most important, however, is that the decision to disclose, and the content of the disclosure, must be determined only after a thorough investigation of the facts.

## CONCLUSION

The authors hope that this chapter sensitizes physicians to a number of the significant legal issues affecting them. ***CAVEAT: The information contained herein is not legal or tax advice, and should not be relied upon as such. Please consult a legal and accounting adviser concerning any particular issue or arrangement.***

## NOTES

[1] Mr. Schabes is with the firm of Benesch, Friedlander, Coplan, & Aronoff LLP in Cleveland, OH, and is the Chairman of the firm's Health Care Practice Group. He is a graduate of Duquesne University, *magna cum laude* (1978) and the Hofstra University School of Law (1981), where he served as an associate editor of the Hofstra University Law Review. His practice focuses on the representation of health-care providers in regulatory matters and transactions, with a particular emphasis on the representation of physicians and long-term care providers.

[2] Mr. Levine is with the firm of Benesch, Friedlander, Coplan, & Aronoff LLP in Cleveland, OH, and is a member of the firm's Health Care Practice Group. He is a graduate of the University of Michigan (1982) and the Boston University School of Law (1986), where he served as an editor of the *American Journal of Law and Medicine*. His practice focuses on the representation of health-care providers in regulatory matters, transactions, and civil and administrative litigation.

[3] The authors have arbitrarily opted to use the male pronouns only.

[4] There are other types of legal entities (the general partnership, limited partnership, limited liability partnership) to which the practice of medicine is not particularly well-suited, which will not be discussed.

# II  PATIENT EVALUATION

# 6  Urologic History, Physical Examination, and Urinalysis

*Mark R. Licht,* MD

**CONTENTS**

    INTRODUCTION
    UROLOGICAL HISTORY
    PHYSICAL EXAMINATION
    URINALYSIS
    SELECTED READING

## INTRODUCTION

Despite the prevalence and availability of high-technology diagnostic tests, the history and physical examination continue to serve as the most important initial clinical tools in assessing a patient's condition. In urology, a urinalysis complements the history and physical examination, and a diagnosis can often be made and others excluded based on these findings alone. In an era of cost containment, an accurate history, physical examination, and urinalysis in the office can speed clinical diagnosis and determine appropriate therapy without the use of unnecessary and sometimes costly testing.

## UROLOGICAL HISTORY

The principles of taking an accurate, complete history are learned in medical school. The patient must be comfortable with the interviewer and the setting, and must be given enough time to communicate his or her problem. A comprehensive history has recently been defined by the Health Care Financing Administration (HCFA) in their Evaluation and Management (E&M) Guidelines. It must include a separate statement of the chief complaint and an extended history of the present illness. To characterize a symptom for diagnostic purposes, the history of the present illness must include a description of bodily location, quality and quantity, chronology, the setting in which it takes place, aggravating and alleviating factors, and associated manifestations. Finally, a review of systems directly related to the chief complaint and a review of all additional body systems plus a complete past, family, and social history must be conducted. Patient medications and allergies must also be listed. This section reviews the most common presenting urological signs and symptoms in the context of forming a differential diagnosis based on a comprehensive history.

From: *Current Clinical Urology: Office Urology: The Clinician's Guide*
Edited by: E. D. Kursh and J. C. Ulchaker © Humana Press Inc., Totowa, NJ

Table 1
Hematuria

| Timing of hematuria | Likely site | Possible causes |
|---|---|---|
| Initial | Urethra | Urethral stricture, urethritis, meatal stenosis, urethral cancer |
| Total | Bladder, ureter, kidney | ADPCKD, hydronephrosis, renal cyst, renal or ureteral stone, glomerulonephritis, exercise, hemorrhagic cystitis, trauma, renal ureteral or bladder tumor, bladder calculus, tuberculosis, sickle cell disease |
| Terminal | Bladder neck, prostate | BPH, regrowth BPH, bladder-neck polyps, tumors |

## *Hematuria*

Hematuria is one of the most dramatic and often ominous signs in urology. Hematuria is defined as a ratio of greater than 3 red blood cells per high-powered microscope field. Both microscopic and gross hematuria require a complete urological evaluation to determine the etiology of the bleeding and rule out a urinary-tract malignancy. Patients with gross hematuria are more likely to have an identifiable source of bleeding, whereas an evaluation is often negative in patients with only microscopic hematuria. Hematuria is often intermittent, and the resolution of bleeding should never serve as a reason to omit an evaluation. A single exception is hematuria associated with a culture-proven urinary-tract infection in women, which resolves after the infection is completely treated.

The timing of hematuria, the patient's age and sex, and the presence of associated symptoms often help to identify the cause of bleeding. Table 1 compares the timing of hematuria with the most likely sites and causes of bleeding. In general, hematuria in younger patients is usually caused by benign conditions, such as a stone or infection. However, even patients in their 20s can have urinary-tract malignancies. Bleeding in older males is often the result of benign prostatic hyperplasia, and urinary-tract infection accounts for most benign cases of bleeding in adult females. Hematuria associated with flank pain or suprapubic pain is often benign in nature, whereas painless hematuria should be considered a sign of malignancy until proven otherwise.

## *Hematospermia*

Blood in the seminal fluid is a frightening sign. However, the underlying etiology is usually benign, and hematospermia often resolves quickly without a need for further evaluation or treatment. The most common cause is infection or inflammation of the prostate or urethra. Older patients with persistent hematospermia should be evaluated to rule out urethral pathology, prostate adenocarcinoma, or transitional-cell carcinoma of the prostatic ducts.

## *Pain*

Genitourinary-tract pain can be caused by obstruction, inflammation, or ischemia. Acute distention of the renal pelvis or ureter causes severe pain that often fluctuates in intensity (colic). Acute bladder distention causes continuous suprapubic pain and

## Table 2
## Genitourinary Pain

| Organ | Sensory innervation | Etiology | Site of pain |
|---|---|---|---|
| Local pain | | | |
| Kidney | T10–12, L1 | Inflammation, obstruction, ischemia, trauma | Ipsilateral costovertebral angle, flank below 12th rib |
| Bladder | T6–L5, S1–4 | Obstruction | Suprapubic region |
| Testicle | S1–4 | Inflammation, trauma, torsion | Ipsilateral testicle |
| Penis | S2–4 | Infection, paraphimosis, Peyronie's disease | Glans, foreskin, or erect shaft or penis |
| Referred pain | | | |
| Ureter | | | |
| Upper | T11–12 | Obstruction | Ipsilateral testicle, inguinal canal |
| Middle | T12–L1 | | Bladder, suprapubic region |
| Distal | T6–L5, S1–4 | | Ipsilateral testicle or labia |
| Bladder | T6–L5, S1–4 | Cystitis | Distal urethra, tip of penis |
| Prostate | S2-4 | Prostatitis | Perineum, rectum, lower groin, back |
| Testicle | S1-4 | Inflammation, trauma, torsion | Ipsilateral groin, lower abdomen, costovertebral angle |

lower-abdominal pain. A chronic obstruction that occurs slowly over a long period of time, however, is often painless. Examples include an impacted stone, ureteropelvic-junction obstruction, tumor, or chronic retention. Pain from inflammation is caused by edema and capsular distention, and is usually constant in nature. Parenchymal infections are usually quite severe, whereas the discomfort associated with cystitis or urethritis is less intense. Renal ischemia caused by vascular disease and testicular ischemia resulting from torsion produce extremely severe, constant pain. Tumors of the genitourinary tract are usually painless unless they are locally invasive or lead to acute obstruction. Genitourinary-tract pain is either experienced locally at the site of the affected organ, or is referred to another site in the body because of a common sensory innervation. Table 2 outlines common sites of local and referred pain for each genitourinary-tract organ.

### *Lower Urinary-Tract Symptoms*

A change in the normal voiding pattern is the most common cause of urological consultation. An average adult voids approx 4–6 times a day, and not at all or once at night. The average voided volume is about 300 cc, and is accomplished with a good stream that leaves the bladder empty at completion. Variations in normal voiding pattern can be caused by medications, fluid status, pituitary function, or habit, as well as neurologic or intrinsic urologic disease. Any change in a patient's "normal" pattern can cause concern and may prompt a referral to a urologist. Classically, voiding symptoms are categorized as either irritative or obstructive. Although some symptoms can overlap, this classification does serve as a useful framework for evaluating voiding

Table 3
Voiding Symptoms

| Irritative symptoms | Definition/ symptoms | Etiology | Possible causes |
|---|---|---|---|
| Frequency | Voiding at 2-h intervals or less | Decreased bladder capacity, compliance | Bladder-outlet obstruction (BPH, cancer, stricture) elevated postvoid residual, neurogenic bladder (spinal-cord injury, multiple sclerosis), inflammation (cystitis, stone, foreign body, tumor), extrinsic compression (sigmoid, uterus, ovary), stress/anxiety |
| | | Increased urinary output | Drugs/diuretics, polydipsia, diabetes mellitus, diabetes insipidus |
| Nocturia | Voiding two or more times a night | Decreased bladder capacity, compliance | See above |
| | | Increased urinary output | Postural diuresis (peripheral edema, congestive heart failure), increased nighttime fluid intake |
| Urgency | Sudden, strong feeling of need to void | Inflammation | Cystitis, carcinoma *in situ* bladder |
| | | Neurogenic bladder | Uninhibited detrusor contractions (diabetes mellitus, multiple sclerosis, stroke, Parkinson's disease) |
| | | Bladder-outlet obstruction Anxiety | BPH |
| Dysuria | Pain on urination | Inflammation of bladder, urethra, or prostate | Cystitis, urethritis, prostatitis |

complaints. Table 3 lists the irritative voiding symptoms, defines them, and outlines the differential diagnosis of possible underlying cause. The obstructive voiding symptoms include decreased force of stream, hesitancy, intermittency, postvoid dribbling, and incomplete emptying. A weak stream is defined urodynamically as a voided flow rate of <20 cc/s if a voided volume of 150 cc or more is achieved. It can be caused by infravesical obstruction from BPH, urethral stricture, or a large cystocele, or be the result of decreased detrusor function from long-standing obstruction, diabetic neuropathy, or central-nervous-system disorders, such as multiple sclerosis and Parkinson's disease. Complete urodynamic evaluation is often needed to determine the true etiology. The other obstructive voiding symptoms whose definitions are self-evident are most often associated with infravesical obstruction resulting from BPH, although diminished detrusor function can also be the cause.

## Urethral Discharge

Fluid other than urine emanating from the urethra requires urological evaluation. The nature of the fluid, and any associated symptoms, help make the underlying diagnosis. Thick, purulent yellow or gray fluid associated with urethral pain is consistent with gonorrhea. Small amounts of watery fluid that may or may not be associated with pain often represent nonspecific urethritis. Urethral-gland fluid for lubrication is a similar fluid that is sticky in consistency and seen prior to ejaculation. Painless bloody discharge from the urethra could be a symptom of urethral cancer, stricture, or a foreign body.

## Pneumaturia

The passage of air through the urethra often represents a pathological state requiring further evaluation. The most common cause is an enterovesical fistula resulting from cancer, diverticulitis, trauma, or a congenital anomaly. Urinary-tract infection with a gas-forming organism can also cause pneumaturia. This is most commonly seen in diabetics or chronically ill individuals. Patients should be questioned about recent genitourinary instrumentation, because those who have been recently catheterized or have had cystoscopy performed will pass air from their urethra. True pneumaturia must also be distinguished from bubbles in the toilet water with urination. In rare cases this is because of proteinuria, but it is usually caused by the mechanical force of urination. The patient can be reassured that this is normal.

## Urinary Incontinence

The involuntary loss of urine is a significant social and hygienic issue that is often emotionally and physically debilitating. Urinary incontinence can be categorized by the nature of the leakage and the mechanisms involved. A thorough history and physical examination are often sufficient to accurately diagnose and treat patients with urinary incontinence. Table 4 lists the different types of urinary incontinence and the most common causes.

## Erectile Dysfunction

Greater awareness of erectile dysfunction (ED) as a common medical problem with many viable treatment options has markedly increased the number of men with this condition who present for urological evaluation. ED is defined as a man's inability to achieve and maintain the rigid erection needed for vaginal penetration. Classically, the urological history focused on distinguishing between psychogenic and organic causes of ED. Such problems as decreased libido, premature ejaculation, and loss of ejaculation or orgasm are often confused with ED by patients. However, a careful history can separate out these complaints and determine the appropriate medical or psychological therapy needed for these patients. Peyronie's disease, or penile curvature resulting from corporal fibrosis, can also cause diminished erections and physical difficulty with penetration because of the angle of the penile bend. Table 5 compares historical clues to either a psychogenic or an organic etiology for true ED.

## Past Medical History

Depending on the nature of the chief complaint, various past medical problems may have an important bearing on current urological care. The clinician should pay special

Table 4
Urinary Incontinence

| Type of incontinence | Definition/symptoms | Causes |
|---|---|---|
| Total | Continuous loss of urine unrelated to activity or position | Urinary-tract fistula (vesicovaginal, ureterovaginal), female ectopic ureter, epispadias |
| Overflow | Increased intravesical pressure from distention overcomes sphincter resistance. Episodic dribbling leak. Often nocturnal. Palpable bladder on examination | Urinary retention, obstruction vs impaired detrusor function, neurogenic bladder |
| Stress | Episodic leakage of urine with increases in intravesical pressure (cough, laugh, exercise) | **Women**: loss of support of bladder neck and proximal urethra (menopause, childbirth, pelvic surgery), intrinsic sphincteric deficiency (trauma, incontinence surgery, radiation, congenital, neurological disease) |
| | | **Men:** decreased urethral length, and sphincteric weakness (postprostatectomy), congenital, neurological disease |
| Urge | Episodic leakage of urine preceded by an uncontrollable urge to void | Inflammation (cystitis, UTI, carcinoma *in situ* bladder, transitional cell carcinoma bladder), infravesical obstruction (bladder outlet obstruction), upper-motor neuron neurogenic bladder (stroke, MS, Parkinson's disease) |
| Mixed | Related or unrelated episodes of urge and stress incontinence | *See above* Intrinsic sphincteric deficiency can exhibit the same symptoms as urge incontinence |
| Nocturnal enuresis | Involuntary loss of urine during sleep | **Primary:** delayed neurological development. **Secondary:** stress/emotional distress, neurological disease, obstruction, infection |

attention to endocrine, cardiovascular, and neurological diseases, which may affect voiding or sexual function. Hematologic disorders may affect the patient's surgical risk. Previous surgeries, current medications, and allergies should be accurately noted. Smoking and excessive alcohol use have important urological sequelae, as does a family history of renal disease, and kidney and prostate cancer.

## PHYSICAL EXAMINATION

A complete physical examination includes the patient's vital signs and a comment on general appearance. The neck, skin, lungs, heart, and breasts should be examined

Table 5
Erectile Dysfunction

| History | Psychogenic | Organic |
|---|---|---|
| Timing of onset | Often acute | Gradual loss of function over time |
| Nocturnal penile tumescence | Usually present | Often absent |
| Erection in response to visual or tactile sensation | Often present | Often absent |
| Medical risk factors | None, or few | Elevated cholesterol, diabetes mellitus, pelvic surgery, vascular disease, smoking |

as well. Edema, gynecomastia, irregular heart rhythm, and truncal obesity can all have associated urological diagnoses. This section focuses on the portions of the physical examination that are most important for the urologist.

## *Abdominal Examination*

Inspection, auscultation, and palpation of the abdomen is an important first step in examining the urological patient. The kidneys and bladder can be assessed during this portion of the examination. Previous abdominal or flank scars from trauma or surgery can be appreciated, as can large abdominal masses, hernias, or a markedly distended bladder. Systolic renal artery bruits resulting from renal artery disease can be heard after either inspiration or expiration anteriorly or over the flank. Diminished or absent bowel sounds may be because of renal or ureteral inflammation or acute obstruction. Percussion of the costovertebral angles of the flank can elicit tenderness associated with renal obstruction or inflammation. Because of the retroperitoneal location of the kidneys, they are often difficult to palpate. The right kidney is normally lower than the left, and its lower pole can be felt in thin, nonmuscular patients. The left kidney can only be palpated if it is enlarged or displaced inferiorly. The kidney is best examined with the patient supine. One hand pushes up from the back while the other presses down firmly on the abdomen during deep inspiration. Renal masses are ballotable between the two hands. Any possibility of a renal mass on examination should prompt further evaluation by an imaging study, such as ultrasound. The kidney can only be transilluminated in an infant.

The ureter is not directly palpable through abdominal examination in either men or women, because of its location in the retroperitoneum. Ureteral obstruction, however, can cause abdominal pain from palpation, depending on the location of the blockage.

The bladder is normally a pelvic organ, but it rises out of the pelvis toward the umbilicus when it is distended to more than 500 cc. Percussion of the lower abdomen demonstrates a change in resonance over a distended urine-filled bladder. The distended bladder is palpable as a firm, rounded mass emanating from the pelvis. Pressure on this mass usually elicits the urge to void. Bimanual abdominorectal or abdominovaginal examination under anesthesia is often useful to determine the local extent of an invasive bladder tumor. While examining the lower abdomen, the groin is checked for inguinal adenopathy.

## Genital Examination

**Men**

The penis is visually inspected for lesions, and skin pigmentation is noted. In uncircumcised men, the foreskin is completely retracted to visualize the entire undersurface. Lesions and inflammatory changes are noted. The location of the urethral meatus is observed and its size assessed, by pinching the glans between the thumb and index finger. With this method, discharge can be expressed and any tumors, warts, or inflammation of the distal urethra can be visualized. The corporal bodies are palpated to evaluate their consistency, and plaques or firm nodules are noted. The urethra is also palpated to check for tumors, thickening caused by inflammation and stricture, or diverticulum.

The scrotum is visually inspected for lesions, sebaceous cysts, or rash. Edema and hemangiomas are noted. The testicles and cord structures are palpated through the scrotal skin. The testicles are pushed between the fingertips of both hands. The entire surface slides between the fingers to judge the consistency and to feel for small, firm nodules, which are considered tumors until proven otherwise. The size of the testicles can be measured with calipers or an orchiometer. The scrotal contents can be transilluminated to distinguish solid from cystic or fluid-filled structures. The epididymis is palpated along its length posterior to the testicle to check for lesions or thickening resulting from inflammation. Primary tumors presenting as firm masses are rare, whereas benign cysts or spermatoceles are common. The vas deferens is easily identified as a thick cord-like structure running within the spermatic cord. If the vas is not palpable, the urologist should confidently determine that it is not present. A varicocele—or dilated cord veins—is best assessed with the patient standing and performing a Valsalva's maneuver. A new-onset varicocele—or one that does not reduce with the patient supine—should prompt evaluation to rule out a retroperitoneal mass. With the patient standing, the scrotum is invaginated with the index finger to reach the external inguinal ring and to feel for bulging with a cough representing a hernia.

A rectal examination is an important part of the urological physical examination. It is best conducted with the patient standing and bending forward over an examination table. Normal perianal sensation and intact sphincter tone are important clues to neurological integrity. Rectal polyps and masses are often palpable. The prostate gland is palpated by sweeping the index finger over the gland, and the size and consistency of the gland are noted. Fluctuance or pain from palpation denotes infection. Firmer rubbery nodules are often felt with benign prostatic hyperplasia, but hard nodules should always be further evaluated by transrectal ultrasound and biopsy to rule out cancer. The lobes of the prostate can be massaged to produce secretions for microscopic evaluation if indicated. The index finger compresses the gland from the lateral border medially down to the apex of the gland until fluid is expressed from the urethra. The seminal vesicles are often not palpable because of their high location. However, firmness of the seminal vesicles may be the result of infection or extension of prostate cancer and cystic dilatation can result from ejaculatory-duct obstruction. Any stool found on the glove after rectal examination should be guaiac tested for occult blood.

**Women**

The pelvic exam is performed with the patient in the lithotomy position. The external genitalia are inspected to note inflammation, atrophy, discharge, or lesions. The urethral meatus is examined for mucosal prolapse, mass, or caruncle. The urethra is palpated along its length to note induration, mass, or diverticulum. With the patient performing Valsalva's maneuver, the vagina is inspected with a speculum. Bladder-neck hypermobility and the degree of prolapse of the bladder, rectum, uterus, or vaginal cuff are assessed. Stress incontinence is noted if present. Bimanual examination of the pelvic organs is then performed to evaluate for masses, and a rectal examination is performed.

## URINALYSIS

A urinalysis should be performed in all patients who present for urological evaluation. A complete analysis of the urine consists of chemical dipstick testing as well as microscopic examination. A fresh sample of urine should be collected and evaluated immediately to ensure accuracy. Men should collect a midstream clean catch of voided urine. Uncircumcised men will retract the foreskin and clean the glans with an antiseptic pad prior to voiding. Women should wipe the vulva front to back, separate the labia, and collect a midstream sample. For women, a catheterized specimen may be necessary to guarantee that contamination has not occurred. Neonates and infants can have a sterile collection bag placed over the genitalia, and rarely a percutaneous suprapubic needle aspiration is needed to avoid contamination. Normal urine color—resulting from the pigment urochrome—ranges from clear to dark yellow depending on the patient's state of hydration and urine production. Hematuria is the most common cause of red urine. However, myoglobin, anthrocyanin (vegetable pigment), phenolphthalein, and phenothiazines can turn urine red. True hematuria can only be determined through microscopy with red blood cells seen. Such colors as orange, green, blue, and bright yellow occur as a result of ingestion of different medications, chemicals, or vitamins, and are not clinically significant. Cloudy urine does not necessarily represent pyuria or infection, and may instead be the result of organic phosphates. Adding dilute acid to the urine to change the pH clears the sample. Similarly, urine with an unusual odor does not always represent infection.

### *Chemical Testing*

Chemical testing of the urine by dipstick can test for specific gravity, pH, protein, bilirubin, glucose, hemoglobin, leukocyte esterase, and nitrites. Specific gravity of the urine reflects the patient's state of hydration. Disease states, such as diabetes insipidis, decreased renal concentrating function, or inappropriate ADH secretion, must be proven by determining urine osmolality. Urine pH can range from 5.0 to 9.0 by dipstick, with an average of 6.0. Urine pH generally reflects serum pH, because the kidneys can excrete or hold onto an acid load to help maintain blood hemostasis. Patients with renal tubular acidosis, however, maintain an alkaline urine ($\geq 6.0$) despite acidemia because of inappropriate urine bicarbonate excretion. Uric acid and cystine stones form in acidic urine, whereas alkaline urine may be caused by an infection with a urea-splitting organism. Normally, individuals show no urinary protein on dipstick testing. However, proteinuria may be benign as a result of fever, physical activity, stress, or postural changes. Conversely, patients with significant proteinuria should be evaluated with further diagnostic testing for intrinsic renal disease. Urinary protein can also be elevated by overflow of filtered proteins from the kidneys, such as Bence Jones protein, myoglobin, and hemoglobin.

Glucosuria reflects hyperglycemia with overflow of the glucose reabsorption capability of the renal tubules. Although it can infrequently and often transiently occur in normal individuals, glucosuria most likely represents a disease state, and a fasting serum-glucose level should be checked. Urinary ketones are observed with diabetic ketoacidosis, pregnancy, or a catabolic state, such as starvation or significant weight loss. Some high-protein and high-fat diets will produce elevated urinary ketones. Conjugated bilirubin only appears in the urine in such disease states as bile-duct obstruction and primary hepatocellular disease. Elevated levels of urobilinogen are seen with hemolysis and gastrointestinal hemorrhage.

The dipstick test for red blood cells is not specific for hematuria. Myoglobin and hemoglobin proteins can yield a false-positive reading. High levels of urinary ascorbic acid can lead to a false-negative result. Microscopic analysis of the urine sediment is the only way to accurately diagnose and quantitate hematuria. Dipstick testing for leukocyte esterase (white blood cells) and nitrites (bacteria) is sometimes helpful in screening for urinary-tract inflammation and infection. However, microscopic evaluation of the urine is always necessary to confirm the clinical validity of these findings.

## *Microscopic Examination*

At least 10 cc of collected urine is centrifuged for 5 min at 200–300 rpm prior to microscopic examination. The supernatant is decanted and the sediment is resuspended in the drop of urine remaining at the bottom of the tube. A drop of urine is then placed on a glass microscope slide and covered with a cover slip. The slide is viewed under the microscope at both low and high power.

Erythrocytes are easily identifiable circular or crenated biconcave cells. Their presence represents bleeding along the length of the urinary tract. More than three red blood cells per high-powered field would be considered significant hematuria. Dysmorphic, misshapen erythrocytes specifically result from glomerular bleeding.

Leukocytes are larger than red blood cells, and represent inflammation or infection of the urinary tract. More than five white blood cells per high-powered field is considered to be significant pyuria, requiring further evaluation. However, a voided sample from a woman can be contaminated with vaginal leukocytes, and a catheterized sample may be needed to prove pyuria.

Squamous epithelial cells are large cells with a smooth but irregular border and a small central nucleus. In the urine, they usually represent contamination from the distal urethra in men and the vagina in women. Transitional cells are rounder, smaller cells with a larger central nucleus, routinely shed from the normal lining of the urinary tract. However, if they appear in clumps or if they are morphologically abnormal, formal cytology should be performed to rule out malignancy.

Casts are oblong, protein-based structures that form in the renal tubular lumen and often represent some degree of renal pathology. Red blood-cell casts denote glomerular bleeding, and white blood-cell casts are seen with glomerulonephritis or pyelonephritis. Hyaline casts containing only Tamm-Horsfall protein are normally secreted, and their presence does not absolutely determine renal disease.

The presence of bacteria in a clean-catch urine sample in a man and a catheterized specimen in a women represents infection. More than 5 bacteria per high-powered field correlates with a colony count of >100,000/mL. Bacteria and vaginal epithelial cells in a voided sample from a woman are likely to represent vaginal contamination of the sample rather than infection. Rod-shaped bacteria and cocci in chains and clusters are easily differentiated under the microscope. Yeasts are also easily identified in the budding phase by their long branch-like hyphae. Trichomonads are rapidly moving single-cell organisms propelled by flagella.

Urinary crystals have distinct shapes which help with identification. Calcium oxalate crystals have an "envelope" shape, whereas uric acid crystals have a "broken tile" appearance. Cystine crystals have a distinctive hexagonal shape, whereas triple-phosphate or struvite crystals have a "flat top" pyramid shape.

## SELECTED READING

Hodges CV, Barry JM (1975) Non-urologic flank pain: a diagnostic approach. *J Urol* 113:644.

Mohr DN, Offord KP, Owen RA, Melton LJ (1986) Asymptomatic microhematuria and urologic disease. A population study. *JAMA* 256:224.

Stamey TA, Kindrachuk RW (1985) *Urinary Sediment and Urinalysis: A Practical Guide for the Health Science Professional.* Philadelphia: WB Saunders Co.

Woolhandler S, Pels RJ, Bor DH (1989) Dipstick urinalysis screening of asymptomatic adults for urinary tract disorders: 1. Hematuria and proteinuria. *JAMA* 262:1215.

# 7 Endoscopy and Instrumentation in the Office

*Steven H. Selman,* MD

**CONTENTS**
    INTRODUCTION
    CYSTOSCOPES
    SOUNDS, BOUGIES, AND DILATORS
    CATHETERS
    ULTRASOUND
    URETHRAL ANESTHESIA
    VASECTOMY
    PROSTATIC NEEDLE BIOPSY
    BIOFEEDBACK
    URODYNAMIC INSTRUMENTATION
    SELECTED READING

## INTRODUCTION

It can be argued that the modern era of urology began with the development of the cystoscope. The introduction of the new technology of endoscopy complemented traditional instruments of urologic treatment: sounds, catheters, and bougies. Endoscopy remains an integral part of urologic diagnosis and treatment planning. The traditional urologic tools have been enhanced by modern imaging techniques, expanding the scope of office urology.

## CYSTOSCOPES

Both rigid and flexible cystoscopes are available for office endoscopy. Adult rigid cystoscopes (*see* Fig. 1)—available in sizes from 17 French to 25 French—consist of an optical element and eyepiece, a sheath and obturator for introduction, and a bridge system. The Albarrán bridge (*see* Fig. 2) is a deflecting system that allows for intravesical manipulation of graspers and forceps. Smaller-diameter instruments can be used for diagnostic examination, but larger-diameter instruments must be used for the introduction of semirigid graspers and forceps.

From: *Current Clinical Urology: Office Urology: The Clinician's Guide*
Edited by: E. D. Kursh and J. C. Ulchaker © Humana Press Inc., Totowa, NJ

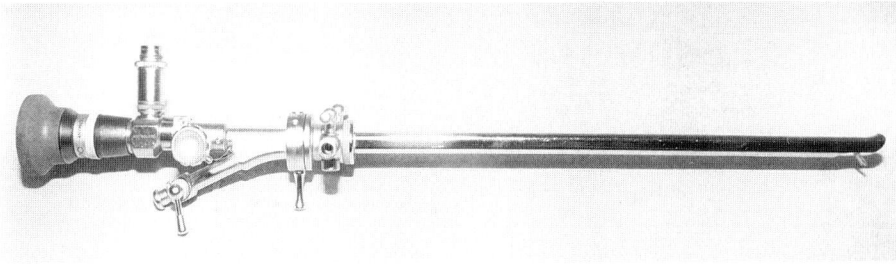

**Fig. 1.** Rigid cystoscope.

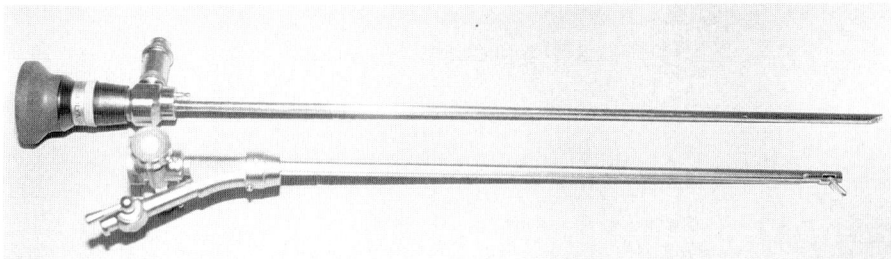

**Fig. 2.** Albarrán bridge and optical element.

Flexible fiberoptic cystoscope (*see* Fig. 3) systems are widely used in office urology. The maneuverability and small caliber of these instruments allows for atraumatic negotiation of the S-shaped male urethra so that complete examination of the bladder and urethra can be accomplished with minimal patient discomfort. (For office endoscopy, a 10-min dwell time of intraurethrally injected xylocaine jelly usually provides excellent anesthesia.) The working channel permits introduction of grasping and biopsy forceps. The flexible cystoscope is passed into the well-lubricated urethra and is negotiated into the bladder by direct visualization of the urethra. It is important to keep the instrument oriented so that the urethral lumen remains in the center of the field of view. Passage of the instrument through the external sphincter and prostate elicits a brief urgency to void. Once past the bladder neck, the entire bladder mucosa can be visualized by rotating the instrument around its central axis in combination with deflection of the tip. Flexible foreign-body forceps (*see* Fig. 4) can also be utilized for stent removal.

Office use of rigid cystoscopy is best suited for the female patient, who generally experiences little discomfort from passage of the instrument into the urethra after local instillation of xylocaine jelly. Because of the natural S-shape of the male urethra, insertion of a rigid cystoscope is usually poorly tolerated. When rigid cystoscopy is necessary in the male patient, the smallest-diameter instrument available should be used.

## SOUNDS, BOUGIES, AND DILATORS

Sounds, bougies, and dilators have traditionally been part of the urologists' armamentarium. Metal Van Buren sounds (*see* Fig. 5) are available from sizes 8F to 30F. They can be used for the urethral dilatation and circumventing an old or newly-created urethral false passage. A set of sounds threaded at the distal tip can be attached to the

Chapter 7 / Endoscopy and Instrumentation

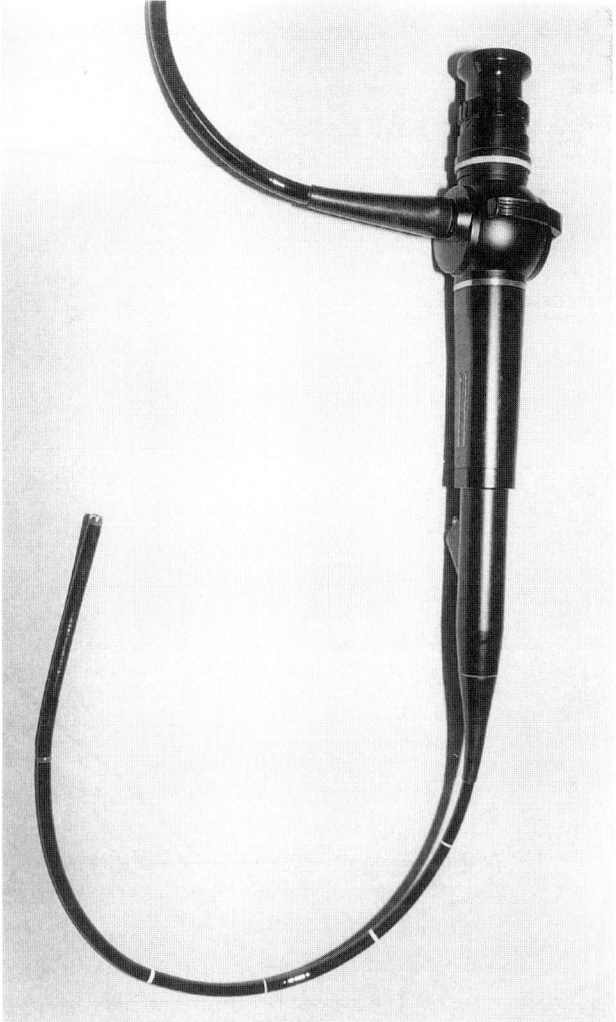

Fig. 3. Flexible cystoscope.

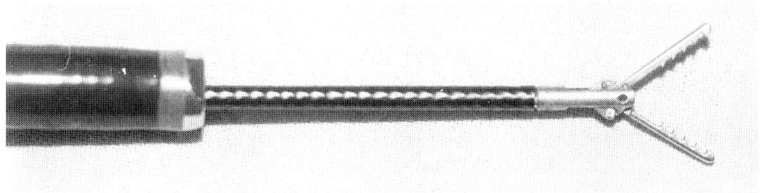

Fig. 4. Flexible foreign-body forceps placed through flexible cystoscope.

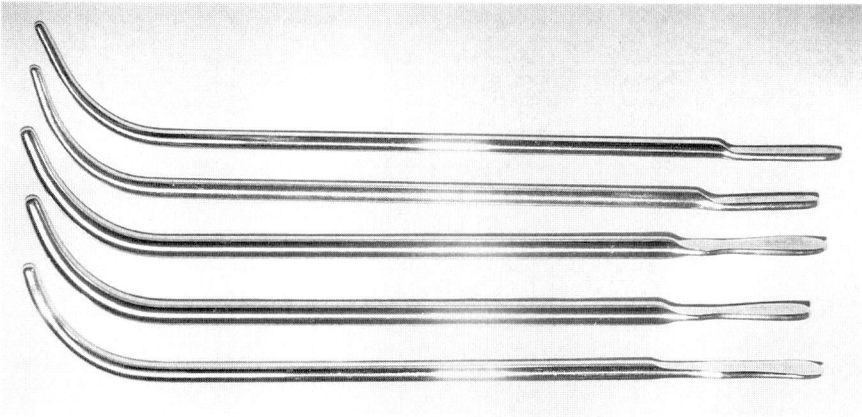

Fig. 5. Van Buren sounds.

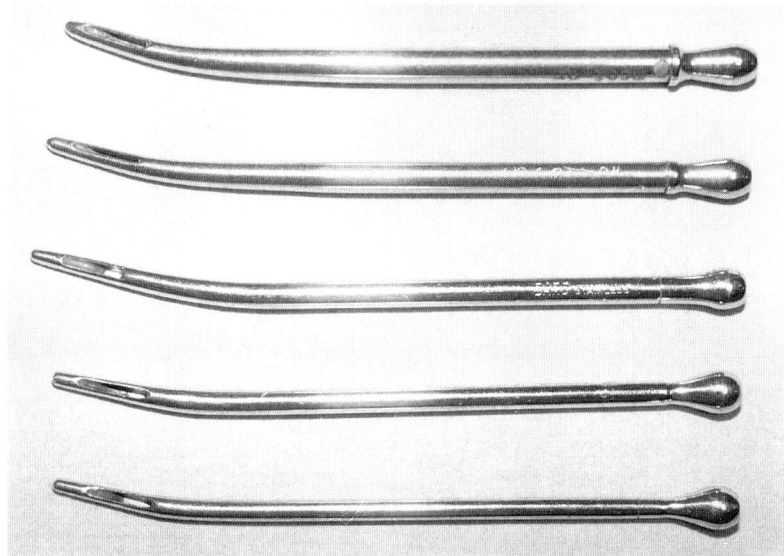

Fig. 6. Walther sounds.

female end of a filiform, and are useful in selected cases. Straight urethral Walther sounds (*see* Fig. 6) as well as olive-tipped bougies (*see* Fig. 7) can be used to gently dilate the female urethra if necessary prior to cystoscopy. A set of filiform and followers (*see* Fig. 8) is essential for the office management of urethral stricture disease. The filiform tips come in a variety of sizes and configurations, and more than one filiform may be placed into the urethra to bypass the strictured site. For difficult urethral strictures, the flexible cystoscope is placed to the site of stricture and a 0.038″ guidewire is threaded under direct vision. Over this wire an open-ended follower can be passed into the bladder.

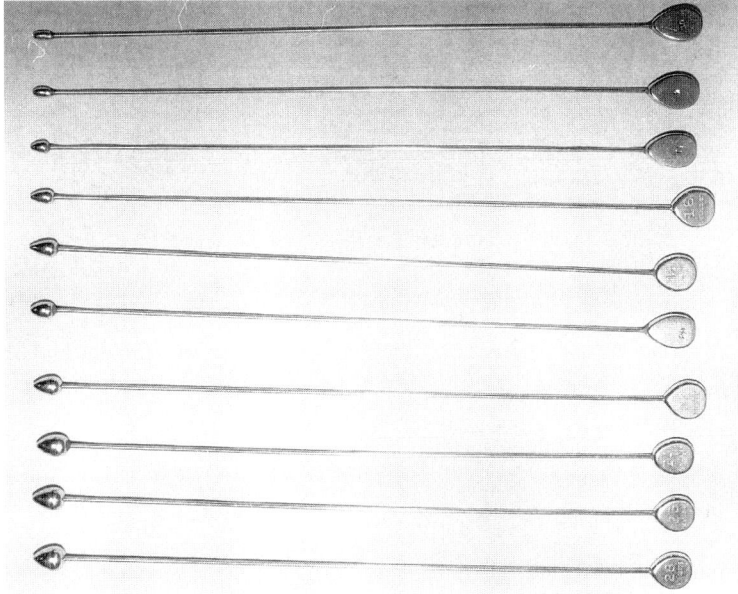

**Fig. 7.** Bougies.

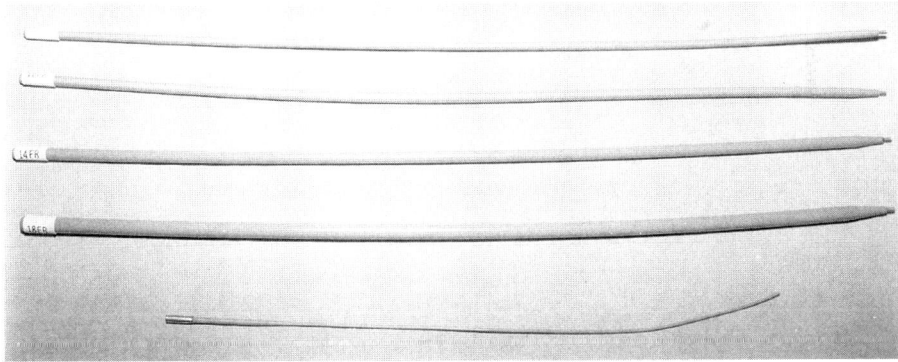

**Fig. 8.** Filiform and follower.

## CATHETERS

A supply of Foley catheters of various diameters is essential for the urologists' office. Nonlatex catheters should be used for patients with latex allergy. Aside from the standard two-way catheter, three-way catheters are useful for patients requiring bladder irrigation in such situations as clot retention. Nonretention catheters (*see* Robinson, Fig. 9) are used for instillation of intravesical antineoplastic agents.

Urethral catheters with a coudé tip should also be available for those patients whose bladder neck may be difficult to negotiate (e.g., status of posttransurethral prostatectomy). A malleable catheter guide provides stiffness for difficult catheter insertion. For

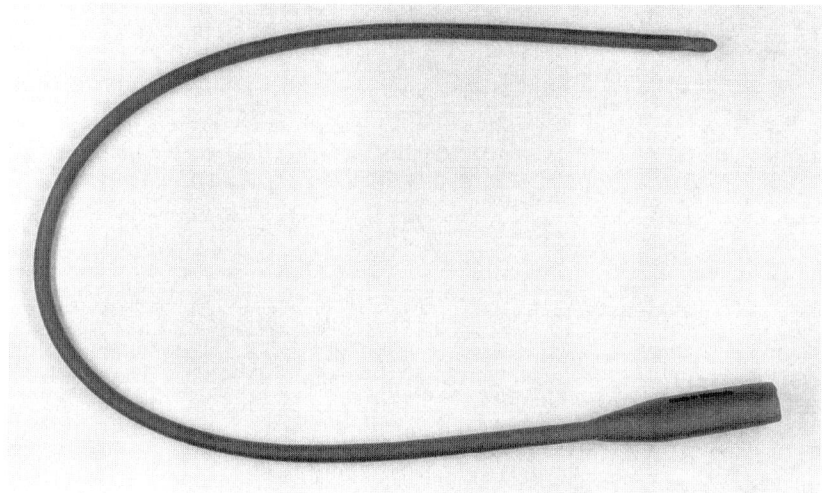

**Fig. 9.** Robinson catheter.

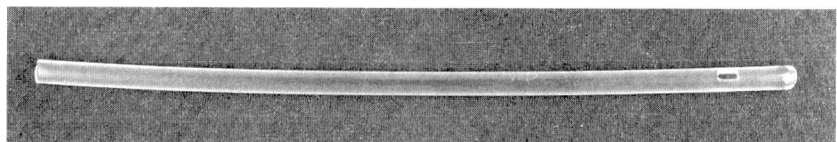

**Fig. 10.** Female "self cath" catheter.

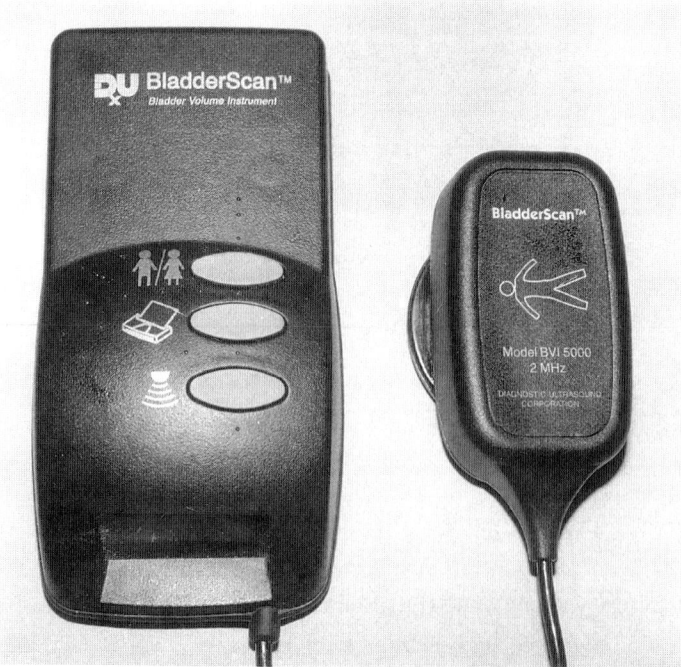

**Fig. 11.** Portable ultrasonic bladder scanner for determination of postvoid residuals.

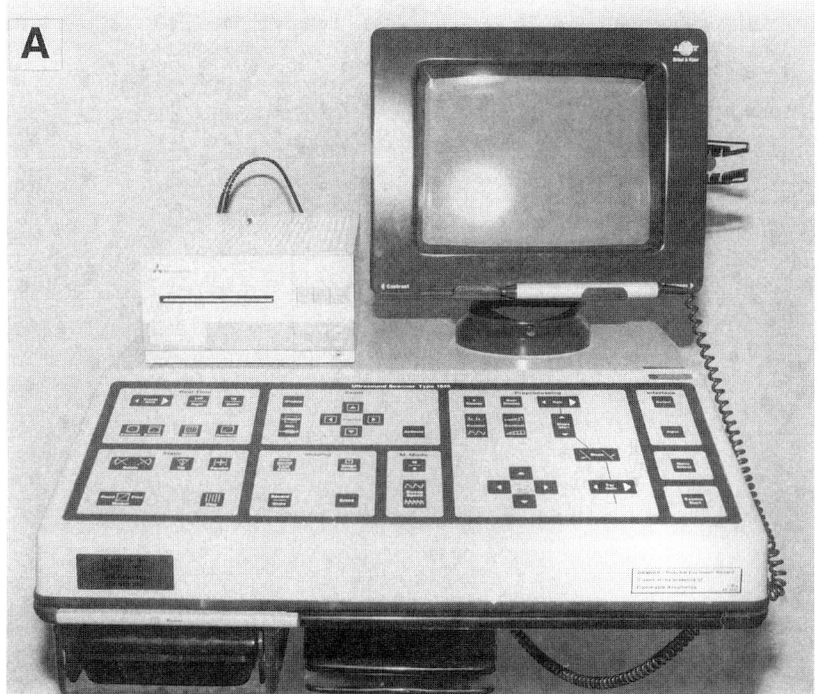

**Fig. 12A.** Office-based ultrasound unit.

the female patient requiring intermittent catheterization, short plastic catheters (*see* Fig. 10) should be available for patient instruction.

## ULTRASOUND

The use of transrectal and transabdominal ultrasound have become an integral part of the urologist's office practice. Office ultrasound equipment is manufactured by a number of commercial vendors.

### *Bladder Ultrasound*

A small, transportable ultrasound unit (*see* Fig. 11) dedicated to the determination of postvoid bladder volumes is useful. The current generation displays results and provides a hard copy for documentation.

### *Prostate Ultrasound*

Prostate ultrasound has evolved over the last two decades. A number of vendors produce instruments (*see* Fig. 12A,B) that produce high-quality gray-scale images of the prostate and seminal vesicles. Prostatic ultrasound is ideal for the guidance of transrectal needle biopsy of the prostate. It is also useful for determination of prostatic volumes for the planning of prostatic surgery and interstitial radiotherapy.

### *Transabdominal Ultrasound*

Transabdominal ultrasound (*see* Fig. 13) can be used to image the kidneys, providing information regarding the presence of stones, hydronephrosis, and renal masses. This

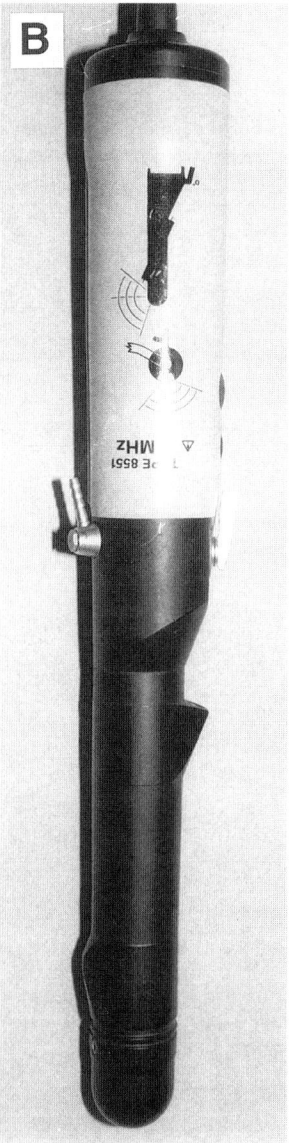

**Fig. 12B.** Rectal probe.

modality is especially useful in the imaging of the transplanted kidney and its surrounding area. Lymphoceles and obstruction are readily deterred with this technology.

## *Testicular Ultrasound*

High-frequency (10 mHz) ultrasound provides excellent imaging of the testicular and paratesticular tissues.

Chapter 7 / Endoscopy and Instrumentation

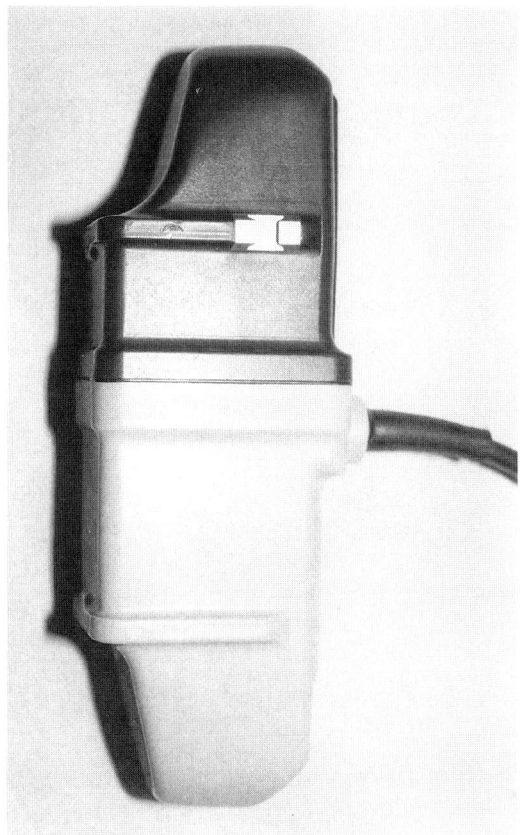

**Fig. 13.** Abdominal ultrasound probe.

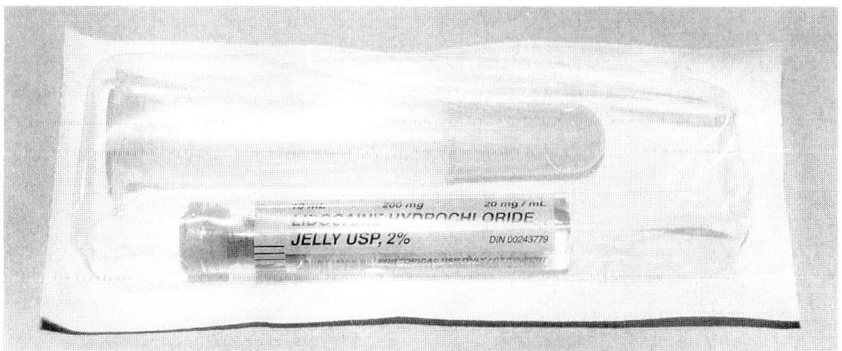

**Fig. 14.** Kit for urethral anesthesia.

## URETHRAL ANESTHESIA

For endoscopic procedures, urethral anesthesia is desirable. A 2% anesthesia gel solution contained in a piston syringe (*see* Fig. 14) is commercially available. The tapered tip of the syringe allows for atraumatic introduction of the anesthetic gel.

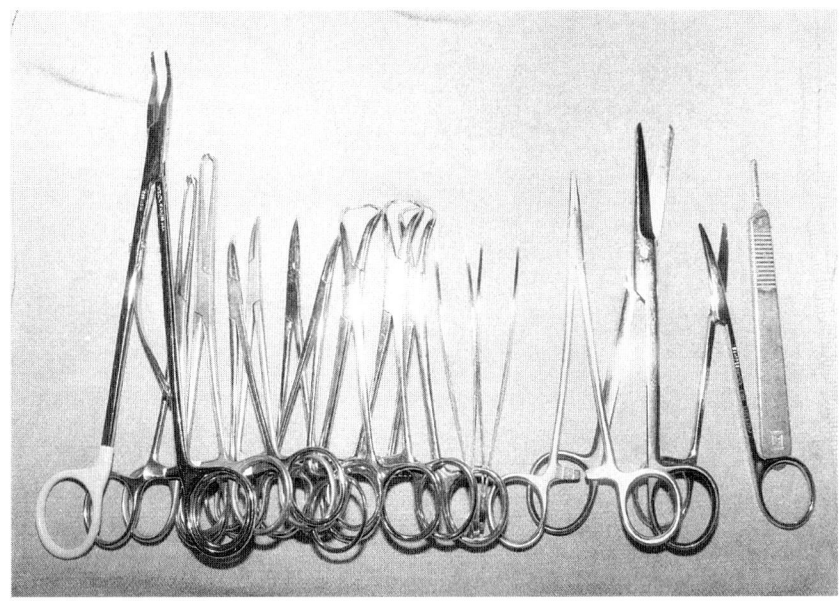

**Fig. 15.** Vasectomy tray.

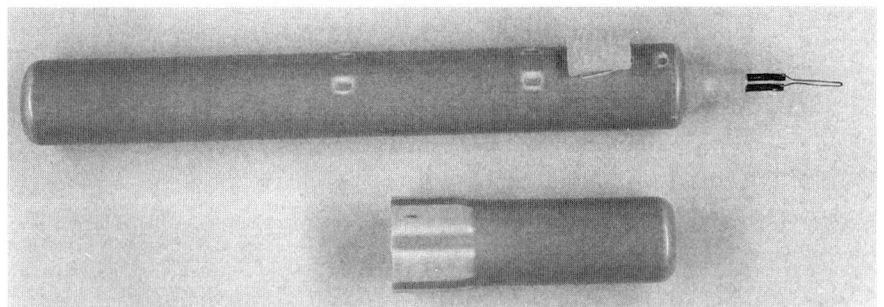

**Fig. 16.** Self-contained cautery unit.

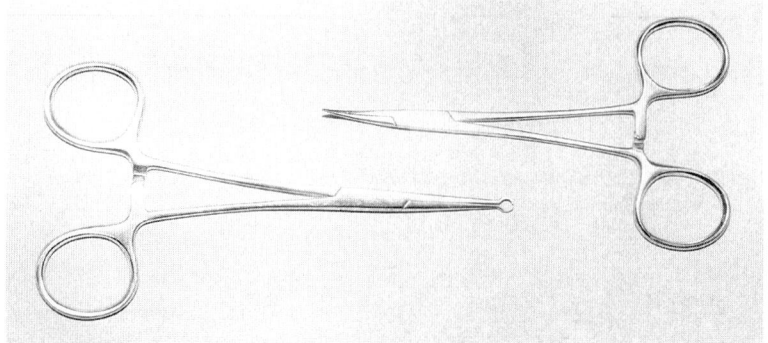

**Fig. 17.** "No-scalpel" instruments.

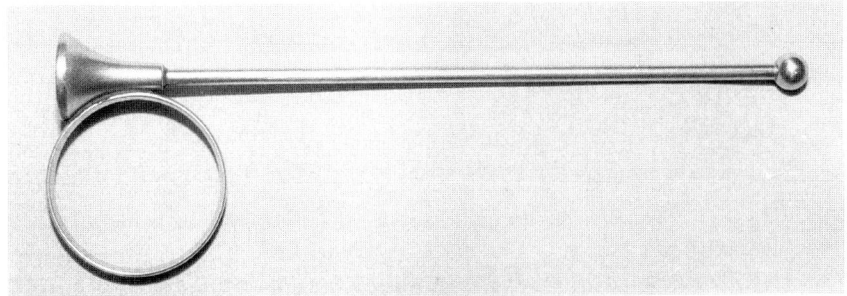

**Fig. 18.** Iowa needle trumpet.

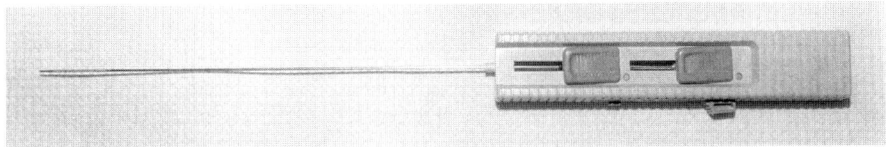

**Fig. 19.** Spring-loaded biopsy needle.

A penile clamp is used to retain the anesthetic within the urethra for an adequate time period.

## VASECTOMY

Vasectomy is one of the most common surgical procedures performed in the urologist's office, and several techniques have been developed. In addition to the standard surgical instruments (*see* Fig. 15), ancillary equipment and instruments may prove helpful. A small disposal hand-held cautery unit (*see* Fig. 16) can be used to obliterate the cut vasal ends. Instruments for the "no-scalpel" vasectomy (*see* Fig. 17) are excellent tools for grasping the vas and dissecting the perivasal tissue.

## PROSTATIC NEEDLE BIOPSY

Transrectal needle biopsy of the prostate is commonly performed in the office. Biopsy-specific sites can be determined with the aid of transrectal ultrasound. The biopsies can be separated and labeled for the site of biopsy. With the use of a long spinal needle, the periprostatic tissues can be infiltrated with Xylocaine to minimize discomfort.

The Iowa needle trumpet (*see* Fig. 18) can be used to direct the biopsy needle transrectally to the suspect area of the prostate in patients with a palpable abnormality within the prostate.

Spring-loaded disposable biopsy needle systems (*see* Fig. 19) allow for rapid and relatively painless biopsies of multiple sites in the prostate and base of the seminal vesicles.

## BIOFEEDBACK

Urinary stress incontinence is a widespread clinical problem. Biofeedback has proven to be successful for the treatment of stress incontinence and urge incontinence, and is

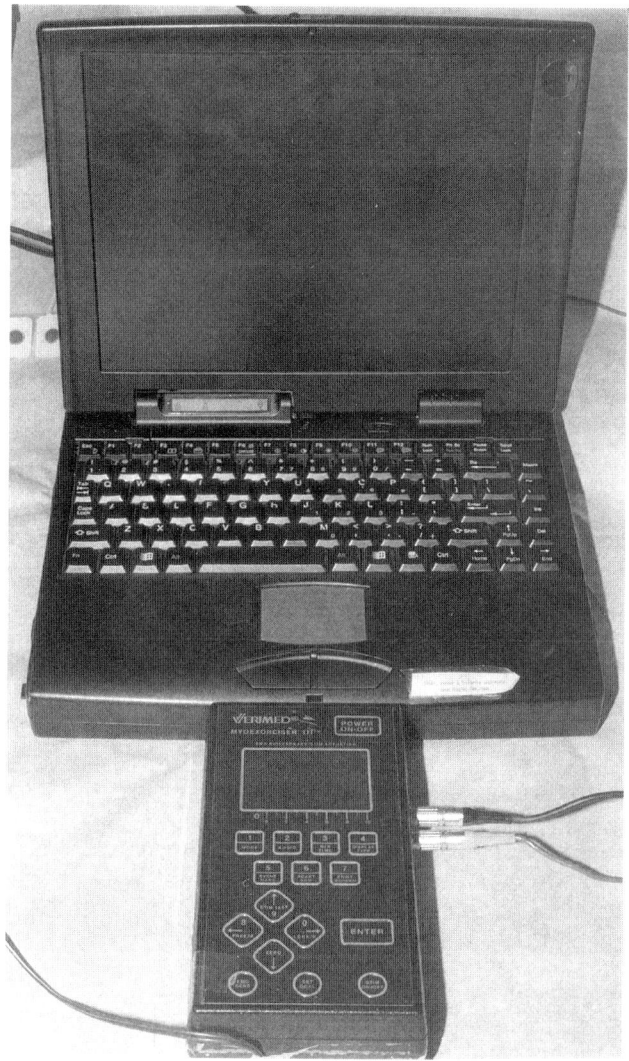

Fig. 20. Office-based biofeedback unit.

currently recommended as a first line of treatment. Anorectal biofeedback permits patients to identify pelvic muscles and teaches patients how to contract and relax these muscles while keeping the abdominal muscles relaxed (*see* Fig. 20).

## URODYNAMIC INSTRUMENTATION

Instrumentation for office urodynamic evaluation is available. Cystometry using either gas ($CO_2$) or water can be performed, providing data on intravesical pressure, compliance, and stability. In addition to cystometry, uroflowmetry (*see* Fig. 21) is easily performed in the office and can provide useful information in the management of bladder-outlet obstruction and response to therapy.

# Chapter 7 / Endoscopy and Instrumentation

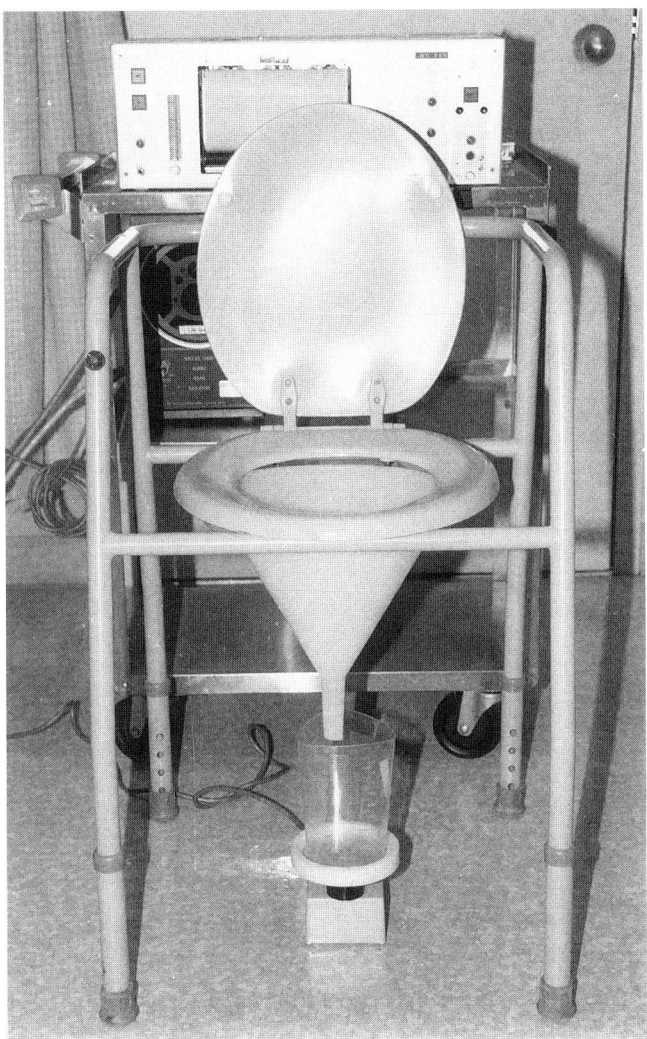

Fig. 21. Office uroflowmeter.

## SELECTED READING

O'Donnell PD, ed. (1997) *Urinary Incontinence.* St. Louis: Mosby.
Resnick MI, Rifkin MD, eds. (1991) *Ultrasonography of the Urinary Tract.* (3rd ed.) Baltimore: Williams and Wilkins.
Walsh PC, Retick AB, Vaughn ED, Wein AJ, eds. (1988) *Campbell's Urology.* (7th ed.) Philadelphia: WB Saunders Co.

# III Infections and Inflammation of the Genitourinary Tract

# 8 Evaluation and Management of Recurrent Urinary-Tract Infections

*Howard B. Goldman, MD*

**CONTENTS**
> INTRODUCTION
> EPIDEMIOLOGY
> DIAGNOSIS
> PATHOGENESIS
> EVALUATION
> TREATMENT
> CONCLUSION
> SELECTED READING

## INTRODUCTION

Urinary-tract infections (UTIs) are among the most common problems seen in medical practice. It is estimated that there are over 6,000,000 office visits per year to physicians for the treatment of this condition.

Most UTI patients are initially evaluated and treated by primary-care physicians but under certain circumstances urologists are asked to assist with their care. Those with recurrent UTIs are especially likely to be referred for further diagnostic and treatment planning. This population makes up a significant proportion of the average urologist's office practice, and recurrent UTIs—and their efficient and cost-effective evaluation and treatment—are of prime importance to all office-based urologists.

## EPIDEMIOLOGY

UTIs affect both men and women of all age groups. They are rare in young and middle-aged men, but become more common in later years and parallel the increase in voiding dysfunction seen in aging males. On the other hand, women have an increased incidence at a young age after the onset of sexual activity. Following menopause, the incidence slowly increases. It is estimated that 20–50% of all women will experience a UTI at some time during their lifetime. In general, most patients who present with

From: *Current Clinical Urology: Office Urology: The Clinician's Guide*
Edited by: E. D. Kursh and J. C. Ulchaker © Humana Press Inc., Totowa, NJ

recurrent UTIs are otherwise healthy women. Recurrent UTIs in the pediatric population are discussed in Chapter 35, and thus will not be explored in this chapter.

## *Classification of UTI*

A UTI can either involve the upper urinary tract (kidneys) or the lower urinary tract (bladder and urethra). Pyelonephritis refers to a UTI involving the kidney. Acute pyelonephritis is a syndrome characterized by fever, chills, and flank pain as well as bacteruria and pyuria. Cystitis refers to an inflammation of the bladder usually associated with dysuria (pain during voiding), frequency, urgency, and suprapubic discomfort. In women, the symptoms of urethritis are very similar to those of cystitis, and it can be difficult to distinguish one from the other. Primary urethritis is relatively rare in women, and more common in men. The most common UTI in adult women is acute bacterial cystitis.

UTIs are either uncomplicated or complicated. The clinical distinction is important, because complicated UTIs can be much more difficult to treat. Uncomplicated UTIs are defined as those in which no underlying structural or functional abnormalities are present. They frequently occur in otherwise healthy adult women and usually respond well to treatment with standard, inexpensive antimicrobial therapy. Complications are rare and the major problem encountered is the morbidity suffered by some women who have recurrent episodes.

In contrast, complicated UTIs are those in which the effectiveness of antimicrobial therapy may be reduced secondary to an underlying structural or functional abnormality. Renal or bladder calculi, urinary obstruction, voiding dysfunction, anatomic abnormalities secondary to previous surgery or of congenital origin, and the presence of an indwelling catheter, as well as other diseases that predispose to infection, such as diabetes mellitus or sickle cell anemia, are among the many abnormalities that can make a UTI "complicated."

UTIs can also be classified as isolated infections, unresolved bacteruria, bacterial persistence, or reinfection. Isolated infections are the first UTI a patient has or a UTI isolated from a previous infection by at least 6 mo. Unresolved bacteruria implies that the urinary tract is not sterilized during therapy. This may be due to the resistance of bacteria to the antimicrobial therapy selected, or secondary to rapid development of resistant bacteria from a previously susceptible population. Unresolved bacteruria may also be secondary to rapid reinfection with another resistant species before the initial species is eradicated. Bacterial persistence refers to recurrence of infection with the same organism after initial sterilization of the urine. It is caused by a site within the urinary tract that has been excluded from the appropriate high level of antimicrobial exposure. Infected stones, urethral diverticula, and enterovesical fistulas are but a few of the common sites that are difficult to sterilize with antimicrobial therapy alone. Reinfections occur when a new UTI infection occurs with a new organism after a previous infection has been eradicated.

Infections are recurrent when there are more than 2 in 6 months, or more than 3 in a year. The vast majority of recurrent infections are caused by reinfection, and the minority indicate bacterial persistence. The importance of this distinction is that patients with reinfection usually do not have any underlying anatomic problems, whereas those with persistence frequently have a remediable underlying problem.

## DIAGNOSIS

The patient with a UTI will usually note a number of the following symptoms: frequency, urgency, dysuria, suprapubic pain, and malodorous urine. A urinalysis is important, and bacteruria with pyuria (leukocytes in the urine) should be confirmed. If pyuria is absent, the diagnosis of a UTI must be questioned. Urine should be carefully collected for culture using a method that reduces the possibility of contamination. In the past it was widely claimed that 100,000 colony-forming units (CFU) had to be present to diagnose a UTI. However, the current thinking is that in the symptomatic patient, as few as 100 CFU per mL represents significant bacteruria.

The vast majority of UTIs are caused by bacteria, although yeasts, fungi, and other infectious agents sometimes cause UTIs. *Escherichia coli (E. coli)* accounts for 80%–90%, *Staphylococcus saprophyticus* for 10%–20%, and other *Enterobacteriaceae*, such as *Klebsiella, Proteus,* and *Enterobacter,* account for most of the remaining uncomplicated UTIs. In complicated UTIs, *E. coli* accounts for only about 20% of cases; *Enterobacteriaceae* and other gram-negative bacilli, such as *Pseudomonas* and *Acinetobacter,* as well as gram-positives like *Staphylococcus aureus,* are more common.

Other conditions that may cause pyuria with bladder irritability include stones and foreign bodies, trauma, bladder tumors, tuberculous, fungal, or viral infections, or infections adjacent to the urinary tract (appendicitis, diverticulitis, and so forth). When a urine culture is negative, these and other etiologies of the patient's symptoms and pyuria should be evaluated.

## PATHOGENESIS

As the male urethra is of considerable length, ascending infections in men with an anatomically and functionally normal urinary tract are unusual. Most older men with recurrent UTIs have an underlying voiding dysfunction that predisposes them to infection, or have acquired an infection after instrumentation. An obstructive process, such as a urethral stricture or enlarged prostate, or a neurogenic cause—all of which lead to poor emptying—may be the underlying cause of recurrent UTIs. Frequently, these men have a significant postvoid residual or bladder stones that act as a reservoir for bacteria and make it difficult to eliminate or prevent recurrent infections. Chronic prostatitis may act similarly, leading to recurrent episodes of cystitis.

In contrast, most UTIs in women represent ascending infections. Bacteria from the fecal reservoir may colonize the perineum, and after ascent to the bladder via the urethra may cause a symptomatic UTI. The relatively short length of the female urethra makes this ascent fairly simple. As noted earlier, most women with UTIs have a urinary tract that is anatomically and functionally normal.

Sexual intercourse may increase the prevalence of infection in otherwise susceptible women, as evidenced by the increase in UTIs once women become sexually active. The theory is that vigorous activity during intercourse "milks" bacteria from the vagina or distal urethra up the length of the urethra and into the bladder. Intercourse may also cause urethral trauma, leaving the urethra more susceptible to infection. Although intercourse may play a role in susceptible individuals, the fact that most sexually active women do not have UTIs argues against its role as a primary mechanism.

A distinct population of women suffer from recurrent UTIs. Research demonstrates that many of these women have an increased adherence of bacteria to vaginal and urethral surfaces as compared to women without UTIs. In addition, these women are more likely to have a nonsecretor blood-group phenotype. Evidently there is a protective effect (fewer UTIs) when secretor blood-group antigens are present. Genetic differences thus influence the ability of the genitourinary epithelium to resist bacterial adherence. Certain bacterial characteristics also increase virulence. Bacteria have cell-surface structures called adhesins that facilitate their binding to epithelial cell-surface receptors. Research demonstrates that certain types of adhesins—in particular pili—may contribute to the virulence of an organism. P pili have been shown to be a particularly important virulence factor in pyelonephritis.

Although the majority of women with recurrent UTIs have uncomplicated infections, some with certain predisposing factors may suffer from complicated UTIs. As with most men with recurrent UTIs, some women may have poor bladder emptying secondary to obstruction, bladder dysfunction, or other complicating factors. The recognition of such factors is important, because the evaluation and treatment of patients with complicated UTIs differs significantly from those with uncomplicated UTIs.

## EVALUATION

Most healthy young women with recurrent UTIs need no additional evaluation beyond a good history, physical examination, urinalysis, and urine culture. A number of studies have evaluated the results of cystoscopy and intravenous urography in these patients. With uncomplicated infections, the number of upper-tract and lower-tract abnormalities identified have been remarkably low. However, if the patient has risk factors for a complicated UTI, further investigation is warranted. Clues in the history may include past nephrolithiasis or congenital urologic malformation, previous urologic surgery or instrumentation, chronic disease states, such as diabetes mellitus or lupus, neurogenic disorders, obstructive voiding symptoms, and hematuria. On physical examination, any flank tenderness or suprapubic fullness should be noted. A thorough pelvic examination and measurement of the postvoid residual are important. Anatomic abnormalities, such as a cystocele or hypersuspended (iatrogenic) urethra, may cause obstruction, whereas a urethral diverticula may serve as a reservoir for bacteria. All of these conditions are indications for a more extensive evaluation. The urine culture may also indicate the presence of a complicated UTI. Infection with unusual organisms—especially urea-splitting bacteria or recurrent infection with the same strain of bacteria—should also prompt a more intensive evaluation. Based on these findings, cystoscopy and upper-tract imaging may be warranted. In certain cases other studies, such as urodynamics, voiding cystourethrography, retrograde ureteral pyelography, or renal scintigraphy, may be indicated.

Other important clues that may help treatment planning should be noted. The degree of estrogenization of the vaginal tissues is important, because lack of estrogen causes marked changes in the vaginal microflora that can predispose to infection. The type of contraception used may also be important, because the use of diaphragms and spermicides have been associated with an increased risk of UTI. The presence of a strong association between sexual activity and UTIs in the individual patient should be noted.

As men are more likely to have an underlying treatable cause for recurrent UTIs, they may require a more extensive evaluation. However, the cornerstone of the work-up remains a good history, physical examination, urinalysis, and urine culture. Many of the risk factors for complicated UTI noted in women may also occur in men, and should be identified.

In male patients, a few specific points deserve particular attention. A history of obstructive voiding symptoms along with physical findings suggestive of obstruction (ie an enlarged prostate, an elevated postvoid residual, induration of the urethra, and so forth) should be identified. A history of sexually-transmitted disease, urethral or perineal trauma, or urethral instrumentation may suggest urethral stricture disease. Symptoms of perineal or lower-back pain or a tender prostate on examination may suggest prostatitis. All of these factors should be noted and may lead to further evaluation with cystoscopy, retrograde urethrography, prostatic-secretion culture, or other imaging studies. Since recurrent UTIs are rare in young men and are frequently associated with treatable abnormalities in older men, most male patients with recurrent UTIs require evaluation of the upper and/or lower urinary tract with cystoscopy, intravenous pyelography, or other studies suited to the particular situation. Finally, any patient—male or female—with breakthrough infections while on therapy who was initially treated without diagnostic studies requires a more extensive evaluation.

In summary, all patients with recurrent UTIs need a thorough history, physical examination, urinalysis, and culture. Healthy women with no signs of a complicated UTI need no further workup. Most males require cystoscopy with or without upper-tract imaging. Patients of either sex with risk factors for complicated UTIs, or with breakthrough UTIs while on therapy usually require cystoscopy and/or upper-tract evaluation with the addition of other diagnostic tests in specific circumstances.

## TREATMENT

The treatment of recurrent UTIs can be divided into complicated vs uncomplicated infections. The key to the effective treatment of complicated recurrent UTIs is the identification and treatment of underlying problems. The relief of obstruction in women through cystocele repair, urethral dilation, or urethrolysis—and in men through repair of urethral-stricture disease or the treatment of BPH—may prevent future infections. Removing or treating reservoirs of infection, such as stones, foreign bodies, urethral diverticuli, or fistulas should prevent UTI recurrence. In patients with poor bladder emptying secondary to a neurogenic or myogenic problem, clean intermittent catheterization can be performed, which should reduce the frequency of infection. Those patients with no treatable abnormalities can be difficult to manage. Pretherapy cultures are important, because many resistant organisms are present in these individuals. Because of the different spectra of pathogenic bacteria seen in these patients, more powerful antibiotics (frequently quinolones) given for longer durations may also be required.

Most patients with uncomplicated UTIs are healthy women. The choice of treatment should take into account the frequency of UTIs and their possible relation to sexual intercourse, as well as the potential side effects and cost of therapy. There are three options for treating women with recurrent uncomplicated UTIs: peri-intercourse prophylaxis, intermittent self-start therapy, and long-term low-dose antimicrobial prophylaxis. Inexpensive oral agents can generally be used. Trimethoprim/sulfamethoxazole (TMP/

sulfa), trimethoprim (TMP) alone, nitrofurantoin, and the fluoroquinolones are all useful. These medications have few side effects when used for short courses of treatment, and have few adverse effects on the normal vaginal flora. Trimethoprim alone has been demonstrated to be as effective as TMP/sulfa in many cases, and is especially useful for long-term prophylaxis. Nitrofurantoin is also particularly effective in the urinary tract, and is remarkable for the low rate of resistance despite years of use, but it is important to note that it is frequently ineffective against *Proteus* and *Pseudomonas*. TMP alone, TMP/sulfa, or nitrofurantoin are all very inexpensive. In some instances, fluoroquinolones may be preferred, although their expense can be prohibitive. A number of recent studies have documented an increasing bacterial resistance to TMP/sulfa. This trend requires close follow-up, because it may change the way UTIs are treated empirically.

### *Peri-Intercourse Prophylaxis*

In those women who note a clear association between sexual intercourse and UTI, a dose of antibiotics either immediately before or after coitus can significantly reduce the rate of reinfection. It is not necessary to take more than one dose per day.

### *Intermittent Self-Start Therapy*

Women with relatively infrequent recurrent UTIs (3–4 per year) may be given a standing prescription for a short course of oral antibiotics that can be started at the first sign of a UTI. Usually 3–5 d of therapy are effective. Some authors have suggested that a urine specimen be collected by the patient prior to starting therapy and brought to the physician's office the next day to assure sensitivity to the antibiotic (some obtain a specimen posttherapy as well to assure eradication of infection.) Although this approach has many merits, it is often impractical. In my practice, I advise patients to start treatment at the first sign of infection, and only when there has been no symptomatic improvement in 48 h do I have them drop off a urine specimen for culture and sensitivity.

### *Low-Dose Long-Term Antimicrobial Prophylaxis*

Women with frequent UTIs may benefit from a daily low dose of an oral antimicrobial agent. This will help prevent infections and may lead to the resolution of colonization of the perineum or urethra with uropathic bacterial species. Numerous studies have shown this to be an effective and well-tolerated mode of therapy, with recurrence decreased by as much as 95%. Prophylactic therapy requires only a low dose of antibiotic at bedtime for a 4–12-mo course. Unfortunately, when prophylactic therapy ends, a significant proportion of women will experience return of UTIs and may need lengthy courses of prophylaxis. TMP 100 mg, TMP-sulfa single-strength tablets, nitrofurantoin 50–100 mg, or a fluoroquinolone at a low dose daily are good choices for long-term prophylaxis. It is important to keep in mind that patients receiving long-term prophylaxis with nitrofurantoin are at risk for developing interstitial pneumonitis and hepatitis, and should be monitored. The risk increases with age and is more common in women over 50.

Other strategies to reduce the rate of reinfection include changes in the method of contraception and estrogen replacement. As noted earlier, women who use a diaphragm and spermicide for contraception are at increased risk for UTIs, and in appropriate circumstances an alternate form of contraception may be considered. Postmenopausal women with loss of estrogenization are also at increased risk for UTIs, and in many cases hormone-replacement therapy, which can be instituted in conjunction with the patient's primary-care physician, may reduce the rate of reinfection.

## CONCLUSION

Patients with recurrent UTIs are frequent visitors to most urologist's offices, and a rapid and cost-effective approach to their management is required. Most patients with recurrent UTIs are healthy women who need only a thorough history, physical examination, urinalysis, and urine culture. It is essential to identify patients with risk factors for complicated UTIs, who require a more extensive evaluation that frequently includes cystoscopy and upper-tract evaluation. These patients must have all abnormalities identified and treated to prevent recurrent infections. On the other hand, those with uncomplicated recurrent UTIs can usually be treated with either peri-intercourse prophylaxis, intermittent self-start therapy, or low-dose long-term prophylaxis with inexpensive oral antibiotics.

## SELECTED READING

Fair WR, McClennan BL, Jost RG (1979) Are excretory urograms necessary in evaluating women with urinary tract infection? *J. Urol* 121:313–315.

Gupta, K, Scholes, D, Stamm, WE (1999) Increasing prevalence of antimicrobial resistance among uropathogens causing acute uncomplicated cystitis in women. *JAMA* 281:736–738.

Kunin CM (1997) Urinary Tract Infections—Detection Prevention and Management (5th ed.), Baltimore: Waverly and Wilkens.

Nickel JC, Wilson J, Morales A, Heaton J (1991) Value of urologic investigation in a targeted group of women with recurrent urinary tract infections. *CJS* 34:591–594.

Schaeffer AJ, Stuppy BA (1991) Efficacy and safety of self-start therapy in women with recurrent urinary tract infections. *J Urol* 161:207–211.

Stamey TA, Condy M, Mihara G (1997) Prophylactic efficacy of nitrofurantoin macrocrystals and trimethoprim sulfamethoxazole in urinary infections: biologic effects on the vaginal and rectal flora. *N Engl J Med* 296:780–783.

# 9 Prostatitis

## *J. Curtis Nickel,* MD

**CONTENTS**

AN IMPORTANT CLINICAL ENTITY
ETIOLOGY AND PATHOGENESIS
DIAGNOSIS
TREATMENT
SELECTED READING

## AN IMPORTANT CLINICAL ENTITY

Urologists and physicians who treat male patients spend a significant percentage of their clinical practice time diagnosing and managing prostate disease. Prostate cancer is the most common malignancy diagnosed in men, and the second most common cause of death by cancer. Benign prostatic hyperplasia clinically affects 50% of men over 50, and half of those require some form of therapy. Is the other significant prostate disease—prostatitis—an important disease in urologic clinical practice?

In the early 1990s, prostatitis accounted for as many office visits per year in the United States as those attributed to BPH or prostate cancer. Urologists in North America follow over 100 prostatitis patients each in their urologic practices. Almost one in ten patient encounters with urologists are billed with a diagnostic code of prostatitis. It is estimated that 35%–50% of males will experience the pain and discomfort of prostatitis during some period in their lives. The prevalence rate has been estimated to be as high as 5%–8% in the United States. The quality of life of patients with chronic prostatitis is significantly worse than that experienced by patients with BPH or localized prostate cancer, and ranks with the quality of life of patients who have just had an acute MI, or have unstable angina or active Crohn's disease. Prostatitis is an important clinical condition, and urologists must become adept at managing these patients.

## ETIOLOGY AND PATHOGENESIS

The primary stumbling block for effective management of the various prostatitis syndromes lies in our lack of understanding of what is actually causing the symptoms and/or inflammation. No one doubts that the acute stage of prostatic inflammation is secondary to a generalized infection of the prostate gland by prostate-pathogenic bacteria. This fulminate, infectious disease—usually associated with generalized urosepsis—

From: *Current Clinical Urology: Office Urology: The Clinician's Guide*
Edited by: E. D. Kursh and J. C. Ulchaker © Humana Press Inc., Totowa, NJ

does not appear to be related to the chronic prostatitis syndromes and is probably an independent disease. It is rare, easily diagnosed, almost never occurs twice in the same patient, and its management (unless the patient develops prostatic abscess) is standard and usually effective.

The chronic prostatitis syndromes, on the other hand, defy such an easily understood pathogenesis that would lead to etiologically-driven management strategies. What does cause chronic prostatitis? As described in the next section, chronic prostatitis (or, as later defined chronic pelvic pain syndrome) is characterized by pain or discomfort associated with variable urinary and sexual symptoms. These patients can present with bacteria localized to the prostate, inflammation localized to the prostate gland, both bacteria and inflammation localized to the prostate gland, or neither bacteria or inflammation associated with the syndrome.

In about 5% of cases, uropathogenic (and supposedly prostate-pathogenic) bacteria can be localized to prostate specific specimens (*see* diagnosis section). These patients experience recurrent urinary-tract infections, but many are asymptomatic between episodes of UTI. The question that must be asked is whether these bacteria actually cause symptoms of chronic prostatitis or chronic pelvic pain, or whether they are just innocent bystanders that occasionally cause lower UTIs such as cystitis? It is intriguing to note that many patients with BPH, without pelvic pain, also have uropathogenic bacteria localized to specific prostate specimens.

Most patients with chronic prostatitis and inflammation localized to the prostate specimens, do not have uropathogenic bacteria localized to their prostate-specific specimens. What causes the inflammation in these patients? The most common and likely theory is a combination of dysfunctional high-pressure voiding and intraprostatic ductal reflux. Whether it is a chemical reaction (ie to uric acid) or an immunologic reaction (to Tamm-Horsfall protein or other substances) has not been established. Other theories with various levels of scientific proof that may account for the inflammation seen in the prostate gland include cryptic nonculturable bacteria, Chlamydia, Ureaplasma, viruses, autoimmune processes, neuropathic etiologies, and so forth. It is also intriguing to know that asymptomatic patients with BPH and prostate cancer can be clearly demonstrated to have a very similar inflammatory pattern in their prostate gland, without experiencing chronic pelvic pain syndrome.

Patients presenting with chronic prostatitis or chronic pelvic pain syndrome without inflammation or bacteria are even more problematic. These patients, who usually have associated urodynamic abnormalities, are thought to have some form of neuromuscular disorder of the pelvic floor and perineum, which evolves into obstruction voiding symptoms and pain.

## DIAGNOSIS

### *Classification*

Historically, urologists have divided the prostatitis syndromes into acute bacterial prostatitis, chronic bacterial prostatitis, chronic nonbacterial (or abacterial) prostatitis, and prostatodynia. This has led to significant confusion in developing management strategies, to such a degree that almost all patients labeled with the clinical diagnosis of prostatitis tend to be treated with a long course of antimicrobial therapy, despite

## Table 1
### Classification of Prostatitis

| Category I | Acute bacterial prostatitis |
|---|---|
| Category II | Chronic bacterial prostatitis |
| Category III | Chronic pelvic pain syndrome (CPPS) |
|    Category IIIA | Inflammatory CPPS |
|    Category IIIB | Noninflammatory CPPS |
| Category IV | Asymptomatic inflammatory prostatitis (AIP) |

## Table 2
### Category I: Acute Bacterial Prostatitis

| Definition | Acute bacterial infection of prostate and bladder |
|---|---|
| | Uropathogenic bacteria and white blood cells in midstream urine specimen |
| Management | Wide-spectrum intravenous antibiotics |
| | Lower urinary-tract drainage |
| | Oral antibiotics for 3–4 wk after fever subsides |

variably poor success. The new NIH classification system of prostatitis syndromes (*see* Table 1) is a step in the right direction in better classifying patients who present with a prostatitis syndrome. Categories I and II are similar to the traditional classification of acute and chronic bacterial prostatitis, respectively. The new categories of chronic pelvic pain syndrome (Category III), inflammatory and noninflammatory, and asymptomatic inflammatory prostatitis (Category IV) address the major problems and omissions of the traditional and historic classification system employed for the last few decades. This new classification system depends on microscopic and culture evaluation of prostate-specific specimens.

## *Clinical Diagnosis*

### Category I

Category I patients present with symptoms of acute cystitis, obstructive voiding symptoms, and generalized symptoms of urosepsis (*see* Table 2). Physical examination reveals a patient in distress, likely to be febrile, with a possible distended bladder and a boggy, tender prostate. A midstream urine specimen will demonstrate leukocytosis and perhaps bacteria on microscopy, and a culture will usually grow a gram-negative uropathogenic bacteria.

### Category II

Patients with chronic bacterial prostatitis typically present with a history of documented recurrent lower urinary-tract infection, such as cystitis (*see* Table 3). Many patients are asymptomatic between episodes. Uropathogenic bacteria and white blood cells are localized to the prostate-specific specimens as described below.

### Category III

The diagnosis of chronic pelvic pain syndrome is based on the "presence of genitourinary pain in the absence of uropathogenic bacteria detected by standard microbiological

Table 3
Category II: Chronic Bacterial Prostatitis

| | |
|---|---|
| Definition | Recurrent UTIs |
| | Uropathogenic bacteria and white blood cells localized to prostate-specific specimens (EPS, VB3, or semen). Patient may be asymptomatic between acute episodes. |
| Management | Oral antibiotic therapy (fluoroquinolones or trimethoprim) for 6 wk (asymptomatic) or 12 wk (symptomatic) |
| | Repetitive prostate massage |
| | Long-term, low-dose prophylactic antibiotic for recurrent episodes |
| | Long-term suppressive antibiotics for relapse |

Table 4
Category IIIA: Inflammatory Chronic Pelvic Pain Syndrome

| | |
|---|---|
| Definition | Chronic genitourinary pain in the absence of uropathogenic bacteria detected by standard microbiological method |
| | White blood cells but no uropathic bacteria in prostate-specific specimens (EPS, VB3, or semen) |
| Management | Trial of antibiotic therapy (6 wk)—fluoroquinolone or trimethoprim and a tetracycline either concurrently or sequentially |
| | Prostate massage |
| | Alpha-blockade (if obstructed) |
| | Theoretical options—finasteride, pentosan polysulfate, antiinflammatory (Cox 2 inhibitors), immune modulation, phytotherapy |

Table 5
Category IIIB: Noninflammatory Chronic Pelvic Pain Syndrome

| | |
|---|---|
| Definition | Chronic genitourinary pain in the absence of uropathogenic bacteria detected by standard microbiological methodology |
| | No bacteria and no white blood cells in prostate-specific specimens (EPS, VB3, or semen) |
| Management | Triple therapy—analgesic (±-amitryptyline), muscle relaxant (diazepam or baclofen), and alpha-blockade |
| | Biofeedback |
| | Lifestyle changes |

methodology." These patients complain of perineal, suprapubic, penile, and testicular pain, dysuria or pain during urination, and pain or discomfort during and/or after ejaculation. Patients also experience variable obstructive and irritative voiding symptoms and sexual dysfunction other than ejaculatory disturbances. Chronic pelvic pain syndrome (Category III) is further divided into an inflammatory category (Category IIIA CPPS; see Table 4) and a noninflammatory category (Category IIIB CPPS; see Table 5) based on the presence (or absence) of white blood cells in the prostate-specific specimens employing the localization procedures described below.

Table 6
Category IV: Asymptomatic Inflammatory Prostatitis (AIP)

| | |
|---|---|
| Definition | Presence of inflammation (white blood cells or histology) and/or bacteria in prostate-specific specimens (EPS, VB3, semen and/or biopsy) |
| | No complaints of genitourinary pain (asymptomatic) |
| Management | No treatment required unless: • Elevated PSA |
| | • Infertile |
| | • Endoscopic manipulation |

Table 7
Lower Urinary-Tract Localization Studies

Meares/Stamey Four-Glass Test

| NIH Classification | Test | Specimen | | | |
|---|---|---|---|---|---|
| | | VB1 | VB2 | EPS | VB3 |
| Category II | WBC | − | ±[a] | + | + |
| | Culture | − | ±[a] | + | + |
| Category IIIA | WBC | − | − | + | + |
| | Culture | − | − | − | − |
| Category IIIB | WBC | − | − | − | − |
| | Culture | − | − | − | − |
| Category IV | WBC | ? | ± | ± | ± |
| | Culture | ? | ± | ± | ± |

Pre- and Post-massage Test (PPMT): A Preliminary Screen

| NIH Classification | Bacteruria | | Leukocytosis | |
|---|---|---|---|---|
| | Pre-M | Post-M | Pre-M | Post-M |
| Category II | ±[a] | + | ±[a] | + |
| Category IIIA | − | − | − | + |
| Category IIIB | − | − | − | − |
| Category IV | ± | ± | ± | ± |

[a]Patients with Category II prostatitis may have recurrent or concurrent bacterial cystitis.

## Category IV

Asymptomatic patients who are noted to have prostatic inflammation and/or bacteria on prostate-specific specimens (including biopsy) are classified as having Category IV prostatitis (*see* Table 6). This is picked up during semen analysis for infertility, biopsy results during evaluation for elevated PSA or prostatic nodules, or histological examination of surgical BPH specimens. The actual relevance of prostatic inflammation in these patients is unknown.

### *Lower Urinary-Tract Localization Studies*

For the past three decades, urologists have been familiar with the Meares-Stamey four-glass test for localization of bacteria and inflammation in the lower male urinary tract (*see* Table 7). This technique, which employs an initial voided urine sample (VB1), midstream or second voided urine sample (MSSU or VB2), an expressed prostatic secretion (EPS) and a third voided urine sample (VB3), remains the gold standard today for lower urinary-tract evaluation in patients with chronic prostatitis. Yet it is rarely used by urologists and almost never used by primary-care physicians. Outside of the research setting, it is cumbersome, expensive, and difficult, and urologists have become frustrated by its very low yield as well as a perceived occurrence of frequent false-negative and false-positive results.

Our group has recently promoted the use of a lower urinary-tract screening technique (the Pre- and Post-Massage Test or PPMT) for patients who present with chronic prostatitis. Patients should be taken off antibiotics for 4–6 wk and urine collected before and after prostate massage is sent for microscopy and culture. If the postprostatic massage urine (post-M) shows excessive leukocytosis and/or bacteria compared to the preprostatic massage urine (pre-M), a presumptive diagnosis into a correct classification can be made. To confirm that diagnosis (if the clinician wishes) in those patients with positive results, an initial stream urine (VB1) can be performed to rule out urethritis, and EPS can be obtained if possible to confirm the diagnosis of category II or IIIA CPPS. This approach to rigorous diagnosis and classification of prostatitis patients will prove invaluable to the subsequent development of management strategies.

## *Other Investigations*

Most patients who present with prostatitis syndromes will only require a good history, focused physical examination, and lower urinary-tract screen before categorization and subsequent management. However, a number of patients require further investigations. We have found it very beneficial to do uroflowmetry. If maximum urinary flow rate is below 20, pressure-flow studies (and even video urodynamics) can be helpful in determining the degree and perhaps the etiology of obstruction. In some cases (but certainly not in all cases of prostatitis) flexible cystoscopy helps to rule out strictures and bladder-neck problems. We have not found transrectal ultrasound to be helpful in management of this syndrome and restrict upper-urinary tract imaging for those patients with recurrent urinary-tract infections or hematuria.

## TREATMENT

### *Category I*

Patients diagnosed with acute bacterial prostatitis should be immediately started on wide-spectrum intravenous antibiotics and if they are in urinary retention, should be gently catheterized with a small-caliber urethral catheter (*see* Table 3). If insertion of the catheter is difficult or causes significant pain, or if it is very uncomfortable *in situ,* percutaneous suprapubic cystotomy should be used for lower urinary-tract drainage. The patient can be switched to a culture-specific oral antibiotic (a fluoroquinolone is preferred) once the fever abates. The oral antibiotic should be continued for 3–4 wk. If the fever, systemic symptoms, and pain do not resolve within 48 h, transrectal ultrasound should be performed to rule out a prostate abscess. If this rare complication arises, it is most effectively treated by transurethral drainage.

## Category II

Patients with bacteria localized to the prostate gland (chronic bacterial prostatitis) should be treated with a long-term course of antibiotics for a period of 6–12 wk (*see* Table 4). If the patients are asymptomatic between recurrent episodes of lower urinary-tract infection, 6 wk is sufficient. If the patient is chronically symptomatic, 12 wk may be better. Either a fluoroquinolone or trimethroprim (with or without sulfamethoxazole) is preferred because of the favorability for pharmacokinetics in the inflamed prostate gland. If a patient with documented chronic bacterial prostatitis remains symptomatic on a long course of a culture-specific antibiotic, the combination of continued antibiotic therapy and repetitive prostate massage (at least twice a week) has proven beneficial. In patients who have recurrent prostatitis, low-dose prophylaxis therapy may be indicated. In patients with relapsing prostatitis (with the same organisms), long-term suppressive antibiotic therapy may be indicated.

## Category III

It has become apparent to most researchers in the field, and to most clinicians, that therapy for the inflammatory (IIIA) CPPS should be tailored differently than that for patients presenting with noninflammatory (Category IIIB) CPPS.

### Category IIIA

Since these patients may have a bacterial etiology (ie, noncultured bacteria, an unculturable microorganism, Chlamydia, or Mycoplasma), they should receive at least one course (6–8 wk) of antibiotic therapy as an empiric trial before abandoning antibiotics altogether (*see* Table 5). Either a fluoroquinolone (with activity against Chlamydia and Mycoplasma) or trimethoprim and tetracycline (concurrently or sequentially) is recommended. If these treatments are unsuccessful and the patient's symptoms persist, repetitive prostatic massage has proven beneficial in some patients. A periodic culture of the expressed prostatic secretion or post M specimen may identify a responsible organism, which should be treated with antimicrobial therapy combined with the continued repetitive prostate massage. If patients have obstructive voiding symptoms (maximum uroflow <15–20 cm$^3$/s) the use of high-dose alpha-blockade has been helpful. Studies assessing the benefits of finasteride, pentosan polysulfate, immune modulators, COX-2 inhibitors, and various plant extracts (phytotherapy) are underway.

### Category IIIB

These patients are usually quite symptomatic and the use of triple therapy, analgesics (potent analgesics ± amitriptyline), muscle relaxants (diazepam or baclofen), and alpha-blockade have proven to be beneficial in a significant number of these patients. The therapeutic strategy begins by starting all three medications concurrently and then decreasing or discontinuing the analgesic and muscle relaxant, while continuing the alpha-blocker. For patients with obstructive voiding symptoms (particularly if urodynamic evaluation has confirmed detrusor-sphincter dyssynergia) various forms of biofeedback and relaxation exercises are helpful.

For many cases of chronic pelvic pain syndrome (and even category II chronic bacterial prostatitis) cure is sometimes impossible. In that case, the goal of therapy is amelioration of symptoms and improvement in quality of life. A caring and empathetic physician with an understanding of the prostatitis syndromes and who is willing to set realistic goals and spend some time educating patients can expect the best management results with this very difficult syndrome.

## SELECTED READING

### *Classic*

Meares EM, Stamey TA (1968) Bacteriologic localization patterns in bacterial prostatitis and urethritis. *Investig Urol* 5:492–518.

Drach GW, Fair WR, Meares EM, et al. (1978) Classification of benign diseases associated with prostatic pain: prostatitis or prostatodynia? *J Urol* 120:266.

### *Epidemiology*

Collins MM, Stafford RS, O'Leary MP, et al. (1998) How common is prostatitis? A national survey of physician visits. *J Urol* 159:1224–1228.

Moon TD (1997) Questionnaire survey of urologists and primary care physicians' diagnostic and treatment practices for prostatitis. *Urology* 50:543–547.

Nickel JC, Nigro M, Valiquette L, et al. (1998) Diagnosis and treatment of prostatitis in Canada. *Urology* 52:797–802.

Moon TD, Hagen L, Heisey DM (1997) Urinary symptomatology in younger men. *Urology* 50:700–703.

### *General Review*

Roberts RO, Lieber MM, Bostwick DG, et al. (1997) A review of clinical and pathological prostatitis syndromes. *Urology* 49:809–821.

Nickel JC (1998) Prostatitis: myths and realities. *Urology* 51:362–366.

### *Management*

Nickel JC (1997) The Pre and Post Massage Test (PPMT): a simple screen for prostatitis. *Tech Urol* 3:38–43.

Nickel JC (1998) Effective office management of chronic prostatitis. *Urol Clin N Am* 25:677–684.

Nickel JC (1995) Prostatitis. In: Mulholland SG, ed. *Antibiotic Therapy in Urology*. Philadelphia: Lippincott Raven, pp. 57–70.

Nickel JC (1996) Rational management of nonbacterial prostatitis and prostatodynia. *Curr Opin Urol* 6:53–58.

### *Textbook*

Nickel JC, ed. (1999) *Textbook of Prostatitis*. ISIS, Oxford.

# 10 Sexually Transmitted Diseases

*Jeannette M. Potts, MD*

**CONTENTS**

>   INTRODUCTION
>   HERPES SIMPLEX VIRUS
>   CHLAMYDIA TRACHOMATIS
>   LYMPHOGRANULOMA VENEREUM
>   PRIMARY AND SECONDARY SYPHILIS
>   GONORRHEA
>   CHANCROID
>   TRICHOMONIASIS
>   GENITAL WARTS
>   SCABIES
>   OVERVIEW OF OTHER SEXUALLY ASSOCIATED INFECTIONS
>   SELECTED READING

## INTRODUCTION

*Primary* prevention through universal safe-sex precautions would eliminate the costly and sometimes tragic consequences of sexually transmitted disease (STD). However, because STD transmission remains prevalent, *secondary* prevention through screening and early diagnosis remains our most valuable weapon against the devastating disease sequelae.

Early detection and appropriate antibiotic therapy have led to decreases in bacterial venereal diseases. For example, the incidence of syphilis in the United States has decreased from 51,000 in 1990 to 15,000 in 1995. Likewise, the incidence of gonorrhea has decreased from one million in 1980 to only 356,000 in 1995. *Chlamydia trachomatis* remains the most common bacterial STD, with an estimated 4.6 million new cases in the United States each year and 50 million worldwide.

Viral infections, for which curative therapy is not available, have been stable or increasing in prevalence. With 500,000 new cases each year, herpes simplex virus (HSV) is one of the most common viral STDs. The prevalence of HSV-2 antibodies observed in the United States ranges from 1% to 46%, depending on the population screened. As many as 80% of serologically positive women have no history of clinical infection and may represent a significant group of asymptomatic viral shedders who

From: *Current Clinical Urology: Office Urology: The Clinician's Guide*
Edited by: E. D. Kursh and J. C. Ulchaker © Humana Press Inc., Totowa, NJ

could transmit the virus. One million new cases of human papilloma virus are diagnosed each year, and the prevalence of this disease is between 24 and 40 million. The virus—particularly DNA types 16, 18, 31 and 45—poses a lifetime risk of malignancy. Human papilloma virus has been proven to cause cervical and penile cancer, and is implicated in some cases of vulvovaginal cancer. More recently, anal cancers have been strongly associated with HPV-16 in both men and women.

People at high risk of contracting sexually transmitted diseases are young adults between the ages of 18 and 28, as well as middle-aged, divorced individuals. It is also important to bear in mind that sexually transmitted diseases rank among the top five risks of international travelers, along with diarrhea, hepatitis, and motor vehicle accidents.

The brunt of the STD burden, both in risk and consequence, falls on women. When exposed to sexually transmitted diseases, women are more likely to become infected and are much more likely to be asymptomatic. STDs can cause pelvic inflammatory disease, with subsequent risks of chronic pain syndromes, ectopic pregnancy, and infertility. Unfortunately, there is very little evidence that treatment will reverse the sequelae.

A urologist should have a high index of suspicion for underlying sexually transmitted disease in women who present with recurrent urinary-tract infections (UTIs) and in those who are symptomatic with sterile urine cultures. Up to 50% of women with signs of UTI during emergency-department examination had subsequent positive cultures for sexually transmitted disease. Physicians should maintain the same level of vigilance when treating lesbians. Genital human papilloma virus has been identified along with squamous intraepithelial lesions among lesbians, and occurs among those who have not have had sexual relations with men.

Proctitis may occur in women and homosexual men. Causative organisms include *Neisseria gonorrhoeae, Chlamydia trachomatis, Treponema pallidum,* and HSV.

A discussion of human immunodeficiency virus (HIV) is beyond the scope of this chapter; however, it is important to remember that STD—especially the ulcerative types—facilitate the transmission and infection of HIV. HSV-2, in particular, may play a role in the transmission of HIV, as it has been identified more frequently than other STD among HIV-concordant couples. Increased risk of HIV concordance has also been observed among couples who both have *Mycoplasma genitalium* antibodies.

The most common sexually transmitted diseases are discussed in the following pages. They include HSV, Chlamydia urethritis/cervicitis, Lymphogranuloma venereum, syphilis, gonorrhea, chancroid, trichomoniasis, human papilloma virus, and scabies. Other sexually associated pathogens, which cause urethritis and vaginitides, will also be discussed briefly.

## HERPES SIMPLEX VIRUS

### *Diagnosis*

Genital herpes infection is caused by HSV-2 in 80–85% of cases. HSV-1 is responsible for 15–20% of cases. The incubation period is 1–26 d. Nongenital infection of HSV-1 during childhood may be somewhat protective against subsequent genital HSV-2 infection in adults. When exposed to HSV-2, women with negative HSV-1 antibodies had a 32% risk of infection per year, whereas women with positive antibodies had only a 10% risk of infection. Silent infection is common and accounts for more than

70% of viral transmission. Asymptomatic viral shedding is greatest in the 3 mo following the primary episode of genital ulceration. Up to 80% of women with HSV-2 antibodies have no history of clinical infection. Primary infection is associated with painful ulcers of the genitalia or anus, and bilateral painful inguinal adenopathy in 80% of cases. The initial infection is often associated with constitutional symptoms. Sacral radiculomyelopathy is a rare manifestation of primary infection that has a greater association with primary anal HSV. Urethral lesions may cause urinary retention in women. Recurrent episodes may be less severe, involving only ulceration of the genital or anal area. Although subtyping is not a standard practice, it may be helpful in determining the natural history and the management of patients with herpetic ulcers. HSV-2 is more likely to recur (80%) than HSV-1 (55%). Asymptomatic shedding is also greater among HSV-2 cases. The diagnosis should be confirmed by ruling out other ulcerative disorders and obtaining a Tzanck smear prepared from the base of the ulcer. Tissue cultures employing M4 transport medium may also be helpful.

### *Treatment*

Primary therapy consists of acyclovir 200 mg (taken five times daily for 7–10 d) or valacyclovir 500 mg (taken twice daily for 7–10 d). For recurrences, acyclovir (200 mg, five times daily for 5 d) or valacyclovir (500 mg twice daily for 5 d) must be initiated during the prodrome or within 1 d of the onset of lesions. Suppressive therapy may be necessary in patients suffering from six or more recurrences per year. The safety and efficacy of daily suppressive therapy has been well-documented (acyclovir 400 mg BID for 6 yr, valacyclovir 500 mg QD for 1 yr).

## CHLAMYDIA TRACHOMATIS

### *Diagnosis*

This is the most common bacterial STD in the United States, caused by serotypes D, E, F, G, H, I, J, and K. The incubation period is 3–14 d. Men will typically experience lower urinary-tract symptoms attributed to urethritis, epididymitis, or prostatitis, and may notice clear or white penile discharge. Up to 85% of women may be asymptomatic until the infection has progressed to pelvic inflammatory disease, which may require hospitalization and parenteral antibiotic therapy. Specimens obtained from urethral or cervical swabs, urine, or prostatic fluid should be cultured. Amplification techniques utilizing polymerase chain-reaction assays for urine have been proven to be a highly sensitive and noninvasive means of screening men and women for Chlamydia infection. This method should not replace pelvic examination or endocervical culture in symptomatic women.

### *Treatment*

Azithromycin (1 g by mouth as a single dose) (1 g sachet is more economical than capsules) or doxycycline (100 mg twice daily for 7 d) are primary treatments. Alternative therapies include erythromycin (500 mg four times daily) or ofloxacin (300 mg twice daily) for 7 d. Erythromycin estolate, doxycycline, and ofloxacin are contraindicated during pregnancy. Erythromycin base or erythromycin ethylsuccinate, amoxicillin, or azithromycin are safe during pregnancy.

## LYMPHOGRANULOMA VENEREUM

### Diagnosis

Lymphogranuloma venereum is caused by *Chlamydia trachomatis* Types L1, L2, and L3, which are rare in the United States. The incubation period is 3–30 d. The initial manifestation of infection is usually a single, painless ulcer on the penis, anus, or vulvovaginal area. However, patients usually present with painful unilateral suppurative inguinal adenopathy that occurs 2–6 wk after resolution of the ulcer. Constitutional symptoms are more likely at that time. Perirectal or deep iliac lymph-node enlargement may occur if the primary lesion arises from the cervix or rectum. Significant tissue damage may occur, leading to labial fenestration, urethral destruction, anorectal fistulas, and elephantiasis of the penis, scrotum, or labia. Compliment-fixation or indirect-fluorescence antibody titers may be necessary to confirm diagnosis, because cultures are positive in only 30–50% of cases.

### Treatment

Antibiotic therapy for 3 wk is required, using one of the following regimens: doxycycline (100 mg twice daily), erythromycin (500 mg four times daily), or sulfisoxazole (twice daily).

## PRIMARY AND SECONDARY SYPHILIS

### Diagnosis

Syphilis is caused by a spirochete, *Treponema pallidum*. Incubation periods vary between 3 and 90 d. A single, clean ulcer that is usually nontender appears on the glans, corona, or perianal area on men and on the labial or anal area on women. It is typically associated with bilateral, nontender, inguinal adenopathy. Secondary syphilis may present up to 24 mo following the initial infection as mucocutaneous lesions and constitutional symptoms. Dark-field examination of specimens obtained from primary or secondary lesions will reveal the spirochete. Sensitivity of serologic testing is 80% for RPR and 70% for VDRL in primary syphilis, and 100% sensitive for both in secondary syphilis. Beware of false-negative serology in the immunocompromised host. HIV testing should be strongly recommended if syphilis is suspected.

### Treatment

Benzthiazide penicillin-G (2.4 million units intramuscularly as a single dose) or doxycycline (100 mg by mouth twice daily for 14 d) are the preferred therapies. If diagnosis is established more than 1 yr following initial infection, penicillin injections should be repeated weekly for a total of three doses, and doxycycline therapy should be extended for a total of 4 wk. In pregnancy, desensitization to penicillin is recommended if patient has a penicillin allergy. Ceftriaxone may be a potential alternative, but insufficient data on its use during pregnancy is available.

## GONORRHEA

### Diagnosis

Gonorrhrea is caused by a gram-negative Diplococcus, Neisseria gonorroeheae. The incubation period is 3–14 d. Risk of infection after one exposure is 10% in men and

40% in women. Men will typically experience lower urinary-tract symptoms attributed to urethritis, epididymitis, proctitis, or prostatitis, with associated mucopurulent urethral discharge. Women may have symptoms of vaginal/pelvic discomfort and dysuria, and may have abnormal vaginal discharge. Manifestations of rare gonococcal dissemination include polyarthralgias, dermatitis, and tenosynovitis. Swabs taken from the urethra and the cervix or rectum should be cultured or tested by means of more sensitive DNA probes.

### *Treatment*

Because of growing concern regarding gonorrhea resistance to quinolones, ceftriaxone (125 mg intramuscularly [IM]) as a single dose remains the preferred treatment. Single oral-dose regimens also include cefixime (400 mg), ciprofloxacin (500 mg), and ofloxacin (400 mg). Azithromycin (2.0 g) is effective, but more costly and associated with greater gastrointestinal side effects. Cephalosporins and Spectinomycin (2 grams IM) can be used during pregnancy.

## CHANCROID

### *Diagnosis*

Chancroid is the most common STD worldwide, and it affects men more often than women (3:1). The incubation period is 1–21 d. It causes a painful, shaggy ulcer on the penis or vulvovaginal area. It spreads laterally by apposition to inner thighs and buttocks, especially in women. It is associated with inguinal adenopathy that is typically unilateral and tender with tendency to fistulize. *Haemophilus ducreyi*—the causative organism—is fastidious and difficult to culture. Gram-staining the specimen obtained from the undermined edge of the ulcer may be more helpful in identifying the short, fine, gram-negative streptobacilli, which are usually arranged in short, parallel chains. Recently, PCR assays have been shown to be a sensitive and specific means of detecting *Haemophilus ducreyi*.

### *Treatment*

The treatment options for chancroid are surprisingly simple: Azithromycin (1 g, single dose), ceftriaxone (250 mg IM as a single dose), ciprofloxacin (500 mg twice daily for 3 d), or erythromycin base (500 mg by mouth, four times daily for 7 d). However, antibiotic susceptibility varies geographically. Symptomatic relief can be provided by needle aspiration of the bubocs. HIV testing is strongly recommended. Ciprofloxacin is contraindicated during pregnancy.

## TRICHOMONIASIS

### *Diagnosis*

Trichomoniasis is caused by the protozoan *Trichomonas vaginalis* and has an incubation period of 1–14 d. The organism is an obligate to the vagina or urethra, and cannot infect the rectum or mouth. Men may have little or no symptoms. Women may notice a foamy white or greenish vaginal discharge and pruritis. On examination the vaginal pH is elevated and a characteristic "strawberry vulva" or "strawberry cervix" may be visualized. Vaginal wet-mount or urine (preferably Voiding Bottle #1) examined microscopically, reveals the flagellated organisms, which are 1–4 times the size of a polymorphonuclear cell.

## *Treatment*

A single 2.0-g dose of metronidazole is effective in most cases and can be used in the 2nd trimester of pregnancy. For nonpregnant treatment failures, 500 mg of metronidazole (twice daily for 7 d) is recommended. Patients must abstain from alcohol during therapy.

## GENITAL WARTS

### *Diagnosis*

Genital warts (*Condylomata acuminata*) are caused by human papilloma virus (HPV). More than 20 HPV types infect the genital area. Low-risk types, such as HPV-6 or HPV-11, are usually associated with proliferative condyloma, and only rare conversion to malignant Buschke-Löwenstein's tumors of the penis. The incubation period may be similar to other viruses, with clinical manifestations occurring years after exposure. HPV may be associated with nonspecific symptoms, such as vulvodynia or pruritus. Malodorous vaginal discharge may also be a presenting sign, and the high rate of coinfection observed in this setting may be a contributing factor. The diagnosis is usually made through the visualization or palpation of nontender papillomatous genital lesions. Aceto-whitening with 3–5% acetic acid may be necessary for the identification of flat warts. High-risk HPVs, types 16, 18, and 31, are associated with invasive cancers of the penis and cervix. These are more commonly identified by means of cervical PAP smears, colposcopy, and androscopy. Among asymptomatic male partners of women with abnormal PAP smears, 22–50% had evidence of HPV on urethral smears. The benefit of evaluating and treating asymptomatic sexual partners of women with genital warts or abnormal PAP smears remains unclear.

## *Treatment*

For few and smaller lesions, patient-applied therapy, such as podofilox (0.5%) solution or gel, is recommended (applied every 12 h for 3 d, then off for 4 d with the option to repeat the treatment cycle three times). This has been proven to be the most cost-effective therapy. Cryotherapy using liquid nitrogen or surgical removal are preferred physician-administered therapies along with podophyllin 10–25% in compound tincture of benzoin, which is applied once and washed thoroughly 1–4 h after treatment, or trichloroacetic acid (TCA) 80–90%, carefully applied only to the warts. Unreacted acid should be removed with baking soda or talc. Podophyllin and TCA may be repeated weekly, if necessary. Podophyllin, imiquimod, and podofilox are contraindicated during pregnancy. Women with genital warts or a history of exposure should seek prompt gynecologic evaluation of the vagina and cervix. Large or extensive lesions surrounding the meatus may herald the presence of urethral or bladder condyloma, warranting cystourethroscopy. Urethral or bladder lesions should be surgically excised. Intraurethral 5% 5-fluorouracil (5-FU) instillations over the course of 2 wk may be necessary to completely eradicate papillomatous lesions. Extensive vulvar lesions may also be treated with 5-FU cream, once weekly for up to 10 wk. Intralesional injection with 5-FU/ epinephrine gel (Accusite) can be used weekly for up to 6 wk, with a 77% success rate. Smoking may increase the risk of dysplastic progression and malignancy in both men and women. Because HPV progresses rapidly in HIV-infected women, cervical cancer is considered one of the AIDS-defining illnesses.

## SCABIES

### *Diagnosis*

This infection is caused by the mite *Sarcoptes scabiei*. Wavy, elongated papules are characteristic of the mite burrow. Eruption with pruritus is caused by an immune reaction to the mites, their eggs, and their feces. Susceptible areas include the penile shaft and glans, areolae, finger webs, and axillary folds. Confirming the diagnosis may require microscopic evidence of the mite (or eggs), which is retrieved by scraping the burrow with a scalpel blade coated with mineral oil.

### *Treatment*

Permethrin cream (5%) should be applied to all areas of the body from the neck down, and washed off 8–14 h later. Lindane (1%) lotion may be applied in a similar fashion and removed after 8 h. If necessary, treatment may be repeated in 1 wk. Lindane should not be used after a bath, and is contraindicated in children < 2 yr of age, pregnant and lactating women, and patients with extensive dermatitis. An alternative for young children or pregnant/lactating women is sulfur (3–6%) applied on three consecutive nights.

## OVERVIEW OF OTHER SEXUALLY ASSOCIATED INFECTIONS

### *Mollicutes*

*Ureaplasma urealyticum, Mycoplasma hominis,* and *Mycoplasma genitalium* have been implicated in up to 40% of nongonococcal urethritis cases. These organisms have also been implicated in cases of chronic prostatitis in men, and urgency/frequency syndromes in women. Although these organisms are considered commensals of the genital tract, they have been isolated as the sole pathogen in symptomatic patients, who respond to antimicrobial therapy targeting these mollicutes. Confirming the presence of the organism from genitourinary specimens requires the visualization of characteristic colonies on specialized agar and color changes of ura broth. Historically, this group of organisms were highly sensitive to tetracycline. Today, however, up to 30% of strains may be resistant, which may explain persistent symptoms in those patients treated empirically for nongonococcal urethritis or presumed Chlamydia infection. As initial therapy, I recommend doxycycline (100 mg twice daily for 2 wk), or a single dose of azithromycin (1-g sachet), which can be repeated after 10–14 d. Other alternatives include erythromycin (500 mg four times daily) or oxfloxacin (300 mg twice daily) for 10–14 d).

### *Bacterial Vaginosis*

Overgrowth of Gardnerella (formerly Haemophilus) vaginalis promoted by anaerobic bacterial activity leads to the liberation of amines, an increase in vaginal pH and inhibition of normal vaginal flora. Patients or their partners may complain of a malodorous vaginal discharge, particularly after sexual intercourse, and nonspecific low-grade

## Table 1
## Genital Ulcer Disease

| Disease | Lesions | Lymphadenopathy | Systemic symptoms |
| --- | --- | --- | --- |
| Primary syphilis | Painless, indurated, clean-based, usually singular | Nontender, rubbery, nonsuppurative bilateral lymphadenopathy | None |
| Genital Herpes | Painful vesicles, shallow, usually multiple | Tender, bilateral inguinal adenopathy | Present during primary infection |
| Chancroid | Tender papule, then painful, undermined purulent ulcer, single or multiple | Tender, regional, painful, suppurative nodes | None |
| Lympho-granuloma | Small, painless vesicle or papule progresses to an ulcer | Painful, matted, large nodes develop, with fistula tracts | Present after genital lesion heals |

[a] Although specificity for clinical diagnosis of genital ulcer disease is good (94–98%), sensitivity is quite low (31–35%). Inguinal lymph-node findings may not contribute to diagnostic accuracy. I strongly recommend confirmatory cultures and serologic testing whenever possible. Because of overlap in disease characteristics, similar ulcerative STDs should be ruled out. Non-STD causes should also be considered: Behcet's syndrome, drug reaction, erythema multiforme, Crohn's disease, lichen planus, amebiasis, trauma, and carcinoma.

genital discomfort. Risk factors for bacterial vaginosis include an increased number of sexual partners, douching, abnormal ureterine bleeding, and contraceptive use. Three out of four of the following factors must be met in order to confirm this diagnosis: thin, grayish vaginal discharge, vaginal pH > 4.5, Clue cells identified via microscopic evaluation of vaginal wet mount, and release of amines (fishy odor) when discharge is tested with potassium hydroxide (KOH). Vaginal cultures are not helpful in this setting; however, I recommend Gram-staining vaginal swab specimens in order to characterize the vaginal flora and identify disruption which would be associated with the pathogenic coccobacilli. Recommended primary therapy includes metronidazole (500 mg twice daily for 1 wk), clindamycin cream intravaginally, (nightly for 1 wk) or Metrogel intravaginally, (twice daily for 5 d). Clindamycin (300 mg, taken by mouth, twice daily for 1 wk) may also be effective. Factors that disrupt the normal vaginal flora, such as douching, should be prohibited. Treatment of the sexual partner may be a consideration in some cases of recurrent bacterial vaginosis.

### *Vulvovaginal Candidiasis*

Vaginitis caused by *Candida albicans* is the most common type seen in the clinical setting. The organism is present in the normal vagina and can also be found in the coronal sulcus of the penis. Sexual transmission with subsequent colonization and infection is possible. Predisposing factors for active infection include hormonal changes resulting from pregnancy or contraception, antibiotic use, systemic corticosteroids, or antimetabolites. Characteristically thick, cheesy vaginal discharge is usually associated with vulvar irritation and itching. The onset is often premenstrual. Over-the-counter antifungal vaginal creams or suppositories are fairly effective, requiring 3–7 d regimens. Treatment agents include: Butoconazole, clotrimazole, miconazole, and terconozole. I also recommend the use of fluconazole (150 mg) as a single oral dose. This is as effective as vaginal preparations and more economical. Recurring infections may require 10–14 d of treatment with vaginal preparations. Oral fluconazole therapy can be repeated 3 d after the initial dose for increased efficacy. Patients suffering from recurrent candidal vulvovaginitis require further evaluation to exclude HIV infection, diabetes, or other immune-compromised states.

## SELECTED READING

Aral SO, Holmes K, Padian NF, Cates W (1996) Overview: individual and population approaches to the epidemiology and prevention of sexual transmitted diseases and human immunodeficiency virus infection. *J Infect Dis* 174(2):127–133.

Baker DA (1997) Diagnosis and treatment of viral STD's in women. *Int J Fertil* 42(2):107–114.

Berg E, Benson DM, Haraszkiewicz P, Grieb J, McDonald J (1996) High prevalence of sexually transmitted diseases in women with urinary infections. *Acad Emerg Med* 3(11):1030–1034.

Bowie WR (1995) Drug therapies for sexually transmitted diseases: clinical and economic consideration. *Drugs* 49(4):496–515.

Cardamakis E, Kotoulas IG, Metalinos K, Mantouvalos H, Relakis K, Scrapari M, Korantzis A, Papathansiou Z (1994) Treatment of urethral condylamata acuminata or flat condylomata with interferon. *J Urol* 152:2011–2013.

DiCarlo RP, Martin DH (1997) The clinical diagnosis of genital ulcer disease in men. *Clin Infect Dis* 25(2):292–298.

Fiumara NJ (1997) Genital ulcer infections in the female patient and the vaginitides. *Derm Clinics* 15(2):233–245.

Frisch M, Glimelius B, van deen Brule AJ, Wohlfahrt J, Meijer CJ, Walboomers JM, et al. (1997) Sexually transmitted infection as a cause of anal cancer. *N Engl J Med* 337(19):1350–1358.

Ginsburg KS, Kundsin RB, Walter CW, Schur PH (1992) Ureaplasma urealyticum and mycoplasma hominis in women with systemic lupus erythematosus. *Arthritis Rheum* 35:4.

Kinghorn GR (1996) Limiting the spread of genital herpes. *Scand J Infect Dis* 100:20–25.

Maeda SI, Tamaki M, Nakanom, Uno M, Dequchi T, Kawada Y (1998) Detection of mycoplasma genitalium in patients with urethritis. *J Urol* 159:405–407.

Marrazzo JM, Koutsky LA, Stine KL, Kuypers JM, Grubert TA, Galloway DA, et al. (1998) Genito human papilloma virus infection in women who have sex with women. *J Infect Dis* 178(6):1604–1609.

Mawhorter SD (1997) Travel medicine for the primary care physician. *Cleve Clin J Med* 64(9):483–492.

McDonald LL, Stites PC, Buntin DM (1997) Sexually transmitted diseases update. *Derm Clinics* 15(2):221–232.

Miller KE (1997) Sexually transmitted diseases. *Primary Care Clinics* 24(1):179–193.

Nuovo J, Melnikow J, Paliescheskey M, King J, Mowers R (1995) Cost-effectiveness analysis of five different antibiotic regimens for the treatment of uncomplicated *Chlamydia trachomatis* cervicitis. *J Am Board Fam Prac* 8:7–16.

Orr DP (1997) Urine-based diagnosis of sexually transmitted infections using amplified DNA techniques: a shift in paradigms? *J Adolesc Health* 20(1):3–5.

Perez G, Skurnick JH, Denny TN, Stephens R, Kennedy CA, Regivick N, et al. (1998) Herpes simplex type II and mycoplasma genitalium as risk factors for heterosexual HIV transmission: report from the heterosexual HIV transmission study. *Int J Dis* 3(1):5–11.

Potts JM, Rackley RR (1997) Ureaplasma urealyticum in men: a commensal or pathogen? [abstract] *J Urol* 157:240.

Pugliesliese A, Klein NC, Cunha PA (1994) Tetracyclines in urogynecology. *Intl Urogyn J* 5:221–227.

Quinn TC, Welsh L, Lentz A, Crotchfelt K, Zenilman J, Newhall J, et al. (1996) Diagnosis by AMPLICOR PCR of *Chlamydia trachomatis* infection in urine samples from women and men attending sexually transmitted disease clinics. *J Clin Microbiol* 34(6):1401–1406.

Rayburn WF (1998) Treatment of sexually transmitted diseases, 1998 recommendations by the Centers for Disease Control and Prevention. *J Reprod Med* 43(6):471–476.

Retiano M (1997) Counseling patients with genital warts. *Am J Med* 102(5a):38–43.

Rosen T, Brown TJ (1998) Genital ulcers: evaluation and treatment. *Derm Clin* 16(4):673–685.

Rosenberg MJ, Waugh MS (1995) Consequences of incomplete antibacterial treatment for chlamydial pelvic inflammatory disease. *Drugs* 49(2):504, 505.

Saxena SB, Jenkins RR (1997) Sexually transmitted diseases in adolescents: screening and treatment. *Compr Ther* 23(2):108–115.

Schwartz MA, Hooton TM (1998) Etiology of non-gonococcal non-chlamydial urethritis *Derm Clin* 16(4):727–733.

Shaffer MA, Pantell RH, Schachter J (1999) Is the routine pelvic examination needed with the advent of urine-based screening for sexually transmitted diseases? *Arch Pediatr Adolesc Med* 153(2):119–125.

Shah KV (1997) Human papilloma virus and anal genital cancers. *N Engl J Med* 337(19):1386–1388.

Sharts-Hopko NC (1997) STD's in women: what you need to know. *Amer J Nurs* 97(4):46–54.

Siegler C, Stary A, Mailer H, Kopp W, Gebhart W, Szotis J (1992) Quinolones as an alternative treatments of chlamydial, mycoplasma, and gonococcal urogenito infections. *Derm* 185:128–131.

Stokes T (1997) Screening for chlamydia in general practice: a literature review and summary of the evidence. *J Pub H Med* 19(2):222–232.

Strauss MJ, Khanna V, Koenig JD, Downs SM, Goldberg SH, Manyak MJ, et al. (1996) The cost of treating genital warts. *Int J Dermatol* 35(5):340–348.

Taylor-Robinson D, Furr PM (1998) Update on sexually transmitted mycoplasmas. *Lancet* 351(3):12–15.

Tchoudomirova K, Mardh PA, Kallings I, Nilsson S, Hellberg D (1998) History, clinical findings, sexual behavior and hygiene habits in women with and without recurrent episodes of urinary symptoms. *Acta Obstet Gynecol Scand* 77(6):654–659.

White C, Wardropper AG (1997) Genital herpes simplex infection in women. *Clin Derm* 15(1):81–91.

Wiener JS, Walther PJ (1995) Human papillomaviruses: biology and role in cervical and penile malignancy. *Infec Urol* 139–147.

# 11 The Diagnosis and Treatment of Interstitial Cystitis

*Kenneth M. Peters, MD*
*and Ananias C. Diokno, MD*

**CONTENTS**
    INTRODUCTION
    DIAGNOSIS
    MULTIMODALITY TREATMENT:
        THE KEY TO EFFECTIVE TREATMENT
    SURGERY
    CONCLUSIONS
    SELECTED READING

## INTRODUCTION

The diagnosis and treatment of interstitial cystitis (IC) has frustrated both clinicians and patients alike. Interstitial cystitis is a bladder disease characterized by urinary frequency, urgency, and pelvic pain, first described more than 80 years ago. Until recently, it has been an ignored disease; patients with IC have been told that their symptoms are imaginary and that there is nothing wrong with them. IC patients have been counseled to seek psychiatric help for their disease, and many patients suffer unduly until a diagnosis is made. Although IC has been considered to be a disease that predominantly affects women, more men are now being diagnosed with this disease. There is evidence that men treated for "chronic abacterial prostatatis"—which is characterized by urinary frequency, urgency, and pelvic/perineal pain—will often have cystoscopic findings suggestive of interstitial cystitis and will respond to standard treatments for IC. The problem with IC is that it is a diagnosis of exclusion, and there are no specific objective tests to definitively diagnosis IC or to monitor disease progression.

A diagnosis of IC means that the disease must be in the health-care worker's differential diagnosis. Too often, patients present to their physicians with symptoms of a urinary-tract infection, and are given multiple antibiotics despite a negative culture—yet their symptoms persist. Many undiagnosed IC patients are managed for years without directed therapy, and often seek evaluations from many different physicians to help determine the cause—and an effective treatment for—their symptoms. Interstitial

From: *Current Clinical Urology: Office Urology: The Clinician's Guide*
Edited by: E. D. Kursh and J. C. Ulchaker © Humana Press Inc., Totowa, NJ

## Table 1
### NIDDK Research Criteria for Interstitial Cystitis

**Inclusion criteria**
1. Glomerulations or Hunner's ulcer on cystoscopic examination after hydrodistension under anesthesia
2. Pain associated with the bladder or urinary urgency

**Exclusion criteria**
1. Awake cystometric bladder capacity > 350 cm$^3$
2. Absence of intense urge to void with bladder filled to 100 cm$^3$ gas or 150 cm$^3$ water during cystometry, at fill rate of 30–100 cm$^3$/min
3. Demonstration of involuntary bladder contractions on cystometry
4. Duration of symptoms < 9 mo
5. Absence of nocturia
6. Symptoms relieved by antimicrobials, urinary antiseptics, anticholinergics, or antispasmodics
7. Frequency of urination, while awake, of less than eight times per day
8. Diagnosis of bacterial cystitis or prostatitis within 3 months
9. Bladder or lower ureteral calculi
10. Active genital herpes
11. Uterine, cervical, vaginal, or urethral cancer
12. Urethral diverticulum
13. Cyclophosphamide or any type of chemical cystitis
14. Tuberculous cystitis
15. Radiation cystitis
16. Benign or malignant bladder tumors
17. Vaginitis
18. Age of < 18 yr

cystitis patients score more poorly on quality-of-life questionnaires than patients on dialysis. Sixty percent of IC sufferers complain of pain with sexual intercourse—in many cases so severe that they abstain altogether. Fifty percent of IC patients are unable to work full-time. On average, $170 million per year is spent for the medical care of IC. Combining lost wages and medical expenses, the economic impact of IC has been estimated to be $1.7 billion per year. The cause of IC is unknown despite a century of study. When a patient is found to have IC, justifying the symptoms by determining the diagnosis is often therapeutic. Once the diagnosis is made, specific therapy can be initiated for this disease.

## DIAGNOSIS

The diagnosis of IC is one of exclusion. There are no standard tests to determine whether a patient has IC. In 1987 and 1988, the National Institute of Arthritis, Diabetes, Digestive and Kidney Diseases (NIDDK) developed research criteria for the diagnosis of IC (*see* Table 1). The purpose of these criteria was to assure that a homogeneous IC population would be included in research studies. The published criteria have often been used to determine the diagnosis of IC in the clinic setting, resulting in selection of a more severe IC patient subset. A recent review from the National Institutes of Health Interstitial Cystitis Database Study demonstrated that 60% of subjects believed by the investigators to have IC failed to meet all of the NIDDK criteria. It is therefore inappropriate in clinical practice to adhere to the NIDDK as the sole means of diagnosing this disease. Many patients with IC do not meet all of these criteria, and excluding the diagnosis of IC in this population will delay initiation of treatment for this difficult disease.

Most patients who present to urologists with IC-type symptoms have been treated with multiple antibiotics without relief of their "recurrent infections." Patients who present with symptoms of urinary urgency, frequency, and/or pelvic pain should undergo a complete history and physical exam. It is appropriate to characterize the degree and the duration of the symptoms, and to determine if a specific event has caused the symptoms. It is a striking characteristic of the IC population that the majority of patients can recall the exact time their symptoms began. There may be an association of IC with documented urinary-tract infections or previous pelvic or bladder surgery. In premenopausal women, endometriosis must be in the differential diagnosis, and if suspected, appropriate evaluation (which may include hormonal manipulation or laparoscopy) should be performed. Dietary factors, such as the amount of caffeine and alcohol consumption, should be established, and removed from the patient's diet. Obtaining a history of back pain or previous bladder or pelvic surgery may lead the physician to suspect a neurologic cause for the symptoms. Obtaining a complete list of medical problems—including diabetes, neurologic diseases, and malignancies—is imperative. Assessing whether the patient has received therapies that may affect the bladder, such as therapeutic radiation or chemotherapies (i.e., Cytoxan), will help the clinician to determine the cause of their bladder symptoms.

Men who present with symptoms of genital pain, perineal pain, frequency, or dysuria are often labeled as having chronic abacterial prostatitis. In fact, the majority of these men have characteristic findings of IC upon cystoscopy and hydrodistension. Interstitial cystitis is more prevalent in men than previously thought, and it is imperative that the health-care worker has a high index of suspicion for IC in the male patient with chronic prostatitis symptoms.

A physical examination that includes a pelvic and neurourologic exam should be performed. A postvoid residual should be obtained to rule out urinary retention. When performing a vaginal exam, vaginal tissues should be carefully inspected to assess the degree of atrophic vaginitis. The anterior vaginal wall, including the urethra and bladder floor, should be carefully palpated. A cotton swab applied to the four corners of the vagina between the labia and hymenal ring may result in a burning sensation suggestive of vulvodynia. Urethral fullness, tenderness, or expression of pus may suggest a urethral diverticulum requiring further work-up. With IC, tenderness to palpation is often noted at the level of the urethra and/or bladder trigone. The patient's ability to contract and relax the pelvic-floor muscles may suggest pelvic-floor dysfunction. The degree of pelvic relaxation and prolapse should be determined. A bimanual exam to detect adnexal or uterine masses should also be performed. In men, a digital rectal exam should be performed to rule out palpable prostatic abnormalities. A urinalysis, urine culture, and cytology may be performed to exclude active infection or evidence of carcinoma *in situ*. Sterile pyuria should prompt the taking of urine TB cultures. If microscopic hematuria is present, a work-up including upper-tract imaging, cystoscopy, and cytology should be performed to rule out bladder cancer or stone disease. A voiding diary with both fluid intake (amount and kind) and urine output—including voided volumes and daytime and nighttime frequency—should be completed. The voiding diary allows the physician to determine the average voiding volume and to document the amount of daytime frequency and nocturia. Validated IC questionnaires are available to monitor other IC symptoms, including pain. Sequential voiding diaries and symptom questionnaires allow the physician to determine the impact of various treatments on IC.

A cystometrogram may be performed to rule out uninhibited contractions and to determine the functional bladder capacity. The usual cytometric finding in IC is a small-capacity bladder of the sensory/urgency type without uninhibited bladder contractions. Once all medical reasons for the bladder symptoms are ruled out and anticholinergics have failed to relieve the symptoms, the physician should consider performing cystoscopy and hydrodistension with bladder biopsy. This procedure is performed under a general or regional anesthetic. A thorough cystourethoscopy is performed, and the bladder is stretched at 80–100 cm/$H_2O$ until no further water flows into the bladder. Women may develop early leakage of fluid around the cystoscope. If this occurs, digital pressure can be applied to the urethra along each side of the cystoscope against the pubic bone, stopping the leakage and allowing for maximal distension. Under no circumstances should the bag of water be squeezed, as this can result in bladder rupture. The bladder is stretched for 2 min and then emptied. The volume instilled is measured, and evidence of bloody effluent is noted. The bladder is stretched a second time in a similar fashion and cystoscopy is repeated. Characteristic findings of IC include glomerulations or petechial hemorrhages seen in areas other than the course of the cystoscope. In approx 10% of IC patients, Hunner's ulcers will be seen as deep cracks or lesions within the bladder. These ulcers suggest the presence of a more severe disease. Treating these ulcers with electrocautery can lead to symptomatic relief. The majority of patients who present with symptoms suggestive of IC will have the cystoscopic findings of this disease, yet glomerulations are not pathognomonic for IC because asymptomatic control subjects can have cystoscopic findings of glomerulations. Biopsies can be performed to rule out cancer or to assess the degree of bladder inflammation. Unfortunately, no classic pathologic findings are associated with IC. Mast cells have been implicated in the pathogenesis of IC by releasing multiple substances that can lead to inflammation in the bladder, such as histamine, kinins, vasoactive peptides, and prostaglandins. Studies have not consistently shown an elevation in bladder mast cells in IC. The role played by mast cells in IC is currently under intense investigation.

After a hydrodistension, bladder symptoms tend to worsen for 1–2 wk, and then either return to their baseline or improve. Approximately 30–40% of IC patients show a marked improvement in their pain and frequency symptoms after a hydrodistension, and this improvement can last for many months.

Some researchers have promoted a potassium chloride (KCl) instillation test to confirm the diagnosis of IC. The assumption is that patients with IC have increased bladder permeability and respond to intravesical potassium by developing bladder pain. The test involves instilling 45–50 $cm^3$ of two solutions in the bladder for 3–5 min. The first solution is sterile water and the second is 400 meq/L KCl. The patient is asked whether the instillation provokes pain on a scale of 0–5. If the water does not provoke symptoms, but the KCl causes a pain rating of 2 or greater on the 5-point scale, the test is considered positive. This theory has not been well-tested, and lacks specificity. In addition, the use of potassium instillation as a definitive test for IC

## Table 2
### Foods to Avoid in IC

| | | | |
|---|---|---|---|
| Apples | Aged cheeses | Corned beef | Saccharine |
| Apricots | Yogurt | Nitrates/nitrites | Aspartame |
| Avocados | Sour cream | Nuts | Tobacco |
| Bananas | Chocolate | Alcohol | Junk food |
| Cantaloupes | Fava beans | Carbonated beverages | |
| Citrus | Lima beans | Cranberry juice | |
| Cranberries | Onions | Caffeinated beverages | |
| Grapes | Tofu | Coffee | |
| Nectarines | Tomatoes | Tea | |
| Peaches | Rye bread | Mayonnaise | |
| Pineapples | Sourdough bread | Spicy foods | |
| Plums | Processed meats and fish | Soy sauce | |
| Pomegranates | Anchovies | Salad dressing | |
| Rhubarb | Caviar | Vinegar | |
| Strawberries | Liver | Citric acid | |

does not afford patients the potential for clinical improvement from the operative hydrodistension, and causes unnecessary pain.

# MULTIMODALITY TREATMENT: THE KEY TO EFFECTIVE TREATMENT

## *Establishing the Diagnosis*

Too often, patients with IC have been told that nothing is wrong with them. Justifying a patient's symptoms by making a diagnosis of IC is often therapeutic. Once the diagnosis is made, the patient should be encouraged to join the Interstitial Cystitis Association (51 Monroe Street, Suite 1402 Rockville, MD 20850; 1-800-HELP-ICA; www.IChelp.org) and local support groups so they can take an active role in treating their disease. Therapies for IC are moderately effective at best and have not been well-researched, leading to a "let's try it and see" treatment regimen. Multimodality therapy is the best approach to managing the IC patient.

## *Dietary Modification*

Some IC patients are very sensitive to various foods. Caffeine and alcohol should be removed from the diet. The effect of diet on IC symptoms is variable, and patients should be instructed to remove certain food items from their diet and assess their symptoms (*see* Table 2). If a particular food item worsens their symptoms, they should avoid this and all similar food items. Adhering to a strict "IC diet" is very difficult for most patients, and identifying specific irritating food items is often more effective. Prelief® (calcium glycerophosphate) is an over-the-counter supplement designed to neutralize the acid in foods. Available in crystals or pill form, it may allow the IC patient greater flexibility with diet.

## Fluid Management

Fluid management is key to the treatment of IC. In general, patients tend to limit their fluid intake in hopes of decreasing their frequency of urination. However, increasing fluid intake may markedly improve IC symptoms. Urine represents the body's waste products, and is very caustic to tissues. The bladder acts as a storage unit and is protected by an intact mucosa layer. In IC, the bladder lining is likely to be damaged and cannot protect the detrusor completely from the urine solutes. Concentrated urine—found in most IC subjects who dehydrate themselves—is more irritating to the bladder. Increasing water intake will deliver more dilute urine to the bladder, and thus causes less irritation, helping to diminish the pain associated with IC and ultimately allowing the patient to retain more urine.

## Physical/Behavioral Therapy

Physical therapy, biofeedback, pelvic-muscle exercises, relaxation techniques, herbal therapy, acupuncture, and behavioral therapy may all help control the symptoms of IC. Many patients have pelvic-floor dysfunction secondary to the chronic pain associated with this disease, and biofeedback and pelvic-muscle exercises can help alleviate pelvic-floor muscle spasms and improve symptoms. Periods of stress tend to worsen IC symptoms, and relaxation techniques and lifestyle changes to reduce stress may help to relieve these symptoms.

## Oral Pharmacotherapy

Once behavioral therapy is optimized, oral medication is a reasonable first-line treatment for IC. The only FDA-approved oral therapy for IC is pentosan polysulfate sodium (Elmiron®). Pentosan polysulfate (PPS) is a glycosaminoglycan that binds tightly to the bladder mucosa. The theory in IC is that the bladder mucosa is "leaky," and PPS may help to rebuild the natural bladder barrier, leading to improvement in symptoms. Elmiron® has been studied in several double-blind, placebo-controlled trials in the United States and in subjects who meet the NIDDK criteria for IC. Thirty-eight percent of those receiving PPS at a dose of 100 mg 3 times per day for 3 mo reported a 50% reduction in bladder pain, compared to 18% of placebo-treated subjects. An open-label physician-usage study that enrolled 2809 patients from 1986 to 1996 demonstrated that 61% of patients on PPS for a minimum of 3 mo demonstrated an improvement in pain or discomfort, and this improvement was sustained while subjects were taking Elmiron®. An IC patient must commit to taking PPS for 3–6 mo before determining that it is ineffective. In addition, if symptom improvement is achieved, Elmiron® may need to be continued indefinitely to maintain the improvement. Elmiron® is a well-tolerated drug, with 1–4% of patients complaining of alopecia (reversible upon discontinuation), gastrointestinal upset, headache, liver-function abnormalities, or abdominal pain. Elmiron® should not be taken in conjunction with routine use of therapeutic doses of aspirin or nonsteroidal anti-inflammatories. Elmiron® appears to help a subset of IC patients and has a good side-effect profile. It is reasonable to give an IC patient a 6-mo trial of Elmiron® and assess the clinical response. Since Elmiron® may require several months before any clinical improvement is seen, it should not be used as a single agent for the treatment of IC.

Antidepressants can aid in the treatment of IC. Patients with chronic pain and sleep deprivation often develop clinical depression. In addition, tricyclic antidepressants have been used for chronic pain disorders by increasing the pain threshold. Low-dose amitriptyline (10–75 mg) taken at night can be very effective in improving sleep and diminishing frequency of urination and bladder pain. Patients should be cautioned that tricyclic antidepressants can cause weight gain and daytime sedation. The sedative side effects will usually diminish with continued usage. The dose should be slowly titrated to minimize symptoms. Some IC subjects will benefit from serotonin uptake inhibitors, such as fluoxetine hydrochloride (Prozac®) or sertraline hydrochloride (Zoloft®). These are nonsedative and should be taken once per morning. Although no definitive controlled clinical trials on the use of antidepressants for IC have been performed, they clearly can provide some symptomatic relief for the treatment of IC.

Hydroxyzine is a mast-cell stabilizer and is used primarily in the treatment of atopic dermatitis, urticaria, and allergic rhinitis. Hydroxyzine can reduce bladder mast-cell degranulation, and anecdotal evidence suggests it may be effective in the treatment of IC. Hydroxyzine may be more effective in IC patients who are found to have increased mast cells on bladder biopsy, or those with seasonal allergies. Hydroxyzine is also sedative and should be started at a dose of 10 mg at night and titrated based on side effects to 75 mg per night. The dose may need to be increased during allergy season. No controlled clinical studies on the efficacy of hydroxyzine for IC have been performed.

An uncontrolled trial using nifedipine (10 mg tid) for IC suggests there may be some efficacy based on smooth-muscle relaxation and cytokine stimulation. A trial of nifedipine is as reasonable as any other treatment for IC.

Some initial reports have suggested that urinary nitric oxide was decreased in the IC population, and that treatment with the amino acid L-arginine (500 mg tid) may increase urinary nitric oxide and improve IC symptoms. This amino acid has minimal side effects, but its utility in treating IC is uncertain.

Hydroxzine along with Elmiran is a good starting oral regimen for the treatment of IC. Hydroxyzine decreases inflammation and Elmiran helps rebuild the protective bladder lining. Other agents, such as Pyridium Plus (1 tablet 3–4 ×/d), can be added to the treatment regimen to decrease bladder irritation.

## *Intravesical Agents*

Intravesical therapies for interstitial cystitis have been a mainstay in treatment for many years. Dimethyl sulfoxide (DMSO) is the only FDA-approved intravesical therapy for this disease. DMSO (RIMSO®) is an unusual compound. It was first developed as an industrial solvent, and may aid in delivering other compounds, such as steroids and heparin, into the detrusor muscle. Clinically, DMSO is thought to have anti-inflammatory properties and mast-cell stabilizing effects. Studies on DMSO have been poorly controlled because of the unique "garlic-like" odor that patients acquire after being instilled with this medication. A "cocktail" of medication comprising 50 mL DMSO, 40 mg Kenalog, and 20,000 U heparin is instilled in the bladder once a week for 6–8 wk and retained 15–20 min. The patient may benefit from the anti-inflammatory effects of the steroid and the coating of the glycosaminoglycan (GAG)-layer from the heparin. This cocktail has not been well-studied, but intuitively it seems reasonable to combine the three agents. Bladder symptoms may initially worsen after DMSO instillation; however, some IC patients will have symptomatic relief from this treatment. The symptom improvement is often short-lived and is best after the first course of DMSO. Subsequent treatments with this medication tend to be less effective.

Intravesical heparin can also be used in the treatment of IC. Heparin is a glycosaminoglycan-type compound that binds tightly to the bladder mucosa. Like pentosan polysulfate, heparin may help rebuild the protective GAG layer of the bladder and improve bladder symptoms. Again, no controlled trials have been performed on this compound. Patients are taught intermittent self-catheterization and to instill 25,000 U of heparin in their bladder in a 15-cm$^3$ volume on a daily basis. The patients hold this medication until their next void. Only 1–3% of oral Elmiron® is excreted in the urine, whereas heparin therapy delivers a large bolus of this GAG compound directly to the bladder mucosa. Daily intravesical heparin can be initiated in conjunction with beginning oral Elmiron®. The heparin can be withdrawn after 8–12 wk, and the patient can be maintained with oral therapy. This treatment has the potential to shorten the time interval required to achieve a therapeutic effect from GAG therapy. If the patient cannot tolerate oral Elmiron®, intravesical heparin can be continued indefinitely. Heparin is not absorbed through the bladder mucosa, so anticoagulation effects are not a concern.

Other intravesical therapies must be performed under a general or regional anesthetic. These include sodium oxychlorosene (Chlorpactin®) and silver nitrate. The utility of these treatments is in question and their use has mostly fallen out of favor. These treatments are highly caustic to the bladder and may lead to destruction of the bladder mucosa and the formation of a new, more intact bladder lining. A voiding cystourethrogram should be performed to rule out vesicoureteral reflux before instilling these medications.

Intravesical Bacillus Calmette-Guérin (BCG) for the treatment of IC is in Phase III clinical trials. A Phase II double-blind, placebo-controlled trial demonstrated a 60% clinical response to TICE® BCG, compared to a 27% placebo response rate. Subjects who received a single 6-wk course of BCG and responded were followed for over 2 yr. Ninety percent of subjects continued to show marked clinical improvement in both pain and frequency symptoms despite no other therapy for their IC. BCG is a weakened strain of the tuberculosis bacteria that has been used effectively for years in the treatment of superficial bladder cancer. The exact mechanism of action of BCG in bladder cancer is unknown, but is thought to act by stimulating an immune response in the bladder. There is some evidence that IC may be secondary to an immune imbalance in the bladder. Intravesical BCG may correct this imbalance, leading to long-term clinical improvement. Fifty milligrams of BCG (1–8 × 10$^8$ CFU) diluted in 50 cm$^3$ of normal saline is instilled in the bladder once a week for 6 wk. Patients are asked to retain the solution for as long as they can for up to 2 hr. Bladder symptoms tend to worsen during the instillation period of BCG because of its irritative effects, and clinical improvement is not usually seen for at least 3–6 mo. Pentosan polysulfate is known to tightly bind to BCG and may prevent attachment of the BCG to the bladder lining; thus patients should not be receiving Elmiron® while being treated with intravesical BCG. Intravesical BCG for the treatment of IC is investigational.

## *Pain Management*

Pain control is a serious problem for the IC patient, and narcotics are often required. Urologists treating IC must be comfortable prescribing narcotics, and if they are not, a referral to a pain specialist is in order. Medications combining both a narcotic and nonnarcotic analgesic, such as codeine plue acetaminophen (Tylenol® #3), hydrocodone plus acetaminophen (Vicodin® Lorcet®, Norco®) or propoxyphene napsylate plus acet-

Table 3
Acetaminophen Levels in Commonly Prescribed Narcotic Compounds

| Trade name | Narcotic | Acetaminophen | Max. pills/d |
|---|---|---|---|
| Tylenol #3 | Codeine 30 mg | 300 mg | 12 |
| Darvocet N-100 | Propoxyphene 100 mg | 650 mg | 6 |
| Vicodin | Hydrocodone 5 mg | 500 mg | 8 |
| Vicodin-ES | Hydrocodone 7.5 mg | 750 mg | 5 |
| Lorcet 10/650 | Hydrocodone 10 mg | 650 mg | 6 |
| Norco 10/325 | Hydrocodone 10 mg | 325 mg | 12 |

aminophen (Darvocet®), can be the initial pain medications used. The total daily dose of acetaminophen should not exceed 4 g/d to prevent liver toxicity. Thus, the physician must be aware of the amount of acetaminophen in each tablet prescribed and be certain that the number of pills taken per day does not exceed the recommended dose (see Table 3). Patients must also be educated on the proper dosage of these medications and cautioned about the sedative and constipating side effects. If patients require higher doses or long-term narcotics to control pain, oxycodone or morphine can be prescribed and carefully titrated until adequate pain relief is achieved. Nonopioid medications, such as acetaminophen or ibuprofen, can be taken concurrently. Long-acting narcotics, such as Oxycontin®, are very effective in controlling pain, have a simple dosing schedule, and remove the peaks and valleys of pain associated with intermittent narcotic use. In patients not previously treated with narcotics, 10 mg of Oxycontin® every 12 h is a reasonable starting dose, and can be titrated up every 2–3 d until the most beneficial dose with minimal side effects is achieved. Patients previously on opiates can be started at a dose of 20 mg every 12 h and titrated accordingly. Patients must clearly understand that under no circumstances should a sustained-release narcotic tablet be broken, crushed, or chewed. This can result in the rapid release of a large dose of opioid, which can be life-threatening. Patients on schedule II narcotics should be seen on a monthly basis to assess side effects and to check vital signs. Narcotics should not be acutely withdrawn, and need to be slowly tapered to prevent withdrawal symptoms. The type and dose of narcotics prescribed must be individualized, and other sedative medications the patients currently take must be considered.

Referral to pain clinics knowledgeable in IC may be beneficial. Various narcotics or neuroleptics can be used, along with nerve blocks or implantable pain pumps, to treat the severe pain that may be associated with IC. In addition, many IC subjects complain of associated problems, such as fibromyalgia, irritable bowel syndrome, and vulvodynia. Referral to the appropriate specialist for treatment of these disorders is recommended.

## SURGERY

Radical surgery for IC is rarely indicated and should be used only as a last resort. Augmenting the bladder or diverting the urine while leaving the bladder in place are often doomed to failure. Removing the bladder with urinary diversion may be effective in very select, end-stage cases; however, this should not be considered the standard of care for IC. Patients who choose this mode of therapy must be aware that this may not resolve the pain associated with IC.

## CONCLUSIONS

An enormous amount of research is now being conducted on this complex disease, and a better understanding of the pathophysiology and new treatments is on the horizon. The clinician must suspect IC to make the diagnosis. In addition, many men with "chronic prostatitis" may in fact have IC. Multimodality therapy is currently the most effective treatment. Education is also extremely important; patients need to understand that this is a chronic disease and that it may take time to find the best treatment combination to alleviate their symptoms. The patient must be involved in determining the treatment course, and a team approach utilizing nursing staff, physical therapists, rheumatologists, pain clinics, and others is often beneficial. Clinicians must continue to seek a treatment or treatment combination to alleviate the suffering of the IC patient.

## SELECTED READING

Baskin LS, Tanagho EA (1992) Pelvic pain without pelvic organs. *J Urol* 147:683–686.
Christmas TJ, Bottazzo GF (1992) Abnormal urothelial HLA-DR expression in interstitial cystitis. *Clin Exp Immunol* 87:450–454.
Fleischmann J (1994) Calcium channel antagonists in the treatment of interstitial cystitis. *Urol Clin N Am* 21:107–111.
Fleischmann JD, Huntley HN, Shingleton WB, Wentworth DB (1991) Clinical and immunological response to nifedipine for the treatment of interstitial cystitis. Interleukin-2 inhibitor was measured using an IL-2 dependent cell line. Urinary IL-2 inhibitor activity was normal in 7 of 9 subjects regardless of symptom severity. *J Urol* 146:1235–1239.
Goin JE, Olaleye D, Peters KM, Steinert B, Habicht K, Wynant G (1998) Psychometric analysis of the University of Wisconsin interstitial cystitis scale: implications for use in randomized clinical trials. *J Urol* 159:1085–1090.
Hanno P, Levin RM, Monson FC, Teuscher C, Zhou ZZ, Ruggieri M, Whitmore K, Wein AJ (1990) Diagnosis of interstitial cystitis. *J Urol* 143:278–281.
Hanno PM (1997) Analysis of long-term Elmiron therapy for interstitial cystitis. *Urology* 49 (5A Suppl):93–99.
Hanno PM, Landis JR, Matthews-Cook Y, Kusek J, Nyberg L, Jr (1999) The diagnosis of interstitial cystitis: lessons learned from the National Institutes of Health interstitial cystitis database study. *J Urol* 161:553–557.
Holm-Bentzen M, Søndergaard I, Hald T (1987) Urinary secretion of a metabolite of histamine (1,4-methyl-imidazole-acetic-acid) in painful bladder disease. *Br J Urol* 59:230–233.
Hunner GL (1915) A rare type of bladder ulcer in women: report of cases. *Boston Med Surg J* 172:660–664.
Joustra B, Karrenbeld A, Mensink H (1996) Specific auto-antibodies in interstitial cystitis patients suggest an auto-immune etiology. *J Urol* 155:431A (Abstract).
Keay S, Zhang C-O, Trifillis AL, Hebel JR, Jacobs SC, Warren JW (1997) Urine autoantibodies in interstitial cystitis. *J Urol* 157:1083–1087.
Keller ML, McCarthy DO, Neider RS (1994) Measurement of symptoms of interstitial cystitis. A pilot study. *Urol Clin N Am* 21:67–71.
Korting GE, Smith SD, Wheeler MA, Weiss RM, Foster HE, Jr (1999) A randomized double-blind trial of oral L-arginine for treatment of interstitial cystitis. *J Urol* 161:558–565.
La Rock DR, Sant GR (1995) Intravesical chlorpactin for refractory interstitial cystitis. *Infections in Urology* September/October:151–157.
Liebert M, Wedemeyer G, Stein JA, Washington R, Jr, Faerber G, Flint A, Grossman HB (1993) Evidence for urothelial cell activation in interstitial cystitis. *J Urol* 149:470–475.
Lotz M, Villiger P, Hugli T, Koziol J, Zuraw BL (1994) Interleukin-6 and interstitial cystitis. *J Urol* 152:869–873.

O'Leary MP, Sant GR, Fowler FJ, Whitmore KE, Spolarich-Kroll J (1997) The interstitial cystitis symptom index and problem index. *Urology* 49 (Suppl 5A):58–63.

Ochs RL, Stein TW, Jr, Peebles CL, Gittes RF, Tan EM (1994) Autoantibodies in interstitial cystitis. *J Urol* 151:587–592.

Parkin J, Shea C, Sant GR (1997) Intravesical dimethyl sulfoxide (DMSO) for interstitial cystitis—a practical approach. *Urology* 49 (5A Suppl):105–107.

Parsons CL (1996) Potassium sensitivity test. *Tech Urol* 2:171–173.

Parsons CL (1997) New concepts in interstitial cystitis. *Int Urogynecol J Pelvic Floor Dysfunct* 8:1, 2.

Parsons CL, Benson G, Childs SJ, Hanno P, Sant GR, Webster G (1993) A quantitatively controlled method to study prospectively interstitial cystitis and demonstrate the efficacy of pentosanpolysulfate. *J Urol* 150:845–848.

Peters K, Diokno A, Steinert B, Yuhico M, Mitchell B, Krohta S, Gillette B, Gonzalez J (1996) The efficacy of intravesical Tice® bacillus Calmette-Guérin (BCG) in the treatment of interstitial cystitis (IC): a double-blind, prospective, placebo controlled trial. *J Urol* 157:2090–2094.

Peters KM, Diokno AC, Steinert BW (1999) A preliminary study on urinary cytokine levels in interstitial cystitis: does intravesical BCG treat IC by altering the immune profile in the bladder? *Urology*, in press.

Peters KM, Diokno AC, Steinert BW, Gonzalez JA (1998) The efficacy of intravesical TICE® bacillus Calmette-Guérin (BCG) in the treatment of interstitial cystitis (IC): long-term follow-up. *J Urol* 159:1483–1487.

Ratner V, Slade D, Greene G (1994) Interstitial cystitis. A patient's perspective. *Urol Clin North Am* 21:1–5.

Sant GR (1987) Intravesical 50% dimethyl sulfoxide (RIMSO-50) in treatment of interstitial cystitis. *Supplement to Urology* 29:17–21.

Sant GR, Theoharides TC (1994) The role of the mast cell in interstitial cystitis. *Urol Clin North Am* 21:41–53.

Silk MR (1970) Bladder antibodies in interstitial cystitis. *J Urol* 103:307–309.

Smith SD, Wheeler MA, Foster HE, Jr, Weiss RM (1996) Urinary nitric oxide synthase activity and cyclic gmp levels are decreased with interstitial cystitis and increased with urinary tract infections. *J Urol* 155:1432–1435.

Smith SD, Wheeler MA, Foster HE, Jr, Weiss RM (1997) Improvement in interstitial cystitis symptom scores during treatment with oral L-arginine. *J Urol* 158:703–708.

Theoharides TC, Sant GR (1997) Hydroxyzine therapy for interstitial cystitis. *Urology 49* (5A Suppl):108–110.

Theoharides TC, Sant GR, El-Mansoury M, Letourneau R, Ucci AA, Jr, Meares EM, Jr (1995) Activation of bladder mast cells in interstitial cystitis: a light and electron microscopic study. *J Urol* 153: 629–639.

Waxman JA, Sulak PJ, Kuehl TJ (1998) Cystoscopic findings consistent with interstitial cystitis in normal women undergoing tubal ligation. *J Urol* 160:1663–1667.

# IV  THE RENAL MASS

# 12 Evaluation of the Renal Mass

*Norm D. Smith,* MD
*and Steven C. Campbell,* MD, PHD

**CONTENTS**

    INTRODUCTION
    DIFFERENTIAL DIAGNOSIS OF THE RENAL MASS
    CLINICAL EVALUATION
    RADIOGRAPHIC EVALUATION
    CYSTIC RENAL MASSES
    RENAL ANGIOMYOLIPOMA
    RENAL ONCOCYTOMA
    RENAL-CELL CARCINOMA
    STAGING EVALUATION OF RENAL-CELL CARCINOMA
    TRANSITIONAL-CELL CARCINOMA
    INFLAMMATORY RENAL MASSES
    PERCUTANEOUS BIOPSY IN EVALUATION OF THE RENAL MASS
    SUMMARY
    SELECTED READING

## INTRODUCTION

The detection and evaluation of renal masses have changed significantly in this era of ubiquitous abdominal imaging for myriad signs and symptom complexes. Currently, the extended use of ultrasonography (US), computed tomography (CT), and magnetic resonance imaging (MRI) has rendered incidental discovery by cross-sectional imaging the most common presentation of a renal mass. The assessment of renal masses is complex, because of the predominance of renal lesions, the vast majority of which are benign in nature. The ultimate goal of evaluation of the patient with a renal mass is accurate diagnosis and staging by clinical and radiographic means, leading to timely treatment and avoidance of unnecessary procedures.

## DIFFERENTIAL DIAGNOSIS OF THE RENAL MASS

The differential diagnosis of renal masses includes (*see* Table 1): cystic lesions, benign neoplasms, such as angiomyolipoma (AML) and oncocytoma, and malignant

From: *Current Clinical Urology: Office Urology: The Clinician's Guide*
Edited by: E. D. Kursh and J. C. Ulchaker © Humana Press Inc., Totowa, NJ

Table 1
Differential Diagnosis of Renal Masses

| | |
|---|---|
| Cystic renal masses<br>　Simple cyst<br>　Complex cystic lesions | Inflammatory renal masses<br>　Acute diffuse or focal pyelonephritis<br>　Renal abscess<br>　Xanthogranulomatous pyelonephritis (XGP) |
| Benign renal tumors<br>　Angiomyolipoma<br>　Oncocytoma | Vascular<br>　Arteriovenous malformation |
| Primary malignant<br>　RCC<br>　TCC of the renal pelvis or calyces | Pseudotumor |
| Secondary malignant<br>　Lung<br>　Breast<br>　GI<br>　Leukemia<br>　Lymphoma<br>　Retroperitoneal sarcoma | |

neoplasms, such as renal cell carcinoma (RCC) and transitional-cell carcinoma (TCC), as well as inflammatory masses like xanthogranulomatous pyelonephritis (XGP) or abscess. Simple cysts are by far the most prevalent renal masses, and easily differentiated from complex cystic lesions and solid masses by routine imaging techniques. Cystic lesions are further assigned malignant risk based on established CT criteria (Bosniak classification). Angiomyolipoma is a benign tumor often distinguished from RCC by various imaging modalities, whereas other benign neoplasms, such as oncocytoma, usually remain pathologic diagnoses. Primary malignant renal tumors include RCC and TCC of the renal pelvis and calyces, as well as rare malignances, such as sarcoma or primary renal lymphoma. Lung cancer is the most common metastatic lesion of the kidney, whereas hematogenous metastases from breast cancer or GI malignancies, direct tumor extension from adjacent organs (such as the colon or pancreas), hematologic malignancies including leukemia or lymphoma, and retroperitoneal sarcoma account for the vast majority of other secondary neoplasms. Inflammatory masses include acute focal or diffuse pyelonephritis, abscess, and XGP; these diagnoses are often suspected by distinct clinical presentations and classic radiographic findings. Vascular lesions that can present as a renal mass include arteriovenous malformations.

## CLINICAL EVALUATION

The history and physical examination are paramount in the evaluation of patients with renal masses (*see* Table 2), as a number of related signs and symptoms have well-established prognostic significance. Important aspects of the history in patients with a known or suspected renal mass include systemic manifestations, pain syndromes, and symptoms related to mass effect or hematuria. Weight loss and general malaise suggest advanced stages of malignancy, but may also occur with large benign tumors or inflam-

Table 2
Signs and Symptoms of RCC

| Historical | Physical exam findings |
|---|---|
| Directly because of the tumor<br>   Hematuria<br>   Flank pain<br>Due to paraneoplastic syndromes<br>   Weight loss<br>   Malaise<br>   Hypercalcemia<br>   Erythrocytosis<br>   Anemia<br>   Hepatic dysfunction<br>   Hypertension<br>Directly because of metastases<br>   Cough<br>   Hemoptysis<br>   Bone pain<br>   Neurologic changes | Palpable mass<br>Lymphadenopathy<br>Lower-extremity edema<br>Nonreducing varicocele<br>Cachexia |

matory masses. Symptoms associated with metastatic disease include cough, dyspnea, hemoptysis, and bone pain from lung and bone metastases, respectively. Classic renal pain is usually present in the flank or costovertebral angle below the twelfth rib, although large masses can produce abdominal pain or gastrointestinal symptoms related to mass effect. Gross hematuria may be intermittent in nature, and should be considered secondary to malignancy until proven otherwise. Symptomatic presentation of RCC is more likely to be associated with advanced stage and compromised survival than incidentally detected disease.

The relevant family history should also be taken, because familial forms of RCC, such as von Hippel-Lindau (VHL) disease, hereditary papillary RCC and familial renal oncocytosis, may account for as many as 4% of all RCCs. These entities should be considered in patients with an early age of onset or multifocal disease. Other findings suggestive of VHL include a family history of brain tumors, blindness, renal tumors, or renal failure; the presence of epididymal tumors (papillary cystadenoma) or adrenal masses (pheochromocytoma); multiple pancreatic or renal cysts; or neurologic or visual changes. Patients suspected of having VHL should be evaluated with MRI of the brain and spinal cord (to evaluate for cerebellar, brain-stem, or spinal-cord hemangiomas) and ophthalmologic consultation (to assess for retinal angiomas), in addition to CT or MRI of the abdomen and pelvis. A molecular screening for VHL gene alterations should also be offered, and all relatives should be appropriately counseled and evaluated.

In the assessment of a renal mass, the physical examination should consist of a focused genitourinary exam, as well as a general survey for lymphadenopathy or other signs of advanced malignancy. Careful examination of the kidneys is essential, and should include inspection, palpation, percussion, and transillumination if feasible. A palpable mass or lymphadenopathy suggests advanced disease. The presence of a nonreducing varicocele or lower-extremity edema implies venous involvement. Despite obvious necessity, the physical examination is usually normal in the evaluation of renal masses because of the sequestered location of the kidneys within the retroperitoneum.

Meticulous evaluation of a renal mass requires judicious use of laboratory testing in an effort to narrow the differential diagnosis, rule out metastatic disease, or diagnose the myriad paraneoplastic syndromes potentially coexistent with RCC. Gross or microscopic hematuria occurs in up to 60% of patients with RCC, making urinalysis mandatory. A urine culture can differentiate inflammatory masses, such as abscess or XGP. Alkaline phosphatase is often elevated in the presence of bony metastases from RCC. Moreover, RCC is associated with a vast array of paraneoplastic syndromes. Laboratory investigation should include analysis for these potential abnormalities, since failure of normalization after radical nephrectomy suggests metastatic disease and heralds a dismal prognosis. More common paraneoplastic syndromes include anemia, erythrocytosis, hypertension, hypercalcemia, and nonmetastatic hepatic dysfunction, or Stauffer's syndrome. Anemia is present in up to 30% of cases of RCC and is an important preoperative consideration. Renal cell carcinoma is the most common cause of paraneoplastic erythrocytosis, which is caused by either tissue hypoxia with production of erythropoietin from adjacent normal kidney or secondary to overexpression or erythropoietin by the tumor itself. Similarly, hypertension can result from elevated renin levels produced by either a tumor or adjacent normal renal tissue. Stauffer's syndrome involves nonmetastatic hepatic dysfunction with abnormalities including hypoalbuminemia, elevated alkaline phosphatase, bilirubin, and prothrombin time, as well as hypergammaglobulinemia. Recent studies suggest that Stauffer's syndrome may be secondary to overexpression of certain cytokines.

The history, physical examination, and laboratory evaluation of a patient with a renal mass are often performed retrospectively by the urologist because of increased fortuitous detection by cross-sectional imaging of the abdomen for various complaints. Nonetheless, these cornerstones of medical practice may provide important insights into differential diagnosis and tumor staging, and often have implications with respect to treatment options and ultimate prognosis.

## RADIOGRAPHIC EVALUATION

A multitude of imaging modalities are now available for the evaluation of renal masses. The ultimate goal of the radiographic evaluation is accurate diagnosis and staging; the clinician's dilemma is selection of the most sensitive, cost-effective, and discriminating noninvasive studies. A brief overview of the imaging armamentarium accentuates the particular strengths and weaknesses of each diagnostic study commonly used in the assessment of renal masses.

Intravenous urography (IVU) with nephrotomograms provides physiologic information about renal function as well as anatomic detail of the renal parenchyma and collecting system. Indications for IVU have diminished, but it retains a primary role for evaluation of urolithiasis, infection, and hematuria. Since hematuria is a presenting sign in up to 60% of patients with RCC, IVU will continue to play a prominent role in diagnosis of renal masses. Nephrotomograms serve as an adjunct to IVU by enhancing imaging of the renal contour and the parenchyma. A distinct advantage of IVU with nephrotomography is the potential to detect abnormalities of the collecting system, such as TCC—but IVU clearly has inferior sensitivity compared to US, CT, or MRI for detecting small parenchymal masses, which often do not alter the morphology of the collecting system or renal contour. Despite its specific limitations, IVU remains an important initial tool in assessment of renal masses because of its utility in evaluating hematuria.

Ultrasonography is often used if a renal mass is suspected on either physical examination or IVU, because it is noninvasive and relatively inexpensive. Renal US offers excellent differentiation of simple cysts from complex cystic lesions or solid masses. Most renal masses detected by IVU with nephrotomograms are benign simple cysts, which can be easily differentiated by US. Findings of a complex cystic lesion or solid mass on US mandate further evaluation with CT.

Computed tomography is presently the gold standard for characterization of complex cystic lesions as well as diagnosis and staging of RCC. Pre- and postcontrast scans are essential for the optimal evaluation of renal masses. Contrast enhancement is a fundamental characteristic in the evaluation of renal masses by CT and is strictly defined as increased attenuation of at least 10 Hounsfield units (HU) after administration of intravenous contrast. Administration of contrast has particular utility in the diagnosis of small, solid tumors or complex cystic lesions in which unequivocal contrast enhancement is invariably indicative of malignancy. Advances in technology, such as spiral CT with multiphasic scanning, permit detection even of very small renal masses. Newer applications of CT, such as 3-D reconstruction, show potential utility as an adjunct to partial nephrectomy.

Currently, MRI is used selectively in the evaluation of renal masses; it is primarily reserved for patients with azotemia, or cases in which diagnosis or staging remain in question despite imaging with CT. MRI is at least as accurate as venacavography in detection and staging of tumor thrombi from RCC, and is presently the premier study for this purpose because it is noninvasive, does not require intravenous contrast, and provides crucial information about both the caudad and cephalad extent of tumor thrombus. The development of paramagnetic contrast agents, such as gadolinium, have improved the MRI evaluation of renal masses because contrast enhancement can then be used to characterize renal lesions similar to contrast-enhanced CT. Gadolinium offers a distinct advantage over iodinated contrast because it has fewer nephrotoxic side effects, making gadolinium-enhanced MRI the diagnostic test of choice for evaluation of renal lesions in patients with previous allergy to iodinated contrast or renal insufficiency. Despite the vast potential and recent increase in use of MRI, CT remains the gold standard for evaluation of renal masses because of its similar sensitivity and specificity, more widespread availability, and lower cost.

The sensitivity of angiography in the diagnosis of RCC is high, as roughly 90–95% of tumors demonstrate classic hypervascularity, but similar patterns are often observed with AML and renal metastases. Angiography is rarely used in the evaluation of renal masses because of discriminating noninvasive modalities, such as US, CT, and MRI. The current role of arteriography in the evaluation of renal lesions includes select cases of RCC for vascular mapping prior to planned nephron-sparing surgery or for angioinfarction of large tumors in either a preoperative or palliative setting. Angiography remains a useful tool in the assessment of renal masses in patients with severe hypertension, vascular disease, or other history when there is a suspicion of concomitant renal-artery stenosis—or to rule out a vascular lesion, such as an arteriovenous malformation, which can sometimes mimic RCC.

The role of nuclear scanning in the evaluation of renal masses is also quite limited. Occasionally, an abnormality on IVU is not seen with US, raising the suspicion of an isoechoic renal mass rather than a pseudotumor. In the past, nuclear renal scans were commonly used in this circumstance because the normal parenchyma of a pseudotumor concentrates radionuclide, whereas a renal cyst or tumor projects a photopenic defect. However, contrast-enhanced CT also distinguishes a pseudotumor from other renal lesions and is presently the diagnostic test of choice to rule out this entity. In the setting of a renal mass, nuclear studies are probably most useful for the determination of differential function in patients with renal insufficiency prior to radical vs. partial nephrectomy.

## CYSTIC RENAL MASSES

The majority of renal cysts are serendipitously detected by cross-sectional imaging for an unrelated process. Simple cysts are the most common renal lesions, and must be readily differentiated from complex cystic lesions and solid masses through imaging to avoid unnecessary procedures. Ultrasound is paramount in the evaluation of renal cystic masses, because lesions that meet strict sonographic criteria for simple cysts require no further evaluation. Complex cystic or solid lesions on US require further examination with CT.

The Bosniak classification of cystic renal masses categorizes lesions based on specific CT findings in an attempt to precisely delineate malignant risk. Bosniak category 1 (*see* Fig. 1A) includes benign simple cysts with sharply defined borders, uniform water density with low attenuation, and absence of contrast enhancement. Lesions that meet the criteria for Bosniak category 1 require no further imaging and essentially present no malignant risk. A Bosniak category 2 lesion, or minimally complex cyst, is characterized by curvilinear calcifications or thin septae (Fig. 1B). Bosniak category 2 also includes the hyperdense renal cyst, which is homogeneously hyperdense (40–90 HU) on noncontrast CT and fails to enhance after administration of intravenous contrast. Although not universal, the vast majority of class 2 lesions are benign in nature. More ominous class 2 lesions are termed 2F and require interval follow-up imaging at 3 mo, 6 mo, and 1 yr to guarantee a stable appearance without progression of CT findings suggesting malignancy. Unfortunately, guidelines for differentiation between class 2 and 2F lesions are not well-established. Bosniak category 3 lesions (*see* Fig. 1C) are complex cystic masses with irregular calcifications, hemorrhage, or complex septae; these lesions often cannot be differentiated as benign vs. malignant despite multimodal imaging. Multiloculated cystic nephroma is one benign mass that often presents as a Bosniak 3 lesion. However, approx 50% of Bosniak category 3 lesions are malignant and clearly warrant surgical exploration. Future directives must try to distinguish Bosniak 3 lesions by radiologic rather than pathologic means. Bosniak category 4 lesions (Fig. 1D) are invariably malignant, and include cystic masses with solid or nodular components, irregular margins, or the presence of unequivocal contrast-enhancement. These lesions are considered RCC until proven otherwise, and thus treated with radical vs. partial nephrectomy.

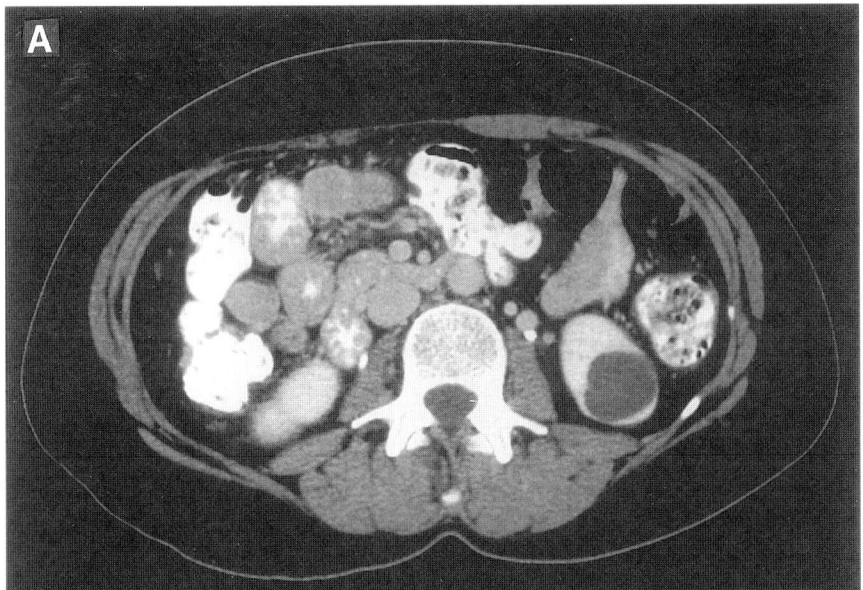

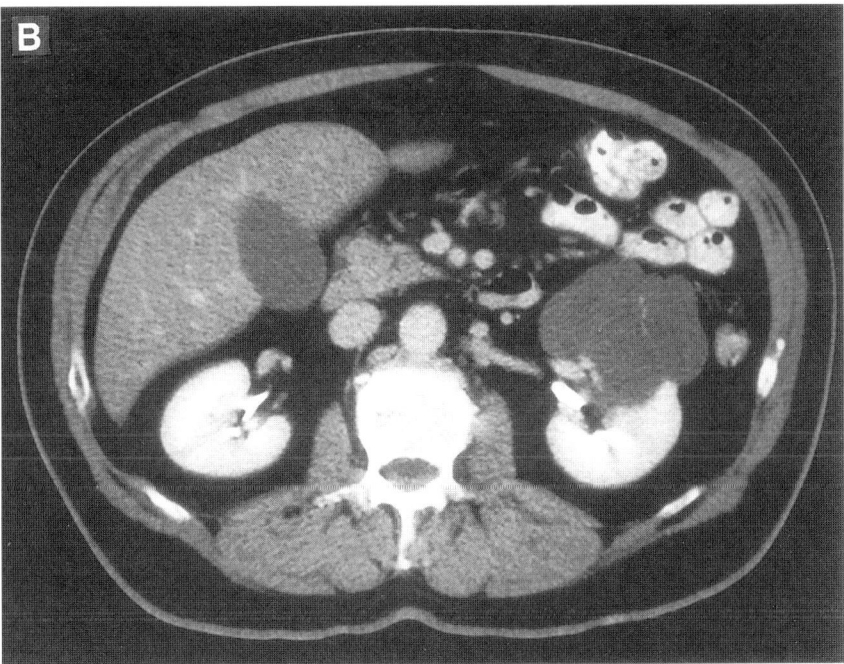

**Fig. 1.** Examples of Bosniak classification 1–4 lesions. **(A)** Postcontrast CT clearly demonstrates a Bosniak category 1 lesion with smooth, almost imperceptible walls, uniform water density, and a lack of internal echoes and contrast-enhancement. **(B)** Minimally complicated cyst or Bosniak category 2 lesion with thin septations. The vast majority of Bosniak 2 lesions are benign and may be managed conservatively with serial imaging. **(C)** Bosniak category 3 lesion with thick, irregular calcifications. These lesions are malignant in roughly 50% of cases and warrant exploration. This particular lesion proved to be RCC on final pathology. **(D)** Bosniak category 4 lesions are cystic masses with CT features, including solid components with unequivocal contrast-enhancement. These lesions are clearly malignant, with a cystic appearance resulting from necrosis, hemorrhage, or liquefaction of a solid tumor.

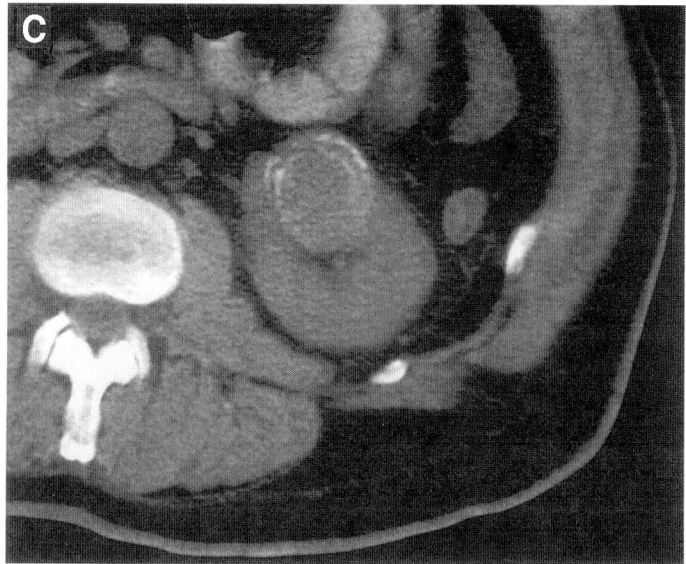

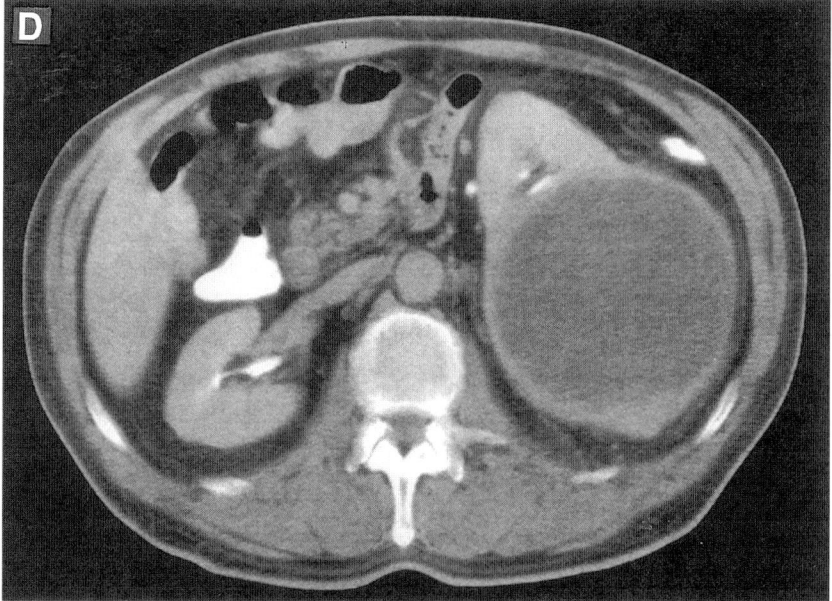

Fig. 1. *Continued*

## RENAL ANGIOMYOLIPOMA

Renal AML is a benign solid tumor characterized by an inconsistent mixture of blood vessels, muscle cells, and fat. A definitive relationship exists between tuberous sclerosis and AML—roughly 80% of patients with tuberous sclerosis ultimately develop AMLs. Renal AMLs are commonly bilateral and multifocal; presentations include mass, abdominal or flank pain, hematuria, or even retroperitoneal hemorrhage and

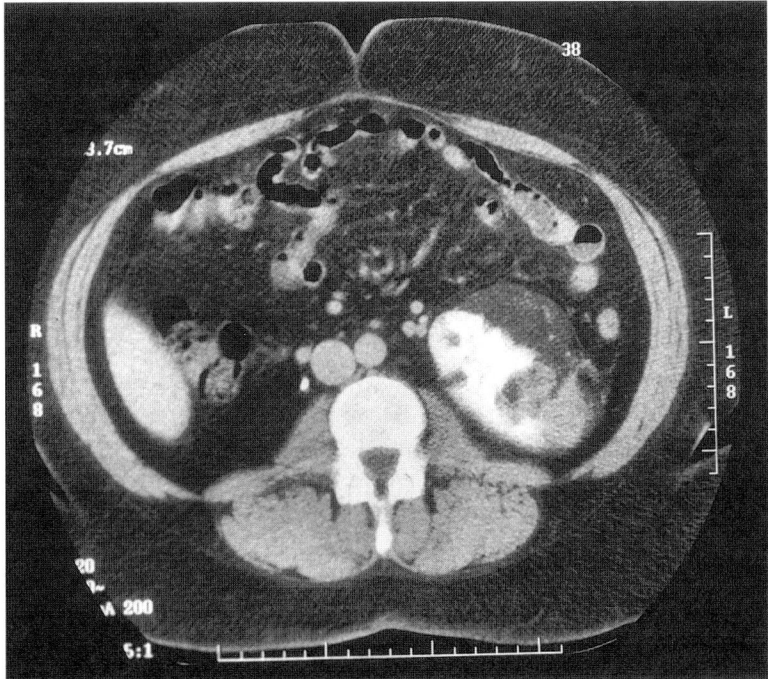

**Fig. 2.** Computed tomography is the radiographic test of choice for the diagnosis of AML, where fat density virtually excludes RCC from consideration. Angiomyolipoma may have a variegated appearance on CT because of a variable admixture of fat, smooth muscle cells, and blood vessels.

hypovolemic shock. Renal AML follows a benign course without metastases, but extracapsular extension and hilar lymph node or venous involvement have all been described in rare instances.

Ultrasonographic differentiation of AML from RCC is often difficult, but characteristics of AML include a sharply defined, uniform mass with increased echogenicity equivalent to the renal sinus complex. Once a diagnosis of AML is established, US is reliable for following small, asymptomatic lesions, as only larger AMLs (>4.0 cm) are overtly prone to hemorrhage. Despite the clinical utility of US in the diagnosis and management of AML, CT or MRI are currently indicated for further evaluation of hyperechoic masses found thorugh US. Fat density (−20 to −80 HU) on CT is essentially diagnostic of AML and excludes RCC from consideration (*see* Fig. 2). Fat saturation techniques display considerable potential for evaluation of AML by MRI because low-signal intensity on fat saturation images confirms the presence of fat and is diagnostic of AML.

The management of AML depends on symptoms, size, and the level of certainty about the radiologic diagnosis. Tumors of <4.0 cm rarely cause symptoms, and can be managed expectantly by serial imaging with US or CT. Symptomatic AMLs and asymptomatic tumors >4.0 cm should be treated with nephron-sparing modalilties, such as angioinfarction or partial nephrectomy, because of frequent bilaterality and multiplicity.

## RENAL ONCOCYTOMA

Oncocytoma is a benign solid tumor accounting for 3–14% of all renal neoplasms and occurs in a similar patient population to RCC, with a M:F ratio of 2:1 and peak incidence at an age of 55 yr. Most renal oncocytomas are serendipitously discovered; a minority of lesions present with pain, mass, or hematuria related to size of the oncocytoma. Radiographic characteristics once thought to be classic for oncocytoma include a solid homogeneous mass with a "central stellate scar" on CT or the so-called "spoke-wheel" pattern on angiography. However, such classic radiologic findings have been observed in only a minority of oncocytomas, and their specificity is also quite low. Open surgical or percutaneous biopsy for diagnosis are not recommended because oncocytoma shares histologic features with granular RCC and is concomitant with RCC in a wide range (7–32%) of reported cases. Unfortunately, oncocytoma cannot be reliably distinguished from RCC by clinical or radiographic means, and surgery is necessary for definitive diagnosis and management. The survival rate for oncocytoma is excellent; a review of cases of metastases and death associated with oncocytoma usually reveals concomitant RCC.

## RENAL-CELL CARCINOMA

Renal cell carcinoma represents approx 90% of primary malignant tumors of the kidney and in 1998 was estimated to account for roughly 28,000 new cancer diagnoses and over 11,000 deaths in the United States alone. It may present in various ways, including the classic triad of flank pain, abdominal mass, and hematuria. This "too late" triad was once considered pathognomonic for RCC, but as few as 10% of patients now present in this manner, mostly in the setting of advanced disease. Hematuria has been supplanted by incidental discovery via cross-sectional imaging of the abdomen as the most common presentation of RCC.

Intravenous urography findings suggestive of a renal mass include abnormalities of renal contour, mass effect, and distortion of the collecting system (*see* Fig. 3). Since the majority of renal masses on IVU are benign renal cysts, US is often next in the imaging armamentarium. Sonographic characteristics of a solid renal mass include irregular shape with indistinct borders, varied echogenicity, and the presence of internal echoes (*see* Fig. 4). Complex cystic or solid renal masses on US require further characterization with CT. The diagnosis of RCC is often difficult despite comprehensive imaging, because of the heterogeneous appearance of various benign and malignant lesions. Nonetheless, the CT scan before and after the administration of intravenous contrast is the gold standard for diagnosis and characterization of renal masses. Computed tomographic characteristics of RCC are manifold and include a solid mass with contrast-enhancement, asymmetric margins with a thick or nodular wall, irregular calcifications, hypervascularity, necrosis, and hemorrhage (*see* Fig. 5). Optimal assessment of small or equivocal renal lesions demands dedicated 5–10 mm sections through the kidneys before and after the administration of intravenous contrast. Computed tomography is also essential in staging RCC, as it allows for assessment of the liver, adrenals, venous structures, and retroperitoneal lymph nodes (*see* Fig. 6).

Other modalities in the imaging armamentarium are best used selectively when diagnosis, staging, or management issues remain in question. Currently, the most appropriate role of MRI in the evaluation of renal masses is as an adjunct to CT when

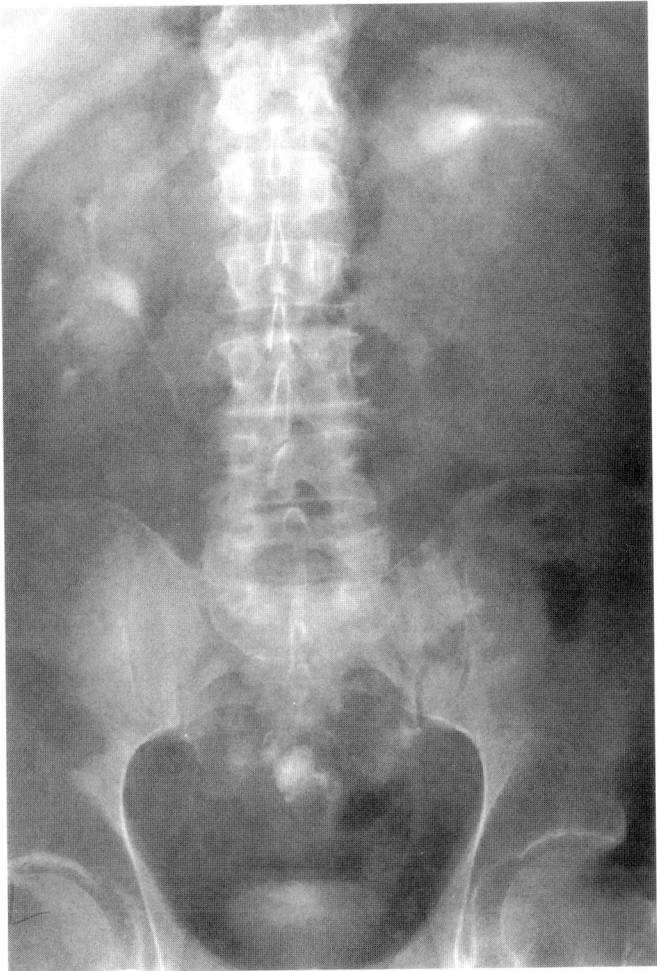

Fig. 3. The classic findings of a renal mass on IVU, including abnormalities in renal contour, mass effect, and distortion or displacement of the collecting system.

the accurate assessment of local invasion or extent of venous involvement is equivocal. The primary role of angiography in patients with RCC is for vascular mapping prior to challenging partial nephrectomy or for tumor angioinfarction (*see* Fig. 7). Nuclear imaging of the kidney has only limited utility in the assessment of RCC, and best serves to provide differential function in patients with borderline renal reserve as a prelude to partial vs. radical nephrectomy.

## STAGING EVALUATION OF RENAL-CELL CARCINOMA

The TNM classificaiton is the preferred staging system for RCC, and has definitively replaced the Robson classification for clinical and pathologic staging. The latest version of the TNM system is represented in Table 3. The cutoff separating T1 and T2 lesions has been changed based on data showing differences in survival rates among patients with 5.0, 7.5, and 10.0 cm lesions, and the 7.0 cm cutoff point was chosen since it represented the mean tumor size in the SEER database. The clinical staging of RCC

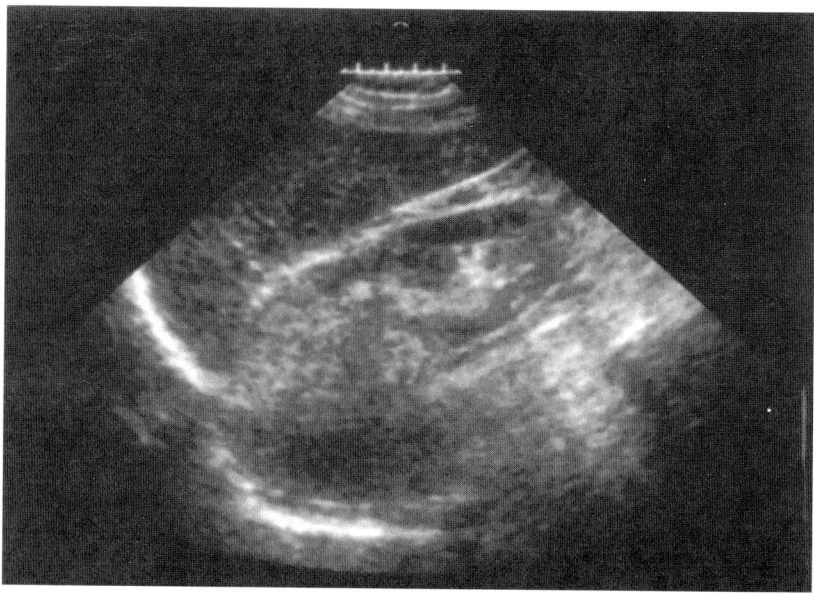

**Fig. 4.** Sonographic features of a solid renal mass include irregular shape with indistinct borders, varied echogenicity, and presence of internal echoes. Complex cystic or solid renal masses on US require further characterization with CT.

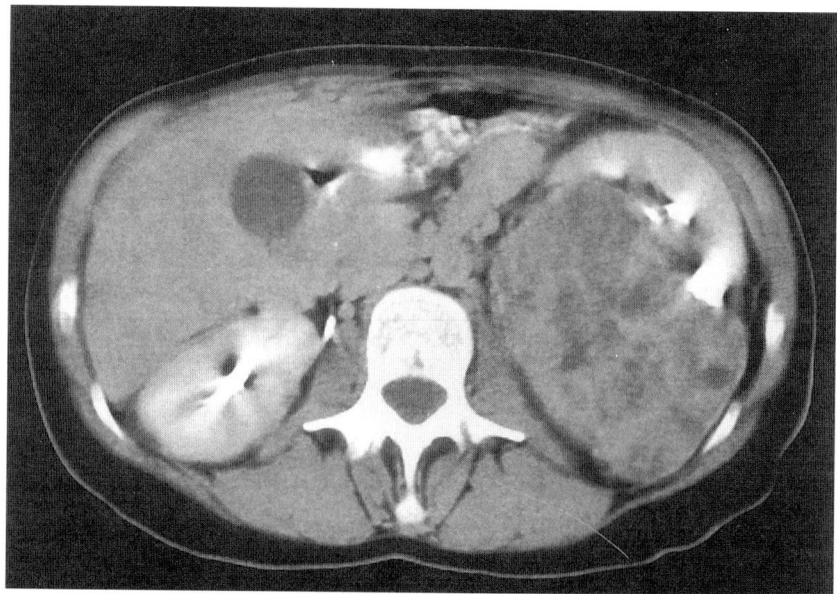

**Fig. 5.** Computed tomographic characteristics of RCC include a heterogeneous mass with obvious contrast-enhancement, obliteration of renal contour or the collecting system, and the presence of areas of central necrosis or hemorrhage.

# Chapter 12 / Evaluation of the Renal Mass

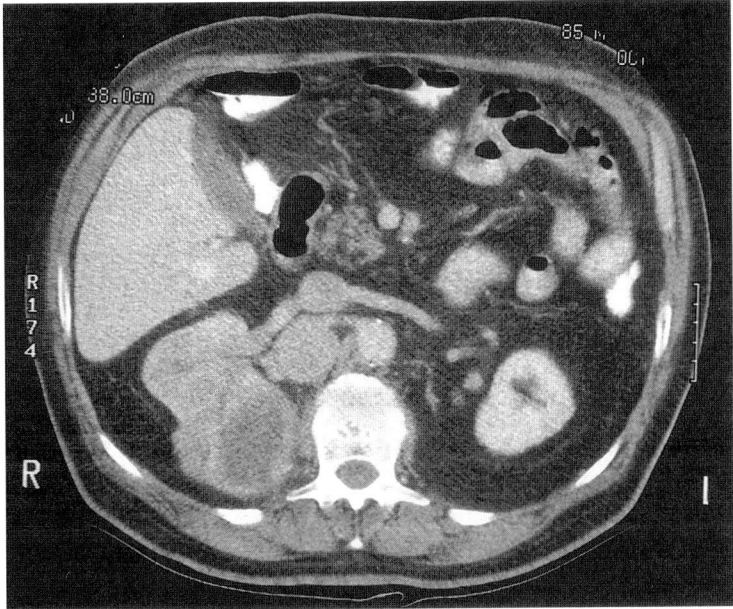

**Fig. 6.** Retroperitoneal lymph-node invasion by RCC, as demonstrated in this patient with enlarged retrocaval nodes, portends a dismal prognosis. Lymph nodes >2 cm on CT scan almost always harbor metastatic disease, whereas those <2 cm are often inflammatory rather than neoplastic.

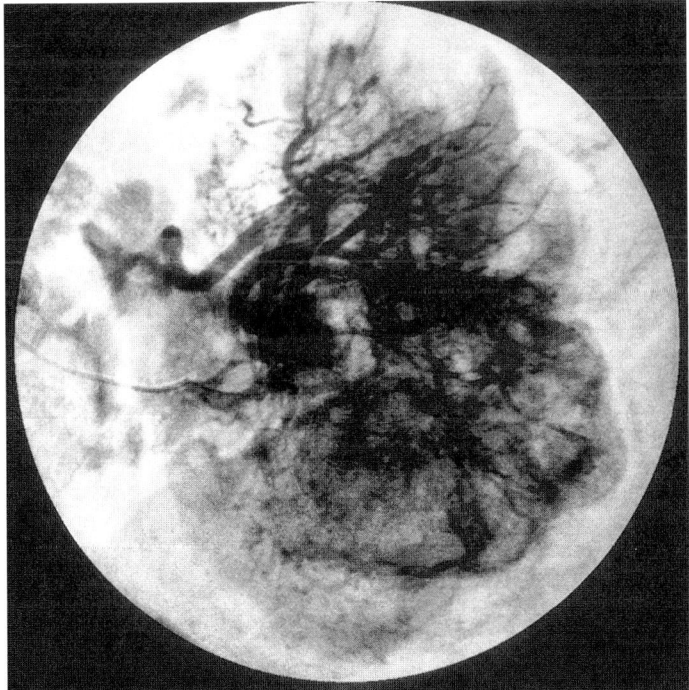

**Fig. 7.** The classic angiographic findings of RCC include hypervascularity, arteriovenous communications, and venous pooling. Angiography can be used as a vascular roadmap prior to nephron-sparing surgery or for embolization of large, advanced tumors in either the preoperative or palliative setting.

Table 3
TNM System for Staging RCC

*T—Primary tumor*
T0:   No evidence of primary tumor
T1:   Tumor < 7.0 cm, confined to kidney
T2:   Tumor > 7.0 cm, confined to kidney
T3a:  Tumor invades perinephric tissues or adrenal gland but is confined to Gerota's fascia
T3b:  Tumor extends grossly into the renal vein or IVC below the diaphragm
T3c:  Tumor extends grossly into the IVC above the diaphragm
T4:   Tumor extends beyond Gerota's fascia

*N—Regional lymph nodes*
NX:   Lymph nodes cannot be assessed
N0:   No regional lymph-node metastasis
N1:   Metastasis in a single regional lymph node
N2:   Metastasis in more than one regional lymph node

*M—Distant metastasis*
MX:   Distant metastasis cannot be assessed
M0:   No distant metastasis
M1:   Distant metastasis

consists of a thorough history, meticulous physical examination, and judicious use of laboratory testing to survey for locally advanced or metastatic disease.

The radiographic staging of RCC can usually be completed with CT scanning of the abdomen and pelvis, and CXR, with selective use of adjunct studies, such as MRI. Computed tomography has specific difficulty with the determination of perinephric tumor invasion, but failure to detect local invasion is not clinically relevant, since most T2 and T3a tumors are similarly treated by radical nephrectomy. Computed tomography findings of venous involvement by RCC include areas of decreased density, changes of intraluminal vein caliber, filling defects, or venous enlargement. Accuracy of CT is approx 78% for renal-vein involvement and 96% for IVC extension of tumor thrombus. Regional lymph-node metastasis by RCC heralds a dismal prognosis, with an approximate survival rate of 10% at 5 years. Lymph-node invasion by tumor is suggested by clustering of normal-sized nodes or the presence of enlarged nodes. Lymph nodes >2.0 cm in diameter almost always harbor metastatic disease. However, lymph-node enlargement of 1.0–2.0 cm may be caused by reactive hyperplasia and must generally be confirmed by surgical assessment. Micrometastatic RCC to the retroperitoneal lymph nodes cannot be determined by any current imaging modality. Compared to CT, staging advantages of MRI include superior definition of tissue planes with better detection of local tumor invasion, as well as improved detection and staging of venous involvement. MRI is especially important in assessment of the cephalad extent of caval thrombus with regard to the diaphragm, veins, and right atrium. Invasion of the caval wall can be determined with an accuracy of about 60%. Overall staging accuracy of MRI ranges from 80 to 90%, with remarkably high specificity (97%) for IVC involvement (*see* Fig. 8).

The metastatic evaluation of RCC at minimum consists of a CXR and liver function tests, including alkaline phosphatase and a CT scan of the abdomen and pelvis. Computed

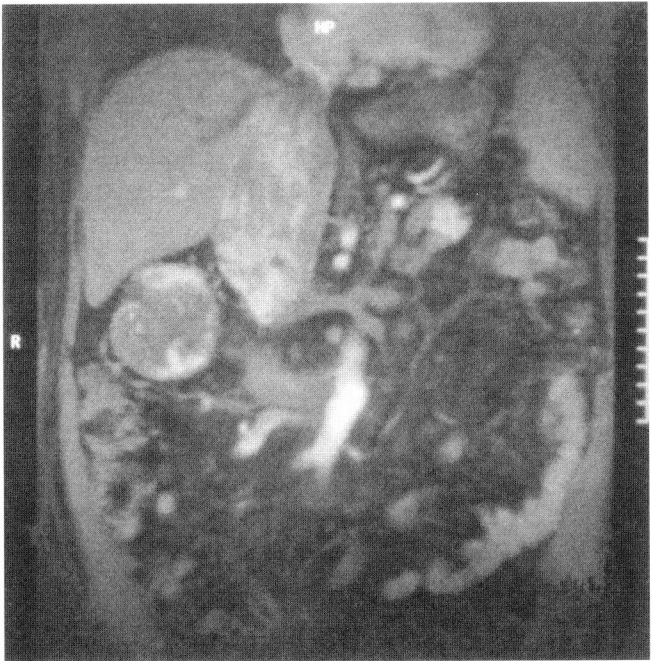

**Fig. 8.** Magnetic resonance imaging demonstrating a right renal tumor with IVC tumor thrombus extending into the right atrium.

tomography of the chest is usually reserved for patients with an abnormality on CXR or symptoms linked to the pulmonary system, whereas a bone scan is reserved for patients with bone pain or an elevated alkaline phosphatase. Magnetic resonance imaging of the abdomen and pelvis can effectively evaluate the extent of local invasion seen with large, locally advanced tumors. Computed tomographic scan or MRI of the brain is reserved for patients with neurologic symptoms, an abnormal neurologic examination, or perhaps prior to attempted curative surgery of a solitary metastatic focus in order to rule out occult CNS metastasis.

## TRANSITIONAL-CELL CARCINOMA

The second most frequent primary malignant renal neoplasm involves the urothelium. Of all urothelial malignancies, over 90% are TCC, with squamous-cell carcinoma (SCC) comprising most of the rest. A small percentage of patients will have bilateral tumors, and 50–75% will also be diagnosed with TCC of the bladder during their lifetimes. Transitional cell carcinoma of the upper tracts is rarely occult, as 75–95% of patients present with gross hematuria. Three to 11% of patients manifest with microscopic hematuria; other rare presentations include pain, palpable mass, obstruction, and pyelonephritis. The most common initial diagnostic test is usually IVU because of its prominent role in the evaluation of hematuria. Most patients display a filling defect on IVU, but inability to visualize the affected renal unit can occur secondary to venous occlusion, parenchymal destruction, or high-grade ureteral obstruction. Cystoscopy with retrograde pyelography (RPG) should be performed when clinical suspicion of a urothelial tumor is high or if there is any contraindication to use of intravenous contrast. Meticulously performed RPG can be diagnostic in up to 85% of upper-tract tumors, and should be complemented with direct ureteroscopic evaluation in most instances.

Computed tomography is paramount in radiographic evaluation of TCC of the upper tracts; it is sensitive for detection of filling defects and can differentiate radiolucent stones from TCC. It can often distinguish TCC from RCC, because TCC is almost always hypovascular. Computed tomographic characteristics of upper-tract TCC include a centrally located hypodense mass that does not disturb the normal renal contour, the presence of filling defects with distortion of the collecting system, and lack of contrast enhancement. CT also has utility in staging TCC of the upper tracts, as it can suggest invasion into the peripelvic fat, renal parenchyma, or adjacent organs, and can be used to evaluate the regional lymph nodes.

## INFLAMMATORY RENAL MASSES

Urinary-tract infection (UTI) in the adult is generally a simple diagnosis based on history, physical exam, and laboratory evaluation. Imaging for presumed acute UTI is most commonly reserved for patients who are unresponsive to appropriate antimicrobials, when urinary-tract obstruction is suspected, or if the patient is severely ill or immunocompromised. Inflammatory masses of the kidney include acute focal or diffuse pyelonephritis, renal abscess, and XGP. Acute pyelonephritis is termed "focal" or "diffuse" based on the extent of renal involvement by imaging. Computed tomographic characteristics of pyelonephritis include poor uptake and excretion of contrast, unilateral renal enlargement, and the presence of wedge-shaped defects. Although a diagnosis of acute focal pyelonephritis can be rendered by clinical presentation and radiographic findings, repeat imaging is usually performed after recovery to verify resolution of the mass. Renal abscess can develop secondary to progression of acute pyelonephritis with CT characteristics, including an irregularly shaped mass with central hypodensity indicative of liquefaction and necrosis. Gas is rarely evident. An abscess can ordinarily be treated with a combination of aggressive percutaneous drainage and broad-spectrum intravenous antimicrobials. Xanthogranulometous pyelonephritis is a rare consequence of chronic urinary-tract obstruction and infection, usually with *Escherichia coli* or *Proteus* species. XGP initially involves the renal pelvis, but may extend to the renal parenchyma or even the retroperitoneum. Patients most commonly present with fevers, chills, unilateral flank or abdominal pain, general malaise, and weight loss. Computed tomographic characteristics of XGP include a heterogeneous, hypodense mass, poor ipsilateral uptake and excretion of contrast, perinephric standing, and the presence of renal calculi, which are commonly staghorn or fragmented (*see* Fig. 9). Focal XGP can mimic RCC, especially in the absence of calculi. Antimicrobials alone are ineffective for the treatment of XGP. Partial nephrectomy is the treatment of choice, but it can be technically demanding, and most patients ultimately require radical nephrectomy because of the extent of parenchymal replacement.

## PERCUTANEOUS BIOPSY IN EVALUATION OF THE RENAL MASS

A confident diagnosis can be made in the majority of renal masses, thanks to the improved sensitivity and specificity of various techniques in the imaging armamentar-

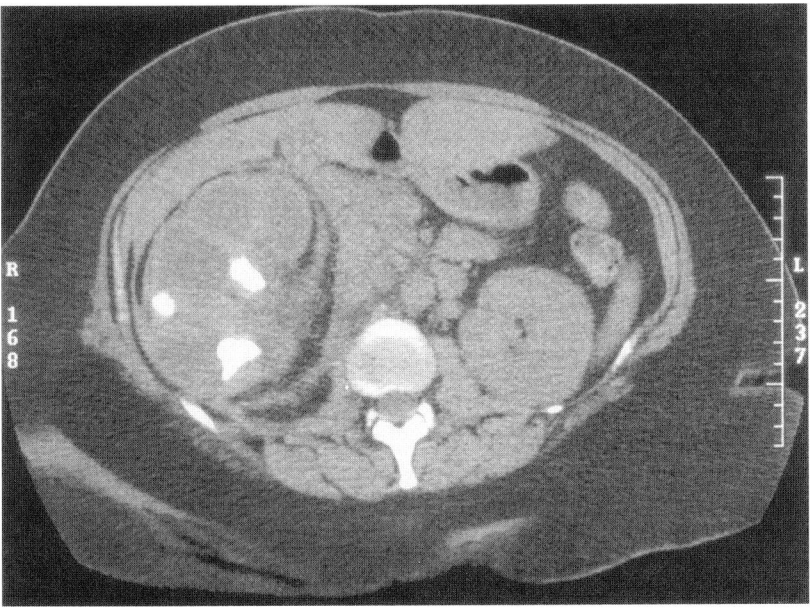

Fig. 9. Computed tomographic characteristics of XGP include a heterogeneous, ill-defined mass with poor function. Staghorn or fragmented calculi are a distinct feature of XGP, occurring in up to 80% of cases.

ium. Even when the diagnosis remains in question, few indications exist for percutaneous renal biopsy, because it will rarely affect patient management.

The currently accepted indications for percutaneous renal biopsy include cases in which abscess, lymphoma, or metastatic disease to the kidney are potential diagnoses. Patients with a febrile UTI and concomitant renal mass may be candidates for percutaneous renal biopsy to evaluate for abscess vs. malignancy. Renal lymphoma usually occurs in the presence of systemic disease and can sometimes be diagnosed by either CT or MRI of the retroperitoneum. Several different patterns of lymphomatous involvement of the kidneys are known. Focal parenchymal disease is often misdiagnosed as RCC, whereas infiltration of the perirenal space with involvement of the kidney, or diffuse infiltration of one or both kidneys with lymphoma, are more readily distinguished from RCC. Finally, massive retroperitoneal lymphadenopathy with engulfment of the kidney is highly suggestive of lymphoma (see Fig. 10). Percutaneous biopsy should be considered for definitive diagnosis, with treatment directed systemically toward the primary pathology.

Multiple tumors in the kidneys usually indicate diffuse metastatic disease, particularly in patients with a history of prior nonrenal malignancies. Renal metastases are present in roughly 12% of autopsies in patients with known cancer, and are most commonly from lung, breast, GI, or malignant melanoma, in decreasing order of frequency. The kidney is a frequent site of hematogenous metastases, with <10% of overall renal metastases secondary to direct invasion or lymphatic spread. CT findings with suspected renal metastases include small, multifocal, and bilateral masses. Percutaneous renal biopsy may be helpful if metastatic disease to the kidney is suspected.

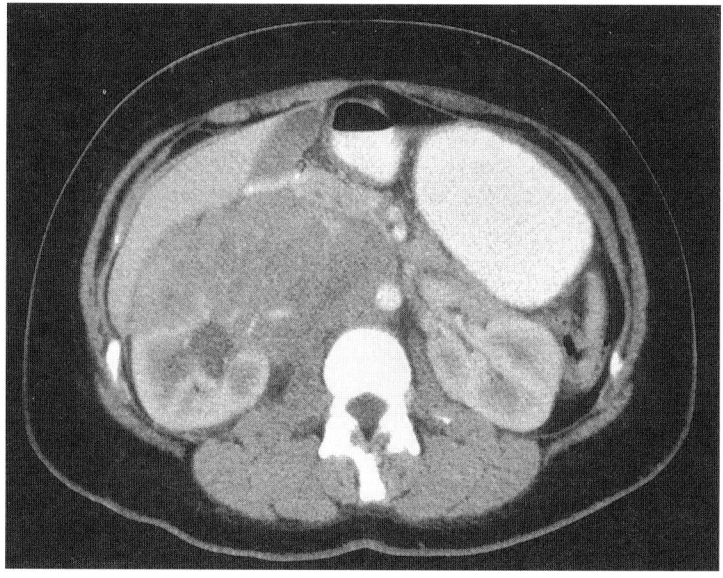

**Fig. 10.** CT findings of massive retroperitoneal lymphadenopathy with invasion or engulfment of the kidney are highly suspect for lymphoma.

## SUMMARY

A careful history and physical examination combined with intelligent use of radiographic and laboratory testing will yield an accurate diagnosis of most renal masses. The complete differential diagnosis should be considered in all cases to avoid missing important clues to the more unusual diagnoses. In the case of RCC, clinical parameters suggesting advanced disease should be taken into account, and meticulous staging and metastatic evaluation should be pursued to facilitate important management decisions.

## SELECTED READING

Baumgarten DA, Baumgartner B (1997) Imaging and radiologic management of upper urinary tract infections. *Uroradiology* 24:545–569.

Bechtold RE, Zagoria RJ (1997) Imaging approach to staging of renal cell carcinoma. *Urol Clin N Am* 24:507–522.

Bosniak MA (1986) The current radiologic approach to renal cysts. *Radiology* 158:1–10.

Bosniak MA, Rofsky NM (1996) Problems in the detection and characterization of small renal masses. *Radiology* 198:638–641.

Buckley JA, Urban BA, Soyer P, et al. (1996) Transitional cell carcinoma of the renal pelvis: a retrospective look at CT staging with pathologic correlation. *Radiology* 201:194–198.

Choyke PL (1997) Detection and staging of renal cancer. *MRI Clin N Am* 5:29–47.

Dimopoulos MA, Moulopoulos LA, Costantinides C, et al. (1996) Primary renal lymphoma: a clinical and radiological study. *J Urol* 155:1865–1867.

Goldfarb DA, Novick AC, Lorig R, Bretan PN, Montie JE, Pontes JE, Streem SB, Siegel SW (1990) Magnetic resonance imaging for assessment of vena caval tumor thrombi: a comparative study with venacavography and computerized tomography scanning. *J Urol* 144:1100–1104.

Jennings SB, Linehan WM (1996) Renal, perirenal, and ureteral neoplasms. In: Gillenwater JY, Grayhack JT, Howards SS, et al. *Adult and Pediatric Urology*, St. Louis: Mosby Year-Book, Inc. 643–694.

Kallman DA, King BF, Hattery RR, Charboneau JW, Ehman RL, Guthman DA, Blute ML (1992) Renal vein and inferior vena cava tumor thrombus in renal cell carcinoma: CT, US, MRI, and venacavography. *J Comput Assisted Tomogr* 16:240–247.

McClennan BL, Deoye LA (1994) The imaging evaluation of renal cell carcinoma: diagnosis and staging. *Radiol Clin N Am* 32:55–69.

Neumann HPH, Zbar B (1997) Renal cysts, renal cancer, and von Hippel-Lindau disease. *Kidney Int.* 51:16–26.

Rabushka LS, Fishman EK, Goldman SM (1994) Pictorial review: computed tomography of renal inflammatory disease. *Urology* 44:473–480.

Rofsky NM, Weinreb JC, Bosniak MA, et al. (1991) Renal lesion characterization with gadolinium-enhanced MR imaging: efficacy and safety in patients with renal insufficiency. *Radiology* 180:85–89.

Silverman SG, Bloom DA, Seltzer SE (1994) The radiological evaluation of renal masses: approach, analysis and new technologies. *AUA Update Series* 13:1–7.

# 13 Selecting the Optimal Treatment for Localized Renal Tumors and Long-Term Follow-Up

*Andrew C. Novick, MD*

**CONTENTS**
RADICAL NEPHRECTOMY
NEPHRON-SPARING SURGERY
FOLLOW-UP AFTER RADICAL NEPHRECTOMY
  AND NEPHRON-SPARING SURGERY
RENAL ONCOCYTOMA
SELECTED READING

Despite recent advances in our understanding of the genetics and biology of renal cell carcinoma (RCC), surgery remains the mainstay of curative treatment for this disease. Nevertheless, the role of traditional radical surgery is changing and nephron-sparing surgery (NSS) now plays an increasing role in the management of localized tumors.

## RADICAL NEPHRECTOMY

Robson et al established radical nephrectomy as the gold-standard curative operation for localized RCC with their report of 66% and 64% overall survival for stage I and stage II tumors, respectively. These results demonstrated better survival rates than those of patients treated with pericapsular nephrectomy. More recent reports indicate 5-yr survival rates of 80% or more following radical nephrectomy for stage I (T1–2) RCC. Radical nephrectomy currently remains the established form of treatment for patients with localized RCC and a normal contralateral kidney.

The concept of radical nephrectomy encompasses the basic principles of early ligation of the renal artery and vein, removal of the kidney outside Gerota's fascia, removal of the ipsilateral adrenal gland, and performance of a complete regional lymphadenectomy from the crus of the diaphragm to the aortic bifurcation. In recent years, controversy has arisen concerning the need for some of these practices in all patients. Performance of a perifascial nephrectomy is of unquestionable importance in preventing postoperative local tumor recurrence, because approx 25% of localized RCCs will manifest perinephric

From: *Current Clinical Urology: Office Urology: The Clinician's Guide*
Edited by: E. D. Kursh and J. C. Ulchaker © Humana Press Inc., Totowa, NJ

Table 1
Results of Nephron-Sparing Surgery for RCC

| Study | No. of patients | Local tumor recurrence (%) | 5-Yr cancer-specific survival |
|---|---|---|---|
| Morgan and Zincke | 104 | 6 (5.8%) | 89% |
| Steinbach et al. | 121 | 5 (4.1%) | 90% |
| Licht et al. | 216 | 9 (4.2%) | 87% |

fat involvement. Preliminary renal-arterial ligation remains an accepted practice. However, in large tumors with abundant collateral vascular supply, it is not always possible to achieve complete preliminary control of arterial circulation. It is now well-established that removal of the ipsilateral adrenal gland is not routinely necessary unless the adjacent upper portion of the kidney is involved with RCC. Finally, the need for performance of a complete regional lymphadenectomy in all cases has not been proven. Although this allows for more accurate staging of the extent of RCC, the therapeutic value of this information is limited because there is no established form of systemic treatment for patients with advanced disease. The therapeutic merits of lymphadenectomy itself have not been conclusively proven, although recent data from Giuliani et al suggest that a subset of patients with micrometastatic lymph-node involvement can benefit. The need for routine performance of a complete lymphadenectomy in all cases is presently unresolved, and a divergence of clinical practice remains among urologists regarding this aspect of radical nephrectomy.

## NEPHRON-SPARING SURGERY

Partial nephrectomy or nephron-sparing surgery has become a successful form of treatment for patients with localized renal-cell carcinoma (RCC) when there is a need to preserve functioning renal parenchyma. Accepted indications for this approach include situations in which radical nephrectomy would render the patient anephric with the subsequent immediate need for dialysis. This encompasses patients with bilateral RCC or RCC involving a solitary functioning kidney. The latter circumstance may be caused by unilateral renal agenesis, prior removal of the contralateral renal function from a benign disorder. Another indication for nephron-sparing surgery is represented by patients with unilateral RCC and a functioning opposite kidney, when the opposite kidney is affected by a condition that might threaten its future function, such as calculus disease, chronic pyelonephritis, renal artery stenosis, ureteral reflux, or systemic diseases, such as diabetes and nephrosclerosis.

The technical success rate with NSS is excellent, and long-term cancer-free patient survival is comparable to that seen after radical nephrectomy, particularly for low-stage RCC (see Table 1). The major disadvantage of NSS for RCC is the risk of postoperative local tumor recurrence in the operated kidney, which has occurred in 4–6% of patients. These local recurrences are most likely a manifestation of undetected microscopic multifocal RCC in the remnant kidney. The risk of local tumor recurrence after radical nephrectomy has not been studied, but it is presumably very low.

We recently reviewed the results of NSS for treatment of RCC in 500 patients managed at The Cleveland Clinic prior to December 1996. A technically successful operation with preservation of function in the treated kidney was achieved in 489 patients (98%). The mean postoperative serum creatinine level in these patients was 1.8 mg/dL. The overall and cancer-specific 5-yr patient survival rates in the series were 81 and 93%, respectively. Recurrent RCC-developed postoperatively in 38 of 473 patients (8.2%) with sporadic RCC. Thirteen of these patients (2.7%) developed local recurrence in the remnant kidney, whereas 26 patients developed metastatic disease. This data confirms that the NSS provides effective therapy for patients with localized RCC when preservation of renal function is a relevant clinical consideration.

### Nephron-Sparing Surgery with a Normal Opposite Kidney

Although radical nephrectomy remains the standard treatment for localized RCC in patients with an anatomically and functionally normal opposite kidney, a growing number of authors have reported excellent results with nephron-sparing surgery in this setting. A recent article detailed the outcome of NSS in 315 reported patients with unilateral localized RCC and a normal opposite kidney. The mean cancer-specific survival rate was 95% at approx 3 yr of follow-up, and there were only two cases of postoperative tumor recurrence. Significantly, the mean tumor size in most of these reports was <3.5 cm. Clearly, patient selection on the basis of small tumor size was a significant factor in the favorable outcome after NSS in these studies.

In a recent study from The Cleveland Clinic, we reviewed the outcome of NSS in 216 patients with sporadic RCC. Our findings confirm that extended cancer-free survival was significantly improved in patients with small (<4 cm) tumors compared to patients with larger ones. Other factors associated with significantly improved survival were unilateral renal involvement, low pathological tumor stage, and the presence of a single tumor. There were no postoperative tumor recurrences, and the cancer-specific 5-yr survival rate was 100% in patients with small (<4 cm), unilateral, stage $T_{1-2}$ RCC.

The aforementioned data suggested that NSS may be an acceptable therapeutic approach in patients who have a single, small (<4 cm) RCC and a normal contralateral kidney. To test this hypothesis, we conducted a subsequent study to evaluate the outcome following radical nephrectomy vs. NSS in 88 patients with a single, small (<4 cm), localized, unilateral, sporadic RCC. The radical ($n = 42$) and nephron-sparing ($n = 46$) surgical groups were well-matched for patient age, sex, renal function, diabetes, hypertension, tumor size, tumor location, and tumor stage. All patients in both groups had low pathological-stage RCC. A single patient in each group developed recurrent RCC postoperatively. The cancer-specific 5-yr survival rates for patients in the radical and nephron-sparing surgical groups were 97 and 100%, respectively. More recently, Lerner and associates from the Mayo Clinic reported the results of a similar study of patients with solitary small (<4 cm) low-stage RCC; the 5-yr cancer-specific survival rates following radical nephrectomy versus NSS were 96 versus 92%, respectively. The data from these two studies affirms that radical nephrectomy and nephron-sparing surgery provide equally effective curative treatment for patients with a single small, unilateral, localized RCC. The patients may now be considered suitable candidates for nephron-sparing surgery even if the opposite kidney is completely normal.

## Nephron-Sparing Surgery in von Hippel-Lindau Disease

Renal-cell carcinoma in von Hippel-Lindau disease (VHLD) differs from its sporadic counterpart because the diagnosis is made at a young age, and there are usually multiple, bilateral renal tumors. Although these are generally low-stage tumors, they are capable of progression with metastasis, and represent a frequent cause of death in patients with VHLD. Histopathologically, RCC in these patients is characterized by both solid tumors and renal cysts that contain either frank RCC or a lining of hyperplastic clear cells representing incipient RCC. Therefore, adequate surgical treatment of localized RCC in VHLD requires excision of all solid and cystic renal lesions.

The surgical options in patients with bilateral RCC and VHLD include bilateral nephrectomy and renal replacement therapy or partial nephrectomy to avoid end-stage renal failure. Although the early results of partial nephrectomy were promising, subsequent studies suggest a high incidence of postoperative tumor recurrence in the remaining portion of the kidney. It is likely that most of these local recurrences were a manifestation of residual microscopic RCC that was not removed at the time of the original partial nephrectomy.

A recent multicenter study has further delineated the outcome following surgical treatment of localized RCC in 65 patients with VHLD managed at eight medical centers in the United States. Renal cell carcinoma was bilaterally and unilaterally present in 54 and 11 patients, respectively. Radical nephrectomy and partial nephrectomy were performed in 16 and 49 patients, respectively. The mean postoperative follow-up interval was 68 mo. The 5- and 10-yr cancer-specific survival rates for all patients were 95 and 77%, respectively. The corresponding rates for patients treated with partial nephrectomy were 100 and 81%, respectively. In the latter group, 25 patients (51%) developed postoperative local tumor recurrence. Yet only two of these patients had concomitant metastatic disease; survival free of local recurrence was 71% at 5 yr but only 15% at 10 yr.

The results of this study indicate that partial nephrectomy can provide effective initial treatment for patients with RCC and VHLD. These patients must be followed closely, since most will eventually develop locally recurrent RCC with the concomitant need for repeat renal surgery. When removal of all renal tissue is necessary to achieve control of malignancy, renal transplantation can provide satisfactory replacement therapy for end-stage renal disease.

## FOLLOW-UP AFTER RADICAL NEPHRECTOMY AND NEPHRON-SPARING SURGERY

In properly selected patients, both radical nephrectomy and nephron-sparing surgery yield excellent long-term cancer-free patient survival, particularly for low-stage RCC. Yet there has been no consensus on a standard surveillance protocol following these operations in patients with localized RCC.

We recently completed a detailed analysis of tumor recurrence patterns after partial nephrectomy for sporadic localized RCC in 327 patients at The Cleveland Clinic. The purpose of this study was to develop appropriate guidelines for long-term surveillance after partial nephrectomy for RCC. Recurrent RCC after partial nephrectomy occurred in 38 patients (11.6%), including 13 patients (4.0%) who developed local tumor recurrence (LTR) and 25 patients (7.6%) who developed metastatic disease (MD). The incidence

Table 2
Postoperative Surveillance After Partial Nephrectomy for Localized RCC

| Pathological tumor stage | History, exam, blood tests | Chest X-ray | Abdominal CT scan |
|---|---|---|---|
| $T_1N0M0$ | Yearly | — | — |
| $T_2N0M0$ | Yearly | Yearly | Every 2 yr |
| $T_3N0M0$ | Every 6 mo for 3 yr, then yearly | Every 6 mo for 3 yr, then yearly | Every 6 mo for 3 yr, then every 2 yr |

of postoperative LTR and MD according to initial pathological tumor stage was as follows: 0 and 4.4% for $T_1N0M0$ RCC, 2.0 and 5.3% for $T_2N0M0$ RCC, and 8.2 and 11.5% for $T_{3a}N0M0$ RCC, and 10.6 and 14.9% for $T_{3b}N0M0$ RCC. The peak postoperative intervals for developing LTR were 6–24 mo (in $T_3$RCC patients) and >48 mo (in $T_2$RCC patients).

The above data indicate that surveillance for recurrent malignancy after partial nephrectomy for RCC can be tailored according to the initial pathological tumor stage. The recommended surveillance scheme is depicted in Table 2. All patients should be evaluated with a medical history, physical examination, and selected blood studies on a yearly or twice-yearly basis. The studies should include serum calcium, alkaline phosphatase, liver-function tests, blood-urea nitrogen, serum creatinine, and electrolytes.

The need for postoperative radiographic surveillance studies after partial nephrectomy varies according to the initial pathological tumor stage. Patients who undergo partial nephrectomy for $T_1N0M0$ RCC do not require radiographic imaging postoperatively because of the very low risk of recurrent malignancy. A yearly chest X-ray is recommended after partial nephrectomy for $T_2N0M0$ RCC, since the lung is the most common site of postoperative metastasis. Abdominal or retroperitoneal tumor recurrence is uncommon in the latter group—particularly early after partial nephrectomy—and these patients require only a recommended follow-up every 2 years of abdominal CT scanning. Patients with $T_3N0M0$ RCC have a higher risk of developing LTR and MD—particularly during the first 2 yr after partial nephrectomy—and they may benefit from more frequent follow-up with chest X-ray and abdominal CT scanning initially. We recommend that both procedures be done every 6 mo during the first 3 yr, followed by a yearly chest X-ray and an abdominal CT scan every 2 years.

Patients who undergo partial nephrectomy for RCC may be left with a relatively small amount of renal tissue. These patients are at risk of developing long-term renal functional impairment from hyperfiltration renal injury. In a study of 14 patients conducted over 17 yr following partial nephrectomy in a solitary kidney, we found that patients with more than a 50% reduction in overall renal mass were at increased risk for developing proteinuria, focal segmental glomerulosclerosis, and progressive renal failure. The development of proteinuria correlated directly with the length of follow-up and inversely with the amount of remaining renal tissue. Renal biopsy results revealed focal segmental glomerulosclerosis in several patients with severe proteinuria. These findings mirror those observed in experimental animal models of partial renal ablation. Since proteinuria is the initial manifestation of the phenomenon, a 24-h urinary protein measurement should be obtained yearly in patients with a solitary remnant kidney to screen for hyperfiltration nephropathy.

Table 3
Postoperative Surveillance After Radical Nephrectomy for Localized RCC

| Pathological tumor stage | History, exam, blood tests | Chest X-ray | Abdominal CT scan |
|---|---|---|---|
| $T_2N0M0$ | Yearly | — | — |
| $T_2N0M0$ | Yearly | Yearly | Every 2 yr |
| $T_{3abc}N0M0$ | Every 6 mo for 3 yr, then yearly | Every 6 mo for 3 yr, then yearly | At 1 yr, then every 2 yr |

Efforts to prevent or ameliorate the damaging effects of renal hyperfiltration have primarily focused on dietary and pharmacologic intervention. Animal studies have suggested that dietary restriction of protein and angiotensin-converting enzyme inhibitor (ACE 1) agents may mitigate this type of glomerulopathy. Preliminary clinical data appear to support this concept. We recently studied 5 patients who had developed proteinuria with stable renal function following partial nephrectomy in a solitary kidney. Four of these patients had documented focal segmental glomerulosclerosis on renal biopsy. All 5 patients had normal renal morphology at the time of surgery. Treatment with ACE inhibition and a low-protein diet decreased the level of proteinuria in 4 patients. Data from other studies have also suggested that ACE 1 therapy can significantly diminish proteinuria in patients with established renal disease. This information suggests that ACE 1 therapy and a low-protein diet may improve the long-term renal functional outcome for patients with a remnant kidney following partial nephrectomy. The optimal time for initiating this regimen is unclear, and it may be best to implement this as early as possible to obviate the maladaptive responses that can lead to progressive sclerosis and renal failure in this setting.

Experimental evidence indicates that nonhemodynamic processes may also contribute to the progression of sclerosis in the remnant kidney. This raises other therapeutic possibilities, such as thromboxane inhibitors, anticoagulants, lipid-lowering agents, and other pharmacologic agents. Future clinical trials will hopefully clarify the potential value of these treatment approaches.

Two recent studies on the outcome of radical nephrectomy for localized RCC have also demonstrated that the risk of postoperative recurrent malignancy is stage-dependent. In a study from the M.D. Anderson Cancer Center, metastatic RCC after radical nephrectomy occurred in 68 of 286 patients (23.8%). The incidence of MD according to initial pathological tumor stage was as follows: 7.1% for $T_1N0M0$ RCC; 26.5% for $T_2N0M0$ RCC; and 39.4% for $T_3N0M0$ RCC. The chance of developing recurrent malignancy was greatest during the first 3 yr postoperatively.

These data indicate that surveillance for recurrent malignancy after radical nephrectomy for RCC can also be tailored according to the initial pathological tumor stage. The recommended surveillance scheme is depicted in Table 3. All patients should be evaluated with a medical history, physical examination, and selected blood studies on a yearly or twice-yearly basis. For patients with $T_1N0M0$ RCC, routine postoperative radiographic imaging is unnecessary because of the low risk of recurrent malignancy. For patients with $T_2N0M0$ RCC, a chest X-ray every year and an abdominal CT scan every 2 yr are recommended. Patients with $T_3N0M0$ RCC have a higher risk of developing recurrent malignancy—particularly during the first 3 yr after radical nephrectomy—and may benefit from more frequent laboratory and radiographic follow-up, as suggested in Table 2.

In patients treated with either partial or radical nephrectomy for RCC, postoperative bone scans, bone-plain films, and head CT scans are necessary only in the presence of related symptomatology. The surveillance schemes outlined in this chapter are cost-effective and allow for early detection of most cases of recurrent RCC following surgical treatment of localized disease.

## RENAL ONCOCYTOMA

Renal oncocytoma is a benign tumor of renal tubular origin. As originally defined by Klein and Valensi, it is a lesion composed of solid sheets of large polygonal eosinophilic cells, usually with no cellular anaplasia. Leiber et al. described higher-grade oncocytomas with the ability to metastasize and cause patient death. However, in their study no patient with a grade-1 oncocytoma experienced metastases or died because of the tumor. Davis et al. recently suggested that nuclear atypia and cellular pleomorphism may not be evidence for aggressive behavior of an oncocytoma, and we have documented one such case. Our patient outcome data support the benign nature of this tumor, with no instances of metastases and a 100% tumor-specific survival rate in all treated patients at The Cleveland Clinic.

A review of the literature reveals renal oncocytoma as an incidental finding in approx 66% of the cases. In a study from our center, renal oncocytoma was found incidentally in 21 of 31 patients (68%) during evaluation for a nonurological disorder. Multifocal and bilateral renal oncocytomas were observed in 5 (16%) and 4 (13%) patients, respectively. Renal oncocytoma and RCC have rarely been found as coexisting lesions within the same or opposite kidney. In a recent review of 166 patients with oncocytoma, RCC was also present in 7.2% of the patients; in 3 RCC was observed as a small focus within an oncocytoma. In our study, we found coexisting oncocytoma and RCC in 10 of 31 patients (32%). Although this high incidence of coexistence of RCC and oncocytoma may partly reflect the unusual nature of our patient-referral population, we believe that this is an important finding with significant clinical implications.

It is presently impossible to establish a preoperative diagnosis of renal oncocytoma through radiographic imaging studies. The CT finding of a central stellate scar or a spoke-wheel appearance on angiography is not specific, and can be seen with RCC. Some investigators have recommended fine-needle aspiration for evaluation of the indeterminate solid renal mass, suggesting that when the cytological findings are consistent with oncocytoma, then conservative surgery or possibly observation may be warranted. Even if a prospective diagnosis of oncocytoma could be established, the large number of patients with concomitant RCC in the same kidney argues against this approach unless a specific indication for nephron-sparing surgery exists.

## SELECTED READING

Butler B, Novick AC, Miller D, et al. (1995) Management of small unilateral renal cell carcinomas: radical versus nephron-sparing surgery. *Urology* 45:34–40.

Davis CJ, Jr, Mostofi FK, Sesterhenn IA, Ho CK (1991) Renal oncocytoma. Clinicopathological study of 166 patients. *J Urogen Path* 1:42.

Giuliani L, Giberti C, Martorama D, et al. (1990) Radical extensive surgery for renal cell carcinoma: long-term results and prognostic factors. *J Urol* 143:468–473.

Hafez KS, Novick AC, Butler B (1998) Management of small solitary, unilateral renal cell carcinomas: impact of central versus peripheral tumor location. *J Urol* 159:1156.

Hafez KS, Novick AC, Campbell SC (1997) Patterns of tumor recurrence and guidelines for follow-up after nephron-sparing surgery for sporadic renal cell carcinoma. *J Urol* 157:2067.

Klein MJ, Valensi QJ (1976) Proximal tubular adenomas of the kidney with so-called oncocytic features. A clinicopathologic study of 13 cases of a rarely reported neoplasm. *Cancer* 38:906.

Lerner SE, Hawkins CA, Blute ML, et al. (1996) Disease outcome in patients with low-stage renal cell carcinoma treated with nephron-sparing or radical surgery. *J Urol* 155:1858.

Levy DA, Slaton JW, Swanson DA, Dinney CPN (1998) Stage specific guidelines for surveillance after radical nephrectomy for local renal cell carcinoma. *J Urol* 159:1163.

Licht MR, Novick AC, Goormastic M (1994) Nephron-sparing surgery in incidental versus suspected renal cell carcinoma. *J Urol* 152:39–42.

Licht MR, Novick AC, Tubbs RR, et al. (1993) Renal oncocytoma: clinical and biological correlates. *J Urol* 150:1380.

Lieber MM, Tomera KM, Farrow GM (1981) Renal oncocytoma *J Urol* 125:481.

Morgan WR, Zincke H (1990) Progression and survival after renal-conserving surgery for renal cell carcinoma: experience in 104 patients and extended follow-up. *J Urol* 144:852–858.

Novick AC (1995) Partial nephrectomy for renal cell carcinoma. *Urology* 36:149.

Novick AC, Gephardt G, Guz B, et al. (1991) Long-term follow-up after partial nephrectomy of a solitary kidney. *N Engl J Med* 325:1058–1062.

Robson CJ, Churchill BM, Anderson W (1969) The results of radical nephrectomy for renal cell carcinoma. *J Urol* 101:297–303.

Sandock DS, Seftel AD, Resnick MI (1995) A new protocol for the follow-up of renal cell carcinoma based on pathological stage. *J Urol* 154:28.

Steinbach F, Stockle M, Muller SC, et al. (1992) Conservative surgery of renal cell tumors in 140 patients: 21 years of experience. *J Urol* 148:24–29.

Steinbach F, Novick AC, Zincke H, Miller DP, Williams RD, Lund G, Skinner DK, Esrig D, Richie JP, deKernion JB, Marshall F, March CL (1995) Treatment of renal cell carcinoma in von Hippel Lindau disease: a multicenter study. *J Urol* 153:1812–1816.

# V BLADDER TUMORS

# 14 Evaluation and Management of Low-Grade, Low-Stage Bladder Cancer

*Michael J. Droller,* MD

**CONTENTS**
    INTRODUCTION
    CLINICAL PRESENTATION
    OFFICE EVALUATION
    SUMMARY
    SELECTED READING

## INTRODUCTION

An estimated 54,000 new cases of transitional-cell cancer of the urinary bladder will be diagnosed in the year 2000. Seventy percent of these will be classified as "superficial" transitional-cell cancers. Of these, 50–75% will recur, whereas only 15–20% overall will progress and create a life-threatening situation. The vast majority of superficial tumors (70%) are low-moderate grade and two-thirds are mucosally confined. Fewer than 5% of these are likely to progress. It is the high-grade (carcinoma *in situ* or CIS) and higher-stage (lamina propria invasive) forms of superficial urothelial cancer that present the greatest risk of progression.

This chapter reviews the manner of presentation of these various forms of superficial urothelial cancer, how they can be treated, whether recurrence of each form can be prevented, and the means by which they can be evaluated for the risk of recurrence and possible progression.

## CLINICAL PRESENTATION

Hematuria is the most common clinical presentation of urothelial cancer. This may occur either as gross or microscopic hematuria, and is usually characterized as "painless" by the patient. Hematuria commonly occurs throughout the urinary stream, but may be grossly and microscopically intermittent.

The degree of hematuria does not correlate with the extent of disease or its potential aggressiveness. The occurrence of hematuria also does not necessarily indicate the presence of a urothelial malignancy, since a variety of nonmalignant conditions (stones, infections, or medical renal disease) may also produce blood in the urinary tract.

From: *Current Clinical Urology: Office Urology: The Clinician's Guide*
Edited by: E. D. Kursh and J. C. Ulchaker © Humana Press Inc., Totowa, NJ

Several studies have suggested that hematuria may be a useful method of screening for urothelial malignancy, and may be particularly valuable in detecting the possible development of urothelial malignancy in specific populations at risk. Since the development of various forms of urothelial cancer has been found to be strongly associated with a number of environmental exposures (such as aromatic amines in the workplace and cigarette smoking), and correlated with certain host factors (enzymatic detoxification or activation of potential genotoxic/carcinogenic agents), testing for hematuria in patients considered at risk has been proposed to permit earlier detection of urothelial malignancies. This testing might make it possible to diagnose potentially aggressive forms of disease earlier, increasing the possibility for cure. Since the majority of superficial urothelial malignancies do not have an aggressive biologic potential, however, some have suggested that screening for hematuria may not be particularly cost-effective, despite the possible (but unproven) clinical benefit of earlier diagnosis.

Occasionally, patients with bladder cancer will complain of irritative voiding symptoms. This is most characteristic of CIS, a form of cancer that displaces the normal urothelium. Its malignant cells grow in the plane of the bladder, undermine the normal urothelium, and often slough to leave behind areas denuded of mucosa. The diffuse form of this entity is often accompanied by irritative voiding symptoms. Papillary forms of a superficial tumor do not usually produce irritative symptoms.

The patient who presents with irritative symptoms (with or without hematuria) is often mistakenly diagnosed as having a urinary-tract infection or "cystitis," (inflammation of the bladder). Since irritative symptoms associated with bacterial, viral, or chemical cystitis and diffuse CIS are indistinguishable from one another, it is important to document or exclude infection when symptoms of urinary frequency, burning on urination (dysuria), and urgency are described, and blood or inflammatory cells are present in the urine. Under these circumstances, both urine culture and cytology are important for diagnosis.

## OFFICE EVALUATION

Since bleeding can originate from any region in the urinary tract, a noninvasive but reasonably productive imaging modality should be performed to assess the kidneys, ureters, and bladder. Abdominal and pelvic sonography can fulfill these requirements. Although not sufficiently sensitive to detect small upper-tract urothelial tumors, this method provides an indication of the possible presence of a renal mass, obstruction of the upper tracts, or the presence of a filling defect representing a tumor in the bladder. Other conditions that may produce hematuria and that can be evaluated with this modality include renal parenchymal disease, kidney stones, and kidney cancers. The diagnosis of any of these conditions does not necessarily exclude the presence of a concomitant urothelial malignancy. This possibility must be considered when nonmalignant causes of hematuria have been successfully diagnosed and treated or excluded, but microscopic hematuria persists.

Another standard imaging study is intravenous pyelography (IVP). In the diagnosis of urothelial malignancy of the upper tracts, IVP is more definitive than sonography, because it can outline the profile of the renal pelvis, the ureter, and the bladder more clearly and without being operator-dependent in order to identify any filling defect suggestive of urothelial malignancy. However, the cystogram phase of the IVP is not a particularly sensitive method of detecting the presence of a small (<1 cm) urothelial malignancy in the bladder. In cases of renal failure or contrast allergy, if urothelial malignancy is suspected, an alternative means of evaluating the upper tracts is by retrograde pyelography. This method is particularly important if cystoscopy is negative, urinary cytology is suspicious, and ureteral obstruction or the presence of a questionable area in the renal pelvis has been visualized on ultrasound.

In addition to the urine culture, which documents or excludes the presence of a urinary infection as a possible cause of the hematuria and irritative voiding symptoms, a urinary cytology is important in the overall evaluation for the presence of urothelial malignancy if the culture is negative. Although urinary cytology has a poor sensitivity in detecting the presence of a low-grade malignancy, it is very effective in detecting the presence of a higher-grade malignancy or CIS. Some have advocated bladder barbotage to increase the sensitivity of cytology in detecting lower-grade urothelial malignancy. However, this may introduce instrumentation artifact, leading to the possibility of a false-positive diagnosis. Generally, several fresh voiding samples may be used to improve the predictive accuracy of urinary cytology, which will also effectively sample the upper tracts.

Recent years have witnessed a growing interest in the assay of substances in urine that might serve as markers to detect urothelial malignancies. These have included nuclear matrix protein (NMP22), bladder tumor "antigen" (BTA), components of human complement factor (BTA stat and BTA trak), fibrin split products (accudif), tumor-associated antigens (immunocyt), telomerase, and hyaluronidase/hyaluronic acid. Of those tests that are currently commercially available, NMP22 and telomerase, appear to have the greatest sensitivity for detecting low-grade urothelial cancers. However, each is affected by inflammation or by instrumentation, and therefore has a lower level of specificity that leads to false-positive results and compromises the negative predictive value of the assay. Various BTA tests have been aggressively promoted because they offer a greater sensitivity than cytology in detecting low-grade urothelial malignancies. Yet their sensitivity is lower than that of other tests for low-grade tumors and lower than cytology and other assays for high-grade tumors and CIS, and similar problems occur with their specificity.

One factor in considering the clinical value of these assays and markers is the question of their high false-positive rate, which could result in the initiation of an extensive but unwarranted evaluation for malignancy. Moreover, the efficacy of their use in monitoring for recurrent cancer must also consider the significant issue of false-negative evaluations.

The *sine qua non* of diagnosis is cystoscopic examination of the bladder, resection of any visible tumor, and biopsy of any abnormal area of the urothelium that suggests the possible presence of CIS malignancy. Although viewed as an invasive and possibly traumatic procedure, the careful and gentle use of a flexible cystoscope or rigid cystoscope provides an examination that is well-tolerated and produces critical information in the assessment of urothelial malignancy of the urinary bladder. Thus, cystoscopy permits visualization of any tumor extending into the lumen of the bladder and also allows for characterization of its configuration (papillary vs. solid or nodular), a determination of whether multiple tumors exist, evaluation of the character of the mucosa (areas of erythema either adjacent to the tumor or at various sites in the bladder) localization of the tumor in proximity to the bladder neck or the ureteral orifices, confirmation of the possible involvement of the proximal urethra, and estimation of the size of the presenting lesion(s).

Transurethral resection of any visible lesion(s) and biopsy of any abnormal area of the flat portion of the mucosa permits histologic characterization of the grade of disease, the extent to which it penetrates the wall of the bladder, and the extent to which the malignant diathesis involves the urothelial mucosa. Each of these characteristics is important in assessing the possibility of recurrence, and more importantly, of potential progression. This in turn will dictate the appropriate form of therapy.

Generally, low-grade, low-stage bladder cancers appear to be papillary, with fronds of proliferative epithelium surrounding a central and usually narrow fibrovascular stalk. Such tumors may be multiple, but the intervening mucosa of the bladder is generally characterized as having a normal appearance. A confluence of dilated vessels may appear adjacent to the tumor, suggesting that angiogenesis has occurred to support the proliferative growth of the epithelial cells. Resection of these lesions, with cauterization of the vessels in the fibrous stalk and of the tumor margin, generally results in effective elimination of that particular tumor.

There is a 50–75% chance that new tumors will subsequently appear (not necessarily at the initial tumor site, but at other sites in the bladder). The presentation of superficial disease in the form of multiple tumors indicates an increased likelihood that tumor recurrence will be seen. Intravesical treatments with various chemotherapeutic agents can be used effectively in preventing or limiting tumor recurrence and minimizing the rapidity with which such recurrence takes place.

Two theories have been proposed to explain the reason for tumor recurrence. One theory suggests the occurrence of field-effect changes that reflect earlier, and the possibility of ongoing processes of carcinogenesis throughout the bladder epithelium. The other theory suggests that clonal (stem cell) implantation from the primary tumor seeds other sites in the bladder for tumor development. Both theories have substantive experimental and clinical support, based on clinical observations and molecular studies that have characterized the genetic nature of the chromosomal defects in multiple concurrent tumors and tumors that have developed over a prolonged interval. Both mechanisms may account for tumor recurrence and must be considered in designing appropriate treatment approaches for both ongoing treatment and prophylaxis.

Generally, low-grade mucosally confined urothelial cancers, even if multiple, have only a 2–4% risk of progressing to a more advanced stage (i.e., more deeply penetrating the bladder wall). No additional treatment is needed for the solitary lesion. Even if recurrence takes place at interval cystoscopic examinations, additional resection or even simple electrocautery can effectively control disease. However, if recurrence is too frequent or if multiple tumors make complete resection and complete elimination of visible disease less feasible, adjunctive intravesical chemotherapy can minimize the rapidity and reduce the multiplicity of recurrence.

The most commonly used (and probably the safest) agents for treatment of low-moderate-grade mucosally confined tumors are thiotepa and mitomycin C. Thiotepa is generally instilled at a concentration of 30 mg/30 cm$^3$ water. The patient is instructed to retain the instilled medication for approx 1 h and then eliminate it through urination. Six weekly instillations are generally used, followed by surveillance cystoscopy 6 wk later. Since the thiotepa molecule is small enough to be absorbed systemically, thiotepa may have a myelosuppressive effect, producing a decrease in platelet and white blood-cell count. However, once treatment is discontinued, the bone marrow generally recovers from any myelosuppressive effect.

Mitomycin C is a larger molecule with limited absorption. It is instilled into the bladder in 6 weekly treatments of 40 mg/40 cm$^3$ water, and the patient is instructed each time to retain this medication for 1 h before expelling it. Surveillance cystoscopy and repeat urinary cytology examination are performed 6 wk thereafter. If extensive resection for multiple tumors has been performed, mitomycin usage may lead to extensive scarring and a contracted bladder, yet this is rare.

Some have suggested instillation of thiotepa or mitomycin in the immediate postresection period to decrease the possibility of recurrence by tumor-cell implantation. Both experimental and clinical evidence appear to support this approach. The potential value of such prophylactic treatment may prompt increased usage in future years, although it has not generally been adopted yet.

The combination of intravesical chemotherapy with periodic resection and electrofulguration is successful in preventing or minimizing recurrence in at least 50–70% of patients with mucosally confined disease. In these patients, the risk of progression is low. In some instances, maintenance therapy with monthly instillation of thiotepa or mitomycin has been used to further reduce the frequency of recurrence. If there is no recurrence for up to 2 yr of such maintenance therapy, the risk of subsequent recurrence is probably <10%. However, with frequent recurrence that is difficult to control, repeat upper-tract evaluation through imaging studies is indicated to exclude upper-tract disease as a possible source of recurrent urothelial tumors in the bladder.

Penetration by the tumor of the lamina propria represents a potentially more aggressive behavior of the cancer than that of the mucosally confined cancer diathesis. Such tumors are generally of higher grade. The cancer cells that have penetrated the basement membrane and the connective tissue matrix of the lamina propria also have the ability to penetrate the microvasculature and lymphatics that lie in the lamina propria. They can then seed (metastasize) to other organs. Such cancers generally appear to be of moderate or high grade rather than the low grade that characterizes mucosally confined disease. Moreover, they are often associated with high-grade flat CIS, immediately adjacent or at distant sites of the urothelium.

When such tumors have not penetrated the lamina propria deeply, their risk for recurrence with progression may still be as high as 30%. However, the risk that such lesions may progress in situations in which they penetrate the lamina propria deeply, or are accompanied by so-called flat CIS, can be as high as 50%. These tumors can appear endoscopically as papillary tumors that are virtually indistinguishable from the lower-grade mucosally confined papillary tumors described above. However, they may also have a somewhat more nodular appearance when more deeply invasive, particularly when accompanied by areas of erythema in the adjacent or distant urothelium that represent marked atypia or flat CIS, indicating a greater risk of progression.

The potentially aggressive nature of such tumors mandates a more aggressive therapeutic approach. Generally, intravesical chemotherapy with thiotepa or mitomycin is ineffective. Instead, an attenuated preparation of the tuberculosis Bacillus Calmette-Guérin (BCG) has been used to control recurrence of such disease and to eradicate CIS from the bladder in as many as 70% of cases. One ampule of attenuated BCG ($10^{9-11}$ organisms or 120 mg) mixed in 60 cm$^3$ of saline is instilled into the bladder, and 6 such weekly instillations are performed. The patient is instructed each time to retain the mixture for 1 h before voiding. Surveillance cystoscopy and repeat urinary cytology are performed 6 wk later. In the absence of a tumor—either endoscopically or by biopsy and urinary cytology—maintenance intravesical BCG can be used in a monthly schedule or in a "booster" schedule of 3 additional weekly instillations every 3 mo for 1 yr and then every 6 mo for another year. Toxicity of BCG may be significant. Bleeding and irritative symptoms are common. Fever is more unusual, but may require isoniazid treatment and cessation of BCG. BCG sepsis and death rarely occur. This is most common following traumatic catheterization or in the circumstance of active bleeding. Considerations of these toxicities have led to a reluctance to use BCG in low-grade mucosally confined "low-risk" disease.

A number of studies have demonstrated an initial efficacy rate as high as 70% for BCG in preventing recurrent disease. Whether ultimate prevention of recurrence and then progression is achieved, however, remains controversial. Certainly, such at-risk patients require compulsive surveillance with urinary cytology (every 3–6 mo), cystoscopy (at least every 6 months after the first 2–3 yr without recurrence), and upper-tract imaging every 2 yr. Patients who may be at risk for developing aggressive disease may express this risk as early as 6 mo after their initial presentation and BCG treatment. Thus, in assessing the grade and extent of penetration of a particular tumor into the lamina propria, it is important to consider whether a failure to respond to an initial course of intravesical BCG warrants a second 6-wk course of intravesical treatment or whether the patient is best served by undergoing cystectomy with the presumption that the disease is likely to progress rapidly, and that a window of opportunity for cure that is available at the time of initial disease presentation may rapidly close. When this type of risk is identified—particularly likely in the setting of high-grade lamina propria disease that is deeply invasive (even if repeat resection shows that it has not penetrated the muscularis propria), is accompanied by diffuse flat CIS, and fails to respond to BCG (with recurrent disease or persistently positive urinary cytology)—prompt cystectomy with inclusion of the distal ureters and possibly of the urethra (depending on the extent of involvement of the bladder neck by CIS) offers the greatest and possibly the only chance for a cure.

Although no successful markers exist for predicting the likelihood of progressive disease, several histologic features of a superficial tumor can be used to indicate an increased likelihood of such progression. For example, high-grade is more commonly associated with lamina propria-invasive disease than it is with mucosally confined disease (found in only 1–2% of cases). In addition, high-grade is often accompanied by diffuse flat CIS, itself an ominous prognostic factor. Invasion of the lamina propria is also an indication of a strong potential for progressive disease, and the depth of penetration may also have prognostic significance. If a tumor has only penetrated in small foci into the superficial component of the lamina propria, the risk of progression of this tumor diathesis is not as great as when a tumor has penetrated the lamina propria deeply and extends almost to the level of the muscularis propria.

A thin muscle layer known as the muscularis mucosae—which may either be well-developed or nearly inconspicuous as only a few wisps of muscle fibers—has been used as a landmark to distinguish between those tumors that are only superficially invasive vs. those that are deeply invasive of the lamina propria. Preliminary observations have suggested a correlation between the depth of penetration by these tumors and the likelihood of their progression. However, this correlation requires further study.

In addition, tumors that have penetrated the lamina propria deeply may have already penetrated the muscularis propria in at least 30% of instances. This represents an entirely different stage of disease, requiring prompt and aggressive surgical intervention.

Although none of the urinary tumor markers discussed previously have been validated to be indicative of the likelihood of progression, several *histological* markers have been studied for their potential value in predicting progression. For example, lamina propria-invasive tumors that have been found to stain positively for the presence of p53 (indicative of a defect in chromosome 17) have been associated with a potentially greater likelihood of progression. Similar observations have been made for muscle-invasive disease and the occurrence of metastases. The absence of expression of the retinoblastoma gene (Rb) in lamina propria-invasive tumors has also been associated with a greater possibility of progression. Other molecular markers that are believed to reflect abnormalities in oncogenes or tumor-suppressor genes are being explored for their usefulness in predicting which cancers are likely to express aggressive behavior and require earlier, more aggressive treatments.

## SUMMARY

The presentation of either gross or microscopic hematuria mandates the need to evaluate a patient for the possible existence of bladder cancer. The standard evaluation includes upper-tract imaging studies to exclude a nonmalignant condition or a urothelial malignancy of the upper tract, urinary cytology to sample cells shed from tumors anywhere along the urinary tract, and cystoscopy to evaluate the bladder for the possibility of a urothelial malignancy. A low-grade, low-stage urothelial malignancy of the bladder will go undetected by urinary cytology in as many as 50–70% of instances. The suggestion that a number of urinary substances may be useful as possible markers for the detection of urothelial malignancy requires validation. The most sensitive of these substances for low-grade disease include NMP22, telomerase, and fibrin-split products. However, each is susceptible to false-positive readings occasioned by inflammatory conditions or instrumentation. Endoscopy and histologic examination, complemented by urinary cytology, therefore remain the diagnostic procedures of choice in assessing a patient for the presence of a bladder tumor and evaluating its biologic potential.

Low-grade tumors generally have a papillary configuration and are mucosally confined. Although these present a substantial risk for recurrence, especially if multiple tumors are present at initial diagnosis, the risk for progression is low. Conservative approaches can therefore be used in their management, both therapeutically and prophylactically. On the other hand, moderate-high-grade tumors, often found to be invasive of the basement membrane and lamina propria, have a 30–50% risk of progressing, especially if associated with adjacent or distant flat CIS. These "superficial" cancers therefore need more intensive vigilance, and possibly aggressive intervention, if the response to conservative measures is incomplete. Assessment of such lesions by urinary cytology (which is sensitive and informative for the higher-grade lesions) and thorough histopathologic evaluation are needed to permit accurate evaluation of the cancer problem and determine appropriate intervention in a timely fashion.

In the future, it will be possible to construct molecular profiles for urothelial tumors on the basis of the detection of chromosomal abnormalities that permit prediction of biologic behavior of a particular tumor diathesis. Ultimately, such information may be translated into effective treatment approaches that may not only prevent tumor recurrence, but also possibly prevent progression.

## SELECTED READING

Abel PD (1993) Follow-up of patients with "superficial" transitional cell carcinoma of the bladder. The case for a change in policy. *Br J Urol* 72:135–142.
Bartsch H, Caporaso N, Coda M, et al. (1990) Carcinogen hemoglobin adducts, urinary mutagenicity, and metabolic phenotype in active and passive cigarette smokers. *J Natl Cancer Inst* 82:1826–1831.
Birch BRP, Harlands J (1989) The pT1G3 bladder tumour. *Br J Urol* 64:109–116.
Bostwick DG (1992) Natural history of early bladder cancer. *J Cell Biochem Suppl* 161:31–38.
Boyd PJR, Burnand KG (1974) Site of bladder tumor recurrence. *Lancet* 2:1290.
Droller MJ (1998) Commentary on Sarosdy, MF et al. Improved detection of recurrent bladder cancer using the Bard BTA test. *J Urol* 159:601.
Engel P, Anagnostaki L, Braendstrup O (1992) The muscularis mucosae of the human urinary bladder: implications for tumor staging on biopsies. *Scand J Urol Nephrol* 26: (Suppl) 249–252.
Gohji K, Nomi M, Okamoto M, et al. (1999) Conservative therapy for stage $T_{1b}$ grade 3 transitional cell carcinoma of the bladder. *Urology* 53:308.
Heney NM, Ahmed S, Flanagan MJ, et al. (1983) Superficial bladder cancer: progression and recurrence. *J Urol* 130:1083–1086.
Herr HW, Wartinger DD, Fair WR, et al. (1992) Bacillus Calmette-Guérin therapy for superficial bladder cancer: a ten-year follow-up. *J Urol* 147:1020–1023.
Holmang S, Hedelin H, Anderstrom C, Johansson SL (1995) The relationship among multiple recurrences, progression and prognosis of patients with stages $T_a$ and $T_1$ transitional cell cancer of the bladder followed for at least 20 years. *J Urol* 153:1823.
Howard RS, Golin AL (1991) Long-term follow-up of asymptomatic microhematuria. *J Urol* 145:335–336.
Huland E, Huland H, Meier T, et al. Comparison of 15 monoclonal antibodies against tumor-associated antigens of transitional cell carcinoma of the human bladder. Submitted for publication.
Jakse G, Loidl W, Seeber G, et al. (1987) Stage $T_1$ grade 3 transitional cell carcinoma of the bladder: an unfavorable tumor? *J Urol* 137:39–43.
Jones PA, Droller MJ (1993) Pathways of development and progression in bladder cancer: new correlations between clinical observations and molecular mechanisms. *Semin Urol* 11:177–192.
Kakizoe T, Matumoto J, Nishio Y, et al. (1985) Significance of carcinoma in situ and dysplasia in association with bladder cancer. *J Urol* 133:395–398.
Kavaler E, Landman J, Chang Y, et al. (1998) Detecting human bladder carcinoma cells in voided urine samples by assaying for the presence of telomerase activity. *Cancer* 82:708–714.
Kaye KW, Lange PH (1982) Mode of presentation of invasive bladder cancer. Reassessment of the problem. *J Urol* 128:31–33.
Lacombe L, Dalbagni G, Zhang ZF, et al. (1996) Overexpression of p53 protein in high-risk population of patients with superficial bladder cancer before and after bacillus Calmette-Guérin therapy: correlation to clinical outcome." *J Clin Oncol* 14(10):2646–2652.
Lamm DL (1992) Carcinoma in situ. *Urol Clin N Am* 19:499–508.
Lamm DL, Crawford ED, Blumenstein B, et al. (1992) Maintenance BCG immunotherapy of superficial bladder cancer: a randomized prospective Southwest Oncology Group Study (meeting abstract). *Proc Annu Meet Am Soc Clin Oncol* 11:A627. Abstract.
Lamm DL, Steg A, Boccon-Gibod L, et al. (1989) Complications of bacillus Calmette-Guérin immunotherapy: review of 2602 patients and comparison of chemotherapy complications. *Prog Clin Biol Res* 310:335–355.
Lamm DL, van der Meijden AP, Akaza H, et al. (1995) Intravesical chemotherapy and immunotherapy: how do we assess their effectiveness and what are their limitations and uses? *Int J Urol* 2 (Suppl 2):23–35.
Landis SH, Murray T, Bolden S, et al. (1998) Cancer statistics. 1998. *CA Cancer J Clin* 48:6–29.
Lokeshwar V, Phan H, Obeck C, et al. (1997) HA-HAase urine test for detecting bladder cancer and evaluating its grade. *J Urol* 157:(Suppl) 321.
Messing EM, Young TB, Hunt VB, et al. (1987) The significance of asymptomatic microhematuria in men 50 or more years old: findings of a home screening study using urinary dipsticks. *J Urol* 137:919–922.

Merz VW, Marth D, Kraft R, et al. (1995) Analysis of early failures after intravesical instillation therapy with bacille Calmette-Guérin for carcinoma in situ of the bladder. *Brit J Urol* 75:180.

Mihara K, Cao XR, Yen A, et al. (1989) Cell cycle-dependent regulation of phosphorylation of human RB gene product. *Science* 246:1300–1303.

Mommsen S, Barfod NM, Aagaard J (1985) N-acetyltransferase phenotypes in the urinary bladder carcinogenesis of a low-risk population. *Carcinogenesis* 6:199–201.

Murphy WM, Beckwith JB, Farrow GM (1994) Tumors of the kidney, bladder, and related urinary structures. In: *Atlas of Tumor Pathology,* Third Series, Fasicle II: AFIP, Washington, DC.

Norming J, Tribukait B, Nyman CR, et al. (1992) Prognostic significance of mucosal aneuploidy in stage $T_a/T_1$ grade 3 carcinoma of the bladder. *J Urol* 148:1420–1427.

Pansadoro V, Emiliozzi P, Defido, et al. (1995) Bacillus Calmette-Guérin in the treatment of stage $T_1$ grade 3 transitional cell carcinoma of the bladder: long-term results. *J Urol* 154:2054–2058.

Pollack MS, Pollack HM (1992) Intravenous urography and retrograde pyelography. In: Droller MJ, ed., *Surgical Management of Urologic Disease,* Mosby-Yearbook, St. Louis: pp. 87–110.

Sarosdy MF, deVere White RW, Soloway MS, et al. (1995) Results of a multicenter trial using the BTA test to monitor for and diagnose recurrent bladder cancer. *J Urol* 154:379–383.

Sarosdy MF, Hudson MA, Ellis WJ, et al. (1997) Improved detection of recurrent bladder cancer using the Bard BTA stat Test. *Urology* 50:349–353.

Schmetter BS, Habicht KK, Lamm DL, et al. (1997) A multicenter trial evaluation of the fibrin/fibrinogen degradation products test for detection and monitoring of bladder cancer. *J Urol* 158:801–805.

Sidransky D, Frost P, Von Eschenbach A, et al. (1992) Clonal origin of metachronous tumors of the bladder. *N Engl J Med* 326:737–740.

Soloway MS, Briggman V, Carpinito GA, et al. (1996) Use of a new tumor marker, urinary NMP22, in the detection of occult or rapidly recurring transitional cell carcinoma of the urinary tract following surgical treatment. *J Urol* 156:363–367.

Varkarakis MJ, Gaeta J, Moore RH, et al. (1974) Superficial bladder tumor: aspects of clinical progression. *Urology* 4:414–420.

Yeh HC (1992) Ultrasonography. In: MJ Droller, ed. *Surgical Management of Urologic Disease.* St. Louis: Mosby-Yearbook. pp. 111–139.

Zlotta AR, Noel JC, Fayt I, et al. (1999) Correlation and prognostic significance of p53, p21 and Ki67 expression in patients with superficial bladder tumors treated with bacillus Calmette-Guérin intravesical therapy. *J Urol* 161:792–798.

# 15 Intravesical Therapy for Superficial Bladder Cancer
*A Practical Guide*

## Michael O'Donnell, MD

**CONTENTS**

INTRODUCTION: ERADICATING THE WEEDS
FORMULATING A DISEASE-RISK ANALYSIS
TOXICITY OF INTRAVESICAL AGENTS
FINANCIAL ASPECTS
GENERAL MEASURES TO OPTIMIZE INTRAVESICAL THERAPY
EFFICACY CONSIDERATIONS
CHEMOTHERAPY FOR TUMOR PROPHYLAXIS
CHEMOTHERAPY FOR RESIDUAL DISEASE
CHEMOTHERAPY FOR CIS
CHEMOTHERAPY CROSSOVER
INTERFERON-ALPHA THERAPY
BCG FOR PROPHYLAXIS
BCG FOR ABLATION OF RESIDUAL DISEASE
BCG FOR CIS
EFFECT OF BCG ON TUMOR PROGRESSION
OPTIMIZING BCG THERAPY
RECOGNIZING AND TREATING BCG TOXICITY
OPTIONS FOR BCG FAILURES
CONCLUSION

## INTRODUCTION: ERADICATING THE WEEDS

If bladder cancer can metaphorically be thought of as weeds in the lawn, then transurethral surgery would be the equivalent of manually pulling out these weeds—an effective treatment as long as the numbers and sizes are relatively limited, the depth of the roots is relatively shallow, and the seeds of recurrence have not already been sown. A lawn rampantly overrun with weeds or one with weeds bearing very deep roots might require a more drastic solution, such as tearing up the lawn. In our metaphor,

From: *Current Clinical Urology: Office Urology: The Clinician's Guide*
Edited by: E. D. Kursh and J. C. Ulchaker © Humana Press Inc., Totowa, NJ

this would translate to the use of radical surgery, radiation, and/or systemic chemotherapy. Yet, as every successful lawn gardener knows, for intermediate situations the judicious local application of a weed-killer—be it chemical or more organic in origin—is superior to manual weeding alone. Analogously, this corresponds to the urologist's use of topical intravesical chemotherapy and immunotherapy for superficial bladder cancer. Just as there is both a science and an art to effective lawn care, so there is an appropriate set of guidelines for the application of intravesical therapy that may differ depending on the specific nature of the disease.

## FORMULATING A DISEASE-RISK ANALYSIS

Ultimately, two major things can go wrong in cases of superficial bladder cancer—it may recur/persist, or it may progress to invasive disease. The former is undoubtedly troubling to the patient and usually a prerequisite for the latter, but ultimately only progression is life-threatening. Thus, before embarking on a particular therapeutic program, the urologist must make an independent risk-assessment for tumor recurrence and progression to determine if it is even worthwhile to begin adjuvant therapy. This decision should be guided by a thorough appreciation of the risk factors associated with the presenting tumor histology (grade, stage, architecture, field effects, size, multifocility), previous tumor history (recurrence rate/year, cumulative years of tumor, recurrence types) as well as newer biochemical and/or genetic markers of aggressivity, many of which are not yet used in routine clinical practice (ploidy, Ki-67, p53, retinoblastoma, p21, E-cadherin, and so forth). As yet no algorithm can accurately define the risk for any single individual, but the confluence of these multiple parameters (*see* Table 1) can help guide the appropriateness and aggressiveness of therapy.

## TOXICITY OF INTRAVESICAL AGENTS

The inherent toxicity of the intravesical agent must also be carefully weighed in selecting and applying topical therapy. Most—but not all—agents cause a self-limiting cystitis that is usually transient but occasionally persists for weeks or months and in rare cases leads to a functionally contracted low-capacity bladder. Unique toxicities also exist for each agent (*see* Table 2). Among the chemotherapeutics, the small molecular-weight alkylating agent thiotepa, for instance, is most likely to lead to myelosuppression because of its more accessible transit through the bladder wall. Adriamycin (Doxorubicin), by contrast, is minimally absorbed but can cause a rare hypersensitivity reaction, whereas mitomycin C may cause a skin rash on the hands and genitalia. Valrubicin (a new lipophilic anthracycline derivative) has evoked no serious systemic toxicity thus far, but it has more limited cumulative clinical experience. The two readily available topical immunotherapeutic agents—Bacillus Calmette-Guérin (BCG) and Interferon-alpha—differ markedly in their side-effect profile. Irritative bladder symptoms are commonplace with BCG, yet remarkably absent with Interferon-alpha. Transient systemic flu-like reactions can occur with both. Because of the live nature of BCG—an attenuated strain of cow tuberculosis—systemic infection, though rare, can be devastating in occasional cases. BCG is thus contraindicated in immunosuppressed patients.

Table 1
Factors Increasing Risk of Tumor Recurence and/or Progression

| Low recurrence, low progression | Mod-high recurrence, increased progression | High recurrence, high progression |
|---|---|---|
| Low-grade | Medium-grade | High-grade |
|  |  | Grade progression during recurrence |
| Stage Ta (mucosal only) | Stage progression Ta to T1 | Stage T1 (submucosal invasion) |
| No dysplasia | Moderate-severe dysplasia | CIS |
| Negative cytology | Abnormal cytology | Highly suspicious or positive cytology |
| Solitary | Multifocal |  |
| Primary (first-time tumor) | Recurrent, especially within 3–6 mo or multi-recurrent |  |
| Papillary configuration |  | Sessile-nodular configuration |
| Size <5 cm | Size >5 cm |  |
| Short disease duration | Long (>4 yr) duration |  |
| Certainty of complete resection | Uncertainty of complete resection |  |
| No prior intravesical therapy | Failed prior intravesical therapy |  |
| Proliferation marker low, eg Ki-67 | Proliferation marker high |  |
| Normal DNA ploidy | Abnormal ploidy | Frank DNA aneuploidy |
| E-cadherin positive |  | E-cadherin negative |
| p53-negative |  | p53-positive |
| RB-positive |  | RB-negative |
| p21-positive |  | p21-negative |

## FINANCIAL ASPECTS

Given the acknowledged limitation of health-care resources and the current realities of medical reimbursement and capitation, it is no longer possible to ignore the financial aspects of intravesical therapy, especially if efficacy among certain agents is near equivalent. Although price-per-unit is a convenient guide for comparison, total cost-per-treatment course must consider the number of treatments for induction and maintenance and the actual dose used. Most agents are typically administered weekly for 6–8 repetitions during induction therapy, but evidence suggests that one single perioperative dose of chemotherapeutic agents may be just as effective. Additional maintenance therapy may be appropriate in some circumstances. What is not usually appreciated is that for all topical agents, once a minimal threshold volume is instilled, the concentration (dose per volume) is more important for efficacy than the actual dose. Thus, 30 mg of thiotepa in 30 cm$^3$ of sterile water (1 mg/mL) provides a surface concentration to the bladder equivalent to 60 mg in 60 cm$^3$. Higher total doses minimize dilution effects

Table 2
Toxicity of Intravesical Agents

| Agent | Toxicity | Frequency | Remarks |
|---|---|---|---|
| Thiotepa | Cystitis | 15–30% | Least irritative of chemotherapeutics |
|  | Myelosuppression | 10–20% | Increased absorption from traumatized bladder |
|  |  |  | Weekly WBC and platelet count recommended; rare leukemia |
| Ethoglucid | Cystitis | 30–40% | 16% require cessation of therapy |
|  | Myelosuppression | 4% | Decreased bladder capacity in up to 20%; rarely permanent |
| Adriamycin | Cystitis | 30–50% | Moderate-severe cystitis not uncommon |
|  | Gross hematuria | 30% | ~10% require cessation of therapy |
|  | Hypersensitivity-anaphylaxis | <0.5% | Rare permanent bladder contracture |
| Epirubicin | Cystitis | <10% | Better tolerated than adriamycin |
| Mitomycin C | Cystitis | 20–40% | ~10% require cessation of therapy |
|  | Rash (genital and palmer) | 5–10% | Decreased bladder capacity in up to 20%; rarely permanent |
|  | Myelosuppression | 1% | Rare death from aplastic anemia |
| Valrubicin | Cystitis | >50% | Local irritative symptoms usually resolve within 7 d |
|  |  |  | ~5% require cessation of therapy |
| BCG | Cystitis–transient | 80–90% | Frequency and intensity increase with longer dosing |
|  | Cystitis–prolonged | 10–20% | ~10% require cessation of therapy |
|  | Gross Hematuria | 30–40% |  |
|  | Systemic effects (fever, chills, malaise) | 30–60% | Usually transient <48 h |
|  | Infectious sequele |  |  |
|  | Local (prostatitis; epid-orchitis) | 1–2% | Histological prostatitis in >40%, often not symptomatic |
|  | Distant (hepatitis; pneumonitis) | 1–2% | Sepsis usually result of trauma |
|  | BCG sepsis | 0.40% | 10 deaths reported/~20 yr |
|  | Reiter's syndrome | <0.5% | Hypersensitivity phenomenon |
| Interferon-alpha | Systemic effects (fever, chills, malaise) | 0–20% | Easily controlled w/acetaminophen, NSAIDs |
|  |  |  | Usually transient <48 h |

Table 3
Dose, Concentration, and Approximate Wholesale Cost of Intravesical Agents[a]

| Agent | Dose | Concentration | Cost/dose |
|---|---|---|---|
| Thiotepa | 30–60 mg | 1 mg/mL | $190/30 mg |
| Adriamycin | 50–90 mg | 1–2 mg/mL | $40/50 mg |
| Mitomycin | 20–40 mg | 1 mg/mL | $200/20 mg[b] |
| Valrubicin | 800 mg | 11 mg/mL | $1200/800 mg |
| BCG | 50–81 mg TICE/Connaught | 1–1.5 mg/mL ~$1 \times 10^{-7}$ CFU/mL | $140/vial |
| Interferon-alpha | 50–100 MU | 1–2 MU/mL | $500/50 MU |

[a]Based on 1999 quote from national distributor in the United States (further bulk reductions may apply).
[b]Recently generic in the United States.

during bladder dwell-time, but could result in higher toxicity in the case of an unrecognized bladder perforation. A listing of approximate unit costs and recommended concentrations is provided in Table 3.

## GENERAL MEASURES TO OPTIMIZE INTRAVESICAL THERAPY

To facilitate catheter placement and produce urine for examination or culture, the patient should be asked to come to the office with some urine in their bladder. To minimize the dilution effects of continued urine production, the patient is advised to limit fluid intake for 6–10 h prior to treatment (which conveniently works out as an overnight fast if treatment is given in the morning) and during the usual 2-h dwell time. Caffeine and alcohol should be avoided, since both have diuretic and irritant properties. Patients with significant baseline bladder instability or low bladder capacity may also benefit from the use of a single application of oral or nasal vasopressin 1 h prior to therapy and/or an anticholinergic, such as sublingual hyoscyamine. In very severe cases, oral narcotics can help with retention time.

Catheters should be appropriate for the individual patient, with the curved-tip coudé style most likely to minimize trauma in the male patient. A generous amount of water-soluble lubricant with or without topical anesthetic facilitates catheter placement, but may impede gravity drainage—a situation easily remedied by gentle aspiration of the catheter. An attempt should be made to completely empty the bladder, using gentle Credé pressure to minimize dilution of the drug by residual urine and flush out residual lubricant. Balloon inflation of the catheter is usually not required.

Instillation of the drug is best performed by gravity at a height of <30 cm. If a plunger syringe must be used, then very slow injection over 2–3 min should be given to avoid high-pressure intravasation or inducing a bladder spasm. Occasionally, despite these precautions, an uninhibited bladder contraction may occur. When this happens, no attempt should be made to restrict outflow, as this can also lead to intravascular delivery.

The practice of rotating patients to different positions during the 2-h detention time has not proven beneficial, and is only of theoretical benefit if there is a significant air bubble in the bladder in the setting of a dome lesion. Normal ambulatory activity is just as likely to disperse the drug evenly. Forced fluid consumption posttherapy may not be beneficial, as it may rapidly dilute out therapeutic drug and/or bioactive immune mediators induced by the treatment. Normal thirst-mediated fluid consumption is preferable.

## EFFICACY CONSIDERATIONS

The ability to keep a patient free from disease over time remains the single most important consideration in selecting the appropriate intravesical agent. In general, intravesical agents have three major indications: prophylaxis for recurrence after the entire tumor has been surgically removed; ablation of residual measurable tumor; and primary therapy for carcinoma *in situ* (CIS). Of course, macroscopic removal of all visible tumor may still leave microscopic foci of viable tumor that requires the ablative effects of the agent. Also, patients with mixed CIS and papillary disease depend on both ablative and prophylactic properties. Nonetheless, these categories form a convenient basis to compare the efficacy results of different agents. A more important consideration is the ability of these agents to prevent disease progression, and ultimately, to improve patient survival.

Ideally, when used for tumor prophylaxis, intravesical therapy should result in the complete elimination of tumor recurrence over a patient's lifetime. However, even extending freedom from disease for several years can be a tangible benefit to the patient in terms of decreasing anesthesia-dependent operations, office procedures, and psychological distress. What is much less clear is whether altering the recurrence rate or the number of tumors per recurrence alone is worthwhile, especially if uncertainty continues to mandate frequent cystoscopies and ultimate progression is not altered. The situation with ablative therapy for either visible tumor or CIS is more straightforward. Generally only a complete response—total cancer elimination with negative cytology— is clinically significant, although conversion of an aggressive subtype such as stage T1, grade 3 to a nonaggressive subtype (stage Ta, grade 1–2) may have some practical meaning. It must also be remembered that all forms of ablative intravesical therapy work best when the tumor burden is minimal. Thus, it is always best to eliminate as much of the visible tumor as possible using transurethral surgery, even if a second cleanup procedure is required.

## CHEMOTHERAPY FOR TUMOR PROPHYLAXIS

### *Modest Net Benefit*

Numerous controlled studies over the past three decades have examined the ability of various intravesical chemotherapeutic agents to prevent or retard the recurrence of the low- to intermediate-grade mucosal (stage Ta) and submucosal (stage T1) papillary tumor after presumed initial definitive transurethral resection of the bladder tumor (TURB). In aggregate, a net benefit vs. surgery alone has been proven, but the degree of benefit has been modest. For the commonly applied chemotherapeutic agents in use in the United States (thiotepa, adriamycin, and mitomycin), Lamm summarized the results of 21 studies involving over 3400 patients, and reported that the net benefit over TURB alone was only 12, 13, and 15%, respectively. Furthermore, when disease progression was examined, no statistical advantage could be shown. Similar results have been reported from a formal meta-analysis involving over 2500 patients participating in six controlled studies conducted by the Medical Research Council (MRC) in Great Britain and the European Organization for Research and Treatment of Cancer (EORTC). At 5 yr, only a 6% difference in freedom from disease for chemotherapy vs. TURB alone was shown, but no clear short-term delay in time to first recurrence. More importantly, no statistical benefit was seen for disease progression, which averaged 12% for the treated group and 9% for the TURB-alone group.

### *No Clear Superiority Among Agents*

As the results from Lamm's bulk-summary analysis indicate, no intravesical chemotherapeutic agent shows a clear advantage over another. Randomized comparative trials have confirmed this with Huland (1983) and Akaza (1992) showing equivalence between mitomycin and adriamycin; Zincke (1985), Flanigan (1986), and Zhang (1995) reporting equivalence between mitomycin and thiotepa; and Llopis (1985), Martinez (1990), and Bouffioux (1992) showing no difference between adriamycin and thiotepa. Valrubicin, a recently approved derivative of adriamycin, has not yet been subjected to comparative trials. The results of two other drugs used in Europe—Ethoglucid and Epirubicin—essentially parallel those of thiotepa and adriamycin, respectively. It is possible that certain subgroups may benefit more from one agent than another. For instance, thiotepa appears to work best on low-grade, low-stage bladder tumors with a low potential for progression. There is some evidence that mitomycin may be marginally superior to thiotepa for higher-grade tumors. However, no strong data currently exists to justify the choice of one chemotherapeutic agent over another based on efficacy considerations alone. Moreover, despite the theoretical appeal of combination chemotherapy, limited studies using both mitomycin and adriamycin have not proven this combination to be more effective than either agent alone.

### *Immediate Perioperative Use*

Although the majority of intravesical chemotherapeutic studies have followed the conventional practice of delaying therapy until at least 1–2 wk following TURB, an emerging body of data suggests that one perioperative dose of chemotherapy (NEVER BCG)—given within 1 h of TURB but up to 24 h later—may be of similar effectiveness. The rationale for this approach is that many recurrences are caused by tumor-cell reimplantation that results from cells released during TURB—a hypothesis supported by the observations of Soloway (1983) on bladder-dome recurrences and the genetic studies of Sidransky (1990) showing that most multifocal tumors are of clonal origin. Not surprisingly, all chemotoxic agents appear to be effective in the perioperative setting, although one large-scale study using more dilute thiotepa failed to show statistical significance (*see* Table 4). Of course, perioperative dosing would be inappropriate if a bladder perforation or significant bleeding occurred. Similarly, considering the enhanced transit of thiotepa through the traumatized bladder wall, this agent might not be ideal in the presence of a large denuded surface where up to 50% absorption of the drug has been documented. A 1-h dwell-time appears sufficient in most cases, and adverse events are infrequent. This author places a three-way Foley catheter that remains clamped for 1 h with the drug while minimizing intravenous fluid administration. After unclamping the catheter and releasing the medication, the bladder is rinsed out with a brisk liter of sterile water and then removed. Patients are discharged home as per the usual routine. The cost advantage to this approach is obvious. Furthermore, once final

## Table 4
## Clinical Trials of Recurrence after Immediate Perioperative Chemotherapy

| Author | Year | Number | Agent | Dose | Initiation | Dwell time | TURB | ChemoRx | Net benefit | Follow-up | Statistics | Toxicity | Remarks |
|---|---|---|---|---|---|---|---|---|---|---|---|---|---|
| Burnand | 1976 | 51 | Thiotepa | 90 mg/100 cm$^3$ | Immediate | 30 min | 97% | 58% | 39% | 2–5 yr | Signif vs. TUR | 5% decr WBC | Additional TT after recurrence not useful |
| Abrams | 1981 | 57 | Adriamycin | 50 mg/50 cm$^3$ | ~24 h | 30 min | 89% | 79% | 10% | 6 mo | NS | 21% cystitis | 33% patients showed improvement vs. TUR |
| Zincke | 1983 | 89 | Thiotepa | 60 mg/60 cm$^3$ | Immediate | 30 min | 71% | 30% | 41% | 3–4 mo | Signif vs. TUR | None | Best for recurrent, multifocal, papillary, lower-grade tumors w/o CIS |
|  |  |  | Adriamycin | 50 mg/50 cm$^3$ | Immediate | 30 min | | 32% | 39% | 3–4 mo | Signif vs. TUR | None | Additional treatment of no benefit |
| Kurth | 1983 | 130 | Ethoglucid | 1.1 g/100 cm$^3$ | ~24 h | 60 min | 96% | 93% | 3% | 4–8 yr | NS | None | Not randomized; lower recurrence rate with treatment; all multifocal or multirecurrent stage Ta, grade 1 tumors |
| M.R.C. | 1985 | 367 | Thiotepa | 30 mg/50 cm$^3$ | I: Immediate- <24 h II: plus q 3 mo × 4 | Not stated | 25% | I: 32% II: 30% | –7% –5% | 1–2 yr | NS | 3% cystitis | All primary; most low-grade and stage |
| Zincke | 1985 | 83 | Thiotepa | 60 mg/60 cm$^3$ | Immediate | 30 min | | 29% | | 16 mo (med) | NS; TT = MMC | 3% cystitis | Included 5 q wk Rxs after initiation |
|  |  |  | Mitomycin | 40 mg/40 cm$^3$ | Immediate | 30 min | | 33% | | | | 10% cystitis | |
| Oosterlinck | 1993 | 431 | Epirubicin | 80 mg/50 cm$^3$ | Immediate- <6 h | 60 min | 41% | 29% | 12% | 2 yr (mean) | Signif vs. TUR | 10% cystitis 3% other | Effective in all subgroups Progression same |
| Bouffioux | 1995 | 834 pooled stats 2 studies | Mitomycin Adriamycin Mitomycin Adriamycin | 30 mg/50 cm$^3$ 50 mg/50 cm$^3$ | Immediate- <24 h 1–2 wk delay | 60 min 60 min 60 min 60 min | Early maintenance (EM) = Early no maintenance (ENM) = Delayed maintenance (DM) –47% vs. delayed no maintenance (DNM) –56% | | | 2.8 yr | NS NS NS Signif worse | 7–9% cystitis 7% other | All received additional q wk × 4; q mo × 5 Additionally randomized +/– q mo × 6 maintenance |
| Tolley | 1996 | 452 | Mitomycin | 40 mg/40 cm$^3$ | Immediate- <24 h + addt'l q 3 mo × 4 | 60 min | 60% | 45% 37% | 15% 23% | 7 yr (med) | Signif vs. TUR NS: 1 vs. 5 Rxs | 0% cystitis 6% cystitis | Effective in all subgroups No progression benefit |
| Rajala | 1999 | 200 | Epirubicin Interferon-A | 100 mg/100 cm$^3$ 50 MU/100 cm$^3$ | Immediate | 2 h | 60% | 44% 63% | 16% None | ~2 yr | Signif vs. TUR NS vs. TUR | 6% cystitis 6% fever | Epirubicin effective in all subgroups |
| Solsona | 1999 | 121 | Mitomycin | 30 mg/50 cm$^3$ | Immediate- <6 h | 60 min | 54% | 40% | 14% | 94 mo (med) | Signif vs. TUR | 4% cystitis | Similar advantage at all time points All solitary, low-grade, low-recurrent |

histology is available, the urologist retains the option of either continuing chemotherapy or initiating alternative therapy, such as BCG, in the usual delayed fashion.

### *Role of Maintenance Chemotherapy*

The utility of extended treatment with chemotherapy remains controversial. Although many clinical studies have employed this strategy, few have actually investigated whether this approach is helpful. From a theoretical standpoint, once surgical and chemotherapeutic ablation is achieved, the addition of further toxic therapy should be unnecessary. Moreover, the intrinsic carcinogenicity of the chemotherapeutic agents themselves has been demonstrated in rodent models although it has not been proven to occur during clinical use. In his comprehensive review of chemotherapy trials, Lamm (1994) found no clear evidence that maintenance therapy has an efficacy benefit. Flamm (1990) and Rubben (1988) found that both short-term and long-term adriamycin courses offered similar efficacy. Huland (1990) and Akaza (1987) demonstrated the same result for mitomycin in prospective multicenter studies. Some clarification is given by a report by Bouffioux (1995) examining the combined results of two separate EORTC chemotherapy studies using mitomycin or adriamycin. He found that maintenance therapy was only beneficial if given after the typical delayed practice of starting chemotherapy 1–2 wk after TURB, but added nothing to therapy initiated at the time of TURB. Simply put: earlier is better than later, and maintenance is unnecessary in the early setting. Bouffioux's report further emphasizes the advantage of perioperative dosing.

## CHEMOTHERAPY FOR RESIDUAL DISEASE

Although the goal should be to surgically ablate all visible disease, this is not always possible because of tumor location, tumor diffuseness, and underlying patient comorbidity. In the therapeutic setting, many intravesical chemotherapeutic agents have demonstrated ablative activity. Complete responses for thiotepa average between 30 and 40%, work best against smaller tumors, and are least effective against tumors that have already failed prior thiotepa. Adriamycin may be slightly more active than thiotepa. It appears to be more effective for recurrent tumors than primary tumors, is equally effective on low- and high-grade tumors, and works against prior thiotepa failures. Interestingly, Epirubicin—a derivative of adriamycin—has been reported to be more effective against primary and chemotherapy naive tumors. Complete response rates with mitomycin have generally been higher than the other agents, averaging ~50%, with even higher responses reported in marker lesion studies. Only a few studies have examined the utility of routine up-front chemoablation with mitomycin prior to an inspection cystoscopy with optional TURB. Unfortunately, early recurrences occurred in nearly 60% of these patients, suggesting that there is no clear advantage to this strategy.

## CHEMOTHERAPY FOR CIS

Short-term complete response rates for chemotherapeutic agents parallel their ablative efficacies against papillary tumors, with thiotepa the least active and mitomycin displaying the greatest efficacy. However, longer-term follow-up suggests that thiotepa and adriamycin should not be recommended as front-line therapy for patients with CIS. Despite intensive therapy with thiotepa, most patients progressed to muscle invasion or metastasis within 3 yr. Studies using adriamycin against CIS have reported median times to recurrence as low as 6 mo, with only 20% of patients disease-free at 3 yr. By contrast, mitomycin—especially when used with at least a 6-mo maintenance regimen—appears to be more effective long-term, with most patients disease-free at 2 yr and 30–40% disease-free at 5 yr.

## CHEMOTHERAPY CROSSOVER

In general, once a patient has failed one chemotherapy drug, there is a reduced likelihood that a different agent will be effective. However, this practice has not been rigorously studied for tumor prophylaxis. Several trials of mitomycin or adriamycin for thiotepa-failure patients in the ablative setting have shown responses in the 30–40% range, suggesting that this strategy may be worthwhile. However, BCG immunotherapy usually becomes the next treatment of choice.

## INTERFERON-ALPHA THERAPY

Although clinical experience using interferon-alpha as an intravesical agent dates back over 13 yr, its high cost and reduced efficacy compared to both chemotherapy and BCG have kept it from achieving widespread use. Comparative trials reveal it to be slightly less active than mitomycin and Epirubicin, and clearly inferior to BCG for prophylaxis in the short term, with most patients relapsing within 1–2 yr. It does not seem to work well against stage T1 tumors and is not effective as a single perioperative dose. Complete responses in CIS approximate 40%, but doses in the range of 50–100 million units are required. Of all the intravesical agents, it has the most favorable local toxicity profile. It may be useful as a salvage agent in chemotherapy and BCG failures, or in combination with BCG.

## BCG FOR PROPHYLAXIS

### *Superiority to Chemotherapy?*

Most studies suggest that BCG is superior to chemotherapy for tumor prophylaxis after TURB. An aggregate analysis of nine contemporary BCG trials involving over 1000 patients with papillary disease randomized to BCG versus TURB alone reveals a net benefit of approx 31%, roughly twice that reported for chemotherapy (*see* Table 5). BCG is also highly effective in patients who have failed prior chemotherapy. Moreover, most trials directly comparing BCG to chemotherapy have also shown a significant advantage to BCG (*see* Table 6). However, mytomycin C remains controversial. Two independent Dutch trials (Vegt, 1995 and Witjes, 1998) in particular suggest the equivalence or even superiority of mitomycin over BCG for recurrent tumors in the absence of CIS. The reason for this discrepancy with the results of several other large-scale studies is not entirely clear. In the Dutch studies, treatment schedules for both BCG and mitomycin were different and patient selection was more biased toward lower-risk patients. The observation that fewer and less severe side effects were found in mitomycin treatment arms has not been disputed. Given the current ambiguity, mitomycin remains an appropriate first-line therapeutic option in low- to intermediate-risk patients.

Table 5
Tumor Recurrence After TURB with or Without BCG (Non-CIS)

| Author | Year | Number | TURB | BCG | Net benefit | Follow-up | Statistics | BCG regimen | Remarks |
|---|---|---|---|---|---|---|---|---|---|
| Lamm | 1985 | 57 | 52% | 20% | 32% | 30 mo | Favor BCG | q wk × 6; late addition maint BCG q 3–6 mo | Crossover for ~1/3 control median relapse 24 vs. 48 mo |
| Rubben | 1990 | 77 | 42% | 35% | 7% |  | NS |  | Biased toward low grade, stage |
| Pagano | 1991 | 133 | 83% | 26% | 57% | 21 mo | Favor BCG | q wk × 6; repeat if NR; q mo × 1 yr; q 4 mo × 1 yr | 1/2 dose BCG Progression 17% vs. 4% BCG |
| Melekos | 1993 | 94 | 59% | 32% | 27% | 32 mo | Favor BCG | q wk × 6 + 4 (high-risk); q 3 mo × 2 yr; q 6 mo | Progression 12% vs. 3% BCG NS |
| Yang | 1994 | 97 | 65% | 34% | 31% | 70 mo | Favor BCG | Not specified |  |
| Zhang | 1995 | 160 | 46% | 18% | 28% | 1–7 yr | Favor BCG | Not specified |  |
| Krege | 1996 | 224 | 46% | 26% | 20% | 20 mo | Favor BCG | q wk × 6; q mo × 4 | Progression 6% vs. 4.5% BCG NS |
| Tkachuk | 1996 | 180 | 43% | 13% | 30% | 3 yr | Favor BCG | q wk × 8; q mo × 1 yr |  |
| Iantorno | 1999 | 146 | 100% | 62% | 38% | 55 mo | Favor BCG | q wk × 6; q mo × 1 yr | 1/2 dose BCG progression 10%, equal, NS |
| TOTAL |  | 1168 | 60% | 29% | 31% |  |  |  |  |

Table 6
Comparative Clinical Trials of Tumor Recurrence After BCG or Chemotherapy (Non-CIS)

| Author | Year | Number | TURB | Thio-tepa | Adr/Epi | Mito-mycin | BCG | Follow-up | Statistics | Remarks |
|---|---|---|---|---|---|---|---|---|---|---|
| Brosman | 1982 | 44 | | 47% | | | 0% | >24 mo | Favor BCG | Intensive 2-yr regimens |
| Tachibana | 1989 | 77 | | | 73% (A) | | 27% | 3 yr | Favor BCG | ? randomized trial |
| Martinez | 1990 | 176 | | 36% | 43% (A) | | 13% | 3 yr | Favor BCG | ~3 × decrease recurrence index |
| Rintala | 1991 | 91 | | | | 62% | 36% | 21 mo | Favor BCG | ~3 × decrease recurrence index |
| Lamm | 1991 | 131 | | | 83% (A) | | 63% | 65 mo | Favor BCG | Median relapse 10 vs. 23 mo |
| Lamm | 1995 | 377 | | | | 54% | 40% | 30 mo | Favor BCG | Median relapse 18 vs. 36 mo |
| Zhang | 1995 | 385 | 46% | 31% | | 30% | 18% | 1–7 yr | Favor BCG | ? randomized trial |
| Melekos | 1993/96 | 161 | 59% | | 46% (E) | | 35% | 33 mo | NS | BCG greatest benefit for T1Gr#3 |
| Krege | 1996 | 337 | 46% | | | 27% | 26% | 20 mo | NS | 2 year Rx w/MMC; 6 mo w/BCG |
| Vegt | 1995 | 387 | | | | 43% | 46% RIVM<br>64% TICE | 36 mo | NS | MMC × 6 mo w/3 Rxs for recurrence |
| Witjies | 1998 | 344 | | | | 47% | 64% | 7.2 yr | Favor MMC | BCG q wk × 6; repeat if recur <6 mo<br>Weighted toward lower stage and grade |
| Malmstrom | 1999 | 187 | | | | 66% | 57% | 64 mo | NS | Intensive 2 yr course for MMC and BCG<br>Greatest benefit for higher-stage and grade |

## BCG FOR ABLATION OF RESIDUAL DISEASE

The ablative effects of BCG on residual papillary tumors range from 55 to 65% as validated by multiple studies. As with chemotherapy, superior responses occur when the total tumor burden is small—usually under 3 cm.

## BCG FOR CIS

BCG has become the treatment of choice for CIS because of its high initial complete response rate (averaging between 70% and 75% if up to two induction cycles are used) and its durability (median duration of response >4 yr). It appears to work equally well for primary and secondary CIS, and is also effective for chemotherapy failures.

## EFFECT OF BCG ON TUMOR PROGRESSION

Although it extends disease-free survival, even BCG has not clearly demonstrated a decrease in tumor progression. Small numbers, low intrinsic progression rates, and insufficient long-term follow-up may be responsible, but it is noteworthy that even in several larger comparative BCG/chemotherapy trials previously mentioned, no absolute differences—or statistical differences—have been observed. Where apparent improvements in progression have been reported, statistical significance was either not achieved (Lamm, 1980; Martinez, 1990; Melekos, 1993), or follow-up was too short (Pagano 1991). The strongest published evidence has come from a study performed by Herr (1988) in a randomized series of 86 patients with aggressive superficial bladder cancers, 88% of which had coincident CIS. In this very high-risk group, BCG therapy delayed tumor progression and prolonged short-term survival. At 5 yr, progression to muscle invasion/metastasis was significantly improved, from 58% in TURB controls to 74% in BCG-treated patients. Survival was also superior: 84 vs. 64%, respectively. Unfortunately, these benefits were ultimately lost because of later recurrence and/or progression occurring over the next 10 yr of follow-up, often outside the bladder vault (Cookson, 1997). Although it can be argued that crossover of TURB controls to BCG treatment and nonoptimized BCG regimens makes definitive conclusions impossible, the evidence that BCG alters ultimate progression and disease-specific bladder cancer survival has yet to be established.

## OPTIMIZING BCG THERAPY

Given the complex immune mechanism underlying BCG efficacy plus the arbitrary foundation upon which the original 6-wk BCG treatment regimen was set up, a substantial potential remains for improving therapy. Percutaneous scarification given simultaneously with intravesical BCG has been shown to be ineffective, and should not be used. Several studies have now shown that a single 6-wk course of BCG is suboptimal; a second course can salvage up to 50–60% of initial nonresponders (Haaff, 1986; Jakse, 1989; Pagano, 1991; Hurle, 1996). However, the mere increase in the number of treatments does not seem to be responsible because 12 sequential weeks is actually less effective than two 6-wk courses separated by 6–12 wk. Along these same lines, prospective studies (Badalament, 1987; Hudson, 1987) specifically investigating monthly or quarterly maintenance therapy failed to demonstrate an efficacy advantage, but toxicity was understandably higher. By contrast, an alternative maintenance schedule

(Lamm, 1999) consisting of sequential minicourses of three weekly treatments given at 3 mo, 6 mo, and then every 6 mo for up to 3 yr has been shown to statistically significantly increase the complete response rate at 6 mo from 68 to 84% for CIS—roughly double the median recurrence-free survival from 36 to 77 mo—and decrease the chance of bladder-cancer related worsening from 76 to 70%. There was also a 5-yr survival improvement trend in favor of maintenance from 78 to 83%. However, only 16% of patients randomized to receive maintenance therapy could complete all planned courses because of toxicity, suggesting less intensive schemes may also be beneficial.

Efforts to decrease BCG toxicity while maintaining or enhancing efficacy are currently being studied. Several recent clinical trials have shown that decreasing the dose of BCG to one-half or one-third in the induction phase will lower the local toxicity, but controversy exists regarding whether efficacy is sacrificed, especially in the more high-risk CIS and stage T1, grade 3 patients (*see* Table 7). This dispute may be partially the result of differences in various patient-population sensitivity to BCG, either genetically or from prior BCG immunization. For instance, US and Canadian populations are rarely vaccinated with BCG, yet this practice was—and is—still commonly used throughout much of the world. The routine use of reinduction courses and extended maintenance regimens may also make up for a weaker induction course. However, until this controversy is resolved, a more sensible approach may be to reduce the dose during the maintenance phase to increase treatment tolerability. Finally, at least one preliminary report (Bassi, 1999) indicates that biweekly (every 2 wk) BCG dosing for low-intermediate risk patients may be as effective as the conventional weekly dosing scheme, but with reduced side effects.

## RECOGNIZING AND TREATING BCG TOXICITY

The toxic effects of BCG may occur both locally and systemically. The vast majority of patients experience a self-limited cystitis associated with marked frequency, urgency, and dysuria that escalates with later treatments. Symptoms usually begin 2–4 h after instillation, peak between 6 and 10 h, and resolve rapidly over the next 24–48 h. Microscopic hematuria and pyuria are common, and occasional gross hematuria and passage of "tissue" (actually white-cell clots) also occur. Systemic manifestation of the inflammatory response follows a similar time course and includes fevers, chills, a flu-like malaise, and occasional arthralgias. During reinduction or maintenance cycles, all of these symptoms tend to be more intense, occur sooner after the instillation, and reach the highest level by the second or third treatment. Most symptoms can be controlled with the appropriate use of acetaminophen, nonsteroidal antiinflammatories (NSAIDs), urinary analgesics, and antispasmodics. The practice of routinely administering antibiotics with catheterization should be discouraged. If clinically indicated for non-BCG infection, penicillins, cephalosporins, trimethoprim/sulfa, and nitrofurantoin are preferable, but fluoroquinolones, azithromycin, and doxycycline should be avoided because they are cidal to BCG and could affect efficacy. Conversely, short courses of anti-BCG-specific antibiotics, such as isoniazid (INH) and rifampin, have not been proven to diminish either the associated symptomatology or the incidence of serious BCG infection.

Clinical signs of a more serious process, such as BCG intravasation into the bloodstream, (BCGosis), include any exaggerated manifestations of the above systemic

## Table 7
## BCG Dose Reduction Trials

| Author | Year | Number | BCG Strain | Standard | Low | Follow-up | Efficacy @ F/U | Toxicity | BCG schedule | Remarks |
|---|---|---|---|---|---|---|---|---|---|---|
| Rintalla | 1989 | 36 Ta/T1<br>10 CIS | Pasteur | | 75 mg (1/2) | 26 mo (mean) | 7-fold decr preRx Recr Rate | Dropout 19%<br>no BCGitis | q wk × 4; q mo × 2 yr | Better than MMC for Ta/T1<br>Not superior to MMC for CIS |
| Blumenstein | 1990 | 136 CIS | Connaught | 120 mg | N/A | 65 mo (med) | 45% NED @ 5 yr | | q wk × 6; q 6 mo × 2 yr | No efficacy difference despite 23-fold variation in lot CFUs |
| Pagano | 1991 | 70 Ta/T1 pap<br>12 T1 nodular<br>44 CIS | Pasteur | | 75 mg (1/2) | 21 mo (mean) | 74% NED vs. 17% TUR<br>33% NED<br>64% NED | Severe cystitis 5%<br>Temp >102 17%<br>No BCGitis | q wk × 6; repeat if NR; q mo × 1 yr | Second course effective in 50–69% of first failures |
| Rivera | 1993 | 108 T1 Gr2,3 | Japanese | | 1 mg | 37 mo (mean) | 81% NED | None severe | q wk × 4; q 2 wk × 4; q mo × 1 yr | Very low dose |
| Mack | 1995 | 25 Ta/T1 "high-risk" | Connaught | | 27 mg (1/3) | 31 mo (mean) | 84% NED | No systemic<br>Occasional severe local | q wk × 6; q mo × 1 yr | |
| Hurle | 1996 | 51 T1 Gr3 | Pasteur | | 75 mg (1/2) | 33 mo (med) | 55% NED | Severe cystitis 4%<br>Fever 14%<br>No BCGitis | q wk × 6; repeat if NR; q mo × 1 yr | Second course effective in 54%<br>14% progression |
| Morales | 1992 | 97 Ta/T1/CIS | Armand-Frappier | 120 mg | 60 mg (1/2) | 21 mo (mean) | 67% NED std dose<br>37% NED low-dose | Decreased toxicity from 33% to 12% w/low dose | q wk × 6 | Low dose especially worse for CIS with T1 |
| Takasi | 1995 | 74 Ta/T1 | Tokyo 172 | 80 mg | 40 mg (1/2) | NS | Untreated BTs-no difference<br>Pretreated BTs-std better | Lower toxicity w/lower dose | q wk × 8 | Retrospective study |
| Martinez | 1995 | 381 Ta/T1<br>33 CIS | Connaught | 81 mg | 27 mg (1/3) | 19 mo (mean) | Std/low 82% vs. 80% NED<br>CIS 92% vs. 69% NED<br>Prog 2.4% vs. 4.8% | Severe local 23% vs. 4%<br>Fever 27% vs. 13%<br>Pulmonary 2.3% vs. 0.4% | q wk × 6; 2 wk × 6 | Caution urged for low-dose BCG used in CIS & Gr3 disease with ~twofold increase in progression |
| Pagano Bassi | 1995<br>1999 (update) | 210 Ta/T1/CIS | Pasteur | 150mg | 75 mg (1/2) | 59 mo (med) | Std vs. low: NED<br>Ta: 58% vs. 56%<br>T1: 44% vs. 53%<br>CIS: 30% vs. 62%<br>($p$=.006 or $p$<0.01) | Std vs. low<br>Cystitis: 57% vs. 32%<br>Fever: 33% vs. 18%<br>Hematuria: 26% vs. 13% | q wk × 6; repeat if NR; q mo × 2 yr | No difference in progression |

effects, particularly if they occur early during the initial course of induction therapy, within 2 h after BCG instillation, or in the setting of traumatic catheterization. Although a fever over 102.5 F associated with rigors is cause for concern, this in itself is not a definite sign of BCGosis, especially if it occurs at the expected peak time and resolves within 24 h. In fact, higher therapeutic responses in such patients have been reported (Luftenegger, 1996). Such patients may be retreated with NSAID prophylaxis (e.g., three doses of 600 mg ibuprofen, taken every 6 h beginning 2 h prior to therapy) and at a reduced dose of BCG. Conversely, fevers that begin after 24 h, persist more than 48 h, or relapse in a diurnal pattern (usually in the early evening) are more indicative of an established BCG infection (BCGitis). Organ-specific manifestations may be present, suggesting epididymal-orchitis, pneumonitis, and hepatitis. These patients usually require hospitalization and the administration of triple-drug therapy, such as INH, rifampin, and ethambutol. A fluoroquinolone may be added, since it covers most gram-negative rods and has moderate activity against BCG. Failure to improve on such therapy, or significant clinical deterioration, should prompt the institution of systemic steroids (e.g., prednisone 40 mg/d tapered over 2–6 wk), which has been shown to be life-saving in such instances. BCG is resistant to both pyrizidimide and cycloserine. Antituberculosis drugs should be continued for 3–6 mo, depending on the severity of the presenting illness.

Prolonged symptomatic BCG cystitis and/or prostatitis (often associated with granulomas) can become a troubling problem during therapy and in the post-BCG observation period. This situation is best avoided by withholding BCG treatment until all significant symptoms from the prior instillation have subsided. A 1–2 wk delay has not been proven to reduce BCG efficacy in such a setting. Reinstitution of BCG at a lower dose, or premature termination of further treatment for this cycle, may also be appropriate. If localized severe cystitis occurs and conservative measures fail, this condition can be treated with oral fluoroquinolones (3–12 wk) or oral INH. A short 2–3 wk oral steroid taper sandwiched between antibiotic coverage has also been shown to be helpful in refractory cases (Wittes, 1999). Rarely, a noninfectious hypersensitivity Reiter's-type syndrome (urethritis, arthritis, conjunctivitis) may occur during BCG treatment, which should prompt the immediate cessation of further treatment (Saporta, 1997).

## OPTIONS FOR BCG FAILURES

Despite the multitude of reports expounding the benefits of BCG, many patients will eventually fail BCG (Nadler, 1994). The decision of how to handle these patients must be individualized based on the intrinsic tumor risk, pattern of failure, comorbidity, and patient preference. For patients at high risk for disease progression—such as those with stage T1, grade 3 tumors that fail even one cycle of BCG—the radical treatment option must be considered early, since up to one-third have unsuspected muscle-invasive disease for which topical therapy is ineffective. Conversely, a patient with recurrences of Stage Ta, grade 1 tumors may explore many other conservative options without great fear of jeopardizing his or her survival. An analysis of the type of BCG failure is also important. Patients who never achieve a disease-free state of greater than 6 mos' duration, or who fail on active maintenance, are unlikely to benefit from additional BCG alone, whereas those who relapse a few years later can be retreated with a reasonably high expectation of success (Bui, 1997). Similarly, relapsers with tumors that have increased in stage, grade, positive cytology, or are p53-positive demand more aggressive action. A positive cytology in the absence of a bladder lesion should also prompt a search for disease in the upper tract or prostate that occurs in up to 20% of patients if followed long enough (Schwalb, 1994). Unfortunately, some patients with locally-advanced superficial disease are not candidates for radical surgery because of comorbid medical illnesses. Others frankly refuse to consider losing their bladders, even after extended discussions of risk. For all these circumstances, alternative and conservative measures may be appropriate.

The utility of chemotherapy or alternative immunotherapy to salvage BCG failures is limited. In one small study of 21 patients, only 4 (19%) were disease-free at 3 yrs with mitomycin (Malmstrom, 1999). In the pivotal trial leading to FDA approval for Valrubicin, of 90 high-risk patients treated once weekly for 6 wk, only 16 (18%) were disease-free at 6 mo. With successive follow-up, less than half have remained disease-free at 2 yr. Interferon-alpha monotherapy has also been used for BCG failures with limited success. In small series, the rough 1-yr disease-free rate is approx 18% for CIS and papillary disease (Belldegrun, 1998). All BCG-refractory patients with CIS relapsed within 6 mo, but half of nonrefractory BCG failures were disease-free at 1 yr. Moreover, four of these five responders have maintained no evidence of disease status for 33+ mo. Anecdotal reports on Keyhole Limpet Hemocyanin (KLH) immunotherapy have been encouraging, but the agent is generally only available in the research setting. A more provocative protocol awaiting confirmation of efficacy is the use of combination low-dose BCG plus interferon-alpha for BCG failures, which has yielded a >50% disease-free rate at 2 yr in a relatively small 37-patient single institution study (O'Donnell, 1999).

External-beam radiation therapy is rarely appropriate for the treatment of superficial bladder cancer because it may cause significant local morbidity and display limited efficacy. CIS is particularly resistant, and low-grade disease responds more poorly than higher-grade disease. Some benefit may be derived for patients with stage T1, grade 3 tumors with 5-yr disease-free survival rates at about 30% (Quilty, 1986). Photodynamic therapy using hematoporphyrin derivatives can achieve a high initial complete response rate, especially against CIS, but generalized cutaneous photosensitivity remains limiting (Nseyo, 1995). Moreover, severe local irritative symptoms that persist for months occur frequently, as well as occasional bladder contractures. These types of therapy are only available at select centers.

## CONCLUSION

Maintaining a disease-free bladder after TURB can be as much work as maintaining an immaculate lawn. For many patients, the judicious use of an appropriate weed-killer combined with surgery can render satisfying results. For less severe cases, low-toxicity chemotherapeutic agents, particularly when delivered perioperatively, are apt to be most helpful. For aggressive cases, the early use of BCG can provide a long-term, meaningful disease-free state. However, in all cases, constant vigilance is required, since progression to more advanced disease can occur even with the best agents available. Superficial bladder cancer is often a lifelong disease, but it does not need to be a life-shortening one as long as a rational approach is taken, accepting and appreciating the practical limitations that exist.

# 16 Selecting and Counseling Patients for Cystectomy or Cystoprostatectomy

*James E. Montie, MD and Robert Marcovich, MD*

**CONTENTS**

INTRODUCTION
INDICATIONS FOR CYSTECTOMY
NONSURGICAL ALTERNATIVES TO CYSTECTOMY
EVALUATION OF THE CYSTECTOMY PATIENT
PREOPERATIVE ASSESSMENT AND SURGICAL CLEARANCE
SELECTION OF PATIENTS FOR URINARY DIVERSION
PREOPERATIVE EDUCATION
SUMMARY
SELECTED READING

## INTRODUCTION

Few would argue that radical cystectomy is the most complicated surgical procedure undertaken by the urologist today. Yet performing the operation may not always be as difficult as deciding which bladder cancer patients need cystectomy. The challenge in selecting the proper candidate for cystectomy involves the ability to distinguish the patient who will benefit from surgery from the patient for whom surgery is either unnecessary or futile.

The purpose of this chapter is to provide a framework for the urologist to use in selecting patients who will benefit from radical cystectomy. This framework will take into account several factors, including the extent of the patient's disease, history of prior treatment, and overall health. The chapter will also serve as a guide for counseling patients on which type of urinary diversion is most suitable for them, and what patients should expect in terms of preparation for the procedure, hospitalization, recovery, and outcome.

From: *Current Clinical Urology: Office Urology: The Clinician's Guide*
Edited by: E. D. Kursh and J. C. Ulchaker © Humana Press Inc., Totowa, NJ

## INDICATIONS FOR CYSTECTOMY

The majority of patients diagnosed with bladder cancer present with their tumors at an early stage. For most patients with low-grade tumors confined to the mucosa (Ta), effective cancer control can be achieved by transurethral resection. Decreasing frequency of recurrence may not be an appropriate goal for those who present with—or progress to—high-grade cancer, carcinoma *in situ* (CIS), or invasion of the lamina propria (Tl). Therapy relying on transurethral resection (TUR) supplemented by adjunctive intravesical therapy is the mainstay in such cases, but the cancer must be eliminated completely and durably. There is no argument that the clearest indication to perform radical cystectomy is the presence of bladder cancer invading the muscularis propria. Muscle-invasive tumors are aggressive by definition, and—if left untreated—will continue to spread locally and soon metastasize, resulting without exception in the death of the patient.

Radical cystectomy can achieve a 50–70% rate of 5-year survival for patients with muscle-invasive (or greater) bladder cancer. It has been noted that in those patients with Tl disease undergoing cystectomy, the survival rate is improved to 80%. Clearly, if the indications for cystectomy were expanded to all Tl tumors, bladder cancer-specific mortality rates would decrease. However, the significant potential morbidity from total cystectomy, both in the perioperative and long-term periods, precludes treating all patients with Tl disease by radical surgery. The challenge is to select those patients who are at higher risk for progression to muscle invasion, and treat them early with the therapy they will eventually need.

Unfortunately, absolute indicators for identifying which Tl tumors are certain to progress are not currently available to the practicing urologist. Several relative "markers" indicative of more aggressive behavior are accessible, including angiolymphatic invasion, presence of multiple Tl tumors, increasing stage or grade in subsequent recurrences, presence of CIS, urethral or prostatic ductal involvement, or rapid recurrence after one or more courses of intravesical therapy. It is important to remember that the rate of clinical *understaging* of Tl tumors approaches 40%. All these factors should be taken into account, and they can be integrated by the urologist and discussed with the patient to determine a course of action. At this point experience must be relied on to suggest an appropriate course, and urologists must at some point accept the potential for treating some cancers too aggressively in order to treat others appropriately. Fortunately, it appears that in the future, such molecular markers as p53 or Rb will become clinically available, and urologists should be aware of their potential to discriminate the aggressiveness of different Tl tumors.

The presence of CIS at any point in a patient's history should alert the urologist to the fact that this patient's disease has serious potential for lethality. Over one-half of patients with diffuse CIS may progress to *metastatic* disease, and 70% of patients with CIS treated only with TUR will almost certainly progress to muscle invasion. In addition, CIS places the patient at a much higher risk for developing carcinoma in the ureter and renal pelvis. Fortunately, intravesical therapy with Bacillus Calmette-Guérin (BCG) has been proven to decrease progression and will probably increase survival in patients with high-grade tumors that do not invade muscle. Recurrence of a noninvasive tumor after an initial 6-wk course of BCG immunotherapy can reasonably be treated with a second 6-wk course. Persistent or recurrent cancer after the second course is a menacing

Table 1
Indications for Radical Cystectomy

Muscle-invasive (T2) tumors
Select "superficial" tumors
   High-grade T1
      Diffuse or not amenable to complete resection
      Recurrent after 2 or more courses of intravesical therapy
   CIS
      Recurrent after adequate intravesical therapy
Intractable symptoms (hematuria, dysuria, urgency, incontinence)
Prostatic ductal involvement

sign, and a patient harboring this type of disease would be well advised to undergo definitive therapy with radical cystectomy. A further indication for cystectomy is the finding of CIS in the prostatic ducts, because cancer in this area is less likely to be adequately treated with intravesical therapy.

Another reason to consider removing the bladder is the presence of extensive, broad-based sessile tumors that at the time of the resection appear to be muscle-invasive. It is reasonable to resect such tumors transurethrally to an extent that allows the pathologist to establish grade and depth of invasion of the tumor, and to then proceed to cystectomy at a later date. In the unlikely event that pathologic analysis has failed to show muscle invasion, a repeat TUR of the residual can be undertaken.

If the patient has a tumor in a bladder diverticulum, partial cystectomy can be considered, as long as three conditions are met. First, the tumor must be solitary. Second, there should be no evidence of urothelial dysplasia or CIS on biopsies of distant mucosal sites, and third, the patient should have no prior history of bladder cancer. These three criteria must apply in any situation in which partial cystectomy is considered.

If the patient has a high-grade papillary tumor (or tumors) which, because of location, are not amenable to effective transurethral resection, cystectomy (radical or partial, depending on extent of tumor and presence of CIS or urothelial dysplasia at other sites) is necessary to ensure elimination of the cancer.

Finally, in the patient with intractable and debilitating local symptoms of bladder cancer—such as refractory hematuria, dysuria, urgency, or incontinence—cystectomy is a reasonable approach for palliation, even if a high likelihood of advanced disease exists. Counseling regarding nonsurgical alternatives to cystectomy should be offered as well. A summary of the indications for cystectomy is presented in Table 1.

## NONSURGICAL ALTERNATIVES TO CYSTECTOMY

A patient under consideration for cystectomy for bladder cancer should be made aware of the alternatives to surgery: radiation therapy (RT) and chemotherapy. No study has reported a 5-yr survival of more than 40% of patients undergoing primary RT for bladder cancer of any stage. For those patients who go on to salvage cystectomy after radiation and are found to have perivesical invasion or nodal metastases, the prognosis is much worse (7–20% rate of 5-yr survival). Studies examining the outcome for patients who had integrated preoperative radiation followed by radical cystectomy found a questionable benefit overall to this course of treatment as well. Therefore, radiation therapy as a single modality cannot currently be recommended as an acceptable alternative to cystectomy for transitional-cell carcinoma of the bladder, and the patient should be made aware of this during discussions regarding treatment.

The patient should also be aware of the option of bladder preservation with chemotherapy and radiotherapy. In appropriately selected patients with muscle-invasive disease, bladder preservation protocols can result in an eradication of cancer in 30–50%. Patients who consider bladder preservation should have had aggressive and complete transurethral resection of their tumor, have no evidence of squamous cell or adenocarcinoma of the bladder, be free of CIS (multiple biopsies throughout the bladder should be performed), and be free of hydronephrosis. Bladder preservation has only been shown to be effective in patients receiving the *full dose* of chemotherapy and radiation, so the patient under consideration for this course of treatment should be otherwise healthy and have good functional status.

## EVALUATION OF THE CYSTECTOMY PATIENT

The potential cystectomy patient may be seen at initial presentation, prior to diagnosis of bladder cancer or, alternatively—and especially in referral-based practices—the patient may present with the diagnosis already in hand. Regardless of presentation, the evaluation should begin with a careful history and physical examination. The inquiry should be directed toward eliciting a history of "local" symptoms of bladder cancer—such as gross hematuria, irritative voiding, and abdominal or pelvic pain—as well as to constitutional complaints, such as fatigue or weight loss, which might indicate the presence of advanced disease.

Patients referred for bladder cancer should undergo a careful review of the history of the disease and past treatments, with attention to time from the original diagnosis, number of recurrences, stage and grade of recurrences, and number of transurethral resections and intravesical treatments. The patient's past medical history should be reviewed, with particular attention to hypertension and to cardiac and pulmonary conditions, which will need to be addressed carefully if the patient is to undergo cystectomy.

The physical examination should be focused on obtaining the most information about the extent of disease and determining how much the cancer has affected the patient's functional status. The patient's general appearance and weight should be noted. Vital signs will alert the physician to potential comorbid conditions, such as hypertension or arrhythmia. The supraclavicular region should be palpated for lymphadenopathy indicative of metastatic disease, and a brief heart and lung examination should be performed. The abdomen should be palpated for masses or tenderness, and a bimanual exam in women and prostate exam in men may provide evidence of locally advanced disease. Inspection of the extremities to rule out peripheral edema and gross vascular insufficiency is also important.

In the patient under consideration for radical cystectomy, the laboratory evaluation should include a complete blood count and serum chemistries, including creatinine, liver function tests, and albumin level. A metastatic evaluation including a chest radiograph and abdominal and pelvic computed tomography (CT) scan should be conducted. If the patient complains of bone pain, or if the serum-alkaline phosphatase level is elevated, a radionuclide scan can exclude the presence of osseous metastasis. Any

## Table 2
### Indications to Refer for Further Preoperative Medical Assessment

Advanced age
Sedentary lifestyle
Cardiac risk
   Prior myocardial infarction
   History of coronary bypass or angioplasty
   Exertional dyspnea or history of congestive heart failure
   Angina pectoris
   Cardiac arrhythmia
   Known valvular disease or valve replacement
Peripheral vascular disease
Uncontrolled hypertension
Chronic pulmonary disease
Cerebrovascular disease
   Prior stroke or transient ischemic attacks
Diabetes mellitus
Obesity
Significant smoking history
Chronic renal insufficiency (unrelated to obstruction from bladder cancer)
Bleeding diathesis
Steroid dependence

specimens from TUR of the bladder tumor, either from the referring institution or from the urologist's own procedure, should be carefully reviewed with a pathologist to assess the tumor's level of invasion.

## PREOPERATIVE ASSESSMENT AND SURGICAL CLEARANCE

Ideally, any patient considered for radical cystectomy should be otherwise healthy and have good functional status. In reality, this is not always the case, especially since cigarette smoking—the major risk factor for developing bladder cancer—is also the cause of most pulmonary, cardiac, and vascular morbidity.

After determining that cystectomy is indicated, it is the urologist's responsibility to ensure that the patient will be able to tolerate surgery without undue risk. The urologist should be equipped to make a preliminary assessment about the patient's overall health, and should be able to determine whether medical appraisal is warranted. In general, any condition (or combination of conditions) that results in a decreased capacity for exertion during a patient's normal daily activities should be viewed as a threat to that patient's ability to tolerate cystectomy. A history of cardiac, pulmonary, or vascular disease, or the presence of diabetes mellitus, renal insufficiency, or nutritional debilitation is important. Yet the presence of such illness should not cause undue delay or cancellation of definitive therapy if the indication for cystectomy exists. It should, however, prompt the urologist to refer the patient for additional medical testing and optimization before surgery is undertaken.

Specific factors that should alert the urologist to a need for further medical assessment are listed in Table 2. Referral of the patient to an internist or medical specialist, and coordination of both the patient's preoperative and postoperative care with this individual, may reduce the occurrence of avoidable, life-threatening complications, and allow for a smoother course for both patient and physician.

## *Cystectomy in the Elderly Patient*

The discussion of preoperative risk assessment leads intuitively to consideration of cystectomy in the elderly. As the population ages, the prevalence of bladder cancer in elderly patients is expected to increase. Even today, the urologist is often confronted with a situation in which a patient who requires cystectomy is also quite elderly and suffers from multiple medical problems that pose a significant threat to surviving a complicated and lengthy surgical procedure. It is tempting to postpone definitive therapy and to avoid the risk of operative morbidity and mortality by pursuing less risky local therapy in such patients. Yet this approach often results later in a patient who definitely requires cystectomy, is now older and perhaps sicker, and is likely to have more advanced disease than if surgery had been performed when it was first indicated.

Advances in surgical techniques and in perioperative care now allow urologists to operate on older and more debilitated patients, with resultant treatment-related morbidity and mortality that—although still greater than in the average 65-yr-old cystectomy patient—are nevertheless quite acceptable in light of the disappointing outcomes after other therapeutic options. Several studies in patients over the age of 80, with multiple comorbidities at the time of the operation, have reported surgery-related death rates of 4–5% (compared to overall rates of 1–3%) and complication rates of 40–50% (compared to overall rates of 20–30%). Thus, the elderly patient with an indication for surgery should be counseled regarding the need for surgery and informed of the somewhat higher risk of death and complications, and also informed of the natural history of bladder cancer and the likelihood for safe recovery after the procedure.

## SELECTION OF PATIENTS FOR URINARY DIVERSION

Once the decision to perform cystectomy has been reached, the physician and patient need to discuss the alternatives for urinary reconstruction. There are three basic choices: noncontinent diversion, continent cutaneous diversion, or orthotopic neobladder. Each variety has advantages and disadvantages that the patient should thoroughly understand before the choice is made.

Noncontinent urinary diversion—generally in the form of an ileal conduit—is advantageous from the standpoint of the surgeon because of the three types of urinary reconstruction, it is the simplest to perform. Conduits also have the lowest rates of short- and long-term complications. As such, they are the most expeditious choice in a patient whose health and overall condition is poor or whose lifestyle is sedentary. Conduits are also ideal for patients who do not have sufficient dexterity or motivation to catheterize a reservoir. A conduit does not require a period of maturation prior to reaching optimal performance, as neobladders and continent reservoirs do as their capacity increases. Since loops conduct urine away from the absorptive intestinal mucosa and result in the least amount of bowel in contact with urine, they are better alternatives for patients with renal dysfunction. Also, because a shorter intestinal segment is removed from the alimentary tract with conduit construction than with either of the other two alternatives, patients with conduits are not at risk for vitamin $B_{12}$ malabsorption. Patients with preexisting intestinal disorders that preclude removal of longer segments will also fare better with conduit formation. Finally, despite the need for an external collecting appliance, patients who elect a noncontinent urinary diversion can expect to return to full participation in all their preoperative activities.

Despite these many advantages, many patients desire an alternative to noncontinent diversion. Some patients may view the need for an external appliance as a threat to body image, and some fear the potential for episodes of massive urinary leakage that may occur without warning because of device malfunction. Stomal complications are rarely a problem with ileal conduits, but stenosis, prolapse, retraction, dermatitis, and parastomal hernias can all occur. These pitfalls may be minimized by an optimal choice of stoma site, surgical technique, extensive patient education in stomal care, and involvement of an enterostomal therapist in the patient's care, education, and routine follow-up.

Continent cutaneous urinary diversion is one alternative for patients concerned with the possible problems of conduits. The most commonly used continent diversion is the Indiana pouch, and as experience with this form of reconstruction has increased, the initially high complication and reoperation rates have decreased substantially. A patient who elects a continent cutaneous diversion must accept the presence of the abdominal stoma and be motivated to catheterize the pouch every 4–6 h, day and night. The patient thus must be dependable and must have normal manual dexterity in order to carry out this function. The patient must also understand that of all three alternatives, the continent diversion carries the greatest risk for metabolic complications, such as acidosis, as well as the highest risk for reoperation—which, even in the best of hands, approaches 10–15%. Because of the marginal benefit of continent cutaneous urinary diversion, it is rarely used in our practice.

The orthotopic neobladder is the most recent form of urinary reconstruction, and attempts to preserve normal volitional voiding. The most important determining factor in deciding to construct a neobladder is location of the tumor. There should be little or no evidence of cancer in the prostatic urethra of males, and none at the urethral margin in men and bladder neck in women. Frozen-section examination of the urethral margin at cystectomy is prudent. A patient who elects neobladder construction must be informed preoperatively of the possibility that an intraoperative decision to perform an alternative diversion might have to be made if findings at surgery indicate the presence of cancer in the aforementioned areas. Thus, the patient should have a stoma site marked prior to the operation.

The candidate for orthotopic neobladder substitution must also be dependable, motivated, and willing and able to perform clean intermittent catheterization if necessary, and must have acceptable renal function (serum creatinine under 3.0 mg/dL). Patients with a history of intestinal disease precluding use of larger bowel segments would be better served with a conduit diversion than a neobladder. A patient should not be discouraged from neobladder substitution solely because of advanced age. The patient's overall motivation and functional ability should be considered much more important than chronological age, and an older patient who is motivated, dependable, and has adequate dexterity will fare better than a younger patient who lacks some or all of these qualities. In addition, the finding of locally advanced or regionally metastatic disease at surgery does not preclude formation of a neobladder, since adjuvant chemotherapy or radiotherapy can be administered whether the patient has a neobladder or some other type of diversion.

The potential neobladder candidate should be counseled realistically about postoperative urinary functioning. Although the ability to void per urethra will be maintained, the patient should understand that the system will not be perfect. The new reservoir will require several months to expand capacity and up to 2 yr to obtain ultimate ideal function. During this time the patient may experience episodes of both daytime and nocturnal incontinence. At the same time, he or she will need to voluntarily void more frequently. In the initial postoperative period, the patient will need to void every 2 h. Gradually, over the next few weeks, the interval will be increased to every 3–4 h, and then to a pattern that keeps voided volumes under 500 cc. The patient should be informed of the occasional need to catheterize in order to check residuals or to irrigate the reservoir free of mucus.

Neobladder patients should be counseled about the potential for incontinence, especially at night. Although the expectation for daytime control is over 90%, approx 20% of patients will continue to have significant nocturnal leakage, and 50% may experience occasional (ie once or twice monthly) leakage of smaller volumes. Men over the age of 70 have more difficulty with continence than younger men or women, and patients who undergo a nerve-sparing cystectomy may fare better overall. In contrast, those who require postoperative chemotherapy will experience a significantly slower return to baseline.

Female neobladder patients should be counseled that although some risk of postoperative incontinence exists, the risk of hypercontinence is more significant. Although the incidence and degree of postsurgical retention can be reduced if the entire bladder neck is resected, there is still about a 25% chance that such a female patient will be unable to void and may require self-catheterization at least once daily to completely empty the reservoir.

## PREOPERATIVE EDUCATION

Effective and thorough preoperative education can serve to empower an individual who has just been informed of the need for a life-threatening and life-changing operation. Since the urologist and patient will discuss the indications and need for cystectomy in the office, this setting is also appropriate for preoperative counseling and education. The urologist's office should be equipped with general written information on bladder cancer as well as literature that can offer a lay explanation of the indications for cystectomy, what the procedure entails, and the alternatives to surgery. This information can be provided to the patient for further review. Patients often have questions and concerns that may not be addressed fully at the office visit, and when these do arise, they can be answered at a subsequent appointment or in a telephone conversation. A nurse who is familiar with urologic practice can also assist with these concerns.

The urologist or a qualified urology nurse should discuss all stages of the planned procedure with the patients, including preoperative, operative, and postoperative phases. In the preoperative phase, the patient may require further radiographic or laboratory testing, or may need to receive medical clearance through consultation with another physician. The patient should be educated about preoperative diet and bowel preparation—which in the majority may be performed at home—as well as the need to have the abdomen marked for the site of the stoma.

The urologist should explain the operation in general terms, and should emphasize to patients who choose an orthotopic neobladder the possibility that an alternative diversion may have to be performed based on intraoperative findings. In addition, risks of cystectomy—both immediate and long-term—should be discussed with the patient, and the possible need for transfusion of blood products during or after the procedure should be noted as well. The discussion of risks should include not only the issue of postoperative continence (as outlined in the previous section) but also the question of postoperative sexual function. Male patients with normal preoperative erectile function should understand that standard radical cystectomy will cause impotence, but that a nerve-sparing procedure may preserve the ability to engage in sexual intercourse in approx 50% of select cases (namely in men younger than 60 yr of age). Patients should be informed that in experienced hands, a nerve-sparing cystectomy will not compromise cancer control by leaving behind positive margins or lymph nodes involved by tumor.

After the urologist has discussed the risks involved, postoperative events and expectations must be addressed in detail. The patient should be informed about the types and numbers of tubes, drains, and stents that will be present after the operation, their purpose, and the time course of their removal. Questions regarding the progression of diet and activity should be answered, and the need for postoperative pulmonary toilet and ambulation should be stressed. Concerns about methods of postsurgical analgesia, medications, and laboratory testing should also be addressed. The patient must be made aware of any plans for discharge with tubes or drains still in place. Procedures that the patient will be expected to perform at home, such as irrigation of a reservoir or neobladder, should be briefly mentioned. The discussion of all these topics may be framed under the guidance of a critical pathway (if one is available at the urologist's institution), which provides a detailed outline of all aspects of postoperative care, as well as expectations and milestones to be achieved by the patient.

Finally, an enterostomal therapy (ET) nurse should be available to meet with the patient to discuss concerns with the planned diversion, even for patients who have elected a neobladder. The ET nurse will be better equipped than the urologist to address questions related to stoma care, lifestyle changes, and both physical and psychological adaptation to the new urinary system. The ET nurse may also choose and mark the site of the ostomy at the preoperative visit. In addition, the ET nurse can refer the patient to either a support group or another individual who has had a similar experience with urinary diversion.

With careful attention to preoperative education and counseling, the urologist and ancillary staff can allay many of the patient's concerns about the upcoming operation. A fully informed patient is more likely to take an active role in his or her recovery, making the experience less alienating and traumatic.

## SUMMARY

The appropriate selection and counseling of patients for radical cystectomy is challenging. The reasons to delay cystectomy are becoming less justifiable—especially for high-grade superficial tumors—despite the fact that there is currently no sure method to determine which cancers may turn out to be lethal. The urologist must depend mainly on clinical judgment gained through experience. Yet factors that may encourage earlier cystectomy include pathologic indicators, such as the presence of high-grade disease, widespread urothelial dysplasia, and angiolymphatic invasion, or other factors, such as resistance to intravesical therapy and rapid recurrence of resected tumors. The development of orthotopic neobladder substitution—which preserves a normal voiding pattern to a higher degree than the previous alternatives—may make the idea of cystectomy less threatening to both patient and physician, and allow for more suitable approaches to certain tumors. Nevertheless, nonsurgical alternatives should be discussed with all patients.

The potential cystectomy patient should be thoroughly evaluated with appropriate history, physical, and laboratory examinations, as well as cystoscopy and aggressive TUR. Advanced age or the presence of comorbid conditions are not valid contraindications to cystectomy. Still, older patients and those with a significant history of underlying disease should be referred for preoperative medical clearance and appropriate optimization before surgery.

The choice of urinary diversion is potentially complex, and since the patient will live the rest of his or her life with this decision, extensive education and counseling about the topic should be the rule. Factors influencing the choice of diversion include location of the tumor; patient considerations, such as motivation, dependability, manual dexterity, and degree of debilitation; and medical history, including the presence of chronic renal insufficiency or preexisting intestinal disorders. The patient should be provided with pragmatic information regarding postoperative functioning with each of the three types of diversions. Realistic estimates of the rates of incontinence, retention, and reoperation will allow the patient to make an informed choice.

The importance of preoperative education for the patient scheduled to undergo cystectomy cannot be overemphasized. In addition to the urologist, appropriate ancillary staff, such as a nurse and an enterostomal therapist, provide invaluable support in addressing the array of questions and uncertainties facing the patient. A patient who is thoroughly aware of all facets of the upcoming procedure will be better prepared physically, mentally, and emotionally, and a smoother course can be expected.

## SELECTED READING

Carlin BI, Rutchik SD, Resnick MI (1997) Comparison of the ileal conduit to the continent cutaneous diversion and orthotopic neobladder in patients undergoing cystectomy: a critical analysis and review of the literature. *Semin Urol Oncol* 15:189–192.

Eagle KA, Brundage BH, Chaitman BR, et al. (1997) Guidelines for Perioperative Cardiovascular Evaluation for Noncardiac Surgery: an abridged version of the report of the American College of Cardiology/American Heart Association Task Force on Practice Guidelines. *Mayo Clin Proc* 72:524–531.

Erwin-Toth P, Calabrese DA (1997) Nursing issues in the management of urinary diversions in women. *Semin Urol Oncol* 15:193–199.

Esrig DE, Freeman JA, Stein JP, Skinner DG (1997) Early cystectomy for clinical stage T1 transitional cell carcinoma of the bladder. *Semin Urol Oncol* 15:154–160.

Hautmann RE (1997) The ileal neobladder to the female urethra. *Urol Clin N Am* 24:827–835.

Montie JE, Park JM (1997) Orthotopic diversion in women. *Semin Urol Oncol* 15:184–188.

Montie JE, Smith DC, Sandler HM (1998) "Carcinoma of the Bladder." In: Abeloff M, Armitage J, Lichter A, Niederhuber J, eds. *Clinical Oncology* (2nd ed.), New York: Churchill Livingstone, Inc., In Press.

Rowland RG (1997) Continent cutaneous urinary diversion. *Semin Urol Oncol* 15:179–183.

Stroumbakis N, Herr HW, Cookson MS, Fair WR (1997) Radical cystectomy in the octogenarian. *J Urol* 158:2113–2117.

Studer UE, Zingg EJ (1997) Ileal orthotopic bladder substitutes: what we have learned from 12 years' experience with 200 patients. *Urol Clin N Am* 24:781–793.

Williams O, Vereb MJ, Libertino JA (1997) Noncontinent urinary diversion. *Urol Clin N Am* 24:735–744.

# VI  Prostate—Benign

# 17 Evaluation of Lower Urinary-Tract Symptoms

*Rasmus H. Krogh, MD
and Reginald C. Bruskewitz, MD*

**CONTENTS**

INTRODUCTION
BASIC EVALUATION
SYMPTOMS
UNEQUIVOCAL INDICATIONS FOR SURGERY
OPTIONAL DIAGNOSTIC TESTS
SUMMARY
SELECTED READING

## INTRODUCTION

Benign prostatic hyperplasia (BPH) is one of the most common causes of morbidity in elderly men, and prevalence increases steadily with age. However, no single diagnostic criterion of BPH has gained wide clinical acceptance, and the prevalence estimates greatly depend on the criteria used. The majority of elderly men develop histologic evidence of BPH, and more than 25% of men over the age of 70 present with moderate-to-severe lower-urinary-tract symptoms (LUTS).

The terminology associated with BPH has changed during the last decade. The term "prostatism" had been broadly used to describe urinary symptoms in elderly men, but in many cases this term was inaccurate because no set of urinary symptoms is diagnostic for BPH. Classic prostatism symptoms may not be caused by prostatic disease. This is clearly illustrated by the fact that these symptoms are not gender-specific. Instead, the term "lower urinary-tract symptoms" (LUTS) has been proposed as a more appropriate expression. "Prostatism" and "LUTS" both fail to recognize that the symptoms may originate in the upper urinary tract or outside the urinary tract (e.g., polyuria, secondary polydipsia, congestive heart failure, and so forth). BPH is now considered a histological diagnosis, and LUTS has replaced the term "prostatism." Bladder-outlet obstruction (BOO) must now be documented with urodynamic investigation. BPH, LUTS, and BOO may coexist. This chapter discusses various diagnostic tools for the male patient with LUTS. Miscellaneous causes of LUTS are outlined in Table 1.

From: *Current Clinical Urology: Office Urology: The Clinician's Guide*
Edited by: E. D. Kursh and J. C. Ulchaker © Humana Press Inc., Totowa, NJ

Table 1
Miscellaneous Causes of LUTS

Benign prostate enlargement
Cancer of the prostate
Cancer of the bladder
Calculi in bladder and urethra
Urethral stricture
Bladder-neck contracture
Urethral foreign bodies
Neurologic dysfunction of the urinary tract
 (e.g., Parkinson's disease, diabetes, and so forth)
Cystitis
Prostatitis
Pelvic masses
Congestive heart failure

## BASIC EVALUATION

The recommended basic evaluation includes a medical history, physical examination, urinalysis, serum creatinine, prostatic-specific antigen (PSA), and assessment of symptoms and bother.

### *Medical History*

A comprehensive medical history is essential to determine whether symptoms are consistent with prostatic disease. Medication history is important, because many drugs can contribute to urinary symptoms, including cold medication, allergy medication, diuretics, anticholinergics, and alpha-sympathomimetics. Special consideration should be given to hematuria, urinary-tract infection, neurological disorders suggesting a neurogenic bladder, history of instrumentation possibly leading to urethral stricture, trauma or sexually-transmitted disease, and urinary retention. A voiding diary may be a useful supplement to the medical history in patients who present with nocturia as a dominant symptom, and it may help identify patients with polyuria or other nonprostatic disorders.

### *Physical Examination*

Evaluation of the patient might suggest uremia, anemia, or edema—all occasionally associated with BPH as well as other medical conditions. Palpation of the abdomen and over the kidneys might suggest bladder distention, in rare cases may identify renal pathology, and is routinely appropriate even if seldom diagnostic. The physical examination includes a digital rectal examination (DRE) and a focused neurological examination. The DRE provides information on anal sphincter tone and prostate asymmetry or induration, which might suggest prostate or colorectal cancer. Although the DRE gives the physician some indication of prostatic size, it does not correlate well with prostatic size as estimated by transrectal ultrasound (TRUS). Prostatic size assessed by DRE also correlates poorly with the severity of LUTS. When the determination of prostatic size is an important factor to guide treatment selection, TRUS (or transabdominal ultrasound) is preferred. The World Health Organization (WHO) guidelines highly recommend that the focused neurological examination include an assessment of the bulbocavernosal reflex and the motor and sensory function of the lower extremities. Manifestations of neurological disease raise the suspicion of a neurogenic bladder, and these patients require more than the standard exam. Urodynamic assessment is also more revealing than in uncomplicated BPH.

### *Urinalysis*

Urinary-tract infection (UTI) and bladder cancer may cause symptoms resembling BPH, and urinalysis is generally recommended to screen for UTI and hematuria in patients who present with LUTS. Urine dipsticks are inexpensive and easy to use, and have largely supplanted microscopic examination of the spun sediment for screening purposes. However, the value of this screening is controversial. There is insufficient evidence to support dipstick screening in the general population and in BPH patients.

UTI alone is not an indication for treating BPH. The urinary symptoms should be reassessed when the infection is treated. UTI prevention by TURP to reduce residual and UTI risk is more presumptive and not factual. Asymptomatic hematuria is a common finding, occurring in approx 13% of the population at some point. The dipstick test itself has a low positive predictive value (PPV) for cancer or other serious urological diseases; in medical literature the PPV varies from 4 to 26% for all entities, and many of these are found inconsequential after evaluation.

A dipstick urine test is only useful in combination with other findings for select patients who require more than the standard workup. Urine cytology can be considered in patients with severe irritable symptoms and a history of smoking.

### *Serum Creatinine*

An elevated serum creatinine level can be expected in more than 10% of BPH patients, and is an indication for imaging studies of the upper-urinary tract. Frequent causes include diabetes mellitus and hypertension leading to vascular disease, and rarely renal insufficiency secondary to obstruction. Studies suggest that the morbidity and mortality of TURP are increased significantly in patients with advanced renal insufficiency. Renal ultrasonography has replaced intravenous urography as the first choice to look for evidence of hydronephrosis.

### *Prostatic-Specific Antigen (PSA)*

Prostatic-specific antigen (PSA) is elevated in conditions that affect the prostate, including BPH. The WHO guidelines strongly recommend a PSA in patients with LUTS with a life expectancy over 10 yr in cases in which the diagnosis of prostate cancer will change the treatment plan. Unfortunately, PSA measurements show substantial intraindividual variability over time and discriminate poorly between BPH and localized prostate cancers. It is also unclear whether patient outcome will improve through early detection and treatment of prostate cancer. When screening for prostate cancer is chosen, the combined use of DRE and PSA is the most effective method. If prostate cancer is suspected, the next diagnostic step is TRUS-guided biopsy of the prostate. Patients treated with finasteride require special attention because the drug lowers serum PSA to an average of 50% after 6–12 mo of treatment. A number of newer PSA assays have been proposed, but their value has yet to be determined.

## SYMPTOMS

The assessment of symptoms is essential for BPH management. The American Urological Association (AUA) symptom index is generally recommended for correct quantification of LUTS. The AUA index is identical to the International Prostate Symptom Score (IPSS) presented in Table 2. Using the IPSS, symptoms can be classified as mild (0–7 points), moderate (8–19 points), or severe (20–35 points). It is important to note that a poor correlation between symptoms and prostatic size or urodynamic measurements and regional and international differences in symptom prevalence or symptom reporting have been found. Symptom scores cannot be used to actually diagnose BPH because of the nonspecificity of LUTS. Symptom scores may be used to establish a baseline of symptom severity and frequency and to monitor BPH patients. When using symptom scores, the physician must still consider the individual patient. Patients with high-baseline symptom scores need a larger numeric change in symptom score to appreciate the improvement than patients with low-baseline scores. Generally, a 30–50% improvement in symptom score—depending on the baseline score after BPH treatment—is considered meaningful.

Traditionally, symptoms of "prostatism" have been divided into "obstructive" and "irritative" symptoms. More recently, LUTS has been classified as voiding and storage symptoms. Voiding symptoms include hesitancy, abdominal straining, intermittency, a weak urinary stream, dribbling, a sensation of incomplete emptying, dysuria, and increased diuria. Storage symptoms include frequency, nocturia, urgency, incontinence, and bladder pain. Cardinal symptoms in BPH include weak stream, hesitancy, frequency, and nocturia.

Men with BPH often present with both voiding and storage symptoms, and the symptoms tend to slowly progress over time. Young patients and patients who present primarily with storage symptoms or rapid onset of symptoms are more likely to suffer from other disorders. Age-related changes in the bladder and other bladder disorders are causes of LUTS that demand attention. In aging men, the bladder capacity decreases and the incidence of detrusor instability increases. The latter might be a physiological energy-saving device in BPH, and prostate surgery has been shown to decrease bladder instability dramatically. Improvement in bladder dysfunction through surgery and pharmaceuticals may have a greater impact on patient well-being than other parameters, such as urinary flow rates. An age-related decrease in the compliance of the prostate is likely to contribute to the decreased urinary flow in elderly men, but has not been studied as thoroughly.

### *Bother*

Different patients with similar symptom scores are bothered to varying degrees. The important consideration for the individual patient is the degree of bother and the impact of the condition on quality of life, rather than a symptom score or other measures. Accordingly, bother is the most important factor in therapeutic decision-making. According to the WHO guidelines, a patient should be evaluated and treated according to the degree of bother caused by his symptoms rather than the symptoms alone. Baseline bother has been shown to be more predictive of TURP outcome than symptom score. There is currently no standard solution for measuring bother. As a supplement to the IPSS, Barry and coworkers developed The Symptom Problem Index (SPI) and the BPH

## Table 2
### International Prostate Symptom Score (IPSS)[a]

| | Not at all | Less than 1 time in 5 | Less than half the time | About half the time | More than half the time | Almost always |
|---|---|---|---|---|---|---|
| **1. Incomplete emptying:** Over the past month, how often have you had a sensation of not emptying your bladder completely after you finished urinating? | 0 | 1 | 2 | 3 | 4 | 5 |
| **2. Frequency:** Over the past month, how often have you had to urinate again <2 h after you finished urinating? | 0 | 1 | 2 | 3 | 4 | 5 |
| **3. Intermittency:** Over the past month, how often have you found you stopped and started again several times when you urinated? | 0 | 1 | 2 | 3 | 4 | 5 |
| **4. Urgency:** Over the past month, how often have you found it difficult to postpone urination? | 0 | 1 | 2 | 3 | 4 | 5 |
| **5. Weak stream:** Over the past month, how often have you had a weak urinary stream? | 0 | 1 | 2 | 3 | 4 | 5 |
| **6. Straining:** Over the past month, how often have you had to push or strain to begin urination? | 0 | 1 | 2 | 3 | 4 | 5 |

| | None | 1 time | 2 times | 3 times | 4 times | 5 or more times |
|---|---|---|---|---|---|---|
| **7. Nocturia:** Over the past month, how many times did you most typically get up to urinate from the time you went to bed at night until the time you got up in the morning? | 0 | 1 | 2 | 3 | 4 | 5 |

**Total IPSS Score =**

### Quality of Life Because of Urinary Symptoms

| | Delighted | Pleased | Mostly satisfied | Mixed (about equally satisfied and dissatisfied) | Mostly dissatisfied | Unhappy | Terrible |
|---|---|---|---|---|---|---|---|
| **Quality of Life:** If you were to spend the rest of your life with your urinary condition just the way it is now, how would you feel about that? | 0 | 1 | 2 | 3 | 4 | 5 | 6 |

[a] Adapted from The WHO Guidelines 1998.

Impact Index (BII). These indices are less popular than the IPSS, but help to objectively assess bother and quality of life in BPH patients.

Our routine approach is to thoroughly review symptoms with the patient to ensure that the symptoms are consistent with prostatic disease, and then ask the patient whether the symptoms are bothersome enough to warrant the various treatments offered.

## UNEQUIVOCAL INDICATIONS FOR SURGERY

Some patients present with unequivocal indications for surgery, and do not require a symptom score or a bother assessment. Both WHO and US guidelines recommend surgery if the patient has refractory urinary retention or any of the following conditions clearly secondary to BPH: recurrent or persistent gross hematuria, bladder stones, and renal insufficiency. Recurrent UTIs and large bladder diverticula are more controversial.

## OPTIONAL DIAGNOSTIC TESTS

In most cases the basic evaluation described above is sufficient. However, in some cases, additional testing may be of value.

### *Urodynamics*

Urodynamics in the form of uroflowmetry, pressure-flow study, postvoid residual urine, or filling cystometry have traditionally been widely used in BPH management. We believe that urodynamics is optional, and usually adds nothing to management. Urodynamics are indicated if the results would make a difference in treatment and when things do not add up—e.g., severe symptoms in younger patients, severe symptoms in patients with normal uroflow, patients with neurological disease, or patients who do not respond to therapy. For men considering surgical treatment, such as TURP, uroflowmetry can be used to estimate a success rate of about 70% if their flow is high (ie, >15 mL/s) or about 90% if their maximum uroflow is low. Pressure-flow studies are usually not warranted because the improvement in predictive value is insignificant compared to uroflowmetry, and the procedure is highly invasive. Some authors attach more importance to urodynamics than we do.

### *Uroflowmetry*

When the results of the basic evaluation conflict, or when surgery is planned, uroflowmetry may be helpful. Uroflowmetry is noninvasive and simple to perform. About 75% of patients with a maximum flow rate ($Q_{max}$) below 15 mL/s are obstructed, and about 25% of patients with $Q_{max}$ >15 mL/s are obstructed. A low $Q_{max}$ may be caused by BOO, a hypotonic bladder, or a combination of both. Similarly, a patient with a normal $Q_{max}$ can still have BOO with good detrusor compensation. The WHO guidelines recommend at least two independent flow-rate recordings because of the intraindividual variability of $Q_{max}$. The maximum flow rate decreases with age from more than 25 mL/s in young men to <10 mL/s in 80-yr-old men.

### *Pressure-Flow Study*

The simultaneous measurement of intravesical pressure and flow rate provides an indication of detrusor function, and pressure-flow study is the best tool to differentiate between patients with BOO and patients with impaired detrusor function. This method be particularly helpful in patients with neurologic diseases or in younger men where BPH is less common and the predictive value of pressure-flow studies is greater.

Intravesical pressure is measured using a small suprapubic or urethral catheter, thereby making pressure-flow study an invasive and more morbid procedure than uroflowmetry. The maximum flow rate ($Q_{max}$) and the maximum detrusor pressure at $Q_{max}$ ($P_{det}$ at $Q_{max}$) are usually plotted on the Abrams-Griffiths nomogram to determine whether the patient is obstructed. However, there is disagreement regarding which numeric values constitute obstruction for pressure and for flow. Furthermore, pressure-flow measurements have shown considerable intraindividual variability, and the fate of untreated obstructed men is unknown.

The prognostic value of urodynamics is still somewhat uncertain. A normal preoperative uroflowmetry or pressure-flow study may predict a slightly increased risk of treatment failure. Available data suggest that both tests are valid and practically identical in predicting the outcome of prostatic surgery. Yet these tests may not be predictive of outcome with medical treatment (alpha-blockers).

### *Postvoid Residual Urine*

Measurements of postvoid residual urine (PVR) show significant intraindividual variability regardless of the techniques used, and correlate poorly with symptoms and other signs of BPH. The clinical value of PVR is thus presumably low, although it has shown some predictive value at baseline toward symptom improvement after treatment. Transabdominal ultrasonography (noninvasive) has now replaced catheterization (invasive) as a routine method for PVR determination.

### *Filling Cystometry*

Filling cystometry is an invasive test that provides information about bladder sensation, capacity, pressure, compliance, and detrusor contractions. An overactive bladder, or involuntary detrusor contractions, is called detrusor hyperreflexia when a neurologic cause is known and detrusor instability (DI) when there is no neurologic abnormality. DI occurs in about 60% of men with BPH, and the prevalence of DI is reduced after prostate surgery to about 26%, but the clinical significance and predictive value of DI are uncertain. Pressure-flow studies provide more specific information, and filling cystometry is usually not warranted but may be performed in patients with suspected primary-bladder or neurological dysfunction who are in urinary retention and cannot urinate for a pressure-flow study.

### *Urethrocystoscopy*

The visualization of the lower urinary tract and the bladder has traditionally been considered helpful, but this invasive procedure has only a limited role in the evaluation of BPH. Cystoscopy cannot be used to identify which BPH patients will require surgery, and it has no predictive value toward the outcome of surgery. The main role of the procedure is to rule out serious alternative pathologies, such as bladder cancer and urethral strictures. Cystoscopy may be performed prior to invasive therapy to guide the urologist in choosing an operative approach.

## *Imaging of the Upper Urinary Tract*

Imaging of the upper urinary tract is not recommended in the routine evaluation of BPH patients, although compromised renal function is the most morbid and potentially fatal complication of BPH. Most patients with LUTS (67–74%) have a normal intravenous excretory urography (IVU), and hydronephrosis is the most commonly reported abnormality (8–13%). Imaging of the upper urinary tract should probably be limited to BPH patients with elevated serum creatinine or other indications of disease in the upper urinary tract. Ultrasonography (noninvasive) is better than IVU (invasive) to detect hydronephrosis, tumors, and stones, and it can safely replace IVU. In patients with elevated serum creatinine, IVU should not be performed because it increases the risk of exacerbating renal failure.

## SUMMARY

The management of men with LUTS is not a matter of accurately diagnosing prostate enlargement, histological BPH, or BOO. The diagnostic objective is to evaluate the patient carefully to find the right treatment and to rule out pathologies other than BPH without exposing the patient to various unnecessary testing. All men who present with LUTS should go through a basic evaluation including medical history, physical examination (including DRE) urinalysis, serum creatinine, PSA, and symptom and bother assessment. Our approach is to review symptoms thoroughly with the patient to ensure that the symptoms are consistent with prostatic disease, and to ask the patient whether the symptoms are bothersome enough to warrant the various specific treatments we offer. Some patients present with unequivocal indications for surgery and might require less than the basic evaluation. Additional diagnostic testing is necessary in other patients. Urodynamics are indicated when things do not add up—e.g., severe symptoms in younger patients, or patients with normal uroflow, patients who present with neurological disease, or patients who do not respond to therapy. Imaging of the upper urinary tract should be limited to BPH patients with elevated serum creatinine, or other indications of disease in the upper urinary tract.

## SELECTED READING

Abrams PH, Griffiths DJ (1979) The assessment of prostatic obstruction from urodynamic measurements and from residual urine. *Br J Urol* 51(2):129–134.

Barry MJ, Fowler FJ, Jr, O'Leary MP, Bruskewitz RC, Holtgrewe HL, Mebust WK, et al. (1992) The American Urological Association symptom index for benign prostatic hyperplasia. The Measurement Committee of the American Urological Association. *J Urol* 148(5):1549–1557.

Barry MJ, Fowler FJ, Jr, O'Leary MP, Bruskewitz RC, Holtgrewe HL, Mebust WK (1992) Correlation of the American Urological Association symptom index with self-administered versions of the Madsen-Iversen, Boyarsky, and Maine Medical Assessment Program symptom indexes. Measurement Committee of the American Urological Association. *J Urol* 148(5):1558–1563.

Barry MJ, Williford WO, Chang Y, Machi M, Jones KM, Walker-Corkery E, et al. (1995) Benign prostatic hyperplasia specific health status measures in clinical research: how much change in the American Urological Association symptom index and the benign prostatic hyperplasia impact index is perceptible to patients? *J Urol* 154(5):1770–1774.

Berry SJ, Coffey DS, Walsh PC, Ewing LL (1984) The development of human benign prostatic hyperplasia with age. *J Urol* 132(3):474–479.

Bosch JL, Hop WC, Kirkels WJ, Schroder FH (1995) The International Prostate Symptom Score in a community-based sample of men between 55 and 74 years of age: prevalence and correlation of symptoms with age, prostate volume, flow rate and residual urine volume. *Br J Urol* 75(5):622–630.

Denis L, Griffiths K, Khoury S, et al. (1998) 4th International Consultation on Benign Prostatic Hyperplasia (BPH). Proceedings. Health Publication Ltd (Referred to in the text as The WHO Guidelines)

Ezz el Din K, Debruyne FM, de la Rosette JJ (1997) Making the diagnosis of benign prostatic hyperplasia. A critical review. *Eur Urol* 31(3):257–262.

Jensen KM (1989) Clinical evaluation of urodynamic investigations in prostatism. *Neurourol Urodyn* 8:545–578.

Jepsen JV, Bruskewitz RC (1998) Office evaluation of men with lower urinary tract symptoms. *Urol Clin N Am* 25(4):545–554.

McConnell JD, Barry MJ, Bruskewitz RC, et al. (February 1994) Benign Prostatic Hyperplasia Diagnosis and Treatment. Clinical Practice Guideline, Number 8, AHCPR Publication No. 94-0582. Rockville, MD: Agency for Health Care Policy and Research, Public Health Service, US Department of Health and Human Services. (Referred to in the text as The USA Guidelines)

McConnell JD (1997) Epidemiology, etiology, pathophysiology, and diagnosis of benign prostatic hyperplasia. In: *Campbell's Urology*, (7th ed), 1429–1452.

# 18 Medical Management of Benign Prostatic Obstruction

*Michael J. Barry, MD
and Claus Roehrborn, MD*

**CONTENTS**

    INTRODUCTION
    PURPOSES OF TREATMENT AND MONITORING RESPONSE
       TO THERAPY
    EFFICACY VS. EFFECTIVENESS OF MEDICAL THERAPY FOR BPH
    ALPHA-BLOCKERS
    5-ALPHA-REDUCTASE INHIBITORS
    ALPHA-BLOCKERS, FINASTERIDE, OR COMBINATION THERAPY?
    PHYTOTHERAPY
    CONCLUSION
    ACKNOWLEDGMENT
    SELECTED READING

## INTRODUCTION

Effective medical therapy for men with clinical manifestations ultimately resulting from the histologic process of benign prostatic hyperplasia (BPH) has changed the practice of urology. For example, despite an aging population, the number of transurethral prostatectomies performed in the United States has fallen from a peak number of 379,000 in 1987 to 145,000 in 1996. This decline has occurred to a large degree because clinicians usually try a course of medical therapy first before resorting to surgical treatment. Also, for better or worse, the availability of medical therapy now allows primary-care physicians to treat men with clinical manifestations of BPH before referring them to a urologist. Effective use of medical therapy for men with symptoms attributed to BPH is a key skill in office urology.

## PURPOSES OF TREATMENT AND MONITORING RESPONSE TO THERAPY

The histologic process of BPH exerts its morbidity primarily through lower urinary-tract symptoms, and secondarily through relatively rare complications, such as acute urinary retention, serious urinary-tract infections, and renal failure resulting from obstructive uropathy. The mechanisms by which the histologic process of BPH eventually leads to lower urinary-tract symptoms is undoubtedly more complicated than formerly known. At one time "voiding" or "obstructive" symptoms (such as a weak stream, hesitancy, straining, intermittency, incomplete emptying, and terminal dribbling) were considered to be directly attributable to bladder-outlet obstruction, whereas "filling" or "irritative" symptoms (such as frequency, nocturia, and urgency) were considered a result of secondary uninhibited detrusor contractions. However, the poor correlation between urodynamic and cystometric measures of the presence and severity of these physiologic phenomena, and measures of the presence and severity of symptoms, casts doubt on these theories. Moreover, some treatments, such as transurethral prostatectomy, appear to reduce symptoms effectively even among men without benign prostatic obstruction, whereas others—particularly transurethral microwave thermotherapy and needle ablation—appear to result in a symptomatic benefit that is disproportionate to their relatively modest impact on parameters that measure the degree of obstruction. Although many experts still feel that the future risk of BPH complications is related to the baseline severity of outlet obstruction, even this common-sense notion has not been rigorously proven.

The goals of treating men with BPH, from the patient's perspective, are to eliminate or reduce lower urinary-tract symptoms and to reduce the risk of future BPH complications. Achieving improvements in other parameters, such as prostate size, postvoid residual urine volume, peak uroflow, or bladder pressure at peak flow, are simply possible means to these ends.

Since lower urinary-tract symptom severity can be measured objectively and directly with such instruments as the American Urological Association (AUA) Symptom Index (*see* Fig. 1), such measurements are the best way to document individual patients' symptom responses to treatment. These measures should be combined with soliciting patients' global impressions of whether their symptoms have improved as a result of treatment. Urologists may also choose to measure other parameters, such as peak uroflow, to assess patients' responses to therapy. However, by monitoring those parameters, the urologist assumes that improvements in the chosen measurement are good proxies for reductions in the patient's future risk of BPH complications. Although such an assumption makes intuitive sense, it is not well-supported by research data.

Whether symptom scores or other measurements are used to objectively assess response to therapy, separating true improvement (or deterioration) from measurement fluctuations attributed to chance alone can be challenging. For example, although men who rate themselves mildly improved on medical therapy for BPH have an improvement in their AUA scores of about 3 points on average, fluctuations of AUA scores of this magnitude may be simply because of chance. When such improvements are larger in magnitude (5 points or greater, consistent with self-ratings of "moderate" improvement), or when smaller changes are persistent over time, they are more likely to represent true changes in the patient's condition. The same principles apply to any other continuous parameter measured serially to assess treatment outcome.

## EFFICACY VS. EFFECTIVENESS OF MEDICAL THERAPY FOR BPH

When interpreting the results of studies of any therapeutic modality, *efficacy* refers to the impact of the treatment in ideal circumstances above and beyond what would

|  | not at all | less than 1 time in 5 | less than half the time | about half the time | more than half the time | almost always |
|---|---|---|---|---|---|---|
| 1. Over the past month or so, how often have you had a sensation of not emptying your bladder completely after you finished urinating? | 0 | 1 | 2 | 3 | 4 | 5 |
| 2. Over the past month or so, how often have you had to urinate again less than two hours after you finished urinating? | 0 | 1 | 2 | 3 | 4 | 5 |
| 3. Over the past month or so, how often have you found you stopped and started again several times when you urinated? | 0 | 1 | 2 | 3 | 4 | 5 |
| 4. Over the past month or so, how often have you found it difficult to postpone urination? | 0 | 1 | 2 | 3 | 4 | 5 |
| 5. Over the past month or so, how often have you had a weak urinary stream? | 0 | 1 | 2 | 3 | 4 | 5 |
| 6. Over the past month or so, how often have you had to push or strain to begin urination? | 0 | 1 | 2 | 3 | 4 | 5 |

7. Over the last month, how many times did you most typically get up to urinate from the time you went to bed at night until the time you got up in the morning?

- 0 none
- 1 1 time
- 2 2 times
- 3 3 times
- 4 4 times
- 5 5 or more times

Score = sum of questions 1-7 = ___ ___

Fig. 1. The American Urological Association Symptom Index for Benign Prostatic Hyperplasia (Barry MJ, Fowler FJ, O'Leary MP, et al. [1992] The American Urological Association Symptom Index for benign prostatic hyperplasia. *J Urol* 148: 1549–1557, with permission from Lippincott, Williams and Wilkins).

be seen with placebo or sham therapy. *Effectiveness* refers to the impact that would be seen in usual clinical practice, which includes the placebo effect. Such authorities as the US Food and Drug Administration tend to focus on the efficacy of a pharmacologic therapy in approval decisions, but clinicians should be more interested in the treatment's effectiveness.

The distinction between efficacy and effectiveness is critical in assessing trials of medical therapies for BPH, because all such studies have shown strong placebo effects on lower urinary-tract symptoms among men thought to have these symptoms because of BPH. In fact, 30–50% of men will rate themselves as improved on blinded placebo therapy in such trials. For example, about 60% of men rated themselves as moderately or markedly improved after 1 yr of treatment with the alpha-blocker terazosin in a large Department of Veterans Affairs (VA) trial, compared to about 40% of placebo-treated patients. These data suggests that for every 10 patients a clinician treats with terazosin for lower urinary-tract symptoms presumably caused by BPH, 6 would feel considerably better—4 from the placebo effect, and 2 more from the direct pharmacologic effect of the drug.

From this example, one can see that much of the benefit seen with medical therapies currently available for BPH represents a placebo effect. However, from the effectiveness perspective, it is unimportant whether a patient who feels better on one of these therapies has improved because of a placebo response or as a result of the true pharmacologic effect of the medication. On the other hand, some clinicians worry that if patients simply feel better because of a placebo effect, they have probably not lowered their risk of BPH complications, another rational goal of therapy.

Another example highlights the clash of the efficacy vs. effectiveness perspectives in clinical decision-making in office practice. In the 4-yr Proscar Long-Term Efficacy and Safety Study (PLESS), comparing finasteride to placebo, the efficacy of finasteride in reducing symptoms was greater for men with larger glands or higher PSA levels (a proxy for gland size). However, this finding did not result from a better finasteride response with larger glands; in fact, the mean symptom-score change from baseline was similar among finasteride-treated men regardless of prostate size. Rather, larger gland size resulted in a poorer response to placebo, and therefore a greater difference in mean-score responses between men in the 2 study arms with increasing prostate size. From an efficacy perspective, finasteride has a greater true pharmacologic impact on symptoms among men with larger prostates. On the other hand, from the effectiveness perspective, it makes no sense to select patients for finasteride therapy based on prostate size in clinical practice (at least when the goal is symptom reduction), because the patient's chance of a good symptom response is no different with a smaller vs. a larger prostate.

## ALPHA-BLOCKERS

The rationale for alpha-blocker therapy for men with lower urinary-tract symptoms presumed to result from BPH is that adrenergic stimulation of alpha$_1$ receptors in the bladder neck, prostatic capsule, and prostate itself cause smooth-muscle contraction and contribute a "dynamic" component to bladder-outlet obstruction. It is currently believed that the alpha$_{1A}$ adrenoreceptor subtype predominates in the prostate, whereas the alpha$_{1B}$ and alpha$_{1D}$ subtypes predominate in vascular smooth muscle. However, the alpha$_{1A}$ adrenoreceptor subtype is not exclusive or specific to the prostate.

The first report of therapeutic responses from alpha-blockers among men presumed to be affected by BPH was published by Marco Caine and colleagues in 1976. Since that time, the use of older, nonselective alpha-blockers, such as phenoxybenzamine, has given way to the use of selective alpha$_1$ antagonists, such as prazosin, terazosin, doxazosin, alfuzosin (outside the United States), and tamsulosin. Terazosin (Hytrin), doxazosin (Cardura), and tamsulosin (Flomax) are long-acting, allowing once-a-day dosing. In general, the impact of the alpha-blockers on lower urinary-tract symptoms has been well-defined, but the impact of these agents on the future risk of BPH complications has been poorly defined.

### *Terazosin and Doxazosin*

Terazosin and doxazosin can lower blood pressure through their effect on vascular smooth muscle; both were initially used in the United States for the treatment of hypertension. As a result, doses must be titrated to check for evidence of orthostatic

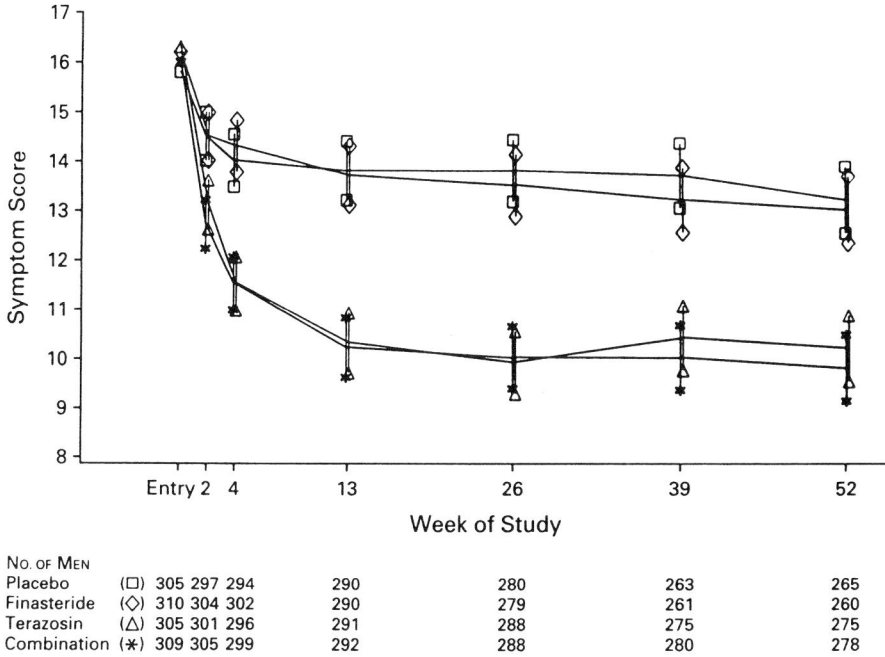

**Fig. 2.** Symptom response to terazosin, finasteride, combination therapy, and placebo in a randomized trial among U.S. veterans with one year follow-up (Lepor H, Williford W, Barry MJ, et al. [1996] The efficacy of terazosin, finasteride, or both in benign prostatic hyperplasia. *N Engl J Med* 335: 533–539, copyright © 1996 Massachusetts Medical Society. All rights reserved).

hypertension, the most troubling side effect of these agents. On the other hand, some patients with both hypertension and BPH can be treated for both problems with alpha-blocker monotherapy. In fact, effects on blood pressure appear to be more dramatic in hypertensive rather than normotensive patients. Terazosin is usually started at 1 mg daily, with dose increases to 2, 5, and 10 mg daily, stopping either for a satisfactory therapeutic effect or the appearance of unacceptable side effects. The analogous dose steps with doxazosin are 1, 2, 4, and 8 mg daily. Most studies suggest a continuing benefit at higher doses for the alpha-blocker, so pushing the dose toward the maximum is reasonable if the patient still sees room for improvement at a lower dose.

Multiple randomized, double-blind trials up to 1 yr in duration have documented the efficacy of terazosin and doxazosin for the treatment of men with lower urinary tract symptoms presumably caused by BPH. In a prototypical trial—a VA trial published by Lepor and colleagues—which randomized men to terazosin, finasteride, placebo, or combination therapy, mean AUA scores dropped from about 16 to 10 points with terazosin (80% of men received the maximum 10-mg daily dose), compared to about 16 to 14 points with placebo, a group mean difference between treatment arms of about 4 points (*see* Fig. 2). From an effectiveness perspective, average AUA scores dropped about 6 points from baseline with terazosin treatment, a change that most men would rate at least "moderately" improved. Terazosin worked quickly, producing a significantly lower symptom-score by 2 weeks into the trial, and maximal responses by 13 wk. The alpha-blockers have also increased peak urinary flow rates to a greater degree than placebo in many trials, but the clinical importance of this effect is not well-defined. The longer-term efficacy of the alpha-blockers is less certain, given the lack of trials with randomized controls with more than 1 yr of follow-up.

Side effects of the selective alpha-receptor blockers, which have consistently occurred more frequently than placebo in clinical trials—aside from postural hypotension—are dizziness and asthenia, which are not necessarily blood-pressure-related. Many clinicians tell patients to take their alpha-blockers at bedtime to reduce these side effects, but the effectiveness of this practice for men with BPH rather than hypertension has been poorly documented. Other side effects noted less consistently include peripheral edema and ejaculatory problems, seen in small percentages of patients. Most patients stay on their alpha-blockers during clinical trials. For example, in the VA trial, over the course of 1 yr, 80% of subjects remained on the maximum dose of terazosin, about 10% reduced their dose because of side effects, and about 10% stopped therapy completely. Whether such adherence could be maintained in usual office practice over longer time periods is unknown. Unfortunately, little data is available even from long-term open-label extension studies regarding the use of alpha-blockers beyond 1 yr. Data from <100 patients, followed for more than 42 mo on either doxazosin or terazosin, suggest that efficacy is maintained, at least in those patients who elected to stay on the drug. Such open-label trials, however, are subject to the problem of responder bias. Alpha-blockers do not change serum prostate-specific antigen (PSA) levels.

### *Tamsulosin*

Tamsulosin was developed to have greater affinity for the prostatic $alpha_{1A}$ adrenoreceptors than the adrenoreceptors that are more prominent in vascular smooth muscle, and it does not appear to affect blood pressure. As a result, tamsulosin is easier to titrate than the other alpha-blockers. Patients can simply begin on a dose of 0.4 mg daily. Although the manufacturer advises a dose increase to 0.8 mg daily if further improvement in symptoms is desired, the symptomatic benefit of increasing the dose appears to be small. At present, tamsulosin is only available in 0.4-mg capsules; patients on the higher dose must take 2 capsules daily, thus doubling the cost of this therapy. The effectiveness of tamsulosin on lower urinary-tract symptoms appears comparable to that of terazosin and doxazosin. Although tamsulosin does not lower blood pressure, side effects still occur, including dizziness, fatigue, and sexual dysfunction. Although tamsulosin was developed to have fewer side effects than the older agents because of its "uroselectivity," it is unclear whether it actually does. In fact, in one head-to-head trial by Buzelin and colleagues comparing tamsulosin with alfuzosin, the therapeutic response and side-effect profile were quite similar between the study arms, although the former agent did have less impact on blood pressure.

### *Which Alpha-Blocker for Which Patient?*

The therapeutic effects of the selective $alpha_1$-blockers appear to be similar, so there is little reason to choose among them on this basis. Although prazosin must be given at least twice a day, it is available generically, and the price may be attractive to some patients. Tamsulosin may be a better choice for patients with marginal blood pressure at baseline, particularly for men on complex drug regimens for cardiovascular disease. It is not yet clear whether tamsulosin offers fewer side effects than the other alpha-blockers—aside from postural hypotension, which is rare. Many clinicians are attracted to tamsulosin's easier dose-titration schedule. The additional costs for men who require two 0.4-mg capsules daily may be a deterrent to some patients.

Investigators have tried to predict which patients will respond best to alpha-blockers, using measurements of prostate size, uroflow, and the presence or absence of urodynamic evidence of bladder-outlet obstruction. In general, none of these measurements have been found to predict therapeutic response.

Some clinicians assume that men with mild to moderate lower urinary-tract symptoms are better candidates for medical therapy than men with severe symptoms (AUA scores of 20 or greater). In fact, for all medical therapies, the higher the symptom score at baseline, the greater the expected fall in score with treatment. Therefore, even men with severe symptoms are reasonable candidates for a trial of medical therapy. Most men with mild symptoms (AUA scores of 7 or below) are usually not troubled enough by their symptoms to accept the potential side effects of medical therapy.

## 5-ALPHA-REDUCTASE INHIBITORS

Finasteride (Proscar) blocks the conversion of testosterone to dihydrotestosterone, the major intraprostatic androgen, by the enzyme 5-alpha reductase. Recent studies have documented two forms of the 5-alpha reductase enzyme in humans. Finasteride is a specific blocker of the Type II enzyme, which appears to predominate in the genitourinary tract. The Type I enzyme appears to predominate in skin outside the genital tract. Although finasteride is the only 5-alpha reductase inhibitor available for the treatment of BPH at present, studies of "dual inhibitors" of both enzyme types are under investigation.

Finasteride is used in the treatment of men with BPH at 5 mg once daily, and no dose titration is necessary. A year's course of therapy with finasteride reduces prostate volume by about 20%. However, because reductions in symptoms do not correlate well with reductions in volume at the patient level, the mechanism by which finasteride affects lower urinary tract symptoms is unclear. Finasteride works more slowly than the alpha-blockers, and 6 mo of treatment may be necessary to observe the full effect on symptoms.

As already noted, the ability of finasteride to reduce symptoms is related to prostate volume, with the greatest efficacy seen among men with prostate volumes of 40 g or more. Its effectiveness is less dependent on prostate size, and size made little difference in symptom-score change from baseline in the 4-yr PLESS trial mentioned earlier. In a meta-analysis of six 1-yr or 2-yr trials of finasteride vs. placebo, mean changes from baseline of 2 (for smaller prostates) to 3 points (for larger prostates) were seen (*see* Fig. 3)—although the symptom index had a range of 1–30, rather than 1–35 for the AUA Index. In the VA trial that did not show that finasteride reduced symptoms more than placebo (*see* Fig. 2), an enlarged prostate was not an entry criterion, and the average prostate volume was relatively low.

Although finasteride's impact on lower urinary-tract symptoms appears to be quite modest, this agent has recently been shown to reduce the subsequent risk of undergoing a prostatectomy and the development of acute urinary retention. These findings were consistent in a meta-analysis of earlier 1–2-yr trials, and in the 4-yr PLESS trial. Approximately 8% of about 1500 PLESS subjects treated with placebo for 4 yr underwent transurethral prostatectomy, compared to about 4% of about the same number of

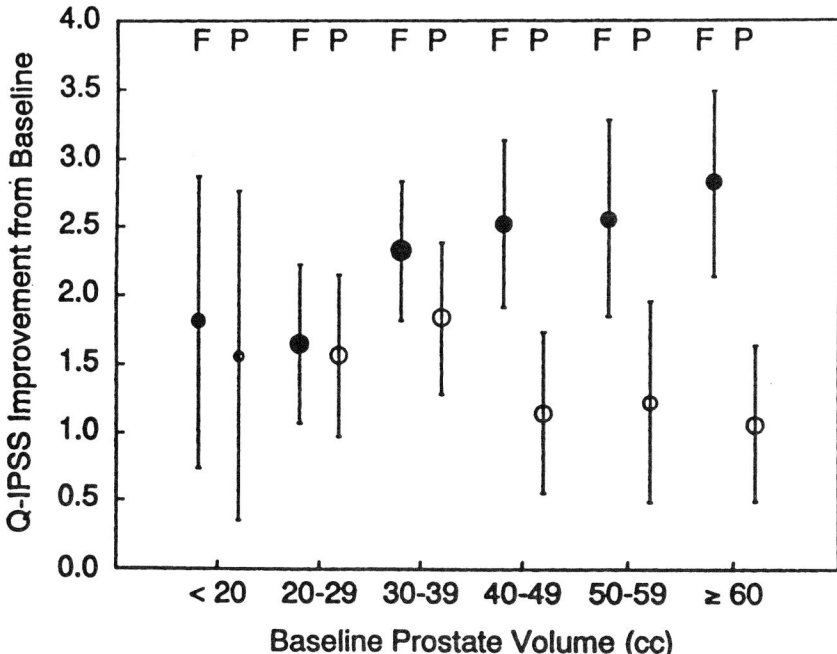

Fig. 3. Improvement in symptom score from baseline in a meta-analysis of six randomized trials of finasteride (F) versus placebo (P), by baseline prostate volume. (Reprinted from *Urology*, vol. 48; Boyle P, Gould AL, Roehrborn CG [1996] Prostate volume predicts outcome of treatment of benign prostatic hyperplasia with finasteride: meta-analysis of randomized clinical trials. pp. 398–405, with permission from Elsevier Science).

finasteride-treated patients. Acute retention occurred in 7% of men on placebo, compared to 3% on finasteride. Thus, about 15 men would have to take finasteride for 4 yr to prevent one event of prostate surgery or acute retention (the "number needed to treat," or NNT).

Both prostate volume and—as a proxy for volume—serum PSA are clinically useful predictors of the risk of urinary retention and/or surgery over time. The risk of either retention or surgery over 4 yr in PLESS was about 8% for men with a baseline PSA of 0–1.3 ng/mL, about 13% for men with a baseline PSA of 1.4–3.2 ng/mL, and about 20% for men with a baseline PSA >3.2 ng/mL. With finasteride treatment, the absolute reduction in risk becomes greater in men with higher PSA values, resulting in more cost-effective therapy (*see* Fig. 4). In PLESS, the NNT to prevent one event of acute retention or surgery over 4 yr was about 29 for men with a baseline PSA of 0–1.3 ng/mL, 18 for men with baseline PSAs of 1.4–3.3 ng/mL, and 9 for men with a baseline PSA >3.3 ng/mL.

The main side effect of finasteride is sexual dysfunction, including loss of libido, erectile dysfunction, and reduced ejaculate. Taken together, about 10–15% of men are affected by these potential problems in the first year of treatment. In clinical practice, these side effects resolve after discontinuation of therapy. Interestingly, the incidence of new onset of sexual dysfunction in yr 2, 3, and 4 of the PLESS trial was identical in the finasteride and the placebo arms, indicating that these delayed effects are probably caused by the normal aging process. Finasteride reduces serum PSA levels by an average

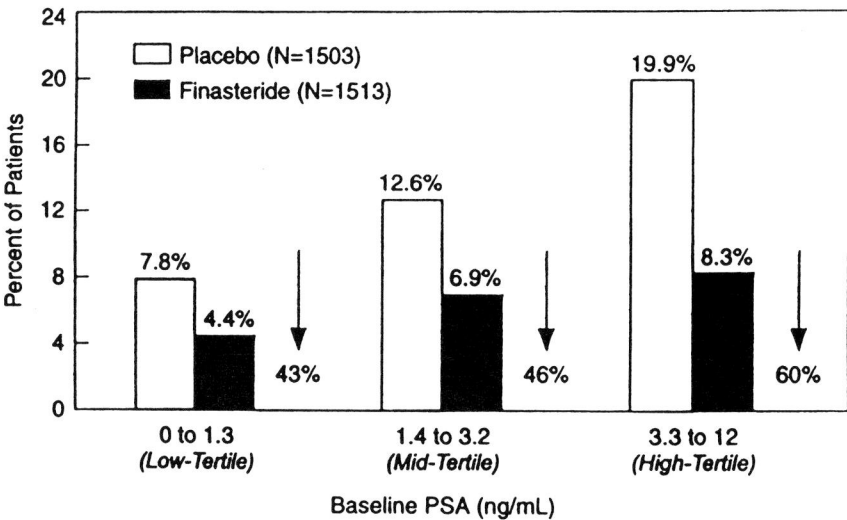

Fig. 4. Four-year cumulative incidences of either acute urinary retention or BPH-related surgery in patients in PLESS treated with finasteride or placebo, stratified by tertiles of baseline PSA levels (Reprinted from *Urology*, vol. 53; Roehrborn CG, McConnell JD, Lieber M, et al. (1999) Serum prostate-specific antigen concentration is a powerful predictor of acute urinary retention and need for surgery in men with clinical benign prostatic hyperplasia. pp. 473–480, with permission from Elsevier Science).

of 50%, and PSA levels must be interpreted differently among men on finasteride. One commonly used strategy is to double the on-finasteride PSA level and interpret the results as usual. In the PLESS trial, rates of detection for prostate cancer were similar in both treatment arms, and there is no evidence that finasteride reduces the detection of prostate cancer, or alters the histology of the prostate enough to complicate the diagnosis of prostate cancer by biopsy.

## ALPHA-BLOCKERS, FINASTERIDE, OR COMBINATION THERAPY?

In a head-to-head comparison of finasteride vs. terazosin—the VA trial published by Lepor and colleagues—terazosin was clearly superior to finasteride at reducing lower urinary-tract symptoms over the course of 1 year of therapy. These findings were duplicated in the 52-wk European PREDICT trial, which randomized over 1000 patients to doxazosin, finasteride, combination, or placebo. A stratified analysis of the VA and PREDICT trials failed to reveal a relationship between symptom improvements and baseline volume or PSA for either drug. This finding, however, may be because of the shorter duration of these trials compared to the PLESS study. Alpha-blockers are clearly the drugs of first choice for reducing lower urinary-tract symptoms in the short to medium term. On the other hand, finasteride has a much stronger track record in terms of preventing BPH complications in the long term—particularly progression to prostatectomy or the occurrence of acute urinary retention—with a more favorable number needed to treat among men with larger prostates or higher PSA levels. Appropriate selection of medical therapy, then, depends on the goals of treatment, which need to be negotiated with each patient.

If alpha-blockers offer better symptom relief and finasteride offers a lower risk of future BPH complications, why not combine both agents, at least for men with larger prostates? This theoretically attractive concept remains to be tested over the long term. In the VA and PREDICT trials, adding finasteride to an alpha-blocker resulted in no greater symptom relief over 1 yr. However, greater symptom relief is not really the goal of combination therapy, and in these trials too few subjects were followed for too little time to determine whether the addition of finasteride would result in fewer symptoms or a reduced rate of complications over a longer time period. The rationale for such combination therapy is attractive enough to consider—pending an adequately powered trial—for men who appear to have a substantially enlarged prostate on digital rectal exam or a baseline PSA >3.3 ng/mL and perhaps even 1.3 ng/mL. Physicians generally underestimate prostate size by up to 30%; if a gland feels big, it probably is.

## PHYTOTHERAPY

Phytotherapy is widely used in Europe for lower urinary-tract symptoms considered attributable to BPH, and plant extracts are frequently prescribed for this purpose by physicians. Patients with lower urinary-tract symptoms in the United States appear to be using plant extracts in increasing numbers as well. The most widely known and best-studied of these agents are extracts of the saw palmetto plant, *Serenoa repens.* In a recently published meta-analysis of randomized trials of various saw palmetto extracts for men with symptoms attributed to BPH—all of which were of relatively short duration—these medications had a small but statistically significant impact on lower urinary-tract symptoms (and peak flow rates as well). Saw palmetto extracts appeared to have a similar impact to finasteride across a number of head-to-head trials of these two treatments. Given finasteride's relatively modest impact on symptoms, such a finding is not particularly impressive. On the other hand, these extracts appeared to have virtually no attributable side effects. Clinicians should question patients about the use of "natural remedies" for their symptoms, and be prepared to answer questions about their effectiveness and side effects. Given the results of the meta-analysis, at least saw palmetto extracts cannot be dismissed as no more than a placebo. However, since these products are not standardized, it is hard to advise a patient on which preparations would yield expected results as reflected in these trials.

## CONCLUSION

Selective alpha$_1$-receptor blockers, such as terazosin, doxazosin, and tamsulosin, provide effective medical therapy for reducing lower urinary-tract symptoms among men presumed to have those symptoms of BPH. There is little reason to choose among the alpha-blockers based on effectiveness; for some men who can afford little if any blood-pressure reduction, tamsulosin will be the preferred agent. Finasteride and saw palmetto extracts also reduce lower urinary-tract symptoms, although they are less effective for this purpose—at least over the short term—than the alpha-blockers. On the other hand, finasteride lowers the future risk of progression to prostatectomy and the occurrence of acute urinary retention; the numbers of patients who need to be treated to prevent one of either event are relatively advantageous for men with larger prostates. Combination therapy with an alpha-blocker and finasteride is a conceptually attractive, though untested, treatment strategy for men with troubling lower urinary-tract symptoms and evidence of considerable prostate enlargement by DRE (or, as a proxy, a high-normal or elevated baseline PSA).

## ACKNOWLEDGMENT

The outcome assessments underlying the content of this chapter were funded by the Agency for Health Care Policy and Research (Grant No. HS 08397).

## SELECTED READING

Andersen JT, Nickel JC, Marshall VR, et al. (1997) Finasteride significantly reduces acute urinary retention and need for surgery in patients with symptomatic benign prostatic hyperplasia. *Urology* 49:839–845.

Barry MJ, Fowler FJ, O'Leary MP, et al. (1992) The American Urological Association symptom index for benign prostatic hyperplasia. *J Urol* 148:1549–1557.

Boyle P, Gould AL, Roehrborn CG (1996) Prostate volume predicts outcome of treatment of benign prostatic hyperplasia with finasteride: meta-analysis of randomized clinical trials. *Urology* 48:398–405.

Buzelin JM, Fonteyne E, Kontturi M, et al. (1997) Comparison of tamsulosin with alfuzosin in the treatment of patients with lower urinary tract symptoms suggestive of bladder outlet obstruction (symptomatic benign prostatic hyperplasia). *Br J Urol* 80:597–605.

Gormley GJ, Stoner E, Bruskewitz RC (1992) The effect of finasteride in men with benign prostatic hyperplasia. *N Engl J Med* 327:1185–1191.

Guess HA, Gormley GJ, Stoner E, et al. (1996) The effect of finasteride on prostate specific antigen: review of available data. *J Urol* 155:3–9.

Jardin A, Bensadoun H, Delauche-Cavillier MC (1991) Alfuzosin for treatment of benign prostatic hypertrophy. *Lancet* 337:1457–1461.

Kirby RS, Pool JL (1997) Alpha adrenoreceptor blockade in the treatment of benign prostatic hyperplasia: past, present and future. *Br J Urol* 80:521–532.

Lepor H, Williford WO, Barry MJ, et al. (1996) The efficacy of terazosin, finasteride, or both in benign prostatic hyperplasia. *N Engl J Med* 335:533–539.

Lepor H, Williford WO, Barry MJ, et al. (1998) The impact of medical therapy on bother due to symptoms, quality of life and global outcome, and factors predicting response. *J Urol* 160:1358–1367.

McConnell JD, Bruskewitz RC, Walsh P, et al. (1998) The effect of finasteride on the risk of acute urinary retention and the need for surgical treatment among men with benign prostatic hyperplasia. *N Engl J Med* 338:557–563.

Narayan P, Tewari A (1998) Overview of alpha-blocker therapy for benign prostatic hyperplasia. *Urology* 51, (Suppl. 4A), 38–45.

Narayan P, Tewari A, Members of United States 93-01 Study Group. (1998) A second phase III multicenter placebo controlled study of 2 dosages of modified release tamsulosin in patients with symptoms of benign prostatic hyperplasia. *J Urol* 160:1701–1706.

Roehrborn CG, Siegel RL (1996) Safety and efficacy of doxazosin in benign prostatic hyperplasia: a pooled analysis of three double-blind, placebo-controlled studies. *Urology* 48:406–415.

Roehrborn CG, Oesterling JE, Auerbach S, et al. (1996) The hytrin community assessment trial study: a one-year study of terazosin versus placebo in the treatment of men with symptomatic benign prostatic hyperplasia. *Urology* 47:159–168.

Roehrborn CG, Girman CJ, Rhodes T, et al. (1997) Correlation between prostate size estimated by digital rectal examination and measured by transrectal ultrasound. *Urology* 49:548–557.

Roehrborn CG, McConnell JD, Lieber M, et al. (1999) Serum prostate-specific antigen concentration is a powerful predictor of acute urinary retention and need for surgery in men with clinical benign prostatic hyperplasia. *Urology* 53:473–480.

Roehrborn CG, Boyle P, Gould AL, Waldstreicher J (1999) Serum prostate specific antigen (PSA) as a predictor of prostate volume in men with benign prostatic hyperplasia. *Urology* 53:581–589.

Wilt TJ, Ishani A, Stark G, et al. (1998) Saw palmetto extracts for treatment of benign prostatic hyperplasia. *JAMA* 280:1604–1609.

Witjes WPJ, Rosier PFWM, Caris CTM, et al. (1997) Urodynamic and clinical effects of terazosin therapy in symptomatic patients with and without bladder outlet obstruction: a stratified analysis. *Urology* 49:197–206.

# 19 The Advent of Minimally Invasive Treatments for Benign Prostatic Obstruction

*Christopher S. Ng, MD,
James C. Ulchaker, MD,
and Elroy D. Kursh, MD*

**CONTENTS**
INTRODUCTION
PRINCIPLES OF THERMAL DAMAGE
MINIMALLY INVASIVE THERAPY FOR BPH
TRANSURETHRAL MICROWAVE THERMOTHERAPY
INTERSTITIAL LASER COAGULATION
TRANSURETHRAL NEEDLE ABLATION
HIGH-INTENSITY FOCUSED ULTRASOUND
PROSTATIC URETHRAL STENTS
TRANSURETHRAL BALLOON DILATION OF THE PROSTATE
SUMMARY
SELECTED READINGS

## INTRODUCTION

The urologic management of benign prostatic hyperplasia (BPH) beyond pharmacotherapy has changed dramatically over the last decade. Open prostatectomy and transurethral resection of the prostate (TURP) have been the mainstays of surgical intervention for BPH. These procedures were initially reserved for patients with obstructive uropathy, prostatic bleeding, or bladder calculi. With improved techniques and lower morbidity, TURP is currently the "gold standard" of treatment for patients with BPH and troubling lower urinary-tract symptoms (LUTS), and patients are being treated prior to the development of these adverse sequelae.

Nevertheless, TURP is still major surgery, requiring either a spinal or general anesthetic and an inpatient hospital stay. Furthermore, TURP is not uniformly successful. Up to 30% of patients report dissatisfaction from the procedure. Complications have been well-described and include bleeding, bladder-neck contracture, erectile dysfunction, retrograde ejaculation, urinary incontinence, and fluid/electrolyte imbalance (post-TUR syndrome). The mortality rate for TURP is approx 2–10/1000 cases. Over the past decade, the number of TURPs being performed has been decreasing as minimally invasive therapies, including alpha-adrenergic blockers, are being used as "first-line" management with increasing frequency and success.

In addition, urologists no longer just treat ill patients in urinary retention. The treatment paradigm has evolved to include patients with persistently troubling symptoms of bladder-outlet obstruction, prior to the development of such adverse sequelae. Furthermore, patients seek the care of a urologist on an elective basis, and they frequently wish to avoid surgery. As described in prior chapters, advancements in our understanding of the pathophysiology of BPH have led to improvements in its medical management and have delayed or precluded surgery in many patients. However, when pharmacotherapy fails, further treatment options need to be discussed. Minimally invasive therapies for BPH have evolved out of this need to "bridge the gap" between medical and surgical management. This chapter describes the current modalities of minimally invasive treatment for benign prostatic obstruction caused by prostatic lobar hyperplasia, and their respective roles in our office practice.

## PRINCIPLES OF THERMAL DAMAGE

In the search for alternative methods of treating BPH, many have investigated the role of cooling or heating the prostate, with the goal of ablating the adenomatous tissue or "shrinking the prostate," thereby mimicking TURP. Such an effect has been well-documented in other tissues using both cryotherapy and thermotherapy. However, the results of cryotherapy in the treatment of BPH have been disappointing.

Hyperthermia of the prostate was initially used experimentally in the 1980s in prostate cancer, and has subsequently been applied to the treatment of BPH. Heating the prostatic interstitium, also called *thermotherapy,* has been shown to produce tissue-ablative effects within the prostate in experimental animal and human models. Intraprostatic temperatures of <45 °C do not cause any significant cellular changes. However, temperatures between 45° and 100°C produce *coagulation necrosis* with irreversible cellular damage and thrombosis of small vessels. These areas of tissue necrosis will undergo liquefaction and subsequent resorption through lymphatic and hematogenous channels, thereby reducing prostatic lobar tissue mass and effectively "shrinking the prostate." Lastly, temperatures >100°C lead to desiccation and carbonization of the tissues, which radically changes the heating properties of the tissue. In this situation, water is boiled off, and the tissue changes color to brown and then black with continued heating. This charred tissue creates an insulation barrier that prevents further propagation of heat. It is therefore evident that heating tissue to temperatures above 100°C is highly undesirable. For all degrees of thermotherapy, the magnitude of the resulting tissue lesion depends directly on the intraprostatic temperatures achieved and the duration of such temperatures.

The beneficial effects of thermotherapy are believed to be twofold. Certainly, reduction of prostatic lobar mass with subsequent widening of the urethral channel will relieve the "static component" to bladder-outlet obstruction. In addition, it has been hypothesized that coagulation necrosis also destroys alpha-adrenergic nerve terminals within the prostate and decreases its sympathetic tone, thus interrupting the "dynamic component" to bladder-outlet obstruction.

## MINIMALLY INVASIVE THERAPY FOR BPH

Most of the minimally invasive modalities for treating BPH available today utilize this concept of thermotherapy to reduce bladder-outflow obstruction and relieve troubling symptoms of prostatism. Such modalities include transurethral microwave thermotherapy (TUMT), interstitial laser coagulation (ILC), transurethral needle ablation (TUNA), and high-intensity focused ultrasound ablation (HIFU). Each modality delivers thermotherapy through different mechanisms, yet they all share a common goal—that is, to raise the intraprostatic temperature sufficiently to induce coagulation necrosis while sparing the surrounding organs, especially the urethra and the rectum. Furthermore, these procedures can be performed in the office setting on an outpatient basis without an anesthesiologist. The advent of these minimally-invasive therapies for BPH over the past decade has clearly added yet another dimension to the practice of office urology, and has enabled urologists to better manage patients with troubling symptoms of bladder-outflow obstruction who have failed conservative measures.

### *Assessment of Treatment Success*

The majority of investigators today use symptom scores and peak urinary flow rates (Qmax) as quantitative measures of outcome for the various minimally invasive therapies for BPH. These same parameters have been used in the assessment of the effectiveness of TURP and pharmacotherapy, and allow for comparison with these standards. The Madsen Symptom Score and the International Prostate Symptom Score (IPSS)—the two main standardized questionnaires used to assess symptoms subjectively—are described in previous chapters. Many authors define treatment success as either a decrease in symptom score or an increase in Qmax of 50% or greater (the "50% rule"). For example, a change in IPSS from 20 to 10 would be considered a treatment success.

## TRANSURETHRAL MICROWAVE THERMOTHERAPY

Transurethral microwave thermotherapy (TUMT) has been investigated in clinical trials for the treatment of BPH since 1991, yet was not approved by the Food and Drug Administration (FDA) until May 1996. This modality uses focused microwaves at frequencies from 900 to 1300 MHz to induce coagulation necrosis within the prostatic adenoma. The intraprostatic temperatures achieved and the resulting lesions created are determined by the depth of penetration of the microwaves, which depends on the wave frequency of the microwaves and the properties of the target tissue. Higher frequencies are less able to penetrate a given medium. Furthermore, tissues with higher water content, such as muscle, reduce the depth of penetration, and tissues with lower water content, such as fat, allow increased transmission of microwaves. Higher frequencies of microwaves have been used to generate more localized treatment because of the lesser magnitude of tissue penetration.

The current commercially available TUMT devices share certain fundamental characteristics. All working elements are contained within a Foley-type catheter design consisting of the antenna probe, water-cooling channel, and balloon channel. There are no protruding needle probes, and the prostatic urothelium is never penetrated (unlike other modalities discussed below). The device is inserted into the bladder per urethra, and the retention balloon is inflated with sterile water. Proper positioning of the balloon at the bladder neck is crucial to the success of the procedure, since the location of the microwave antenna is fixed and cannot be altered. Furthermore, the entire procedure is performed in the absence of cystourethroscopic guidance. Therefore, the position of the balloon must be confirmed by bladder ultrasound. The balloon is composed of material that is more echogenic than the typical drainage catheter in order to aid in its detection.

The microwave antenna is located at the core of the catheter device just below the retention balloon, so it rests within the prostatic urethra. The antenna is surrounded by channels through which cool water (20°C) continuously flows. This feature was specifically designed to reduce the ambient urethral temperature and thus minimize urethral trauma through conductive heat dissipation. Urethral temperatures are monitored by sensors within the device. Furthermore, anterior rectal-wall temperatures are also continuously monitored by fiberoptic thermosensors contained in a rectal probe. The system will automatically shut down temporarily if certain urethral or rectal temperature thresholds are exceeded, thus resulting in potential lapses in therapy. The urethral temperature threshold is 44.5°C, and the rectal temperature threshold is 42.5 or 43.5°C, depending on which software program is used. Since the entire program is computer controlled, the specific version of software used alters the amount of energy and heat delivered.

The most widely used and reported TUMT device is the Prostatron (Edap Technomed, Burlington, MA). This machine, like the others, is regulated by a portable computer with corresponding computer software. The original software version, Prostasoft 2.0, delivers a standard energy level with a maximum of 60 W at an average of 103 kJ per treatment. This TUMT device features a 0.5-cm monopolar antenna located 1 cm below the catheter balloon within the prostatic urethra. In December 1997, a new software program (Prostatron 2.5) which delivers up to 70 W of energy and an average of 157 kJ per treatment was approved by the FDA. The Prostasoft 2.5 software has also been termed the "high-energy" program as opposed to the original "low-energy" software. In addition, this software features a shorter monopolar microwave antenna that is located immediately below the catheter balloon, thus specifically targeting the bladder neck. Furthermore, it uses an increased rectal temperature threshold of 43.5°C as opposed to 42.5°C, allowing more heat to be delivered to the prostate with fewer rectal shutdowns.

Another microwave unit that has been developed more recently is the Targis, formerly called T3 (Urologix, Minneapolis, MN), TUMT device, which features a helical dipole microwave antenna that delivers high-energy thermotherapy primarily to the anterolateral regions of the prostate gland. The difference between monopolar and dipolar microwave antennae has been well documented by Larson and associates. The dipole antenna supposedly delivers symmetric patterns of heat confined to a 23-mm zone around the antenna. Conversely, the monopole antenna creates an asymmetric heating pattern, with noticeable "back heating" along the catheter axis toward the power-source generator. Clinically, this translates into more frequent power shutdowns, with resultant interruptions in therapy caused by overheating of the urethra or rectum. Blute and associates noted that rectal shutdowns occurred in 76% of cases using the Prostatron compared with 4% of cases using the T3. As described above, the T3 preferentially targets the anterior and lateral aspects of the prostate gland, well removed from the rectal wall, and this probably contributes substantially to these findings.

Using the T3 system, Larson and associates compared temperature mappings during TUMT to corresponding prostatectomy specimens obtained in the same patient at an average of 42 wk post-TUMT. Intraprostatic temperatures reached a maximum of 80°C. Histopathologic examination revealed a sharply circumscribed, well-demarcated lesion of hemorrhagic necrosis with minimal inflammation. The border between necrotic and viable tissue was merely 1 mm thick. Urethral mucosae were uniformly intact and uninjured. Tissue temperature mappings recorded at the time of TUMT correlated well with the histologic specimens. In areas of necrosis, the average temperature was 55°C. Border areas measured 45.7°C, and viable areas measured 42°C on average.

## *Patient Selection*

Patients undergo a relatively standard pretreatment evaluation consisting of completion of several forms, including the AUA Symptom Score and Quality of Life Scale, urinary flow study, and measurement of postvoid residual (PVR) using abdominal ultrasound. If the patient chooses to undergo TUMT after a thorough discussion of the risks, benefits, and treatment alternatives, a few additional studies are required. Cystoscopy is performed to establish the anatomy of the prostate and to evaluate the bladder. Patients with trilobar hypertrophy of the prostate with middle-lobe enlargement extending intravesically are not candidates for TUMT, since the device is unable to target or induce coagulation necrosis in this region of the prostate. Finally, pretreatment transrectal ultrasonography of the prostate is performed to determine the prostate size and to specifically measure the length of the prostatic urethra—which is data required to enable use of the software program.

## *Anesthetic Requirements*

TUMT is administered without the need for general or spinal anesthesia. Nevertheless, most patients experience some discomfort during the procedure. The most common complaints are the feeling of heat in the penis (usually near the distal end of the penis); a strong urge to void, or heat in the rectum. Therefore, it is advisable to provide some analgesia and/or sedation prior to treatment. A variety of alternative premedicaiton programs have been used by various investigators. Our own preference is to administer meperidine HCl (Demerol) 100 mg intramuscularly (im), hydroxyzine pamoate (Vistaril) 75 mg im, and diazepam (Valium) 10 mg po 1 h before the procedure. Lower doses are used for more frail elderly individuals. This concept of preemptive analgesia has been well-studied, and has been shown to markedly reduce or eliminate postoperative analgesic requirements.

Other urologists use varying amounts of nonsteroidal antiinflammatory drugs, such as ketorolac (Toradol), and anticholinergic agents. Additionally, we have been inserting a heparin lock prior to therapy to administer small doses of meperidine intravenously if the patient experiences discomfort. Finally, prior to inserting the urethral catheter, topical anesthesia is also employed by injecting xylocaine 2% jelly intraurethrally. In addition, methods of distraction and repeated vocal reassurance seem to alleviate what is mainly anxiety in some patients. Interruptions in therapy may also allow pain to subside; however, this may adversely affect the efficacy of the procedure.

## Post-TUMT Management

Following treatment with the Prostasoft 2.0 software, 12–36% of the patients require an indwelling catheter or intermittent self-catheterization for approx 1 wk. Conversely, almost all of the patients managed with the Prostasoft 2.5 software require a catheter for 1–2 wk after therapy. We habitually remove the catheter 1 wk following high-energy therapy and start the patient on intermittent self-catheterization if he is unable to void. Antibiotics are administered perioperatively. Postoperative narcotic analgesics are usually not required. Varying degrees of hematuria are expected, but the degree of bleeding is usually mild and easily managed by increasing fluid intake.

## Results

The widest experience with TUMT has been with the Prostatron device using the 2.0 software package. In an analysis by De La Rosette summarizing the treatment of 1527 patients from multiple series, the Madsen Symptom Scores decreased from a baseline of 13.2 to 5.2, representing a 61% decrease. Peak urinary flow rate (Qmax) improved from a baseline of 9.2 to 12.9 mL/s, representing a 42% increase. Furthermore, 62% of patients exhibited more than a 50% improvement at the 12-mo follow-up, compared to 18% of patients treated with a sham procedure. Dahlstrand and associates reported 2-yr follow-up data on 69 candidates for TURP who were randomized to either TUMT or TURP. Eleven percent (4 of 37) of patients treated with TUMT required re-treatment. Of the remaining 89% of patients, 84% noted more than a 50% improvement in Madsen Symptom Score. Conversely, only 1 of 32 patients treated with TURP needed further therapy, and 97% of patients noted more than a 50% improvement at 2 yr. Although the results following TURP were obviously superior, there was no statistical difference between the two groups. In general, the mean symptom score decreases by 40–70%, and the Qmax increases 35–40% following treatment with the Prostasoft 2.0 software.

In the past 2 yr, long-term follow-up results of patients treated with the Prostatron using the 2.0 software have become available. Hallin and associates reported that only 23% of patients were satisfied with their treatment after 4 yr of follow-up. Furthermore, 66% required additional treatment. Of these, 71% needed only the addition of medical therapy (alpha-adrenergic blockers or finasteride), 27% underwent TURP, and 2% underwent a secondary TUMT. Median time to re-treatment was 45 mo. The patients who received no further treatment over 4 yr were found to have a 37% reduction in Madsen Symptom Scores (12.2 to 7.7). Keijzers and colleagues reported 5-yr follow-up data on 231 patients. The re-treatment rate was 57%, representing 41% with invasive therapy (open prostatectomy, TURP, or repeat TUMT), and 17% with medication only. The cohort that required no further treatment similarly exhibited a 37% improvement in Madsen Symptom Scores.

Patients treated with the higher-energy Prostasoft 2.5 software achieved greater objective improvement than those treated with the lower-energy Prostasoft 2.0 version, with peak flow-rate improvement ranging from 50 to 70%. Symptom scores decreased by approx 60%, a similar result to the changes observed following treatment with the 2.0 software. Some investigators also report an improved cystoscopic appearance with a nonobstructing prostatic fossa in some patients following high-energy TUMT. Clearly, the results are better following high-energy TUMT, yet at the expense of increased morbidity. Almost all patients require a urethral catheter for 1–2 wk. There is an increased risk of hematuria, and patients experience varying degrees of irritative voiding symptoms during the recovery period. Edap Technomed recommends that the 2.5 protocol be indicated for patients with prostatic lengths of 25–50 mm, in whom the benefits of obstructive improvement outweigh the intendant risks. In other words, the high-energy program is advisable for patients with larger-volume prostates and higher degrees of bladder-outflow obstruction. Because of this well-established greater efficacy, we employ the high-energy program in the overwhelming majority of patients.

Similar results are being reported with the use of the T3 or Targis TUMT system. Blute and colleagues compared T3 to sham, with 6-mo follow-up data. IPSS decreased from 21.3 to 8.8 (59%) in the T3 group vs. 21.3 to 14.5 (32%) in the sham group. Qmax increased from 7.5 to 13.2 mL/s (76%) after treatment with T3 vs. 8.8 to 10.7 mL/s (22%) after the sham procedure. Larson and associates reported data from a randomized prospective multicenter study on the use of Targis TUMT for symptomatic BPH. In the treatment group, IPSS decreased from 20.8 to 10.5 and 10.2 (51%) at 6 and 12 mo, respectively, and Qmax increased from 7.8 mL/s to 11.8 and 11.6 mL/s (50%) at 6 and 12 mo, respectively. Conversely, in the sham group, IPSS decreased by 32% and Qmax increased by 26%. At 6-mo follow-up, 98% of patients treated with the T3 needed no further treatment vs. 83% in the sham group. At 12 mo, approx 11% of patients treated with T3 required further treatment.

## *Adverse Events*

Urinary retention is more frequently seen with the high-energy systems because of the increased prostatic edema that occurs after thermotherapy. With the Prostasoft 2.0 software, one can expect 12–36% of patients to require an indwelling catheter or intermittent catheterization, usually for 1 wk and rarely for 1 mo. Conversely, all patients treated with the Prostasoft 2.5 software require a urethral catheter for approx 2 wk and will experience irritative voiding symptoms for 3 wk thereafter. Similarly, all patients treated with the Targis (T3) system require immediate postoperative catheterization; however, 90% will be able to void within 24 h, and 98% will be able to void in 1 wk. Discussion has been raised regarding the temporary placement of a prosthetic urethral stent at the time of TUMT to avoid catherization during the initial lag phase. The timing, morbidity, and cost issues of a second procedure to remove the stent need to be examined. Nevertheless, this "combination" modality is intriguing.

The low rate of reported morbidity after TUMT is the main attraction of this minimally invasive procedure. Transient hematuria is reported in 5% of patients after Targis TUMT, yet is seen in up to 75% of cases after Prostatron 2.5. Minor urethral bleeding and discharge is expected with TUMT, and approx 50% of patients experience irritative voiding symptoms—yet these events are self-limited. The vast majority of men report no change in erectile function postoperatively. However, retrograde ejaculation can occur in 0–4% of patients treated by T3, 0–11% after Prostasoft 2.0, and up to 44% after Prostasoft 2.5.

Long-term symptomatic improvement after one treatment of TUMT can be expected in less than half of all patients, although only long-term data on low-energy TUMT are currently available. There is considerable variation in individual responses to TUMT, in part because of the heterogeneity of the prostatic tissue and prostatic vascularity and the inconsistent intraprostatic temperatures achieved. Most authors report no observable difference between successes and failures regarding age, baseline symptom scores, uroflow parameters, PVR, or prostate volume. However, Keijzers and associates found that patients with Madsen Symptom Scores >15, Qmax <10 mL/s, and/or age >65 yr were more likely to fail TUMT. Certainly, patients with more severe bladder-outlet obstruction are less likely to benefit from low-energy TUMT. Whether these parameters will change our indications for low-energy TUMT has yet to be determined.

## *Summary*

The goal of TUMT is to duplicate the impressive symptomatic improvement achieved with surgery in an outpatient or office-based setting and in a cost-effective manner. TUMT fills the gap between medical and surgical therapy for BPH, and is easily tolerated, without the side effects of medicine or risks of surgery. Reported trials suggest a benefit of standard TUMT in a subset of patients, and we await the long-term results of high-energy TUMT. With this low-risk minimally invasive armamentarium becoming more readily available in our offices, we may begin treating patients earlier in the course of the disease when symptoms are less severe, and thus attract younger, more motivated patients. Perhaps this population is best suited for low-energy TUMT, where sexual function is less likely to be affected.

## INTERSTITIAL LASER COAGULATION

Laser-beam technology in the treatment of BPH is nothing new. Over the past 6 yr, various contact and free-beam lasers in either straight or side-firing configurations have been used in human trials to treat symptomatic bladder-outlet obstruction. Prostatic tissue is ablated by one of two mechanisms: vaporization with deeper coagulation necrosis, or coagulation necrosis alone. The neodymium yttrium-aluminum-garnet (Nd:YAG) laser has been used almost exclusively. All devices approach the prostate transurethrally, but none of them spare the urethra. In the majority of reports, patients required general or regional anesthesia and stayed overnight in the hospital. The results of video or endoscopic laser ablation of the prostate (VLAP or ELAP), which employ contact vaporization of the prostate, are similar to those of TURP and are safe, with relatively fewer complications than TURP. In contrast, there are more side effects following VLAP or ELAP, particularly a prolonged need for an indwelling Foley catheter and irritative voiding symptoms. Also, like TURP, VLAP/ELAP is not an office procedure.

The strong interest in developing more minimally invasive laser therapies spawned the TULIP (transurethral laser-induced prostatectomy) device. The device consists of a transurethral probe containing a 7.5 MHz ultrasound imager and a side-firing Nd:YAG laser to induce coagulation necrosis. Targeting is done solely under ultrasound guidance. Like the aforementioned laser treatments, this modality does not spare the urethra, and significant prostatic and urethral mucosal edema is the rule. Patients still require hospitalization in the majority of cases, and either urethral or suprapubic catheters are needed for up to 2 wk. Nevertheless, TULIP is safe and approaches the efficacy of TURP. Two-year follow-up data from the United States Cooperative Study revealed an improvement in symptom score of 69% and in Qmax of 68%. European studies confirmed these data. TULIP is now used primarily in Europe and Asia.

Currently, the most promising minimally invasive laser therapy utilizes laser-diffusing fibers inserted directly into the prostatic interstitium beneath the urethral surface through transurethral, transrectal, or transperineal approaches to transmit focal thermotherapy with resultant coagulation necrosis to selected areas of the prostate, including the median lobe. This minimally invasive modality—called interstitial laser coagulation (ILC)—was first described by Hofstetler in 1991 and reported by Muschter in 1992. Laser-energy wavelengths in the range of 800–1100 nm are most effective for tissue thermotherapy caused by deep water penetration and efficient volumetric tissue heating. Currently, two types of lasers fall into this category, including the Nd:YAG laser (1064 nm) and the diode laser (830 nm) (Indigo Medical, Inc.). Diode lasers are particularly appealing, since they utilize solid-state semiconductors that use the same technology found in compact disc and video disc players, and are cheaper to build and maintain.

The Indigo 830e Diode Laser System (Indigo Medical, Inc.) is the most widely used and reported ILC device in the United States. The Indigo laser fibers deliver volumetric or 3-dimensional heat deposition at low power (20 W), as opposed to the point-source heating used by some of its competitors. Photons are propagated a distance of 5–6 mm in all directions from the fiber prior to being absorbed, and the heat travels approximately another 4 mm by diffusion. Therefore, an olive-shaped area of coagulation necrosis approx $2 \times 2.5$ cm occurs, which translates into a volume of approx 4 cm$^3$ of tissue destruction. The generator's wattage output is regulated by computer software to deliver a smooth rise in intraprostatic temperature to 85°C, and this temperature will be maintained for the remainder of the 3-min cycle for sustained coagulation necrosis. The generator receives feedback from an optical sensor at the tip of the laser fiber, which monitors intraprostatic temperatures during treatment. The Indigo Laser System is also equipped with a "blackbody monitor system" that detects heating above 100°C, signifying carbonization or charring. The system is based on the principle that all energy is conserved—if the fiber cannot transmit energy to the target, the energy will be reflected back up the fiber. The Indigo power generator detects carbonization and immediately shuts off the system. In addition, this monitoring system immediately shuts off treatment if the fiber is damaged or broken.

### *Preoperative Assessment*

Before laser therapy, patients undergo standard preoperative evaluation. If the patient has a PVR larger than 200–300 cm$^3$, a pressure-flow study is usually performed to better quantify the degree of voiding dysfunction. Prior to performing ILC, we recommend performing transrectal ultrasound of the prostate to measure prostate volume, since this study is the most accurate means of estimating prostate size. This information is useful in determining the approximate number of punctures to employ when performing ILC.

We do not recommend performing ILC of the prostate if the patient has a motor paralytic bladder from long-standing outflow obstruction. These patients generally have very large residual urine volumes and relatively hypotonic bladders. We believe it is preferable to perform a TURP in these instances in order to ensure that all of the obstructing tissue has been removed, rather than performing a procedure that results in reduction in size of the prostate and resorption of tissue over time.

### *Anesthesia Requirements*

ILC is primarily done in an ambulatory surgical setting. Some investigators are also performing this procedure in the office with sedation. Topical anesthesia with a prostate block and monitored anesthesia care (MAC) provides adequate anesthesia for most patients. We recommend using general or spinal anesthesia in patients with larger glands that require more than six or seven punctures. In our series, approximately one-third of patients tolerate topical anesthesia with prostate block, another third require spinal anesthesia, and a third undergo general anesthesia. Postoperative analgesics are usually unnecessary.

### *Technique*

The transurethral approach under cystoscopic guidance with the patient in dorsal lithotomy position is the most widely used method. The laser fiber can be passed through the working port of any standard cystoscope sheath. Proper laser eyewear is required during the procedure. Under direct vision, the fiber is inserted into the prostate at the complete discretion of the surgeon. A 3-min cycle of thermotherapy is administered per puncture. Temperatures are measured at the tip of the fiber and displayed every second on the device's digital monitor. Wattage delivery and temperature shutdown are regulated by the device itself.

We prefer to proceed in a systematic fashion similar to performing a TURP, in that the median lobe is treated first, followed by one complete lateral lobe, then the contralateral lobe. Our experience has shown that it is unnecessary to treat the floor of the prostatic urethra if the middle lobe is not enlarged. Initial cases in which the prostatic floor was treated resulted in a high incidence of postoperative irritative voiding symptoms and retrograde ejaculation.

The number of punctures per lobe depends on the size of the lobe. A small lobe can be completely treated with one puncture, and a large lobe may require five or more punctures. The estimated volume of thermal damage per puncture is 4 $cm^3$. Some investigators, such as Muschter, advocate high-volume treatment, employing one puncture per half centimeter of prostate length. Others recommend low-volume treatment with no more than one puncture per centimeter of prostate length. Our preference is somewhere between these two approaches. Furthermore, we advocate performing "test punctures" after completion of treating one entire lobe to ascertain the ambient temperature in that lobe—a residual temperature of >40°C within the prostate suggests adequate treatment of that lobe. Lastly, since the laser fiber delivers heat in a three-dimensional area around the fiber, it is crucial to direct the fiber as far away from the urethra as possible. An angle of at least 30° into the prostate is needed to spare the urethral mucosa from thermal damage and subsequent sloughing. The entire procedure takes approx 20–60 min, depending on the number of punctures performed. All patients require a urethral catheter, usually for 5–7 d, and are instructed in intermittent self-catheterization preoperatively, since prolonged urinary retention may occur in a small percentage of patients.

## Results

We have shown a 60–75% improvement in Qmax at various intervals of evaluation. Approximately 40%–45% of patients achieve >50% improvement in Qmax, and another 20%–30% achieve >100% improvement in Qmax. A summarization of 370 patients from various series with follow-up data to 12 mo revealed decreases in AUA Symptom Scores from 25.7 to 5.9 (77%), and increases in Qmax from 8.0 to 15.8 cm$^3$ (97.5%). Furthermore, studies using magnetic resonance imaging revealed an 8.2–41.6% reduction of prostatic volume. These results indicate that a fair number of patients are achieving a satisfactory outcome according to objective criteria, but the results are not uniformly successful.

Interestingly, in a multivariate analysis of a large single-surgeon series of patients treated with ILC, Muschter revealed that the only independent predictor of success or failure was the prior experience of the surgeon. Furthermore, the incidence of postprocedure morbidities decreased in each subsequent series by the same investigator. There is indeed a steep learning curve to any new procedure, as seen in the laparoscopy literature. ILC is certainly not as "automated" as TUMT, and is subject to much more interoperator discrepancies.

ILC has been successful in patients with acute urinary retention and satisfactory bladder function. Conversely, poor results have been noted in patients with long-standing urinary retention and large postvoid residuals—most require prolonged intermittent catheterization, and therefore ILC is not recommended for these patients.

## Adverse Events

Twenty-four percent of our patients developed urinary-tract infection following ILC of the prostate. Early in our series when the prostatic floor was treated, the incidence of irritative voiding symptoms was 26%, and retrograde ejaculation occurred in 7.5% of patients. Both symptoms now rarely occur when the prostatic floor is spared. These values correspond to those in other large series. In a series of over 60 cases, we have observed one instance of incontinence and one instance of impotence following ILC, but others have not reported clinically significant incontinence.

Secondary operative procedures were required in 7.5% of our patients. Two patients required a transurethral resection of the bladder neck. After cystoscopy it is interesting to note that these patients revealed a hollowed-out prostatic fossa similar to post-TURP defects. One patient required TURP and another underwent repeat ILC, with an eventual positive result. The literature reveals retreatment rates ranging from 0 to 15.4% among a variety of investigators.

## Summary

ILC is a safe and effective minimally invasive therapy for BPH. There is bona fide tissue ablation, with resultant defects that resemble TURP. An increasing percentage of cases are being performed in the office. Higher success rates and fewer complications can be expected as the physician performs more of these procedures.

# TRANSURETHRAL NEEDLE ABLATION

Radiofrequency technology has also been used in thermotherapy of the prostate. Low-level frequencies around 490 kHz have been found to achieve intraprostatic temperatures

>45°C and therefore induce coagulation necrosis in the prostatic adenoma. This minimally invasive modality—called transurethral needle ablation (TUNA) of the prostate (VidaMed, Menlo Park, CA)—consists of two treatment electrodes or antennae in the form of protruding needles that penetrate the urethral mucosa to enter the prostate gland. Only the tissue that is in direct contact with the needle electrode is heated. Thus, there is minimal distance dissipation of the thermal effect, and well-circumscribed areas of coagulation necrosis are created. This allows for more accurate localized treatment zones, with little damage to surrounding organs, including the urethra and rectum.

The device consists of a 22-Fr molded catheter containing two radio-frequency-emitting antennae or needles at approx 60–90° to each other, which are hidden within the tip of the catheter until deployed by the operator. A 0° cystoscope lens can be passed through the device for direct visual positioning of the needles, which are deployed at 90° angles to the catheter tip into the prostate interstitium through the urethral mucosa by the surgeon from the handle of the device. The needles are not actually seen, and thus the proper length of deployment is determined preoperatively by transrectal ultrasound. Teflon sheaths are then passed over the proximal portions of the needles in order to protect the urethra from thermal damage. Furthermore, intraprostatic and urethral temperatures are recorded by thermosensors at the tips of the protective sheaths and at the tip of the catheter, respectively, and anterior rectal-wall temperature is recorded by a rectal probe. The device is connected to the radiofrequency generator and is regulated by computer software. Shutdown occurs when urethral or rectal temperature exceeds 45°C, or when the tissue impedance exceeds 400 $\Omega$.

Each puncture into the prostate receives a 3–5-min cycle of radio-frequency thermotherapy, reaching intraprostatic temperatures up to 100°C. This produces a focal area of coagulation necrosis between 7 and 14 mm in diameter. Only one lateral lobe can be done per puncture. Multiple punctures are thus required, usually one in each lateral lobe for every 1 cm of prostate length. It has been estimated that one puncture is required per 20 g of prostate tissue. TUNA is not indicated for treatment of an enlarged median lobe. Total time of the procedure takes approx 30–40 min and is performed under local anesthesia (lidocaine 2% jelly per urethra), although some men require intravenous sedation.

In one series of patients treated with TUNA, IPSS improved from 21.0 to 8.8 at 1-yr follow-up and to 9.2 at 2 yr; Qmax increased from 9.8 mL/s to 17.0 mL/s at 1 yr and 16.8 mL/s at 2 yr. However, this exceptional series represents the best possible results after TUNA, and most other reports are much less optimistic. In a large multicenter prospective, randomized investigation comparing TUNA to TURP, significant improvements in symptom score and Qmax were noted in both groups at 1-yr follow-up. Furthermore, TUNA was associated with fewer and less severe side effects than TURP. In the TUNA cohort, there were no cases of retrograde ejaculation, erectile dysfunction, urinary incontinence, or blood transfusion, and 40% of patients required catheterization for only 24 h after the procedure. All TURP patients required catheters for 24–48 h.

TUNA is another safe and effective minimally invasive therapy for symptomatic BPH that can be performed in the office setting. Although initially comparable to TURP, long-term follow-up data after TUNA is needed.

## HIGH-INTENSITY FOCUSED ULTRASOUND

In the early 1990s, experiments were performed with dogs using high-intensity focused ultrasound (HIFU) to ablate prostatic tissue. A single transrectal probe contained both an ultrasound imager and an ultrasound therapeutic transducer. It was shown that a pulse of 4 MHz for 4 s could produce a $2 \times 2 \times 10$-mm cylindrical area of coagulation necrosis. Commercial devices were then developed for trials in humans. The Sonoblate HIFU device (Focal Surgery, Milpitas, CA) uses a 4-MHz imaging frequency and a 4-MHz therapeutic transducer. The tip of the probe moves linearly to reach from the prostate base to the apex. The probe also rotates along this axis to target different areas within one transverse plane. The Ablatherm HIFU device (Technomed International, Lyon, France) uses a 7.5-MHz imager and a 2.25-MHz therapeutic transducer within a single transrectal probe.

In 1994, Madersbacher and colleagues reported 12-mo follow-up data in 50 patients treated with HIFU using the Sonoblate device. Qmax improved from 9 to 13 mL/s (44%), and AUA Symptom Score decreased from 25 to 11 (56%). Importantly, there were no rectal injuries and no reports of urethral discomfort. However, most of these patients required at least epidural anesthesia, and suprapubic catheters were used in patients who developed urinary retention. In 1996, these same investigators provided urodynamic evidence of improvement in voiding patterns after HIFU. Minimum voiding pressure decreased from 70 to 51 cm $H_2O$, and detrusor pressure at maximum flow decreased from 74.2 to 57.0 cm $H_2O$.

In 1997, Nakamura and associates reported similar results using the second-generation Sonoblate 200 device. At 6-mo follow-up, Qmax improved by 54%, and IPSS improved by 56%. Interestingly, coagulation necrosis defects within the prostate were confirmed by magnetic resonance imaging in their study. Approximately 20% of patients developed transient retention, and 25% developed hematuria. Mulligan and colleagues reported significant improvements in symptom scores of approx 70% at 2 yr after HIFU, yet there was no sustained improvement in flow rates.

HIFU is a safe thermotherapeutic modality with reasonable short-term efficacy, yet its long-term durability remains in question. Furthermore, the majority of patients require at least regional anesthesia for the procedure. We await long-term follow-up data in randomized trials, as well as newer devices or protocols, that will allow for more routine usage in the office setting.

## PROSTATIC URETHRAL STENTS

Prosthetic stents were originally used in peripheral and coronary vessels, and have now been used in renal and iliac arteries, inferior vena cava, trachea and bronchi, cervical os, and even lacrimal ducts. Temporary stents have been used in the prostatic urethra since the early 1980s. Stainless-steel spiral stents and polyurethane stents have been shown to restore voiding immediately in patients with urinary retention. However, these stents do not become epithelialized, are prone to migration and encrustation, and are associated with increased urinary-tract infections and severe frequency, urgency, and incontinence.

Epithelializing wire-mesh stents, such as the UroLume Wallstent (American Medical Systems, Minnetonka, MN), and the Titan Intraprostatic ASI Stent (Boston Scientific,

Boston, MA), have recently been under investigation. The UroLume endoprosthesis was approved by the FDA for urethral strictures in April 1996. Its indications were extended to include BPH in May 1997 and for detrusor-external sphincter dyssynergia for investigational trials only in the United States.

The UroLume Wallstent is composed of a flexible metal superalloy that is self-expanding to 42 Fr once deployed in the prostatic urethra. The placement procedure begins with dilation of the urethral meatus to 26 Fr as needed. A marked catheter is used to measure the distance of the prostatic urethra from the bladder neck to the midverumontanum. The proper prosthesis size is determined by subtracting 0.5 cm from the measured length. One of six available stents ranging from 1.5 to 4.0 cm in length can be selected. The stent is placed under direct vision, using its own deployment device under local anesthesia in the office as an outpatient procedure. Some patients may require intravenous sedation and/or analgesia. A urethral catheter should not be placed, and any transurethral procedures should be postponed for at least 8 wk. The stent becomes completely epithelialized by 6 mo, at which time cystoscopy or catheterization may be performed. The stent may be removed endoscopically at any time with minimal difficulty or trauma to the urethra. More than one stent may be placed in the same patient—the proximal stent should be placed first, and any distal stents should overlap as much as possible.

This technique was initially reserved for the elderly debilitated patient in either acute or chronic urinary retention, with poor surgical risk, and as an alternative to chronic indwelling urethral catheterization. However, recent trials have included healthy patients with symptomatic BPH who were candidates for TURP, including patients in urinary retention. The National UroLume Study Group showed that at 4 yr of follow-up, Madsen Symptom Score decreased from 14.5 to 6.7, and Qmax increased from 9.2 mL/s to 14.7 mL/s. All patients in urinary retention resumed spontaneous voiding after placement of the stent, although the UroLume has not yet been officially approved for the indication of urinary retention. By 12 mo, nearly all stents were completely epithelialized. The overall removal rate was 15.8%. The main postoperative complications included migration (3.2%), encrustation (27.7%), postvoid dribbling (61.5%), urge incontinence (53.8%), urgency (65.6%), sexual dysfunction (25.8%), and retrograde ejaculation (18.2%). Primary candidates for treatment with the UroLume stent appear to be patients with BPH and moderate to severe obstruction, and those with lateral-lobe hyperplasia only. Current contraindications to the use of the UroLume include active infection, median prostatic-lobe hyperplasia, conditions requiring transurethral access within 8 wk, known or suspected cancer of the bladder, prostate, or urethra, prior BPH procedures, prostatic urethral length <2.5 cm, bladder calculi, and neurogenic bladder.

Foreshortening of the length of the stent after deployment within the prostatic urethra is a well-known shortcoming with these stents. A large European multicenter study investigated a modified version of the UroLume Wallstent, named the "less-shortening" or "LS" stent, which featured an increased wire diameter, decreased wire-crossing angle, and decreased rigidity. However, at 18-mo follow-up, approx 38% of patients experienced complications and over 15% of stents had to be removed. This version of the stent was subsequently taken off the market. The Titan ASI stent is composed of a titanium alloy and is not self-expanding. It requires high-pressure balloon inflation to expand the stent to its maximum diameter of 33 Fr. Improvements in symptom scores from 16 to 9 (44%) and in Qmax from 9 mL to 11 mL/s (22%) are modest compared to the UroLume. Currently, studies comparing prostatic stents to TURP are underway. Prostatic stents should be reserved for the older patient with lateral-lobe hyperplasia and moderate to severe lower urinary-tract symptoms, and they continue to be a safe option for patients with poor surgical risk. There may be a role for these stents in combination with TUMT or ILC to overcome the initial postoperative prostatic edema and keep the patient catheter-free, but absorbable stents are under development and would be preferable in this setting.

## TRANSURETHRAL BALLOON DILATION OF THE PROSTATE

Akin to the evolution of prostatic stents from the successes of cardiovascular interventions, balloon dilation of prostatic urethra and bladder neck up to 90 to 120 Fr has been performed. The mechanism of success—when it occurs—is unknown, but may be the result of either physical stretching or tearing of tissues or from alpha-adrenergic nerve damage. Balloon dilation of the prostate appears to be a safe modality; however, early flow-rate improvements have not been sustained. Although symptom scores tend to improve, they are not significantly better than placebo. Therefore, balloon dilation is no longer recommended.

## SUMMARY

The management of BPH has indeed changed dramatically over the past decade, and will continue to evolve over the next decade. The advent of minimally invasive therapies for BPH has added yet another dimension to the practice of office urology by bridging the gap between medicine and surgery. The current modalities will continue to improve, and certainly new modalities will arise. Nevertheless, the realm of minimally invasive treatment is still in its infancy. Long-term durability remains in question, and we have yet to match the results of our gold standard, TURP. Furthermore, these therapies may not be cost-effective if multiple sessions are required and if patients inevitably progress to TURP. The challenge remains to achieve more consistent delivery of thermotherapy to the appropriate areas of the prostate and to eliminate the variability in patient response to treatment. The wide benefit-to-risk ratio in patients who undergo these treatments will sustain efforts to improve this technology and better define a place for minimally invasive procedures in the management of BPH.

## SELECTED READING

Beduschi MC, Oesterling JE (1998) Transurethral needle ablation of the prostate: a minimally invasive treatment for symptomatic benign prostatic hyperplasia. *Mayo Clin Proc* 73:696–701.

Blute ML, Larson TR, Hanson KA, King BF (1998) Current status of transurethral thermotherapy at the Mayo Clinic. *Mayo Clin Proc* 73:597–602.

Dahlstrand C, Walden M, Geirsson G, Pettersson S (1995) Transurethral microwave thermotherapy versus transurethral resection for symptomatic benign prostatic obstruction: a prospective randomized study with a 2-year follow-up. *Br J Urol* 76:614–618.

De La Rosette JJMCH, D'Ancona FCH, Debruyne FMJ (1997) Current status of thermotherapy of the prostate. *J Urol* 157:430–438.

Defalco AJ, Oesterling JE, Epstein HB (1993) The North American experience with the UroLume endourethral prosthesis as a treatment for BPH: three year results. *J Urol* 143:829.

Djavan B, Larson TR, Blute ML, Marberger M (1998) Transurethral microwave thermotherapy: what role should it play versus medical management in the treatment of benign prostatic hyperplasia? *Urology* 52:935–947.

Hallin A, Berlin T (1998) Transurethral microwave thermotherapy for benign prostatic hyperplasia: clinical outcome after 4 years. *J Urol* 159:459–464.

Keijzers GBJM, Francisca EAE, D'Ancona FCH, Kiemeney LALM, Debruyne FMJ, De La Rosette JJMCH (1998) Long-term results of lower energy transurethral microwave thermotherapy. *J Urol* 159:1966–1973.

Larson TR, Blute ML, Bruskewitz RC, Mayer RD, Ugarte RR, Utz WJ (1998) A high-efficiency microwave thermoablation system for the treatment of benign prostatic hyperplasia: results of a randomized, sham-controlled, prospective, double-blind, multicenter clinical trial. *Urology* 51:731–742.

Larson TR, Bostwick DG, Corica A (1996) Temperature-correlated histopathologic changes following microwave thermoablation of obstructive tissue in patients with benign prostatic hyperplasia. *Urology* 47:463–469.

Larson TR, Collins JM, Corica A (1998) Detailed interstitial temperature mapping during treatment with a novel transurethral microwave thermoablation system in patients with benign prostastic hyperplasia. *J Urol* 159:258–264.

Muschter R, de la Rosette JJMCH, Whitfield H (1996) Initial human clinical experience with diode laser interstitial treatment of benign prostatic hyperplasia. *Urology* 48:223–228.

Neal DE, Ramsden PD, Sharples L, et al. (1989) Outcome of elective prostatectomy. *Br Med J* 299:762–767.

Oesterling JE, Issa MM, et al. (1997) Long-term results of a prospective, randomized clinical trial comparing TUNA to TURP for the treatment of symptomatic BHP. *J Urol* 157 (Suppl):328.

Oesterling JE, Kaplan SA, Epstein HB, Defalco AJ, Reddy PK, Chancellor MB (1994) The North American experience with the Urolome endoprosthesis as a treatment for benign prostatic hyperplasia: long-term results. *Urology* 44(3):353–362.

Perlmutter AP, Muschter R (1998) Interstitial laser prostatectomy. *Mayo Clin Proc* 73:903–907.

Schulman CC, Zlotta AR (1996) Transurethral needle ablation (TUNA) of the prostate: clinical experience with two years follow-up in patients with benign prostatic hyperplasia (BPH). *Eur Urol* 30 (Suppl 2):263.

Walsh PC, Retik AB, Vaughan ED, Wein AJ, eds. (1998) *Campbell's Urology* (7th ed.) Philadelphia: Saunders Co., pp. 1479–1509.

# VII Prostate—Malignant

# 20 Evaluation of Prostate Cancer

*Robert L. Grubb III,* MD
*and Gerald L. Andriole,* MD

**CONTENTS**
  SCREENING FOR PROSTATE CANCER
  CURRENT RECOMMENDATIONS FOR SCREENING
  DIAGNOSIS OF PROSTATE CANCER
  SUMMARY
  SELECTED READING

Over the last decade the introduction of prostate specific antigen (PSA) testing and the increased awareness of prostate cancer as a significant public-health problem has resulted in an explosion of new information. In this chapter, a contemporary approach to prostate cancer screening, diagnosis, and staging is presented.

## SCREENING FOR PROSTATE CANCER

Prostate cancer is the most commonly diagnosed malignancy in males and is the second-leading cause of cancer death in men (the first is lung cancer). An estimated 40,000 prostate cancer-related deaths occurred in 1998. Population-based studies from Olmstead County, MN, showed a 3.4-fold increase in the age-adjusted incidence of prostate cancer between 1983 and 1992, coincident with the introduction of widespread PSA testing in the late 1980s. Since 1992, however, the incidence of prostate cancer appears to be declining toward that of the pre-PSA era.

PSA screening has been associated with a significant downward-stage migration for prostate cancer at the time of detection. From 70 to 80% of cases detected on the basis of repetitive PSA-based screening are pathologically organ-confined, whereas in the pre-PSA era, when digital rectal examination (DRE) was the predominant means of screening, only 20–30% of prostate cancers were organ-confined at the time of detection.

Critics of routine screening for prostate cancer have pointed out that no large randomized studies demonstrate that PSA-based early diagnosis coupled with current treatment of prostate cancer has decreased prostate-cancer mortality. Critics have also voiced concern that asymptomatic cancers detected by PSA screening are not apt to be clinically significant. Finally, the human and economic cost of screening and treatment of prostate

From: *Current Clinical Urology: Office Urology: The Clinician's Guide*
Edited by: E. D. Kursh and J. C. Ulchaker © Humana Press Inc., Totowa, NJ

cancer may be significant. These concerns have spawned some opposition to widespread screening for prostate cancer.

In response to these concerns, it is important to note that randomized trials evaluating the effectiveness of routine screening are underway. The National Cancer Institute has initiated the Prostate, Lung, Colorectal, Ovarian (PLCO) screening trial and the European Randomized Study of Prostate Cancer (ESPRC) is in progress. Because these are prospective trials, conclusive data may be many years away. Current data suggests that most cancers discovered on the basis of PSA-based screening are clinically significant. Finally, some preliminary evidence suggests that prostate-cancer screening may contribute to reduced prostate-cancer mortality. In 1996, the National Center for Health Statistics reported a 6.3% reduction in prostate cancer mortality in the United States—the first time that such a reduction has occurred. Since implementation of screening and aggressive therapy were the only major changes, it is reasonable to infer that these approaches contributed to the mortality reduction. Also, a randomized trial of 46,289 men from Quebec has shown a fivefold decrease in prostate-cancer deaths among the men in its screening arm; however, methodological concerns about this study preclude it from being considered definitive.

## CURRENT RECOMMENDATIONS FOR SCREENING

The American Urological Association (AUA) and the American Cancer Society (ACS) have recommended offering annual DRE and PSA testing for males age 50 and older when life expectancy exceeds 10 yr. Because of the higher incidence of prostate cancer in African Americans, and its potential for more aggressive behavior in these men, it is recommended that African Americans begin screening at age 40. Men with two or more first-degree relatives with prostate cancer have a relative risk of prostate cancer two to three times higher than the general population. Moreover, some studies suggest that these cancers may have a more aggressive course than sporadic cancers. Because of these findings, men with a family history of prostate cancer should begin screening at the age of 40.

These guidelines for initiating screening are fairly well-accepted among urologists and many primary-care physicians. The precise interval of PSA testing, however, is less clear. Longitudinal studies have suggested that a man's initial PSA is a strong predictor of his risk of eventually developing prostate cancer, and that those with an initial PSA of 0–2.5 ng/mL have a 1% risk of developing cancer within the next 4 yr. That risk increases to 12% for males with an initial PSA of 2.5–4.0 ng/mL, and increases to 38.4% for males with an initial PSA of 4.1–10.00 ng/mL. It has been suggested, therefore, that men with a normal DRE and PSA <2.0 ng/mL could safely increase the screening interval to every 2–3 yr. Using similar considerations, it may be reasonable to stop testing among elderly men with a normal DRE and a PSA <1.0 ng/mL.

## DIAGNOSIS OF PROSTATE CANCER

### *Medical History*

The medical history is often unrevealing for men with prostate cancer. Since 70% of prostate cancers occur in the peripheral zone, away from the urethra, most men have no urinary symptoms from prostate cancer.

Symptoms, when present, may be indicative of locally advanced or metastatic disease. Urinary symptoms of locally advanced prostate cancer are usually obstructive in nature, but irritative symptoms and hematuria or hematospermia may occur.

Patients with widely metastatic disease may complain of skeletal pain. Widespread infiltration of the bone marrow may lead to anemia. Prostate cancer infiltrating the pelvic lymph nodes may cause edema of the lower extremities.

## *Physical Examination*

In the past DRE has been the primary method of detecting prostate cancer. Its sensitivity varies from 2 to 20%, and its specificity is approx 80%. The positive predictive value of DRE varies from 10 to 50%, depending on the examiner's threshold to define a suspicious finding. Despite these shortcomings, DRE remains an essential diagnostic test for prostate cancer, since PSA levels will be "normal" in 10–20% of men with prostate cancer.

The general physical examination should search for signs of metastatic disease (palpable lymphadenopathy or bony tenderness) or renal obstruction (CVA tenderness).

## *PSA Testing*

PSA is a serine protease produced by the prostatic epithelium and periurethral glands and is secreted into the seminal fluid where it is involved in liquefaction of the seminal coagulum. PSA is metabolized by the liver and has a serum half-life of approx 2–3 d.

PSA has been found to be the single best test for prostate cancer. However, it is nonspecific: up to three-quarters of men with an abnormal PSA reading may not have prostate cancer. Numerous factors can alter the serum PSA level and interfere with its reliability as a test for cancer. Increases in serum PSA levels are caused by disruption of the prostatic epithelium by disease processes, such as malignancy, benign prostatic hyperplasia, and prostatitis. Manipulation of the prostate by DRE and ejaculation may lead to transient increases in the PSA. Transrectal needle biopsy can significantly increase the PSA for up to 1 mo after biopsy. These effects are usually transient, and are not of clinical significance unless the PSA is on the border of a cutoff point. PSA measurements may also be decreased by hormonal therapies, including finasteride (a 5-alpha-reductase inhibitor), which may decrease serum PSA by approx 50%.

The ideal cutoff point to define normal serum PSA levels has not been determined. Currently PSA values of <4.0 ng/mL are considered normal, but recent studies have shown that up to 25% of men with prostate cancer have a PSA value of <4.0 ng/mL and that about 20% of men with PSA levels between 2.5 and 4.0 ng/mL have prostate cancer. Moreover, our understanding of certain "PSA derivatives" is progressing, and current evidence suggests that the algorithm in Fig. 1 is appropriate. The following are practical considerations for using PSA derivatives.

## *PSA Velocity*

PSA velocity (or slope) is defined as the change in PSA value over a period of time. It is hypothesized that PSA will rise more rapidly in men with significant cancers than in men with benign prostatic hyperplasia. However, because of the variability of PSA—even among men with benign prostate cancer—at least three measurements separated by at least 18 mo are needed to reliably calculate PSA velocity. The acceptable rate

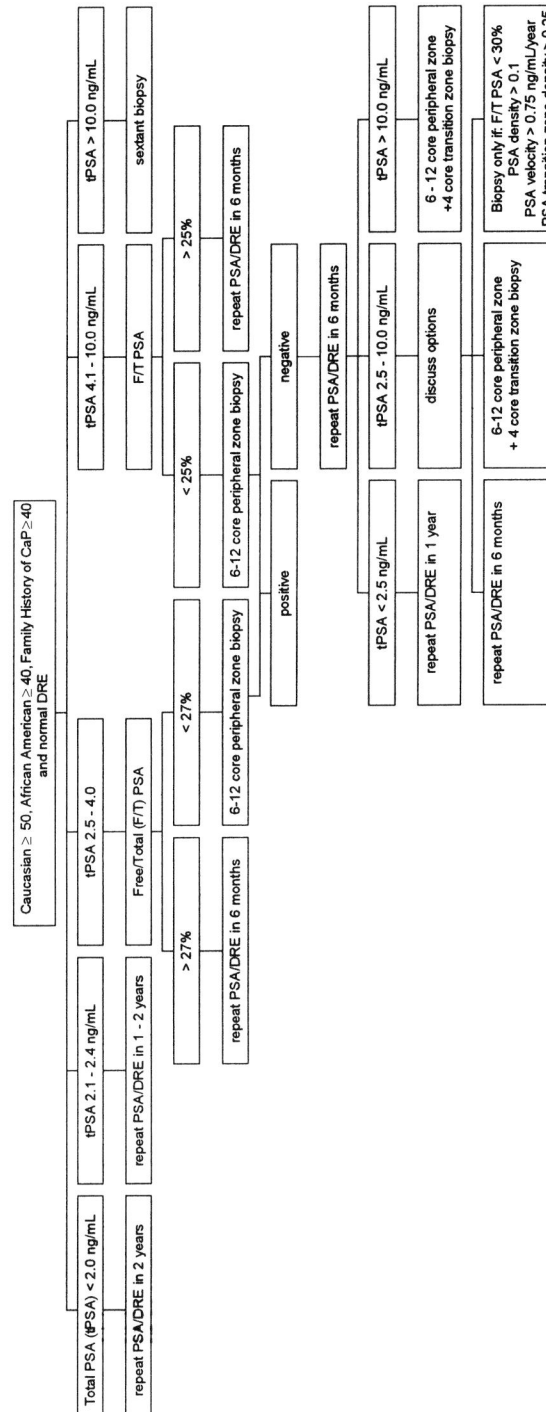

**Fig. 1.** Proposed prostate cancer screening algorithm.

of change has not been determined; a value of 0.75 ng/mL/yr in one study yielded a sensitivity of nearly 80% and a specificity of 66% for men with PSA values <4.0 ng/mL. Use of PSA velocity may save 10–30% of biopsies among men with elevated serum PSA and prior negative biopsy, but it may miss 5–20% of cancers.

### *PSA Density*

PSA density is calculated by dividing the serum PSA (ng/mL) by the prostate volume (in cm$^3$). It is conjectured that PSA density adjusts for increases in serum PSA that are caused by benign prostatic enlargement. A value of 0.1 retains the sensitivity of the test, but reduces the number of biopsies by 24–42%. In men with a total PSA of 4.0–10.0 ng/mL and a prior negative biopsy, the performance characteristics may be even better. Thirty-one percent of rebiopsies may be prevented but 10% of prostate cancers may be missed.

Because prostatic enlargement occurs in the transition zone and most serum PSA comes from the transition zone, calculating a PSA density using the transition-zone volume (PSA transition-zone density) may be more predictive of prostate cancer than using the total prostate volume. A cutoff of 0.3 ng/mL for PSA transition-zone density in men with normal DRE reduced the number of biopsies by 51%, but detected 7 of 8 cancers. Sensitivity and specificity were 88% and 57%, respectively. A cutoff of 0.25 ng/mL/cm$^3$ has been suggested to maintain a 95% cancer-detection rate while avoiding the largest number of biopsies (53%). The transition-zone PSA density performed better for prostate glands with a volume of 30 cm$^3$ or more. These studies were based on referral populations, and studies of screening populations have failed to show a significant benefit of transition-zone PSA density in the detection of prostate cancer.

Total PSA density and transition-zone PSA density are not ideal primary-screening modalities because they require TRUS, an invasive and costly procedure. Additionally, TRUS-calculated volumes are imprecise, which may limit the accuracy of the calculated PSA densities. PSA density seems to be most useful for patients with an elevated PSA who have had a previous negative biopsy.

### *Age-Specific PSA Range*

Age-specific PSA reference ranges were established based on the assumption that PSA increased with age, regardless of whether cancer was present. The 95th percentile for PSA levels among age-stratified cohorts of men without prostate cancer was determined. By raising the upper limits of "normal" for older men, it was hypothesized that the number of biopsies in this population would be reduced without compromising prostate-cancer detection among younger men. This concept has not been borne out; studies have shown that in the PSA range of 4.0–10.0 ng/mL, older men are *more* likely to have detectable prostate cancer. For men in the 60–69 age group, age-adjusting the PSA cutoff from 4.0 to 4.5 ng/mL would eliminate 15% of biopsies but miss 8% of cancers. Among men aged 70–79, 44% of biopsies could be prevented, but at the expense of missing 47% of cancers. These findings indicate that age-adjusted PSA reference ranges seem to have limited clinical utility.

### *Free PSA*

Most PSA in the serum is complexed to other serum proteins such as alpha$_1$-antichymotrypsin or alpha$_2$-macroglobulin. Men with prostate cancer tend to have a lower proportion of unbound or "free" PSA than men without prostate cancer. Conventional serum PSA assays measure both the bound and free PSA, but assays that specifically detect free PSA have been developed. These have been used to increase the specificity of PSA testing. The percentage of free PSA assay results—like total PSA values—may be affected by factors other than the presence of malignancy. The percentage of free PSA tends to correlate with increasing age and larger prostate size. The percentage of free PSA has an inverse correlation with tumor aggressiveness; a lower percentage of free PSA may suggest a more aggressive form of prostate cancer.

The optimal cutoff point for free PSA has not been determined. To achieve the goal of minimizing the number of benign biopsies in older men without compromising cancer detection in younger men several different cutoff points have been suggested. Using a cutoff of 25% for the percentage of free PSA among men with total PSA between 4 and 10 ng/mL eliminates 34% of unnecessary biopsies in men aged 69–75, 19% in men aged 60–69, and 11% in men aged 50–59. This system works at the cost of missing 2% of cancers in men aged 50–59, 6% among those age 60–69, and 9% among men aged 69–75. Another system recommends using a higher cutoff point for the percentage of free PSA in men with a total PSA of 2.5–4.0 ng/mL. For these men, a cutoff point of 27% for percentage of free PSA eliminated 18% of biopsies and missed 10% of cancers. Table 1 provides a summary of the use of PSA derivatives.

## *Transrectal Ultrasound and Needle Biopsy*

Transrectal ultrasound (TRUS), combined with needle biopsy of the prostate, has become the favored method for obtaining a tissue diagnosis of prostate cancer. Random systematic sextant biopsies are the most widely used technique today. Only 5% of cancers were missed by systematic sextant biopsies as compared to biopsies directed at hypoechoic lesions. Seventeen percent of cancers were missed using biopsies directed only at specific hypoechoic areas.

Approximately 20% of cancers may require a second set of biopsies for detection using the sextant technique. The utility of further biopsies decreases in patients who have no DRE abnormalities. Studies have shown that cancer detection rates improve with repeated biopsies, especially among men with larger glands.

The 5-region technique for prostate biopsy increased prostate-cancer detection over the traditional sextant method by 35%. In addition to systematic sextant biopsies, two biopsies are taken from the lateral aspect of each side of the gland and three biopsies from the middle of the prostate, for a total of 13 cores. The 5-region technique most significantly improves cancer detection in patients with serum PSA <10.0 ng/mL. Potential disadvantages of this technique include the detection of insignificant tumors and increased morbidity resulting from the additional biopsies. Tumors detected by sextant techniques and the 5-region technique demonstrated similar pathologic characteristics.

The 20% incidence of prostate cancer arising in the transition zone has led some authors to advocate directing additional biopsies toward the transition zone. Transition-zone biopsies showed the greatest yield in men with a persistently elevated PSA and previous negative peripheral-zone biopsies. Cancer detection was also improved in patients with a normal DRE and elevated PSA without previous biopsies. This utility has not been uniformly demonstrated. Clearly, the optimal number of biopsies to be

Table 1
Use of PSA Derivatives to Determine the Need for Re-Biopsy in Men Being Screened
for Prostate Cancer Who Have Previously Undergone Negative Prostate Biopsy

| PSA derivative | Total PSA range (ng/mL) | Suggested cutoff-point | Approximate biopsies avoided (%) | Approximate cancers missed (%) |
|---|---|---|---|---|
| Velocity | ≤ 4.0 | 0.75 ng/mL/yr | 40 | 40 |
| Total PSA density | 4.0–10.0 | 0.1 ng/mL | 30 | 10 |
|  |  | 0.08 ng/mL | 10 | 5 |
| Transition zone density | 4.0–10.0 | 0.25 ng/mL | 53 | 5 |
| Percent free PSA | 4.0–10.0 | 30% | 10–20 | 5–10 |

taken, and the pattern in which they should be directed, has not been definitively demonstrated.

## *Clinical Local Staging of Prostate Cancer*

Currently used clinical staging systems include the Whitmore-Jewett and TNM system, base local, or T staging on the DRE. As mentioned above the DRE is limited by its low (2%–20%) specificity. DRE understages locally advanced prostate cancer in up to 50% of cases. Urologists have evaluated a number of modalities to improve the accuracy of T staging. Most commonly used is TRUS, which had a sensitivity of 66% and a specificity of 46% for predicting localized disease. This is not a significant improvement over DRE. Traditional body-coil MRI has performed similarly to TRUS, with a sensitivity of 65% (range 37%–80%) and a specificity of 69% in a combined series (range 57%–100%). The development of endorectal-coil MRI has improved results, increasing sensitivity to 87% (range 63%–90%) and specificity to 81% (range 77%–92%). False negative results are usually caused by microscopic foci of capsular penetration. Poor resolution limits the usefulness of computed tomography (CT) for local staging. CT and MRI rarely provide additional useful information for assessing the T stage of prostate cancer to justify local staging beyond a carefully performed DRE and TRUS.

Clinical stage, serum PSA levels, and the Gleason score have been used independently to predict the final pathologic stage. Results were improved by combining the three variables. A variety of nomograms based on multivariate logistic regression analysis can be used to help urologists predict the final pathologic stage of patients with clinically localized prostate cancer. These data can be used to guide the distant staging and treatment of prostate cancer.

## *Clinical Distant Staging of Prostate Cancer*

Distant clinical staging of prostate cancer begins with accurate local clinical staging to determine those patients at higher risk for positive pelvic lymph nodes and distant metastases. For these patients, the judicious use of bone scintigraphy or cross-sectional imaging (CT/MRI) may be indicated. All patients with newly diagnosed prostate cancer should have complete blood work, including hematologic screening and serum electrolytes, blood urea nitrogen (BUN), creatinine and liver function tests. Chest radiograph is mandatory, although the incidence of thoracic involvement is thought to be low.

Bone is the second most common site of metastasis for prostate cancer; lymph nodes are the most common. Bone scintigraphy is the imaging modality of choice in patients at risk for bony metastases. In a series of 521 patients newly diagnosed with prostate cancer, none of the 118 patients with a serum PSA of <10.0 had a positive bone scan for metastatic disease. The investigators concluded that a bone scan was unnecessary in patients with no skeletal symptoms and a serum PSA <10.0 ng/mL. Despite these findings, many urologists obtain bone scans at the time of diagnosis, as a baseline study, in case the patient develops metastatic disease in the future.

In a review of studies with pathological staging correlation of lymph-node status, CT and MRI had a sensitivity of approx 35% and a specificity of approx 96% for predicting lymph-node positivity. The low sensitivity of CT and MRI for detecting pelvic nodal metastases limits their usefulness in patients in whom the suspicion of nodal metastasis is low. Wolf and colleagues used decision analysis to determine that a pretest probability of pelvic lymph-nodal metastases of 32–45% was required before pelvic cross-sectional imaging became useful and cost-effective.

CT or MRI may be helpful in specific instances of abnormal liver-function tests, endocrine anomalies, or other signs of intra-abdominal metastasis. CT and MRI may be used to delineate the extent of spread in patients with obvious extracapsular extension.

There is a recent resurgence of interest in radioimmunoscintigraphy (RIS) using In-111 capromab pendetide as an imaging modality. In a small study, RIS was found to have a sensitivity of 75% and a specificity of 86% for detecting metastases compared with 20% and 68% for CT/MRI in the same group of patients. False-positive studies with this modality are a particular problem, because biopsy or surgical exploration of remote locations may become necessary to rule out extraprostatic disease. Other potential drawbacks include side effects from the use of antibodies and technical difficulty in interpreting the study. Despite these problems, RIS using In-111 capromab pendetide appears to be a promising new modality, but must be tested in a larger series of patients to more clearly define the parameters for its use. An algorithm for distant staging of prostate cancer is proposed in Fig. 2.

## SUMMARY

Prostate cancer diagnosis and staging have undergone a rapid evolution since the use of PSA screening has become more widespread. Although the benefit of early detection and treatment has not been proven in studies showing diminished disease-specific mortality, the impressive stage migration and early results of treatment suggest inroads are being made. Based on the current literature, the most widely used screening protocol offers DRE and annual PSA testing, beginning at age 40, for patients at high risk for developing prostate cancer (African Americans and those with a family history), and at age 50 for all others. History and physical examination should be directed at accurate local staging and screening for the presence of distant metastatic disease.

PSA has been found to be the single best screening test for prostate cancer, but it is nonspecific. PSA derivatives have been developed to increase the specificity of PSA for diagnosing prostate cancer. Free PSA appears to be the most helpful of the PSA

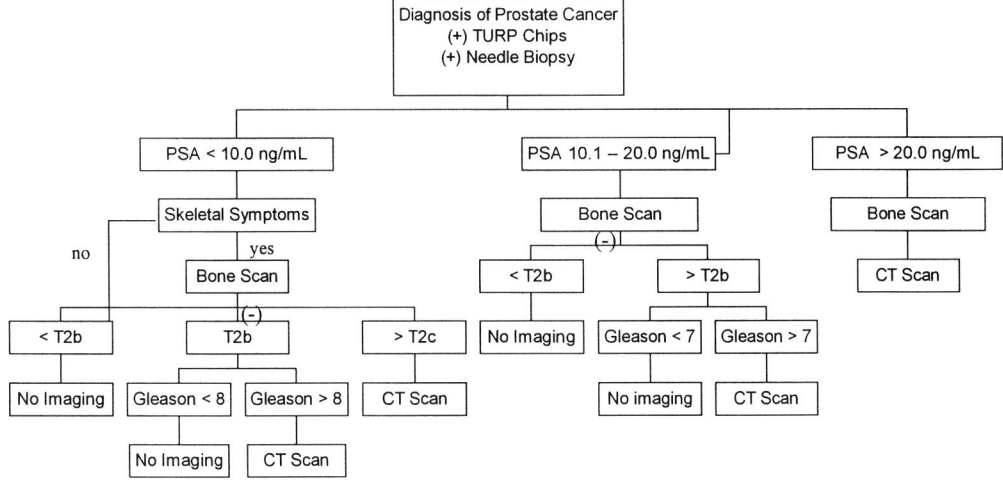

**Fig. 2.** Algorithm for staging prostate cancer.

derivatives, especially in men with glands measuring <30 cm$^3$ in size. Theoretically, PSA transition-zone density may be most useful among men with glands >30 cm$^3$ in size.

TRUS with needle biopsy is used to obtain a pathologic diagnosis of prostate cancer. The ideal pattern for biopsy and the number of biopsies needed have not been definitively determined.

Once prostate cancer is diagnosed, the local staging evaluation consists of DRE to determine clinical T stage, the Gleason score (pathologic analysis of biopsy specimen), and the total PSA. The potential for metastatic disease can be predicted using logistic regression tables based on these parameters. Patients with a PSA >10.0 ng/mL should have a bone scan to rule out osseous metastases. Cross-sectional imaging is of limited utility and should not be used as a routine procedure in staging of prostate-cancer patients.

The state-of-the-art regarding prostate cancer screening, diagnosis, and screening is constantly changing and this chapter should provide the basis for a current, logical, and straightforward approach to the evaluation of prostate cancer.

## SELECTED READING

Badalament RA (1998) Multicenter radioimmunoscintigraphic evaluation of patients with prostate carcinoma using indium-111 capromab pendetide. *Cancer* 83(4):739–747.
Carter HB, Partin AW (1998) Diagnosis and staging of prostate cancer. In: *Campbell's Urology* (7th ed.): 2519–2537.
Catalona WJ, Richie JP, Ahmann FR, Hudson MA, Scardino PT, Flanigan RC, DeKernion JB, Ratliff TL, Kavoussi LR, Dalkin BL, Waters WB, MacFarlane MT, Southwick PC (1994) Comparison of digital rectal examination and serum prostate specific antigen in the early detection of prostate cancer: results of a multicenter clinical trial of 6,630 men. *J Urol* 151:1283–1290.
Catalona WJ, Smith DS, Wolfert RL, Wang TJ, Rittenhouse HG, Ratliff TL, Nadler RB (1995) Evaluation of percentage of free serum prostate-specific antigen to improve specificity of prostate cancer screening. *JAMA* 274:1214–1220.
Chelsky MJ, Schnall MD, Seidmon EJ, Pollack HM (1993) Use of Endorectal surface coil magnetic resonance imaging for local staging of prostate cancer. *J Urol* 150:391–395.
Djavan B, Zlotaa AR, Byttebier G, Shariat S, Omar M, Schulman CC, Marberger M (1998) Prostate specific antigen density of the transition zone for early detection of prostate cancer. *J Urol* 160:411–419.

Eskew LA, Bare RL, McCullough DL (1997) Systematic 5 region prostate biopsy is superior to sextant method for diagnosing carcinoma of the prostate. *J Urol* 157:199–203.

Eskew LA, Woodruff RD, Bare RL, McCullough DL (1998) Prostate cancer diagnosed by the 5 region biopsy method is significant disease. *J Urol* 160:794–796.

Hinkle GH, Burgers JK, Neal CE, Texter JH, Kahn D, Williams RD, Maguire R, Rogers B, Olsen JO, Ikonen S, Karkkainen P, Kivisaari L, Salo JO, Taari K, Vehmas T, Tervahartiala P, Rannikko S (1998) Magnetic resonance imaging of clinically localized prostate cancer. *J Urol* 159:915–919.

Hodge KK, McNeal JE, Terris MK, Stamey TA (1989) Random systematic versus directed ultrasound guided transrectal core biopsies of the prostate. *J Urol* 142:71–75.

Keetch DW, Catalona WJ (1995) Prostatic transition zone biopsies in men with previous negative biopsies and persistently elevated serum prostate specific antigen values. *J Urol* 154:1795–1797.

Keetch DW, Catalona WJ, Smith DS (1994) Serial prostatic biopsies in men with persistently elevated serum prostate specific antigen values. *J Urol* 151:1571–1574.

Lee CT, Oesterling JE (1997) Cancer of the prostate: diagnosis and staging in *Urologic Oncology*. 357–377.

Lui PD, Terris MK, McNeal JE, Stamey TA (1995) Indications for ultrasound guided transition zone biopsies in the detection of prostate cancer. *J Urol* 153:1000–1003.

Maeda H, Arai Y, Ishitoya S, Okubo K, Aoki Y, Okada T (1997) Prostate specific antigen adjusted for the transition zone volume as an indicator of prostate cancer. *J Urol* 158:2193–2196.

O'Dowd GJ, Veltri RW, Orozco R, Miller MC, Oesterling JE (1997) Update on the appropriate staging evaluation for newly diagnosed prostate cancer. *J Urol* 158:687–698.

Oesterling JE (1993) Using PSA to eliminate the staging radionuclide bone scan. Significant economic implications. *Urol Clin N Amer* 20:705–711.

Oesterling JE, Martin SK, Bergstralh EJ, Lowe FC (1993) The use of prostate-specific antigen in staging patients with newly diagnosed prostate cancer. *JAMA* 269:57–60.

Ornstein DK, Andriole GL. Screening for prostate cancer in 1999. AUA Update Series, Lesson 1, Vol. 18.

Partin AW, Yoo J, Carter HB, Pearson JD, Chan DW, Epstein JI, Walsh PC (1993) The use of prostate specific antigen, clinical stage and gleason score to predict pathological stage in men with localized prostate cancer. *J Urol* 150:110–114.

Rietbergen JBW, Kranse R, Hoedemaeker RF, Boeken Kruger AE, Bangma CH, Kirkels WJ, Schroder FH (1998) Comparison of prostate-specific antigen corrected for total prostate volume and transition zone volume in a population-based screening study. *Urology* 52(2):237–246.

Schiebler ML, Schnall MD, Pollack HM, Lenkinski RE, Tomaszewski JE, Wein AJ, Whittington R, Rauschning W, Kressel HY (1993) Current role of MR imaging in the staging of adenocarcinoma of the prostate. *Radiology* 189:339–352.

Tempany CM, Zhou X, Zerhouni EA, Rifkin MD, Quint LE, Piccoli CW, Ellis JH, McNeil BJ (1994) Staging of prostate cancer: results of radiology diagnostic oncology group project comparison of three MR imaging techniques. *Radiology* 192:47–54.

Wolf JS, Cher M, Dall'era M, Presti JC, Hricak H, Carroll PR (1995) The use and accuracy of cross-sectional imaging and fine needle aspiration cytology for the detection of pelvic lymph node metastases before radical prostatectomy. *J Urol* 153:993–999.

Zlotta AR, Djavan B, Marberger M, Schulman CC (1997) Prostate specific antigen density of the transition zone: a new effective parameter for prostate cancer prediction. *J Urol* 157:1315–1321.

# 21 Transrectal Ultrasound and Prostate Biopsy in the Office

*Christopher A. Haas, MD*
*and Martin I. Resnick, MD*

**CONTENTS**
>INTRODUCTION
>PHYSICS OF ULTRASOUND
>ULTRASONOGRAPHIC CHARACTERISTICS OF THE
>    NORMAL PROSTATE
>EFFICACY OF TRUS
>EFFICACY OF TRUS-GUIDED BIOPSIES
>TECHNIQUE OF EXAMINATION: PATIENT PREPARATION
>PROCEDURE
>COMPLICATIONS
>REPEAT TRANSRECTAL ULTRASOUND BIOPSY
>CONCLUSIONS
>SELECTED READING

## INTRODUCTION

The medical application of ultrasonography is a relatively recent development that stems from advancements made in sonar technology during World War II. Initial ultrasound images of the prostate were of poor quality, and only with the introduction of transrectal B-Mode ultrasound did prostate imaging improve. Further advancements, including hand-held probes, gray-scale imaging, high-frequency biplanar transducers, and real-time imaging, have led to the development of the modern portable ultrasound unit. Today, ultrasound has become a critical part of the modern urologists' office-based practice as a method for evaluating the prostate and guiding transrectal needle biopsies of the prostate.

## PHYSICS OF ULTRASOUND

Ultrasound is a form of mechanical radiation that consists of acoustic vibrations generated by a transducer composed of crystalline substances. The piezoelectric proper-

From: *Current Clinical Urology: Office Urology: The Clinician's Guide*
Edited by: E. D. Kursh and J. C. Ulchaker © Humana Press Inc., Totowa, NJ

ties of the crystals within the transducer allow for the conversion of electrical energy to sound energy and vice versa. The application of an electrical voltage generates high-frequency sound waves from these crystals. The waves are reflected back to the transducer after encountering two tissues with different acoustic impedances. In order to prevent interference from intervening air pockets, a gel is used as a coupling medium between the transducer and tissue interface. When these reflected sound waves return to the transducer, a voltage potential is generated and amplified to produce an image. Therefore, the transducer acts as both ultrasound generator and detector.

The resolution of images produced by ultrasound depends on the frequency and wavelength of the sound waves generated. The higher the frequency of sound waves generated, the greater the absorption by soft tissues and less the degree of penetration. The higher the wavelength of sound waves generated, the less image resolution. Since frequency and wavelength are inversely related, as the wavelength decreases to provide a sharper image the frequency is increased, causing less tissue penetration. In order to provide a balance between image resolution and tissue penetration, most transrectal ultrasound (TRUS) transducers utilized for prostate imaging and biopsy have frequencies from 6.0 to 7.5 MHz (1 million cycles/s).

## ULTRASONOGRAPHIC CHARACTERISTICS OF THE NORMAL PROSTATE

To accurately evaluate the prostate gland with ultrasound, the characteristic appearance of the normal prostate should be familiar to the examiner. First, in the transverse plane the prostate appears as a symmetrical, ellipsoid structure surrounded by a continuous capsule (*see* Fig. 1). The normal gland has a homogenous echo pattern with the capsule appearing more echogenic and free from any distortion. In the longitudinal or sagittal plane, the prostate appears round in the midline, with a similar acoustic pattern. In the longitudinal plane, the relationship of the prostate to the bladder neck, urethra, and seminal vesicles can be identified. The seminal vesicles normally appear as paired, crescent-shaped structures that are less echogenic than the prostate and are separated from the prostatic base by highly echogenic fatty tissue (*see* Fig. 2).

The internal architecture of the normal prostate corresponds to its zonal anatomy as originally described by McNeal. The glandular elements are divided into three zones: the central, transition, and peripheral. The central zone surrounds the ejaculatory duct as it runs from the seminal vesicle to the verumontanum. It normally comprises about 25% of the glandular tissue of the prostate, and approx 10% of carcinomas originate in this zone. The transition zone surrounds the proximal urethra, and in the normal young male patient it comprises 5–10% of the glandular tissue. However, the transition zone is the site for the development of benign prostatic hyperplasia, where it can comprise up to 90% of the glandular tissue. About 20% of prostatic carcinomas originate in the transition zone. The peripheral zone encompasses the glandular tissue in the posterior, lateral, and apical portions of the gland, and in the normal young male patient it comprises 70–75% of the glandular tissue. About 70% of prostatic carcinomas originate in the peripheral zone. In the transverse plane the transition zone can be identified as slightly hypoechoic, whereas peripheral and central-zone tissue has a fine, homogenous echo pattern. A distinct layer of fibrous tissue separating the transition

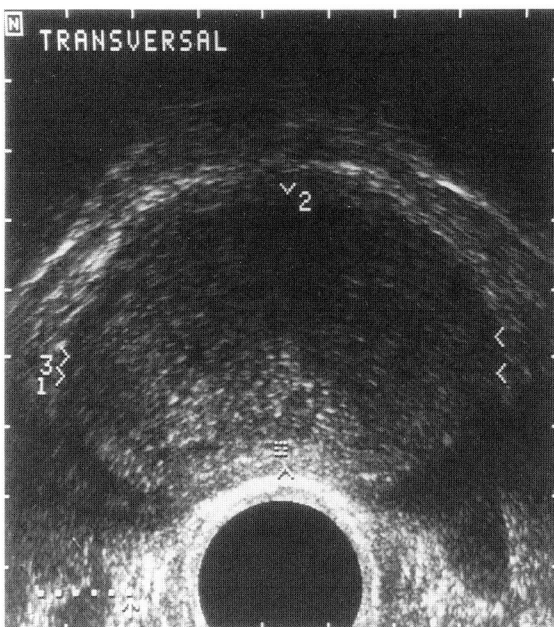

**Fig. 1.** Transverse transrectal ultrasound (7.5 MHz) of a normal prostate. Notice its smooth contour and relative homogenous sonographic appearance.

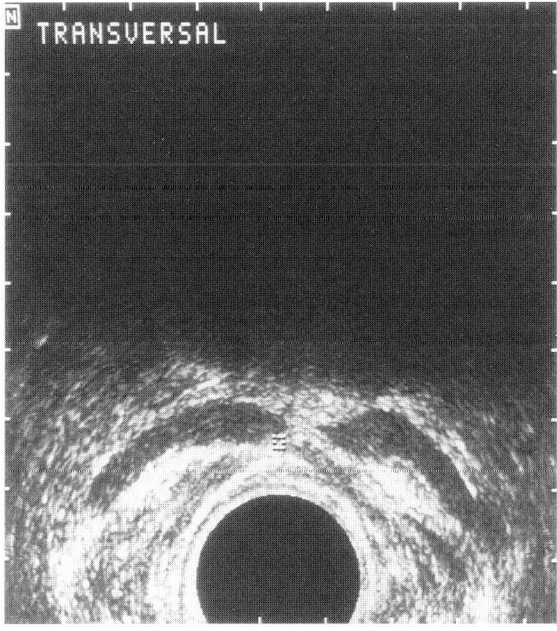

**Fig. 2.** Transverse transrectal ultrasound (7.5 MHz) of normal appearing seminal vesicles. Notice the crescent-shape and relative hypoechoic internal pattern of these structures.

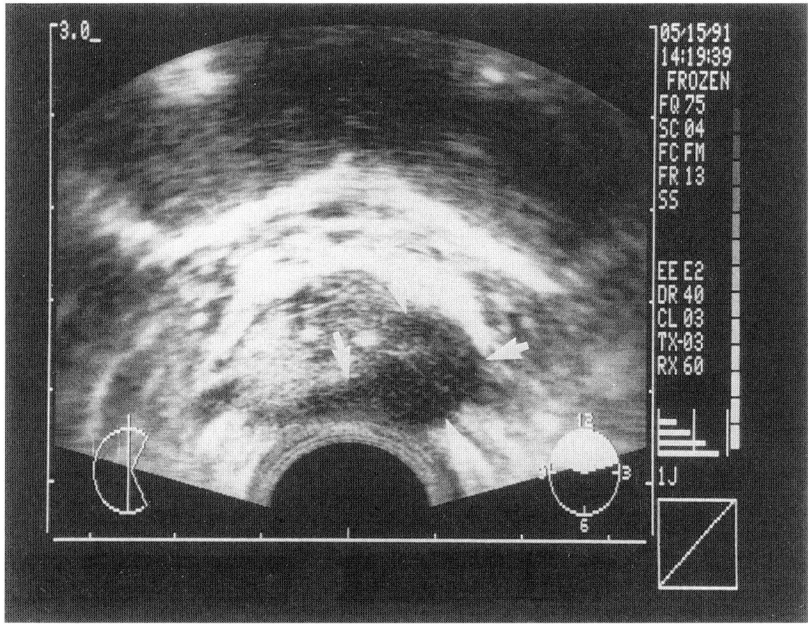

**Fig. 3.** Transverse transrectal ultrasound (7.5 MHz) of the prostate demonstrating a large hypoechoic lesion (arrows) typical of prostate cancer (from Hoffman DM, Gazelle GS, Seftel AD, Haaga JB, Resnick MI (1995) Atlas of Urologic Imaging, Williams and Wilkins).

zone from the peripheral zone and central zone (surgical capsule) can sometimes be identified, but is usually more prominent in patients with benign prostatic hyperplasia.

## EFFICACY OF TRUS

The sonographic appearance of prostate cancer is variable, and initial studies using low-frequency transducers have indicated that prostate cancer appeared hyperechoic or isoechoic when compared to the normal peripheral-zone pattern. Later evaluations using higher-frequency transducers have demonstrated that the majority of prostate cancers appeared hypoechoic with irregular margins (*see* Fig. 3). Despite this pattern, about one-third of prostate cancers will appear isoechoic, whereas others may appear hyperechoic. There are several possible reasons for these varied sonographic patterns besides differences in interpretation.

The size and grade of the tumor may have an effect on its sonographic appearance. For example, smaller lesions tend to be isoechoic when compared to the surrounding normal tissue, whereas larger tumors tend to be more hypoechoic. Well-differentiated cancers with a low Gleason's grade tend to appear isoechoic, which also makes these lesions difficult to identify on ultrasound. Several types of benign lesions can also appear hypoechoic, including benign prostatic hypertrophy, cysts, blood vessels, inflammatory lesions, prostatic infarction, and postbiopsy hematomas. Because of these limitations, the current role of TRUS is to guide the performance of prostate biopsies in those patients suspected of having prostate cancer.

## EFFICACY OF TRUS-GUIDED BIOPSIES

The indications for prostate biopsy are an abnormality on digital rectal examination (DRE) or an elevated serum-prostatic-specific antigen (PSA) level (>4.0 ng/mL). The targeted biopsy of TRUS-suspicious lesions and the systematic sextant biopsies of areas without suspicion are the standard techniques for diagnosing prostate cancer. This process entails a systematic approach in which biopsies are taken from 6 sectors of the peripheral zone, including the base, midgland, and apex on each side of the prostate. If a hypoechoic lesion is noted in any of these sectors, separate biopsies are obtained. Hodge et al demonstrated the importance of this systematic sector approach by showing that in a cohort of 136 men who had both systematic and directed TRUS-guided biopsies, only 3 of the 83 detected cancers would have been missed if no directed biopsies were performed. In a retrospective review of 941 men undergoing 1001 sextant biopsies, Ellis et al analyzed TRUS and biopsy results from individual prostatic regions and found that 37.6% of the cancers diagnosed were in isoechoic regions. Furthermore, 24.6% of these patients would have been misdiagnosed if only the hypoechoic regions had been biopsied. Although others have also demonstrated the importance of a systematic approach in obtaining biopsy specimens, recent debate has centered around such issues as the optimal location and number of biopsies needed to maximize the detection of clinically significant prostate cancer.

Studies of radical prostatectomy specimens clearly indicate that cancers are commonly found laterally in the midportion of the gland, and unless a sonographic abnormality exists in this area, sextant biopsies will miss these tumors. In a cohort of 512 patients with suspected prostate cancer, Norberg et al demonstrated that by substituting TRUS-guided biopsy samples from the middle of the midgland for samples taken more laterally, the sensitivity of the sextant protocol increased from 85% to 94%. Eskew et al performed TRUS-guided biopsies in a 5-region systematic fashion that included sextant biopsies with additional biopsies taken from the far lateral and midregion of the prostate (see Fig. 4) in 119 patients with an abnormal DRE and/or an elevated PSA (>4.0 ng/mL). Pathologic findings of these additional biopsies demonstrated that 35% of patients with prostate cancer only demonstrated it in these additional regions. It was also determined that in a subgroup of patients with PSA ranging from 4.0 to 10.0 ng/mL, the 5-region biopsy method detected 54% of cancers that would have been undetected with the sextant method, but offered no further advantage for those with a PSA >10 ng/mL. Although these findings suggest that biopsy location may alter cancer detection rates, the number of biopsies also plays a role—especially when taken in the context of the larger-volume gland.

Levine et al performed two consecutive sets of sextant biopsies under TRUS guidance in a single office visit in 137 men with an abnormal DRE or an elevated PSA based on age-specific ranges. Thirty percent of the total cases of prostate cancer were detected exclusively in the second biopsy set, a finding that supports the idea that the number of biopsies is most important in maximizing cancer detection. Furthermore, the cancer detection yield was increased by 63% for glands larger than 50 cm$^3$ using this 2-sextant biopsy technique. This volume relationship was also confirmed by Epstein et al, who performed sextant and transition-zone biopsies on 193 radical prostatectomy specimens from men with nonpalpable cancer (T1c) detected through needle biopsy. On repeat

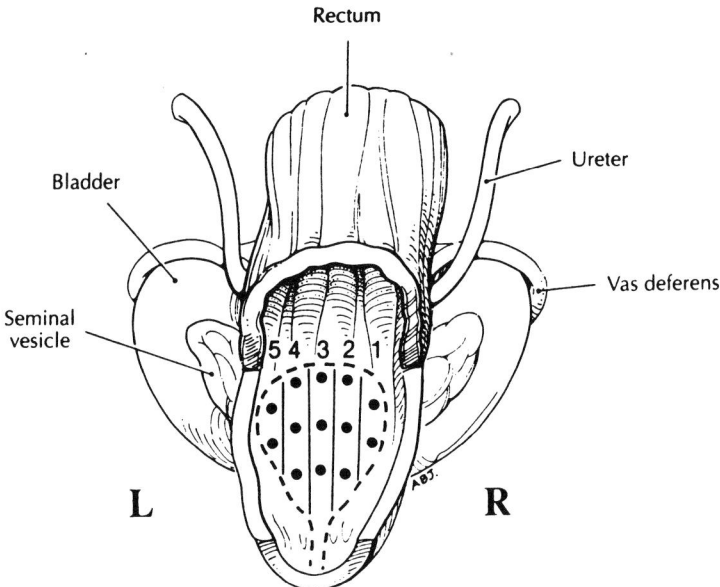

**Fig. 4.** Posterior view as seen through the rectal wall demonstrating the five regions for prostate biopsy (from Eskew LA, Bare RL, McCullough DL, (1997) Systematic 5 region prostate biopsy is superior to sextant method for diagnosing carcinoma of the prostate. J Urol 157: 199).

biopsy, 31% showed no cancer, despite the fact that cancer was present in all pathologic specimens. A multivariate analysis demonstrated that decreased tumor volume, decreased radical prostatectomy grade, and increased gland size were each independent predictors of a negative repeat biopsy.

In sum, these data suggest that traditional sextant biopsies may not maximize cancer detection rates, especially in the subgroup of patients with larger-gland volumes and PSAs in the 4.0–10.0 ng/mL range. Until these issues are evaluated in a prospective fashion, it is our practice to perform TRUS-guided biopsies in a sextant fashion with biopsies directed to sonographically suspicious areas.

The issue of whether routine seminal-vesicle and transition-zone biopsies should be performed in all patients undergoing TRUS-guided prostate biopsy has been recently addressed. Terris et al compared 736 men undergoing sextant biopsies to 161 men undergoing combined sextant, transition-zone, and seminal-vesicle biopsies and found that only 1 patient (1.8% of men with cancer) had cancer only in the transition zone, but 6 patients (10.9%) had cancer in the seminal vesicles. The authors concluded that routine transition-zone and seminal-vesicle biopsies in all men undergoing TRUS-guided sextant biopsies are not warranted. Although we also follow these recommendations, some data suggests that seminal-vesicle biopsies should be considered for men at risk for pathologic upstaging, such as in those with clinical stage T2b or greater disease, or in those with a PSA of >20 ng/mL or a Gleason score of 7 or greater. We limit the potentially more painful transition-zone biopsies to men with a persistently elevated PSA and previously negative systematic sector biopsies.

## TECHNIQUE OF EXAMINATION: PATIENT PREPARATION

After obtaining informed consent, the routine patient preparation for TRUS-guided prostate biopsies includes a cleansing enema usually given 1–2 h prior to biopsy and broad-spectrum antibiotic prophylaxis. This is usually accomplished with a Fleet enema, and an oral fluoroquinolone administered 1–2 h prior to biopsy and continued for 24–48 h after biopsy. Before the biopsy is performed, a thorough medical history is taken to identify any factors that may modify the routine patient preparation for prostate biopsy. Factors that need to be addressed include a history of valvular heart disease or prosthetic heart valves, artificial joints, and the current or recent use of aspirin, nonsteroidal antiinflammatory medications (NSAIDs), or oral anticoagulants.

Patients with cardiac valvular disease or prosthetic valves should receive bacterial endocarditis prophylaxis as outlined by the American Heart Association Guidelines. These guidelines categorize patients into high, moderate, and negligible risk groups. Those in the high-risk group include patients with prosthetic heart valves and require 2.0 g of ampicillin intramuscularly (im) or intravenously (iv) plus intravenous gentamicin at a dose of 1.5 mg/kg (not to exceed a total dose of 120 mg) within 30 min of starting the procedure. Six hours after the procedure, 1 g of im/iv ampicillin or 1 g of oral amoxicillin is required. Those in the moderate-risk group require 2.0 g of oral amoxicillin 1 h prior to the procedure or 2.0 g of im/iv ampicillin within 30 min of starting the procedure. Those in the negligible-risk group include patients with physiologic or innocent heart murmurs, and these patients require no prophylaxis. Dajani et al provided a more detailed description of these recommendations, describing alternate antibiotic combinations in patients with penicillin allergies. Patients with artificial joints should receive a high dose of an oral fluoroquinolone 1 h prior to biopsy, which is then continued for at least two more doses.

Patients who are taking aspirin or NSAIDs should have these discontinued at least 1–2 wk prior to biopsy or have a normal bleeding time prior to performing prostate biopsy. Patients taking oral anticoagulants, such as coumadin, should have these stopped at least 3 d prior to the planned biopsy, with normal coagulation studies documented prior to performing the biopsy. Patients may then resume these medications on the evening of the biopsy. If the patient cannot safely stop the oral anticoagulant—as is the case in patients with prosthetic heart valves—then intravenous heparin is administered while the oral anticoagulant is discontinued. The intravenous heparin is discontinued 4–6 h prior to the planned biopsy and again resumed 4–6 h after biopsy. Using these guidelines, the significant complication rate for TRUS-guided prostate biopsy can be minimized.

## PROCEDURE

Once the patient has changed into a hospital gown, he can be placed in one of several positions, including the knee-chest, kneeling, lithotomy, or left-lateral decubitus. The position usually depends on the examiner's preference, and whether other procedures are also necessary. For example, the lithotomy position is most useful when the patient also requires cystoscopy. No matter which position is used, prior to performing the procedure a DRE is performed to detect any anorectal abnormalities, which may contraindicate transducer insertion, and to palpate the prostate for irregularities. Next, the well-lubricated ultrasound probe is guided into the rectum 8–10 cm above the anal verge under sonographic guidance. Using real-time imaging, a systematic examination of the prostate and seminal vesicles is performed in both the transverse and sagittal planes, using the biplanar capabilities of most modern ultrasound transducers. All relevant images should be recorded and appropriately labeled.

Imaging of the prostate is initially performed in the transverse plane, starting at the level of the bladder base and then gradually moving caudal in order to scan from prostate base to apex through the urogenital diaphragm. The seminal vesicles are located in a more cephalad position, and each should be thoroughly evaluated for any change in its normal crescent-shaped appearance or distortion of its normal hypoechoic internal sonographic pattern. These types of findings may modify the biopsy strategy to include directed sampling of the seminal vesicles. Next, the remaining transverse imaging of the prostate is completed, with special attention given to the peripheral zone and its border with the transition zone, noting any hypoechoic regions. An evaluation for glandular asymmetry is also important, since large tumors can replace the entire peripheral zone. The prostatic capsule and area between the seminal vesicles and prostate should be examined, since irregularities or distortion may represent tumor extension. Next, a similar systematic evaluation of the prostate is performed in the sagittal plane, with appropriate images recorded.

The prostate volume should be calculated, because it may help guide biopsy strategy, increase diagnostic specificity when used to calculate PSA density, guide treatment planning as in the case of prostate brachytherapy, or be used to monitor prostate-cancer treatment effectiveness. Prostate volume is calculated by measuring the gland in three planes using the largest transverse image to obtain the anterior–posterior (AP) diameter and transverse diameter (TR), and then changing to the midline sagittal plane to obtain the superior–inferior (SI) diameter. These measurements are then used to calculate the prostate volume by employing the formula for a prolate ellipse $\{\pi/6\ (AP \times TR \times SSI)\}$, which is an automated function in most modern ultrasound units.

After this systematic examination is completed, biopsies can be performed by localizing the area of planned biopsy in both the transverse and sagittal planes. A sterile 18-gage biopsy needle placed into a spring-driven biopsy device is advanced through a biopsy guide attached to the ultrasound probe. Using the marker line available with most modern ultrasound view screens, any suspicious lesions can be biopsied so that the sample will include the largest possible diameter of the lesions (*see* Fig. 5). Next, systematic biopsies should be taken of the peripheral zone and transition zone if indicated. The strategy of random peripheral-zone biopsies was addressed earlier, and if transition-zone biopsies are to be taken, two to four random samples are usually obtained with an explanation to the patient that these are usually more painful. Our practice is to send individual specimens separately to pathology with appropriate identification.

After completion of the biopsies, the patient is gradually assisted off the examination table in order to minimize any vasovagal episodes. We perform a postbiopsy interview to explain our examination findings, discuss what the patient may possibly experience after the biopsy, and determine what complications require immediate medical attention.

## COMPLICATIONS

TRUS-guided prostate biopsy is a well-tolerated procedure with a T<2% reported incidence of major complications requiring hospital admission. However, other minor

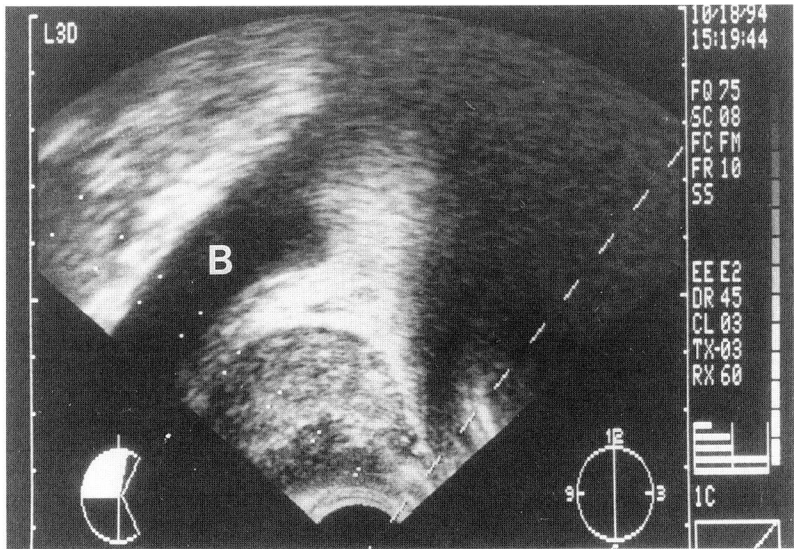

Fig. 5. Transrectal ultrasound (7.5 MHz) of the prostate in the sagittal plane demonstrating the biopsy marker line that defines the proposed area of prostate biopsy. Note the relationship of the prostate to the bladder (B) in this plane.

complications commonly occur, with an incidence rate ranging as high as 60–70%. Historically, the main complications related to prostate biopsy have been caused by hemorrhage and infection. Today, many of these complications can be avoided if the appropriate preventative measures are employed, as previously outlined.

Current estimates on the incidence of biopsy-related hemorrhagic complications range from 12–58% for hematuria, 5–45% for hematospermia, and 3–37% for hematochezia. In a recent prospective series of 128 men undergoing prostate biopsy, Rodriguez et al estimated the incidence of biopsy-related complications and found the incidence of hematuria, hematospermia, and hematochezia to be 47, 9.5, and 10%, respectively. The amount of rectal bleeding was associated only with the total number of biopsies performed, but not associated with the site of biopsy, prostate volume, cancer diagnosis, or history of aspirin or NSAID use prior to biopsy. The presence of hematuria and hematospermia was not statistically related to the total number or site of biopsies or to the previous use of aspirin or NSAIDs. These findings suggest that the recent use of aspirin or NSAIDs may not be an absolute contraindication to the performance of a prostate biopsy, yet this finding needs further confirmation.

Current estimates on the incidence of biopsy-related infectious complications are as high as 53% for urinary-tract infections, up to 6% for fever, and since the advent of routine antibiotic prophylaxis, remain <1% for sepsis. Although some investigators recommend the use of metronidazole along with a fluoroquinolone, or recommend a longer course of antibiotics for routine prophylaxis, the overall rate of infection remains low regardless of the prophylactic regimen.

Other complications associated with TRUS-guided biopsy include difficulty in voiding in up to 14% of patients, with urinary retention occurring in <1% of patients. In the study by Rodriguez et al., 8% of men experienced a vasovagal episode at the time of biopsy; of this number, 5% required treatment with intravenous fluids. In the same study, the discomfort experienced during examination was estimated by the patient after biopsy, and 25% of men were found to have moderate to severe discomfort during the TRUS-guided biopsy procedure. It was statistically determined that older men tolerated the procedure with less discomfort, and the amount of discomfort was proportional to the amount of rectal bleeding during biopsy. Other factors, such as ethnicity, prostate volume, or number or site of biopsy, were not statistically associated with discomfort. This age relationship is important, because younger patients can be advised before biopsy about possible discomfort and may benefit from analgesics or local anesthetics.

## REPEAT TRANSRECTAL ULTRASOUND BIOPSY

The selection criteria for patients who should undergo a repeat TRUS-guided biopsy of the prostate have recently become better defined. Today, general indications for a repeat biopsy include a pathologic diagnosis of atypia or high-grade prostatic intraepithelial neoplasia (PIN). Several contemporary series estimate the risk of diagnosing prostate cancer on subsequent biopsy in patients with high-grade PIN to range from 40 to 100%. We recommend repeat TRUS-guided sextant biopsies within 3 mo on all men found to have high-grade PIN on original biopsy.

One issue that remains poorly defined is selecting which patient with a previously negative prostate biopsy and a persistently elevated PSA or abnormal DRE should undergo repeat biopsy. Several recent series have demonstrated a false-negative rate for initial prostate biopsy as high as 30%. In a study by Fleshner et al., 130 men underwent a repeat biopsy for either a persistently elevated PSA (4.0 ng/mL or greater), elevated age-specific PSA, or abnormal DRE in order to define any predictors for positive repeat biopsies. It was determined that the overall baseline risk of a positive repeat biopsy was sufficiently high that a subset of patients who did not require repeat biopsy could not be identified. In conclusion, they recommend that a repeat biopsy be performed in all patients who meet the criteria for TRUS-guided biopsy and in whom the initial biopsy is negative. We repeat TRUS-guided biopsies in all men with a persistently elevated PSA (4.0 ng/mL or greater) and/or and abnormal DRE within 6 mo of a negative initial biopsy. We routinely perform both sextant and systematic transition-zone biopsies for patients with a persistently elevated PSA because of studies demonstrating up to one-third of patients harboring cancer only in the transition zone on repeat biopsy.

The false-negative rate for repeat biopsy is in the 7–8% range, with 96% of cancers detected on the first two sets of biopsies. We reserve a third biopsy for those men with a high clinical suspicion of prostate cancer, such as those with a rapidly rising PSA velocity.

## CONCLUSIONS

TRUS-guided prostate biopsy is a well-tolerated procedure associated with little morbidity, and is ideally suited as an office-based procedure. As outlined in this chapter, no matter how the practicing urologist performs the procedure, a systematic approach to maximize cancer detection and minimize complications should be the primary objective.

## SELECTED READING

Allepuz Losa CA, Sanz Velez JI, Gil Sanz JG, et al. (1995) Seminal vesicle biopsy in prostate cancer staging. *J Urol* 154:1407.

Brawer MK, Chetner MP (1998) Ultrasonography of the prostate and biopsy. In: Walsh PC, Retik AB, Vaughan ED, Wein AJ, eds., *Campbell's Urology* (7th ed.) Philadelphia: WB Saunders Co.

Dajani AS, Taubert KA, Wilson W, et al. (1997) Prevention of bacterial endocarditis. *JAMA* 277 (22):1794.

Egawa S, Wheeler TM, Greene DR, et al. (1992) Unusual hyperechoic appearance of prostate cancer on transrectal ultrasonography. *Br J Urol* 69:169.

Ellis WJ, Chetner MP, Preston SD, et al. (1994) Diagnosis of prostatic carcinoma: the yield of serum PSA, DRE, and TRUS. *J Urol* 52:1520.

Epstein JI, Walsh PC, Sauvageot J, et al. (1997) Use of repeat sextant and transition zone biopsies for assessing extent of prostate cancer. *J Urol* 158:1886.

Eskew LA, Bare RL, McCullough DL (1997) Systematic 5 region prostate biopsy is superior to sextant method for diagnosing carcinoma of the prostate. *J Urol* 157:199.

Fleshner NE, O'Sullivan M, Fair WR (1997) Prevalence and predictors of a positive repeat transrectal ultrasound guided needle biopsy of the prostate. *J Urol* 158:505.

Haas CA, Resnick MI (1997) Office-based ultrasound for urologists. *AUA Update Series,* 16(31):242–247.

Hodge KK, McNeal JE, Terris MK, et al. (1989) Random systematic versus directed ultrasound guided transrectal core biopsies of the prostate. *J Urol* 142:71.

Levine MA, Ittman M, Melamed J (1998) Two consecutive sets of transrectal ultrasound guided biopsies of the prostate for the detection of prostate cancer. *J Urol* 159:471.

Lui PD, Terris MK, McNeal JE, et al. (1995) Indications for transrectal ultrasound guided transition zone biopsies in the detection of prostate cancer. *J Urol* 153:1000.

Norberg M, Egevad L, Holmberg L, et al. (1997) The sextant protocol for ultrasound-guided core biopsies of the prostate underestimates the presence of cancer. *Urology* 50:562.

Rodriguez LV, Terris MK (1998) Risks and complications of transrectal ultrasound guided prostate needle biopsy: a prospective study and review of the literature. *J Urol* 160:2115.

Terris MK, Pham TQ, Issa MM, et al. (1997) Routine transition zone and seminal vesicle biopsies in all patients undergoing transrectal ultrasound guided prostate biopsies are not indicated. *J Urol* 157:204.

Wilson TM, Gburek BM (1996) Transrectal ultrasonic-guided prostate biopsy. *AUA Update Series* 15(27):214.

# 22 Selecting and Counseling Patients on Appropriate Treatment of Prostate Cancer

*Faiyaaz M. Jhaveri, MD, and Eric A. Klein, MD*

**CONTENTS**

INTRODUCTION
TREATMENT FOR CLINICALLY LOCALIZED DISEASE
TREATMENT FOR CLINICALLY ADVANCED DISEASE
SUMMARY
SELECTED READING

## INTRODUCTION

It has been estimated that in 1998, physicians will have diagnosed prostate cancer in approximately 200,000 American men, who will be offered a variety of treatments to cure or control the progression of their disease. The lack of data from large, randomized trials with long-term follow-up has caused considerable controversy and confusion regarding the treatment options of newly diagnosed localized prostate cancer. In the absence of such controlled trials, it becomes difficult to compare treatment outcomes because of differing pretreatment risk characteristics and different specific therapeutic techniques. Adding to the confusion are the various endpoints used to gauge the success or failure of a particular treatment. Many prostatectomy and radiation therapy series use prostate-specific antigen (PSA) recurrence-free survival, defined a variety of ways, as an outcome parameter that may not translate into overall and prostate-cancer specific survival within the lifetime of a patient. Also, because of the profound downward-stage migration to more organ-confined disease during the PSA-screened era, improved outcomes reported from recent prostatectomy, external-beam radiation therapy, and interstitial brachytherapy series may not be related only to improvements in specific therapeutic techniques.

As a result of this controversy on cancer control with various treatments, issues regarding quality of life, morbidity, patient satisfaction, and the cost of these options have come into focus. Multiple reports in the literature document results of continence,

From: *Current Clinical Urology: Office Urology: The Clinician's Guide*
Edited by: E. D. Kursh and J. C. Ulchaker © Humana Press Inc., Totowa, NJ

potency, bowel toxicity, and other complications of radical prostatectomy and radiation therapy, with each treatment offering distinct advantages and disadvantages.

Which treatment is right for an individual with prostate cancer? Several factors must be considered, such as life expectancy and overall health, characteristics of the cancer, and the potential benefits and side effects of the various treatments. The main treatment options are:

1. Observation;
2. Radical prostatectomy;
3. External-beam radiation therapy;
4. Interstitial brachytherapy;
5. Cryotherapy; and
6. Hormone ablation therapy.

The three issues to consider when choosing a therapy are cancer control, morbidity and side effects, and salvage of treatment failures. Patient satisfaction and cost of treatment also need to be addressed.

## TREATMENT FOR CLINICALLY LOCALIZED DISEASE

### *Observation*

Prostate cancer is most frequently diagnosed in older men. During its usual long, protracted course, many investigators question whether any treatment is actually necessary. Data from long-term prospective, randomized trials comparing early diagnosis and active treatment vs no treatment (watchful waiting)—such as that being addressed by the Prostate Cancer Intervention Versus Observation Trial (PIVOT)—will not be available for several years. To provide guidance to urologists and patients facing prostate cancer today, data from long-term studies on the natural history of untreated, localized prostate cancer needs to be evaluated.

**Cancer Control**

Several investigators have evaluated long-term outcomes associated with conservative management of localized prostate cancer. In 1997, Johansson et al. reported the 15–yr results of a population-based cohort of 642 men who had initial observation for newly diagnosed prostate cancer. Only 300 of these patients had disease localized to the prostate, and only 85 were younger than 70 yr. The number of patients with moderate-grade or high-grade tumors was small, with approximately half of the men with well-differentiated tumors. Despite these limitations, their results showed that 6% of their patients with well-differentiated cancer, 17% with moderate-grade disease, and 56% with poorly differentiated disease died of prostate cancer.

Several investigators have confirmed a decreasing survival rate with worsening tumor histology. In a pooled analysis of 828 men included in six nonrandomized studies describing the natural history of localized prostate cancer, Chodak et al. reported that men with well-differentiated and moderately differentiated tumors had an 87% 10-yr disease-specific survival. This rate compared to only a 34% 10-yr disease-specific survival in men with poorly differentiated disease.

However, tumor histology alone cannot be used to counsel men with newly diagnosed prostate cancer who are contemplating watchful waiting. Two other important factors—patient's age and competing medical risks—were taken into account in the analysis

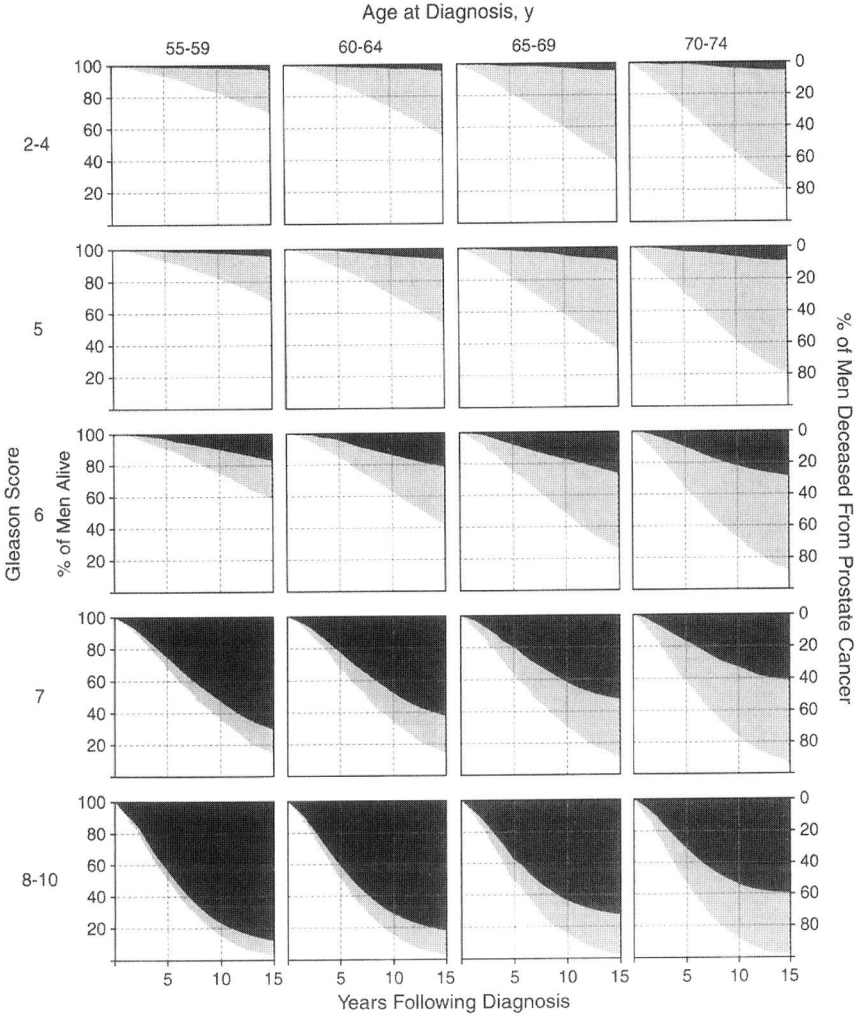

**Fig. 1.** Probability of dying of prostate cancer compared to Gleason score and age at diagnosis.

performed by Albertsen et al. in 1995 and updated in 1998. Their earlier study showed that the age-adjusted survival for men with tumors having a Gleason score of 2–4 was not different from that of the general population, but the maximum estimated lost life expectancy for men with Gleason score of 5–7 was 4–5 yr, and for men with Gleason score of 8–10 was 6–8 yr. In addition, they showed that tumor histology and patient comorbidities were powerful independent predictors of survival. Their 15-yr data estimated the probability of dying from prostate cancer or competing causes given a patient's tumor histology and age at diagnosis (*see* Fig. 1). The survival curves in their study provide evidence for two important concepts. First, men with tumors that have a Gleason score of 5 or less—especially older men—have a minimal risk of dying from prostate cancer, as compared to their risk of dying of other competing causes (*see* Table 1). However, even in men over 70, the risk of dying of prostate cancer is substantial for tumors with a Gleason score of 7 or greater. These curves are useful

Table 1
Estimated Percentages of Patients Managed Conservatively Who Died From Prostate Cancer by Age and Gleason Score at Diagnosis[a]

| Gleason Score | 55–59 yr | 60–64 yr | 65–69 yr | 70–74 yr |
|---|---|---|---|---|
| 2–4 | 4% | 5% | 6% | 7% |
| 5 | 6% | 8% | 10% | 11% |
| 6 | 18% | 23% | 27% | 30% |
| 7 | 70% | 62% | 53% | 42% |
| 8–10 | 87% | 81% | 72% | 60% |

[a]Data from Albertsen et al. (1998) *JAMA* 280: 975–980.

when counseling men with newly diagnosed, localized prostate cancer considering observation.

## Morbidity and Side Effects

Few studies have compared general and disease-specific health-related quality of life of patients who undergo active treatment for prostate cancer with control groups, and even less have reported outcomes longitudinally. Those who used controls found that men who underwent radical prostatectomy or pelvic irradiation had more urinary and sexual impairment, but no differences were noted in general health-related quality of life.

When counseling patients on the side effects of active treatments, health-related quality-of-life changes must be analyzed in the context of any impairment that may have been present at baseline. A recent study by Litwin presented general and disease-targeted health-related quality-of-life outcomes of a statistically valid population-based control sample of older men without prostate cancer. They reported that approximately one-third of men had some degree of urinary leakage, one-third had some degree of rectal dysfunction, and nearly two-thirds claimed significant difficulty with erection. Therefore, if "normal" is defined as the absence of any dysfunction, prostate-cancer treatment groups may be held to too high a standard. The psychological effect of having untreated cancer must also be taken into consideration.

### *Radical Prostatectomy*

In the United States, the most common treatment offered to patients with localized prostate cancer and a 10-yr or greater life expectancy is radical prostatectomy (RP). Because of the profound downward-stage migration to more localized and organ-confined disease, more patients are candidates for this form of treatment. However, radical prostatectomy should be offered to men who are likely to be cured and will survive long enough to benefit from the cure.

## Cancer Control

The results of long-term studies show a great disparity between overall cause-specific and biochemical disease-free survival following RP. The 10-yr PSA progression-free likelihood has ranged from 47 to 73% from several retropubic prostatectomy series. However, the 10-yr overall actuarial cause-specific survival rates are approx 90% in these large long-term series. This suggests that although the use of a PSA-free survival rate may be used as an endpoint and indicator of the success of surgery, the clinical significance of this endpoint needs to be evaluated with longer follow-up of these patients.

Several investigators have shown that higher preoperative PSA levels are often associated with advanced pathological features, such as extracapsular extension, seminal-vesicle invasion, and positive lymph nodes. However, Stamey et al. have shown that some patients with large transition-zone cancers confined to the prostate can still produce highly elevated serum PSA levels. Therefore, PSA alone cannot be used to predict the stage of the cancer, and should not solely be used as a contraindication to definitive treatment.

Many investigators have identified tumor histological grade as the most powerful prognostic variable in men with prostate cancer. A large population-based study by Lu-Yao et al. found a 10-yr prostate-cancer-specific survival rate of only 45% in patients with GS >7 prostate cancer managed conservatively. Furthermore, 5 yr after diagnosis, the relative survival compared to age-matched cohorts was only 0.61 in men with high-grade cancer managed conservatively, compared to 0.98 after prostatectomy.

The presence of extracapsular extension and positive margins has been implicated as predictors of disease progression. In a recent study by Ohori et al., extracapsular extension was found to be the most important independent predictor of time to PSA progression, with a relative risk ratio of 4.3 (95% CI: 1.9–9.4). However, we recently reported the 10-yr overall actuarial survival rates of those patients with extracapsular extension—with or without PSA recurrence—and found it was nearly identical, at 88% and 89% respectively. In addition, patients with positive margins with or without PSA failure had an identical 10-yr survival rate of 86%. Although a detectable PSA with regard to extracapsular extension and/or positive margins may represent recurrent disease, we found no impact on overall survival at 10 yr. Seminal-vesicle invasion was also found to be an independent predictor of PSA progression, and patients with locally advanced disease (stage T3) have a 20–50% chance of lymph-node metastases. Fortunately, the widespread use of PSA has enabled early detection, and the incidence of pelvic lymph-node metastases has fallen from 20% to 5% in more recent series.

Although neoadjuvant hormone-ablation therapy reduces the incidence of positive surgical margins, this effect is thought to be artifactual. No long-term benefit on disease control or survival has been demonstrated in men who received neoadjuvant androgen ablation prior to prostatectomy.

Radical prostatectomy appears to offer excellent cancer control and survival rates. However, it should be considered only for men in general good health who have a 10-yr or greater life expectancy. Furthermore, from studies on the natural history of low-grade prostate cancer, the risks of death from competing causes may outweigh that of a cancer death, especially in the elderly population. The risk of short- and long-term complications of radical prostatectomy may not outweigh the small benefit of a cancer cure in such patients.

**Morbidity and Side Effects**

Radical prostatectomy can be performed safely and with short hospital stays. At our center, patients routinely spend two nights or less in the hospital, with high satisfaction rates. The most common intraoperative early complication, historically, has been blood loss. However, with improvements in surgical technique and the delineation of precise anatomy, a substantial reduction in blood loss has resulted, with most centers reporting an average of <1000 mL. Operative mortality has been reported to be only 0.3% when combining several large series. The incidence of deep venous thrombosis (1.1%) and pulmonary embolism (1.3%) are also very low in patients who undergo radical prostatectomy. Anastomotic stricture has been found to be between 0.5 and 9% in contemporary series.

Late complications are more common. Urinary incontinence has ranged from 5 to 20%, depending on the center and definition of incontinence. Interestingly, series reporting surveys of patients questioned anonymously show increased incontinence rates ranging from 19 to 31%. However, severe total incontinence is relatively rare (<4%). It is important to note that incontinence improves with time up to 2 yr following surgery. Older age, presence of an anastomotic stricture, or baseline bladder dysfunction can contribute to incontinence following prostatectomy.

Erectile dysfunction following radical prostatectomy has been shown to correlate with increasing age, and is dependent on the ability to preserve the neurovascular bundles. Potency following bilateral nerve-sparing prostatectomy has ranged from 20 to 90%, depending on the age of the patient, the method used for data collection, the definition of potency, and the surgical technique used. Most patients will experience at least temporary erectile dysfunction after RP, and many never regain full potency. However, it is important to note the potency status of the patient before the procedure. The use of sildenafil citrate (Viagra) following radical prostatectomy has recently been shown to enhance erections in men with erectile dysfunction after bilateral nerve-sparing prostatectomy. Other minimally invasive treatments for impotence, such as the vacuum-erection device and penile injection therapy, offer excellent patient and spousal satisfaction rates. Although the number of patients receiving penile prosthetic implants has decreased because of these oral and minimally invasive treatments, penile implants remain a valid option in refractory cases, with high patient satisfaction rates.

**Salvage of Treatment Failures**

Three treatment options exist for a rising PSA after radical prostatectomy: observation, androgen ablation, and pelvic irradiation. Since observation and androgen ablation are not curative, radiation therapy is usually considered as salvage therapy. For radiation therapy to be curative, the recurrent tumor must be localized to the prostatic fossa and be sensitive to radiation therapy. Some investigators report that Gleason 8 or greater tumors—and those involving the seminal vesicle or lymph nodes—are not amenable to irradiation. Distant metastases are usually suspected in patients with elevated PSA within 1 yr of radical prostatectomy, and with PSA doubling times of <6 mo. However, for patients with recurrences without these features, salvage radiation therapy of 60–70 gy has resulted in a PSA response of >1 yr in more than 60% of patients with or without the use of preradiation therapy hormones. However, the long-term durability is uncertain. Pelvic radiation therapy in this setting appears to be well-tolerated, with less severe toxicity than in patients undergoing primary radiation therapy and with no increased risk of incontinence.

### *External-Beam Radiation Therapy*

Historically, in surgical series, patients tend to be younger, healthier, and have smaller tumors, whereas in past radiation-therapy series, patients usually have been deemed noncandidates for surgery. In addition, radiotherapy patients tend not to be surgically staged. Although several attempts have been made, radiotherapy and surgical series are incomparable retrospectively, and cannot generally be matched in terms of prognostic characteristics. As a result of the ongoing controversy in cancer control, many patients may choose radiation therapy to avoid the side effects and morbidity of radical prostatectomy.

**Cancer Control**

Although many pathological prognostic parameters—such as extracapsular extension, seminal-vesicle invasion, and pelvic lymph-node status—cannot be used to compare radiotherapy to surgical outcomes, it is important to at least estimate similar pretreatment characteristics when comparing efficacy of different therapies. Using a variety of definitions of disease freedom, investigators of recent radiotherapy series claim excellent 5-yr disease-free survival rates, and many describe treatment results equal to or better than radical prostatectomy. In a recent study by Keyser et al. of patients with a pretreatment PSA of <10 ng/mL, and using the definition of a PSA failure of two consecutive rising PSA values, 5-yr biochemical relapse-free survival of 75% was achieved, compared to 76% from radical prostatectomy. In a recent study by Zelefsky et al., patients with favorable-risk prostate cancer (pretreatment PSA ≤10 ng/mL, clinical stage ≤T2b, and Gleason score ≤6) who underwent three-dimensional conformal radiotherapy (median dose of 70.2 gy) had a biochemical failure rate (defined as three successive PSA elevations observed from the posttreatment nadir PSA value) of only 8%, with a median follow-up of 36 mo. Similar short-term results in contemporary patients with early-stage disease are seen from other centers. Yet 10-yr results are generally lower, because of the relatively more advanced tumors treated during the earlier period.

In a recent multi-institutional pooled analysis, Shipley et al. evaluated outcome data on 1756 men treated with external-beam radiotherapy from 1988 to 1995 from six medical centers. Only patients with clinical-stage T1b, T1c, and T2 tumors were included. The PSA failure-free rates at 5 and 7 yr after treatment for patients with a pretreatment PSA of <10 ng/mL were 78 and 73%, respectively. The PSA failure-free rate at 5 yr for patients with Gleason scores 5–6 was also favorable at 73%; however, it was significantly lower for Gleason score ≥7, at only 53%. This series needs to mature for a few more years to determine the durability of these rates at 10 yr and beyond. In addition, a rising PSA value has not been validated as an early surrogate endpoint for progression or death caused by prostate cancer.

The issue of nadir-level PSA following radiation therapy was recently addressed in a study from Critz et al. They evaluated 354 men following radiation therapy, and correlated 10-yr disease-free survival with nadir PSA levels. They concluded that men must achieve a nadir PSA of at least 0.5 ng/mL or less to be cured of prostate cancer by irradiation. In addition, the prognostic value of this nadir level depends on most men achieving a nadir of 0.2 ng/mL or less, where the 10-yr disease-free survival rate rises from 62 to 89%. Therefore, treatment outcomes between surgery and radiation therapy may be more realistic when using essentially the same definition of disease freedom for both treatments. Investigations using three-dimensional conformal-beam radiation with higher doses of 7100–8100 cgy have been shown to improve nadir levels postradiation, and may ultimately lead to improved cancer control. The effect of hormonal cytoreduction before radiotherapy to improve local control is awaiting phase III trials.

**Morbidity and Side Effects**

The typical radiation treatment requires 35 sessions (5 d/wk for 7 wk). The acute side effects of pelvic irradiation are usually self-limiting, and include diarrhea, rectal irritation, dysuria, and frequency. A chronic complication rate of only 5% can be expected overall. The late complications can include chronic rectal and bladder injury, enteritis, and urethral stricture. Impotence (40–70%) and rarely, severe incontinence (1%), can also occur. Treatment-related mortality is low at 0.2%, as are severe complications, such as intractable hematuria and rectal bleeding. With the wider use of bladder- and rectal-sparing three-dimensional conformal techniques, higher doses of radiation can be delivered to the prostate with fewer side effects.

As mentioned previously, using different measures, Litwin et al. found no differences between radical prostatectomy and radiation therapy for patients in general health-related quality of life. However, there were marked differences in urinary control, sexual function, and bowel function between these groups, with urinary and sexual function better in the radiation group and bowel function improved in the radical prostatectomy group. Despite these problems, Fowler et al. showed that the overwhelming majority of patients reported that they would choose the same therapy again, although slightly more radical prostatectomy patients than radiation therapy patients felt that way (92 vs 87%). In addition, radical prostatectomy patients were more certain about cure and less worried over cure than radiotherapy patients.

**Salvage of Treatment Failures**

Salvage prostatectomy should be reserved for patients who are likely to have local recurrence picked up early after radiation therapy, and low-risk factors such as low initial PSA values and failure levels of <10 ng/mL. Rogers et al. showed that if the preoperative PSA was <10 ng/mL, only 15% of patients had advanced pathological features, compared with 86% if the PSA was >10 ng/mL.

It is also important to rule out distant metastasis. When faced with a patient with a rising PSA level following radiation therapy, the urologist has several parameters to help determine local vs distant recurrence, which may ultimately help guide therapy. The higher the pretreatment PSA, biopsy Gleason score, and clinical stage, the more likely it is that a patient may have occult metastatic disease. The timing, rate of rise, and doubling time of PSA after therapy appear to be helpful in predicting the site of recurrence. When local recurrence is suspected, TRUS with guided biopsies may be indicated to diagnose local recurrence. If distant disease is suspected, bone scans have a limited role unless the PSA rises to above 30 ng/mL. Finally, the role of immunoscintigraphy has yet to be determined, with future study still evolving.

The complication rate of prostatectomy is considerably higher following radiation therapy vs primary radical prostatectomy in nonirradiated patients. After salvage prostatectomy, there is virtually no chance of potency, a 30–60% chance of significant urinary incontinence (usually requiring an artificial sphincter), and a much higher rate of rectal injury (potentially requiring a temporary colostomy) in up to 15% of patients.

Overall, Rogers et al. reported a 55% actuarial undetectable PSA rate at 5 yr after salvage RP. Organ-confined disease was highly likely if salvage surgery was performed when the failure PSA was <10 ng/mL, but this has not been confirmed in all series. Thus in selected individuals, salvage prostatectomy can offer a chance of cure despite substantial morbidity.

### *Interstitial Radioactive Seed Implants*

Advances in imaging and technique during the last decade have resulted in a new interest in brachytherapy for localized prostate cancer. As a monotherapy, brachytherapy is attractive because it offers the potential advantages of a single and safe outpatient procedure with a reduced risk of incontinence and impotence than is typical with surgery. In addition, recent reports claim that brachytherapy yields intermediate-term results comparable to RP with respect to cancer control. However, similar to RP and external-beam radiation therapy series, these results have been criticized for comparing cohorts of patients with different pretreatment characteristics from different institutions. In addition, different definitions of recurrences, as mentioned earlier, make studies comparing these modalities potentially flawed and misleading.

**Cancer Control**

Ragde et al. has reported favorable results for $^{125}$iodine interstitial radiotherapy in a select group of prostate-cancer patients comprised largely of men with Gleason scores of 6 or less, and serum PSA of <10 ng/mL (80%). He reported a 7-yr actuarial recurrence-free survival of 79%, with tumor recurrence defined as PSA of >0.5 mg/mL. Even with the significant limitations of retrospective comparisons at different centers, Polascik et al. reported a 7-yr recurrence-free survival of 98% in radical prostatectomy patients matched by Gleason score. However, recently Ramos et al. reported a 7-yr recurrence-free survival of 84% in a group of patients matched even more closely with that of the brachytherapy series reported by Ragde et al. Similarly, D'Amico et al. showed that low-risk patients (stage T1c, T2a, and PSA≤10 ng/mL and Gleason score≤6) had similar estimated 5-yr PSA outcome after treatment with RP, external-beam radiation therapy, or seed implant. The intermediate- and high-risk patients treated with RP or external-beam radiotherapy did better than those treated by implant. However, because of the severe limitations of such retrospective comparisons, the answers to which therapy offers the superior cancer control await prospective trials comparing 10- and 15-yr actual survival data.

**Morbidity and Side Effects**

Because of the ongoing controversy on long-term cancer control, many patients—especially those with the favorable characteristics of Gleason score of 6 or less and PSA levels of <10 ng/mL—may opt for the less morbid procedure. Common side effects are self-limiting, and include bladder or rectal irritation, urinary retention (which may require a temporary catheter or intermittent self-catherization) and rarely, persistent hematuria. Incontinence, impotence, and bladder-neck contractures are also rare.

In a recent study by Zelefsky et al. a comparison of morbidities of three-dimensional conformal radiotherapy (3-D CRT) vs transperineal permanent iodine-125 implantation (TPI) for early-stage prostatic cancer were accessed. The 5-yr PSA relapse-free outcome was similar at 88% vs 83%, respectively. Urinary symptoms that required medications for relief (grade 2) were observed in 42% of the 3D-CRT patients, but resolved within 4–6 wk after completion of therapy, with 5-yr actuarial likelihood of late-grade-2 urinary toxicity of only 8%. Protracted grade-2 urinary symptoms were more prevalent among the TPI group, persisting for more than 1 yr in 31% with a median duration of 23 mo. Acute urinary retention was seen in 3% of TPI patients, but not found in the 3D-CRT group. Urethral strictures developed in 1% in the 3D-CRT group vs 7% in the TPI group. The 5-yr likelihood of grade-2 late-rectal toxicity was similar for the 3D-CRT (6%) and TPI (11%) groups. No patient in either group developed grade 3 or higher late-rectal toxicity. The 5-yr likelihood of posttreatment erectile dysfunction among patients who were potent before therapy was 43% for the 3D-CRT group and 53% for the TPI group.

**Salvage of Treatment Failures**

Unfortunately, there is a shortage of data for salvage prostatectomy following the contemporary brachytherapy techniques. Because of the limited tissue reserves for healing and repair in postradiation therapy patients, salvage prostatectomy following brachytherapy may have high morbidity rates, although the amount of radiation to surrounding tissues may be less than with external-beam radiotherapy.

## *Cryotherapy*

Cryotherapy is the destruction of tumors through the application of freezing temperatures. Historical data on cryotherapy suffers from the same uncertain comparisons of different patient populations, different outcome definitions, and variations of technique over time. No randomized data is available for any current cryotherapy regimens for prostate cancer, and therefore this technique should be considered investigational.

Crawford et al. performed whole-mount analyses after salvage RP after failed TRUS-guided cryotherapy. The whole mounts revealed areas of unaffected adenocarcinoma and normal prostatic parenchyma, although intraoperative TRUS predicted that the entire prostate would show freeze-destruction. This finding suggests that the entire prostate is not lethally frozen when its boundaries are included within the hypoechoic ice ball seen on TRUS.

Cryotherapy has been suggested as a less invasive and potentially less morbid alternative to salvage RP. The overall experience is still limited, with one report showing only 3 of 10 patients not on androgen ablation therapy followed for a minimum of 1 yr after surgery having a PSA of <0.4 ng/mL. Tissue slough (15%) and incontinence (10%) were not uncommon. In another report, only 14% of patients with 1-yr follow-up had a PSA of <0.3 ng/mL, and 100% of the 23 patients had complications, including significant lower urinary-tract symptoms. Fifty-five percent of patients required transurethral resection for tissue slough. This therapy is presently associated with significant morbidity and a limited chance of cure, and should be considered investigational.

## TREATMENT FOR CLINICALLY ADVANCED DISEASE

### *Hormone Ablation Therapy*

In patients with prostate cancer, medical or surgical castration has been shown to be effective palliation, and is commonly applied to either locally advanced or metastatic prostate cancer. However, recent studies do not reveal a survival advantage of any effective androgen ablation-treatment regimen.

## Cancer Control

Cure of prostate cancer by means of androgen ablation therapy is extremely unlikely. Some men with prostate cancer die of competing causes, and thus cannot be considered cured. Objective and subjective responses vary between 40 and 80%, depending on the criteria used for evaluation and stage of disease at initiation of therapy. Response to treatment is seen with pain relief, improvement with obstructive symptoms resulting from shrinkage of the primary tumor, and improvement of the performance status. A complete response with disappearance of all clinically identifiable disease and normal PSA levels is only seen in 5–10% of patients. In patients with metastases, time to clinical progression and death varied from 18 to 24 and 30 to 36 mo. These periods may be longer in patients with locally extensive disease.

Multiple randomized studies have addressed the issue of surgical vs. medical castration and the exclusion of adrenal androgens by maximal androgen blockade. The EORTC GU group studied newly diagnosed metastatic prostate cancer in which patients were randomized to bilateral orchiectomy compared with 1 mg of diethyl-stilbesterol (DES) and orchiectomy with cyproterone acetate. In 1995, Robinson et al. reported in the final analysis that no difference in progression or survival rates was found between the treatment arms. Similarly, results of an overview analysis by Dalesio et al. of data from 5600 patients randomized to 21 studies, and the largest study of 1378 patients by the SWOG Intergroup 0105, provide evidence that there is no significant difference in the rates of progression or survival among surgical castration, leutinizing hormone-releasing hormone (LH-RH) agonist therapy, or maximal androgen blockade. Castration remains the gold standard of androgen ablation therapy.

Although the question of whether early vs delayed androgen ablation therapy provides an overall survival advantage remains unanswered, early androgen ablation appears to delay progression in patients with lymph-node metastases. Also unanswered is the issue of intermittent androgen ablation therapy that provides a cyclic form of endocrine treatment. A small pilot study by Horwich et al. showed that temporary cessation of hormone therapy can be associated with significant periods of therapy with a high chance of a second hormone response. The advantage may be an increase in quality of life and lower cost during the nontreatment intervals, but whether cancer control is equivalent to continuous treatment awaits the results of a phase III trial.

## Morbidity and Side Effects

Quality-of-life measurements should be taken seriously in treatments that are palliative in nature. Instruments to measure quality-of-life issues are being developed. The most frequent side effects of androgen ablation therapy are loss of libido and potency, hot flashes, osteoporosis, fatigue, loss of muscle mass, anemia, and weight gain. Although the clinical advantage of pure antiandrogen monotherapy is the maintenance of libido and potency, equal effectiveness with castration has not been proven in regard to cancer control.

## SUMMARY

The difficult decision of treatment faced by patients with clinically localized prostate cancer involves many factors. The current health status and life expectancy of patients must be addressed, apart from the fact that they have prostate cancer. When comparing the various treatments, patients need to be counseled on cancer control, morbidity, patient satisfaction with therapy and quality of life, and ease of salvage of treatment failures. Although short-term outcomes of many contemporary surgical and radiation therapy series may appear similar, long-term cancer control remains uncertain. Different organ systems are affected by each therapy, resulting in different acute morbidity and functional outcomes, although the majority of patients would choose the same treatment again. The toxicity of salvage radiation therapy after RP appears to be less substantial than for salvage prostatectomy or salvage cryotherapy, although long-term data on cure rates are not yet available. All of these issues must be discussed with patients to help them choose which factors are most important for their individual circumstances.

## SELECTED READING

Alberston PC, Hanley JA, Gleason DF, et al. (1998) Competing risk analysis of men aged 55 to 74 years at diagnosis managed conservatively for clinically localized prostate cancer. *JAMA* 280:975–980.

Albertson PC, Fryback DG, Storer BE, et al. (1995) Long-term survival among men with conservatively treated localized prostate cancer. *JAMA* 274:626–631.

Bales GT, Williams MJ, Sinner M, et al. (1996) Short-term outcomes after cryosurgical ablation of the prostate in men with recurrent prostate carcinoma following radiation therapy. *Urology* 46:676–680.

Catalona WJ, Basler JW (1993) Return of erections and urinary continence following nerve sparing radical retropubic prostatectomy. *J Urol* 150:905–907.

Catalona WJ, Smith DS (1998) Cancer recurrence and survival rates after anatomic radical retropubic prostatectomy for prostate cancer: intermediate-term results. *J Urol* 160:2428–2434.

Catalona WJ, Smith DS, Ratliff TL, et al. (1993) Detection of organ-confined prostate cancer is increased through prostate-specific antigen based screening. *JAMA* 270:48.

Chodak GW, Thisted RA, Gerber GS, et al. (1994) Results of conservative management of clinically localized prostate cancer. *N Engl J Med* 330:242–248.

Critz FA, Levinson AK, Williams WH, et al. (1999) Prostate specific antigen nadir achieved by men apparently cured of prostate cancer by radiotherapy. *J Urol* 161:1199–1205.

Dalseo O, Schroeder FH, Peto R (Writing Committee), and the Prostate Cancer Trialists' Collaborative Group (1995) Maximal androgen blockade in advanced prostate cancer: an overview of 22 randomized trials with 3289 deaths in 5710 patients. *Lancet* 346:265–269.

D'Amico AV, Whittington R, Malkowicz B, et al. (1998) Biochemical outcome after radical prostatectomy, external beam radiation therapy, or interstitial radiation therapy for clinically localized prostate cancer. *JAMA* 280:969–974.

Dillioglugil O, Leibman BD, Kattan MW, et al. (1997) Hazard rates for progression after radical prostatectomy for clinically localized prostate cancer. *Urology* 50:93–99.

Forman JD, Meetze K, Pontes JE (1997) Therapeutic radiation for patients with an elevated post-prostatectomy PSA level. *J Urol* 157:1251A (suppl).

Fowler FL, Jr, Barry MJ, Lu-Yao G, et al. (1995) Effect of radical prostatectomy for prostate cancer on patient quality of life: results from a Medicare survey. *Urology* 45:1007–1015.

Fowler FJ, Jr, Barry MJ, Lu-Yao G, et al. (1996) Outcomes of external-beam radiation therapy for prostate cancer: a study of Medicare beneficiaries in three surveillance, epidemiology, and end results areas. *J Clin Oncol* 14:2258–2265.

Frazier HA, Robertson JE, Humphrey PA, et al. (1993) Is prostate specific antigen of clinical importance in evaluating outcome after radical prostatectomy? *J Urol* 149:516–518.

Gong M, Ferrari M, Stamey TA (1996) Combined androgen deprivation and radiation therapy for treatment of residual prostate cancer following radical prostatectomy. *J Urol* 155:645A (suppl).

Grampas SA, Miller GJ, Crawford ED (1995) Salvage radical prostatectomy after failed transperineal cryotherapy: histologic findings from prostate whole-mount specimens correlated with intraoperative transrectal ultrasound images. *Urology* 45:936–941.

Horwich A, Huddart JG, Boyd PJ, et al. (1998) A pilot study of intermittent androgen deprivation in advanced prostate cancer. *Br J Urol* 81:96–99.

Jhaveri FM, Klein EA, Kupelian PA, et al. (1999) Declining rates of extracapsular extension in radical prostatectomy: evidence for continued stage migration. *J Clin Oncol* (in press).

Jhaveri FM, Klein EA (1999) How to explore the patient with a rising PSA after radical prostatectomy: defining local versus systemic failure. *Semin Urol Oncol* (in press).

Jhaveri FM, Zippe CD, Klein EA, et al. (1999) Biochemical failure does not predict overall survival after radical prostatectomy for localized prostate cancer: 10 year results. *Urology* (in press).

Johansson JE, Holmberg L, Johansson S, et al. (1997) Fifteen-year survival in prostate cancer: a prospective, population-based study in Sweden. *JAMA* 277:467–471.

Keyser D, Kupelian PA, Zippe CD, et al. (1997) Stage T1–2 prostate cancer with pre-treatment PSA level 10 ng/mL or less: radiation therapy or surgery? *Int J Radiat Oncol Biol Phys* 37:351–358.

Klein EA (1992) Early continence after radical prostatectomy. *J Urol* 148:92–95.

Klein EA (1998) Radiation therapy versus radical prostatectomy in the PSA era: a urologist's view. *Semin Rad Oncol* 8:87–94.

Kupelian P, Katcher J, Levin H, et al. (1996) Correlation of clinical and pathological factors with rising prostate-specific antigen profiles after radical prostatectomy alone for clinically localized prostate cancer. *Urology* 48:249–260.

Landis SH, Murray T, Bolden S, Wingo PA (1998) Cancer statistics, 1998. *CA Cancer J Clin.* 48:6–29.

Leandri P, Rossignol G, Gautier JR, et al. (1992) Radical retropubic prostatectomy: morbidity and quality of life: experience with 620 consecutive cases. *J Urol* 147(3 pt 2): 883.

Litwin MS (1999) Health related quality of life in older men without prostate cancer. *J Urol* 161:1180–1184.

Litwin MS, Hays RD, Fink A, et al. (1995) Quality-of-life outcomes in men treated for localized prostate cancer. *JAMA* 273:129–135.

Lu-Yao GL, Yao S (1997) Population-based study of long-term survival in patients with clinically localised prostate cancer. *Lancet* 349:906–910.

McCarthy JF, Catalona WJ, Hudson MA (1994) Effect of radiation therapy on detectable serum prostate specific antigen levels following radical prostatectomy: early versus delayed treatment. *J Urol* 151:1575–1578.

Miller RJ Jr, Cohen JK, Shuman B, et al. (1996) Percutaneous, transperineal cryosurgery of the prostate as salvage therapy for post radiation recurrence of adenocarcinoma. *Cancer* 77:1510–1514.

Partin AW, Pound CR, Clemens JQ, et al. (1993) Serum PSA after anatomic radical prostatectomy: the Johns Hopkins Experience after 10 years. *Urol Clin N Am* 20:713–725.

Patel A, Dorey F, Franklin J et al. (1997) Recurrence patterns after radical prostatectomy: clinical usefulness of prostate specific antigen doubling times and log slope prostate specific antigen. *J Urol* 158:1441–1445.

Polascik TJ, Pound CR, DeWeese TL, et al. (1998) Comparison of radical prostatectomy and iodine 125 interstitial radiotherapy for the treatment of clinically localized prostate cancer: a 7-year biochemical (PSA) progression analysis. *Urology* 51:884.

Ragde H, Blasko JC, Grimm PD, et al. (1997) Interstitial iodine 125 radiation without adjuvant therapy in the treatment of clinically localized prostate carcinoma. *Cancer* 80:442.

Ramos CG, Carvalhal G, Smith DS, et al. (1999) Retrospective comparison of radical retropubic prostatectomy and 125-iodine brachytherapy for localized prostate cancer. *J Urol* 161:1212–1215.

Robinson MRG, Smith PH, Richards B, et al. (1995) The final analysis of the EORTC Genito-Urinary Group phase III clinical trial (protocol 30805) comparing orchidectomy, orchidectomy plus cyproterone acetate and low dose stilbesterol in the management of metastatic carcinoma of the prostate. *Eur Urol* 28:273–283.

Rogers E, Ohori M, Kassabian VS, et al. (1995) Salvage radical prostatectomy: outcome measured by serum prostate specific antigen levels. *J Urol* 153:104–110.

Rogers R, Roach M, Presti J, et al. (1997) Radiation therapy for the management of biopsy-proven local recurrence after radical prostatectomy. *J Urol* 157:1131A (suppl).

Shipley WU, Thames HD, Sandler HM, et al. (1999) Radiation therapy for clinically localized prostate cancer: a multi-institutional pooled analysis. *JAMA* 281:1598–1604.

Shipley WU, Zietman AL, Hanks GE, et al. (1994) Treatment related sequelae following external beam radiation for prostate cancer: a review with an update on patients with stages T1 and T2 tumor. *J Urol* 152:1799–1805.

Soffen EM, Hanks GE, Hunt MA, et al. (1992) Conformal static filed radiation therapy of early prostate cancer versus nonconformal techniques: a reduction in acute morbidity. *Int J Radiat Oncol Biol Phys* 24:485–490.

Stamey TA, Donaldson AN, Yemoto CE, et al. (1998) Histological and clinical findings in 896 consecutive prostates treated only with radical retropubic prostatectomy: epidemiologic significance of annual changes. *J Urol* 160:2412–2417.

Stamey TA, Ferrari MK, Schmid HP (1993) The value of serial prostate specific antigen determinations 5 years after radiotherapy: steeply increasing values characterize 80% of patients. *J Urol* 150:1856–1859.

Stein A, deKernion JB, Smith RB, et al. (1992) Prostate specific antigen levels after radical prostatectomy in patients with organ confined and locally extensive prostate cancer. *J Urol* 147:942–946.

Steiner MS, Morton RA, Walsh PC (1991) Impact of anatomical radical prostatectomy on urinary continence. *J Urol* 145:512–514.

Wilt TJ, Brawer MK (1995) Early intervention or expectant management for prostate cancer. The Prostate Cancer Intervention Versus Observation Trial (PIVOT): a randomized trial comparing radical prostatectomy with expectant management for the treatment of clinically localized prostate cancer. *Semin Urol* 13:130–136.

Zagars GK (1993) Serum PSA as a tumor marker for patients undergoing definitive radiation therapy. *Urol Clin N Am* 20:737–747.

Zagars GK, Pollack A (1995) Radiation therapy for T1 and T2 prostate cancer: prostate-specific antigen and disease outcome. *Urology* 45:476–483.

Zagars GK, Sands ME, Pollack A, et al. (1994) Early androgen ablation for stages D1 (N1 to N3, M0) prostate cancer: prognostic variables and outcome. *J Urol* 151:1330–1333.

Zelefsky MJ, Wallner KE, Ling C, et al. (1999) Comparison of the 5-year outcome and morbidity of three-dimensional conformal radiotherapy versus transperineal permanent iodine-125 implantation for early-stage prostate cancer. *J Clin Oncol* 17:517–522.

Zietman AL, Coen JJ, Shipley WU et al. (1994) Radical radiation therapy in the management of prostatic adenocarcinoma: the initial prostate specific antigen value as a predictor of treatment outcome. *J Urol* 151:640–645.

Zincke H, Oesterling JE, Blute ML, et al. (1994) Long-term (15 years) results after radical prostatectomy for clinically localized (stage T2c or lower) prostate cancer. *J Urol* 152:1850–1857.

Zippe CD, Kedia AW, Kedia K, et al. (1998) Treatment of erectile dysfunction after radical prostatectomy with sildenafil citrate (Viagra). *Urology* 52:963–966.

# 23 Prostate Cancer
## Endocrine Therapy

*Hamed A. Daw, MD*
*and David M. Peereboom, MD*

**CONTENTS**
    INTRODUCTION
    ENDOCRINOLOGY OF THE PROSTATE GLAND
    PRIMARY HORMONAL TREATMENT OPTIONS
    COMBINED ANDROGEN BLOCKADE
    EARLY OR DELAYED ENDOCRINE THERAPY
    INTERMITTENT ANDROGEN BLOCKADE
    HORMONAL THERAPY AS AN ADJUNCT TO
        PRIMARY TREATMENT
    SECOND-LINE HORMONE THERAPY
    CONCLUSIONS
    SELECTED READING

## INTRODUCTION

Prostate cancer is the most frequently diagnosed noncutaneous malignancy in men, and thus is becoming a major public health problem in the United States. After a peak incidence of 334,500 new cases in 1996, the American Cancer Society predicts a drop to approx 179,300 new cases of prostate carcinoma in this country for 1999. However, the death rate will be essentially unchanged, at approx 41,800 deaths each year, making prostate cancer the second leading cause of death among men in the United States. Despite increasing understanding of the biology of this disease and continuous research, strategies for diagnosis and management remain controversial. In this chapter, we will explore the various modalities of endocrine therapy of prostate cancer, their physiologic basis, and their contribution to the management of patients with prostate cancer.

## ENDOCRINOLOGY OF THE PROSTATE GLAND

It is generally accepted that the growth of the prostate gland depends largely on androgen stimulation. However, the prostate gland is sensitive to a variety of hormones, including estrogens, growth hormone, prolactin and various tissue-growth factors. Prostatic tissue growth and differentiation is therefore rather a complex process involving regulatory mechanisms acting at the level of the central nervous system (CNS), hypothalamus, pituitary gland, adrenal glands, and testes. It is essential to understand this process for the optimal application of the currently available treatment agents.

## *Androgens*

Androgens are derived from the testis and the adrenal gland. The testes are the primary source of testosterone, which is released by the Leydig's cells under the effect of luteinizing hormone (LH) secreted by the pituitary gland. LH secretion is itself triggered by a pulsatile release of luteinizing hormone-releasing hormone (LHRH). The testes secrete approx 5–10 ng of testosterone in the bloodstream each day, and also contribute about 30% of the plasma androstenedione levels. Testosterone is converted into dihydrotestosterone (DHT) in the peripheral tissues and in the prostate itself by the activity of 5-alpha-reductase. Once in the cytoplasm, DHT binds with high affinity to a specific androgenic receptor, which is a nuclear receptor. The DHT-receptor complex finally binds to an acceptor chromatin site to induce protein synthesis and the specific response at the cellular level, such as production of growth factors and programmed cell death. Testosterone may also bind to the receptor, but with a much lower affinity (fourfold to fivefold less). Finally, human prostatic tissue can also utilize adrenal androgens directly.

Under the influence of pituitary adenocorticotropin (ACTH), the adrenal glands secrete small amounts of testosterone (5–10% of the total amount of circulating androgens), and other compounds, including dehydroepiandrosterone (DHEA), dehydroepiandrosterone sulfate (DHEAS), and androstenedione. These undergo a multistep conversion to testosterone and DHT in the peripheral tissues and the prostate itself.

At the prostate level, androgens appear to function primarily as survival factors. When prostatic cells are deprived of androgens, they rapidly involute with histologic features characteristic of apoptotic death. However, only glandular epithelial cells but not basal-stromal cells undergo apoptosis when subjected to androgen deprivation. This observation has led to the conclusion that even in normal prostatic tissue, a population of "androgen-independent" cells remains after androgen deprivation, capable of regrowth if a supply of androgen is available. This marked contrast with the response of glandular prostate-cancer cells to androgen deprivation suggests that the androgen-independent cells are not glandular and that basal-stromal cells are involved in the evolution of androgen-independent prostate cancer.

## *Estrogens*

Estrogens are synthesized by aromatization of androgens and by a negative feedback mechanism, and they control the release of LHRH and gonadotropins. Estrogens also exert a trophic role on the prostate gland, although the exact mechanism is unclear. The implications of these findings for the treatment of patients with prostate cancer will be discussed later in this section. Other substances, including growth hormone (GH), prolactin, epidermal growth factor, fibroblast growth factor, and nerve growth factor, may play a role in the growth of prostate tissue. However, the details of their possible participation in carcinoma of the prostate are not fully understood.

## PRIMARY HORMONAL TREATMENT OPTIONS

The importance of androgens in prostate cancer became known with the seminal work of Huggins, who first described the effects of castration on advanced carcinoma of the prostate in the 1940s. As a result, the disruption of the hypothalamic-pituitary-gonadal axis by medical or surgical means has been used extensively in the therapy of metastatic prostate cancer (stage D), and more recently in locally advanced prostate cancer (stage C). The various options for endocrine therapy of prostate cancer are based on the level of action of the different agents used on the hypothalamic-pituitary-gonadal-adrenal action. Four major methods of androgen deprivation can be used in the treatment of prostate cancer:

1. Removal of the primary androgen-producing organs: i.e., bilateral orchiectomy.
2. Reduction of LH production: e.g., estrogens, LHRH agonists.
3. Inhibition of androgen action at the target organs level: e.g., antiandrogens.
4. Combined androgen blockade (CAB).

### *Bilateral Orchiectomy*

Surgical castration is considered the "gold standard" for androgen ablation. It results in a 95% reduction of circulating testosterone to a level of approx 10–50 ng/100 mL 3 h after surgery. Nearly 75% of patients experience a significant reduction in pain after orchiectomy. Radiographic objective responses occur in up to one-half of patients. Advantages of this procedure, when compared to LHRH agonists, include improved patient compliance, low cost, and the rapid depletion of testosterone. This safe outpatient procedure achieves lifetime androgen deprivation. Because lifetime androgen deprivation is recommended for patients with metastatic disease, orchiectomy represents a major cost savings over LHRH agonists over the life of these patients, who have an expected survival of 30–50 mo. Furthermore, the immediate androgen depletion provides more rapid relief of symptoms but avoids the initial testosterone surge associated with LHRH agonists. Up to 72% of patients included in recent clinical trials achieved a significant subjective benefit from surgical castration, as manifested by a significant decrease in pain. Objective response to orchiectomy as measured by complete or partial regression of objectively documented disease was less frequently reported (20–57%). Bilateral orchiectomy is an appropriate choice for patients with significant pain and impending complications of paralysis by metastatic disease. Side effects of bilateral orchiectomy are secondary to androgen withdrawal (loss of libido, impotence, hot flushes, bone-mineral loss, and anemia), and local complications that may occur at the site of orchiectomy eg, infection and postoperative hematoma. Measurement of serum testosterone alone is not a reliable indicator of the impact of androgens in an individual patient. Although bilateral orchiectomy leads to a 95% reduction in serum testosterone concentration, a much smaller effect is seen on the only meaningful reflection of androgenic action at the prostatic level—namely, the intraglandular concentration of dihydrotestosterone (DHT).

### *Estrogens*

In the treatment of prostate carcinoma, estrogens act primarily through negative feedback at the hypothalamic-pituitary level to reduce LH secretion and testicular androgen synthesis. This effect, as reflected by a castration level of testosterone (<50 ng/mL) for patients who receive a daily oral dose of 3 mg of diethylstilbestrol (DES), was achieved in 20–60 d. Interestingly, if the treatment with estrogens is discontinued after 3 yr of uninterrupted exposure, serum testosterone may remain at castration levels for up to another 3 yr. This prolonged suppression is thought to result from a direct effect of estrogens on the Leydig's cells. DES has been the standard synthetic estrogen used in the treatment of carcinoma of the prostate, although it is no longer generally available. In the past, high doses of DES (10–20 mg daily) were given. Five milligrams of DES daily is associated with significant atheroembolic toxicity (pulmonary embolism, deep venous thrombosis, cerebrovascular accidents, and myocardial infarction) and is no longer used. Cardiovascular complications are thought to be secondary to the metabolic effects of estrogens at the liver level, leading to increased triglyceride levels, increased LDL levels, and increased activity of factors VI, VIII, and fibrinogen. Other side effects include gynecomastia, impotence, and hot flashes. The generally accepted optimal dose of DES is 3 mg daily. A large prospective trial confirmed that this dose is sufficient to induce regression of prostate cancer in up to 46% of patients, but as many as 13% must discontinue therapy because of toxicity. DES given at a dose of 1 mg daily will lower testosterone to castration levels in nearly 80% of patients, but this effect is variable, often stabilizing above the castration range. Despite this observation, a recent European trial has confirmed the equivalence of orchiectomy and DES at a dose of 1 mg daily.

### *Luteinizing Hormone-Releasing Hormone Agonists (LHRH)*

Soon after the structure of LHRH was elucidated in 1971 by Schalley et al., it was noted that continuous exposure to these agents leads to downregulation of pituitary receptors. This downregulation abolishes LH secretion, leading to castration levels of testosterone. The administration of LHRH agonists initially causes stimulation of LH production, with a surge in the plasma concentration of testosterone to approx 150% of basal levels within few days. Testosterone levels fall within 1–2 wk and castration levels are obtained in 3–4 wk.

Numerous phase II and III trials have compared the LHRH agonists with orchiectomy or estrogen therapy. In general, subjective responses were noted in 80–90% of the patients and objective responses in 35–50% of cases. Thus, no evidence suggests that LHRH monotherapy is superior to orchiectomy or estrogen therapy in terms of response rate, time to progression, or survival. A transient worsening of signs and symptoms ("tumor flare") within the first 1–8 d of therapy is a well-documented side-effect of LHRH analogs, and is the result of LH and testosterone surge. The peak increase in serum testosterone level usually occurs within 72 h. Clinical manifestations of this phenomenon may include worsening of bone pain, worsening ureteral obstruction, and worsening neurologic symptoms for patients with spinal-cord or nerve-root compression. It has been estimated that the "tumor flare" phenomenon is responsible for the death of up to 2% of all patients with acute deterioration after the initiation of treatment. For this reason, antiandrogens are often added at the beginning of LHRH agonist therapy. If used in this setting, antiandrogens should be started at least 3 d before the administration of the LHRH agonist and continued for the first month. Asymptomatic patients who are selected for LHRH agonist monotherapy can safely avoid this temporary antiandrogen therapy. Long-term side effects of LHRH agonists may include hot flashes, loss of libido, impotence, gynecomastia, accelerated bone loss, and anemia. The currently available LHRH agonists available in the United States include:

1. Leuprolide (Lupron): The half-life is 3–4 h. The recommended dose of leuprolide is 7.5 mg of the depot im preparation given monthly, or 22.5 mg im every 3 mo.
2. Goserelin (Zoladex): The half-life is 4.2 h. The recommended dose is 3.6 mg injected into the upper abdomen area every 28 d, or 22.5 mg every 3 mo.

## *Antiandrogens*

An antiandrogen is a compound that blocks the effects of androgens at the prostate-tissue level. These drugs interfere with the binding between androgens and their receptors in the presence of normal or even increased target-tissue levels of DHT. They were initially introduced in an attempt to avoid the psychological effects of orchiectomy and the cardiovascular toxicity of estrogen therapy. Antiandrogens consist of two types: nonsteroidal agents and antiandrogens with progestational activity.

### Steroidal Antiandrogens

1. Megestrol acetate: This progestational agent suppresses serum testosterone to near castration levels in 4–6 wk, but testosterone levels rapidly "escape" toward the normal range. This can be avoided by the addition of low-dose estrogen therapy to the progestin regimen.
2. Cyproterone acetate: This synthetic hydroxyprogesterone derivative appears to be as effective as estrogen therapy, but with a lower cardiovascular toxicity. It has been extensively studied in Europe, but is not available in the United States.
3. Ketoconazole: This imidazole derivative inhibits the cytochrome P450-dependent enzymes, and therefore inhibits both testicular and adrenal androgens. This drug is usually well-tolerated, with side effects limited to nausea, pruritus, and abdominal pain. A commonly used regimen consists of 400 mg orally three times a day in combination with 30 mg of hydrocortisone daily to compensate for adrenal suppression.

### Nonsteroidal Antiandrogens

These agents act directly on the prostate-cancer cells by competitively blocking the binding of DHT to the nuclear androgen receptor. However, LH secretion is not suppressed, and androgen levels tend to rise for patients who are chronically treated with these agents. This mechanism explains why libido and potency are preserved for patients who receive these drugs. As single agents, these drugs have objective response rates of 38–55%. In general, these drugs have proved inferior to castration in both time to progression and survival. Therefore, antiandrogens as single agents are not recommended for initial hormone therapy. Antiandrogens have three main uses: 1) prevention of LHRH-induced flare; 2) second-line therapy for patients with progressive disease after orchiectomy or LHRH agonists; and 3) combined androgen blockade (*see* Table 1). The following antiandrogens are currently available in the United States:

1. Bicalutamide (Casodex) has a longer half-life, and the recommended dose is 50 mg orally, once a day. It is a well-tolerated agent with no significant hepatotoxicity, pulmonary toxicity, or gastrointestinal toxicity, and is probably the drug of choice because of its convenience and low side-effect profile.
2. Flutamide (Eulexin) is usually given at a dose of 250 mg orally every 8 h. The toxicity of flutamide has been manageable, with nausea, diarrhea, hot flashes, and breast tenderness being the most common side effects. Of concern is the risk of severe and sometimes fatal cases of hepatotoxicity; fortunately these are rare (<1%).

Table 1
Antiandrogens and LHRH Analogs

| Agent | Dosage | Side effects |
|---|---|---|
| Flutamide | 250mg tid | diarrhea, hot flashes, liver toxicity. |
| Nilutamide | 300mg po qd | hot flashes, nocturnal visual disturbances, alcohol withdrawal. |
| | For 30 days, then 150 mg Po qd. | |
| Bicalutamide | 50mg po qd | No gastrointestinal or hepatic toxicity. |
| Megestrol acetate | 40-320 mg daily in divided doses. | depression, weight gain, jaundice. |
| Ketoconazole | 400 mg tid. | Nausea, abdominal pain, pruritus. |
| Leuprolide | 7.5mg IM q mo, Or 22.5mg IM q 3 mo, Or 30mg IM q 4 mo. | hot flashes, "flare," diarrhea. |
| Goserelin | 3.6 mg subcutaneously q mo. Or 10.8 mg subcutaneously q 3 mo. | Hot flashes, "flare," sexual dysfunction. |

3. Nilutamide (Nilandron) has a longer half-life, and the recommended starting dose is 300 mg once a day for 30 d followed by a total daily dose of 150 mg. Reported side effects include nausea, hot flashes, visual disturbances (especially nocturnal), alcohol intolerance, and occasional cases of interstitial pneumonitis.

## COMBINED ANDROGEN BLOCKADE

The concept of combined androgen blockade (CAB) stems from the observation that a small but significant percentage of circulating androgens is derived from the adrenal glands. Residual androgens remaining after castration (surgical or medical) may contribute to progression of metastatic prostrate cancer. A large number of randomized clinical trials have compared CAB with monotherapy. Overall, the trials do not show a substantial survival benefit from CAB. However, a subgroup of patients seems to benefit from CAB. This includes patients with minimal disease (limited to axial skeleton) and good performance status. In this good prognosis subgroup, CAB (leuprolide+flutamide) achieved a median time to progression of 48 mo as compared with 19 mo for patients receiving monotherapy (leuprolide alone). Overall survival was also significantly better for the CAB group (median, 61 vs 42 mo, $p = 0.03$). This benefit, however, was not confirmed in a recent large randomized trial using orchiectomy with or without flutamide. For reasons that remain unclear, LHRH agonists and orchiectomy appear to act differently when combined with nonsteroidal antiandrogens. For men with stage D prostate cancer who elect LHRH agonists over orchiectomy, those with good performance status and minimal disease as defined above may benefit from the addition of nonsteroidal antiandrogens. CAB continues to be evaluated in regimens of intermittent androgen blockade and in conjunction with radiation therapy for locally advanced disease.

## EARLY OR DELAYED ENDOCRINE THERAPY

The finding that CAB is of benefit mainly for patients with low tumor burden has led some investigators to institute CAB early in the course of the disease.

A Vetarans Administrative Cooperative Research Group trial revealed a survival benefit in younger patients with stage D prostate cancer (Gleason scores of 7–10) when endocrine therapy was started at diagnosis. Several studies have suggested a modest benefit for institution of early hormone therapy. A recent trial suggested a survival benefit mainly for patients without radiographically detectable metastases. For the patient with a rising PSA and no radiographic evidence of disease, the timing of hormone therapy is controversial. The benefits are modest and require treatment of a large number of men with potential toxicities, including fatigue, anemia, accelerated bone loss, impotence, and hot flashes. The economic consequences of such an approach should not be underestimated. A cost analysis of CAB estimated the cost per life-year gained to be between $20,000 and $32,000.

## INTERMITTENT ANDROGEN BLOCKADE

Animal experiments suggest that intermittent androgen therapy delays the time to androgen independence and results in lower serum PSA when compared to continuous treatment. Initial clinical experience with this mode of treatment has demonstrated prolonged therapy-free intervals with no obvious survival disadvantage. A commonly studied protocol uses continuous CAB for an initial period of 6 mo, followed by withholding treatment until the PSA increases to a predetermined level (usually around 10 ng/mL). A current Intergroup trial of intermittent vs continuous CAB will compare survival and quality of life for patients with stage D2 prostate cancer. If proven equivalent to continuous CAB, intermittent CAB would afford a substantial cost savings. The role of intermittent monotherapy has not been evaluated.

## HORMONAL THERAPY AS AN ADJUNCT TO PRIMARY TREATMENT

The role of hormonal therapy for patients treated primarily with prostatectomy or radiotherapy has been evaluated.

### *Hormonal Therapy as an Adjunct to Prostatectomy*

Randomized clinical trials have addressed the use of hormonal therapy in the neoadjuvant setting. Three such clinical trials have randomized patients to 3 mo of CAB, or observation. In these studies, there was a decrease in the incidence of positive margins at surgery, but no difference in time to treatment failure or overall survival. Thus, hormonal therapy should not be used in this setting.

### *Hormonal Therapy as Adjunct to Radiotherapy*

The role of hormonal therapy for patients receiving definitive radiation therapy for locally advanced prostate cancer has been studied in several randomized trials with varying schedules and regimens. Several trials have shown improved local control and relapse-free survival, and one trial demonstrated improved overall survival for patients treated with hormone therapy and radiation. Although several regimens have shown promise, two regimens with proven benefits are as follows: 1) CAB begun 2 mo before radiation and continued during radiation, and 2) goserelin begun concurrent with radiation therapy and continued for 3 yr. With the latter regimen, patients receive a nonsteroidal antiandrogen for 1 mo beginning 1 wk before the initiation of goserelin.

## SECOND-LINE HORMONE THERAPY

Patients with metastatic prostate cancer eventually develop hormonal resistance as manifested by rising PSA levels, progressive disease on imaging studies, and ultimately, worsening symptoms. Significant advances have been made in the treatment of hormone refractory prostate cancer. Available options for second-line hormonal therapy are described in this section.

### *Antiandrogen Withdrawal*

The antiandrogen withdrawal syndrome was initially identified in the early 1990s. It has been postulated that the androgen receptor allows antiandrogens to act as agonists through a mutation in the steroid-binding domain. Withdrawal responses occur in 15–30% of patients treated with flutamide, bicalutamide, or nilutamide. Antiandrogen withdrawal should be the first therapeutic approach for patients who progress on primary hormonal therapy, which contains antiandrogens.

### *Adrenal Antiandrogens*

Adrenal antiandrogenens include aminoglutethimide and ketoconazole. Aminoglutethimide with hydrocortisone in combination with flutamide withdrawal has a 48% PSA response, which is higher that the response rate seen with flutamide withdrawal alone. When ketoconazole and hydrocortisone were combined with flutamide withdrawal, 62% of the patients in one study had a decrease in PSA >50%. Prior response to flutamide withdrawal did not affect response to ketoconazole, and the median duration of response was 3.5 mo.

### *Glucocorticoids*

These agents are usually used in combination with agents that cause a medical adrenalectomy and with a number of chemotherapeutic agents. Glucocorticoids have modest response rates for patients who have failed androgen deprivation.

## CONCLUSIONS

Metastatic prostate cancer remains an incurable disease, and hormone therapy is the mainstay of treatment. Unfortunately, patients who undergo complete androgen deprivation will progress within 12–16 mo after initiating therapy. Patient survival after failure of hormone therapy averages 9–18 mo. Continued research may yield protocols capable of delaying the onset of hormone-refractory disease. Table 2 shows an algorithm for the management of prostate cancer.

Newer approaches may include genetic therapy, which takes advantage of genetic changes that have been noted in prostate cancer (e.g., overexpression of bcl-2, mutations of the p53 gene, and deletion of the retinoblastoma gene, angiogenesis inhibition, and methods using peptide-based and dendritic cell vaccines. Suggested endpoints for future

Table 2
Algorithm for the Management of Prostate Cancer

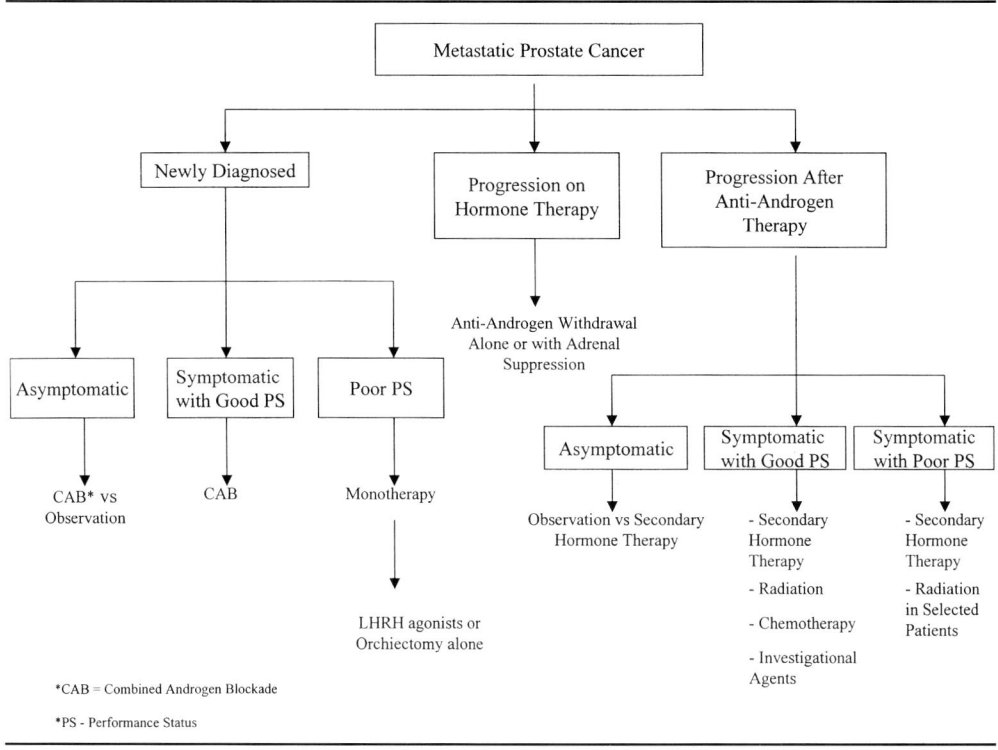

clinical trials should include validated quality-of-life assessments to document net benefit to patients, not just surrogate measurements, such as a fall in PSA. Inclusion of eligible patients in such clinical trials should be strongly encouraged.

## SELECTED READING

Akakura K, Bruchovsky N, Goldenberg SL, et al. (1993) Effects of intermittent androgen suppression on androgen-dependent tumors. Apoptosis and serum prostate-specific antigen. *Cancer* 71:2782–2790.
Berges RR, Furuya Y, Remington L, et al. (1993) Cell proliferation, DNA repair, and p53 function are not required for programmed death of prostatic glandular cells induced by androgen ablation. *Proc Natl Acad Sci USA* 90:8910–8914.
Boccardo F, Pace M, Rubagotti A, et al. (1993) Goserelin acetate with or without flutamide in the treatment of patients with locally advanced or metastatic prostate cancer. *Eur J Cancer* 29A:1088–1093.
Bolla M, Gonzalez D, Warde P, et al. (1997) Improved survival in patients with locally advanced prostate cancer treated with radiotherapy and goserelin. *N Engl J Med* 337:295–300.
Byar DP, Corle DK (1988) Hormone therapy for prostate cancer: results of the Veterans Administrative Cooperative Urological Research Group Studies. *NCI Monogr* 165–170.
Cox RL, Crawford ED (1995) Estrogens in the treatment of prostate cancer. *J Urol* 154:1991–1998.
Crawford ED, Eisenberger MA, McLeod DG, et al. (1989) A controlled trial of leuprolide with and without flutamide in prostatic carcinoma. *N Engl J Med* 321:419–424.
Denis L (1993) Prostate cancer: primary hormonal treatment. *Cancer* 71:1050–1058.
Dowling AJ, Tannock IF (1998) *Cancer Treatment Reviews* 24:283–301.
Eisenberger MA, Blumenstein BA, Crawford ED, et al. (1999) Bilateral orchiectomy with or without flutamide in metastatic prostate cancer. *N Engl J Med* 339(15):1036.

Ferrari P, Castagnetti G, Ferrari G, et al. (1993) Combination treatment in M1 prostate cancer. *Cancer* 72:3880–3885.

Geller G (1993) Basis for hormonal management of advanced prostate cancer. *Cancer* 71:1039–1045.

Geller J (1991) Megestrol acetate plus low-dose estrogen in the management of advanced prostatic carcinoma. *Urol Clin N Am* 18:83–91.

Geller J, Albert J, Yen SSC (1978) Treatment of advanced cancer of the prostate with megestrol acetate. *Urology* 12:537–541.

Goldenberg SL, Bruchovsky N (1991) Use of cyproterone acetate in prostate cancer. *Urol Clin N Am* 18:111–122.

Goldenberg SL, Klotz LH, Srigley J, et al. (1996) Randomized, prospective, controlled study comparing radical prostatectomy alone and neoadjuvant androgen withdrawal in the treatment of localized prostate cancer. Canadian Urologic Oncology Group. *J Urol* 156:873–877.

Harper ME, Pike A, Peeling WB, Griffiths D (1974) Steroids of adrenal origin metabolized by human prostatic tissue in vivi and vitro. *J Endocrinol* 60:117–125.

Hillner BE, McLeod DG, Crawford ED, et al. (1995) Estimating the cost effectiveness of total androgen blockade with flutamide in M1 prostate cancer. *Urology* 45:633–640.

Jacobo E, Schmidt JD, Weinstein SH, et al. (1976) Comparison of flutamide (SCH-13521) and diethylstilbestrol in untreated prostatic cancer. *Urology* 8:231–233.

Kelly WK, Scher HI (1993) Prostate specific antigen decline after antiandrogen withdrawal. *J Urol* 149:607–609.

Klijn JGM, de Voogt HJ, Studer UE, et al. (1993) Short term versus long term addition of cyproterone acetate to buserelin therapy in comparison with orchidectomy in the treatment of metastatic prostate cancer. *Cancer* 72:3858–3862.

Klotz LH, Herr HW, Morse MJ, Whitmore WF (1986) Intermittent endocrine therapy for advanced prostate cancer. *Cancer* 58:2546–2550.

Kuhn JM, Billebaud T, Navrath H, et al. (1989) Prevention of the transient adverse effects of a gonadotropin-releasing hormone analog (buserelin) in metastatic prostatic carcinoma by administration of an antiandrogen (nilutamide). *N Engl J Med* 321:413–418.

Kyprianou N, Isaacs JT (1988) Activation of programmed cell death in the rat ventral prostate after castration. *Endocrinology* 122:552–562.

Labrie F, Belanger A, Simard J, et al. (1993) Combination therapy for prostate cancer: endocrine and biologic basis of its choice as new standard first-line therapy. *Cancer* 71:1059–1067.

Landis SH, Murray T, Bolden S, et al. (1999) Cancer statistics, 1998. *CA Cancer J Clin* 49:8–31.

Leuprolide Study Group (1984) Euprolide versus diethylstilbestrol for metastatic prostate cancer. *N Engl J Med* 311:1281–1286.

Lin BJ, Chen KK, Chen MT, et al. (1994) The time for serum testosterone to reach castrate level after bilateral orchiectomy or oral estrogen therapy in the management of prostatic cancer. *J Urol* 151:238A.

Lindle R, Doelle GC, Alexander N, et al. (1981) Reversible inhibition of testicular steroidogenesis and spermatogenesis by a potent gonadotropin-releasing hormone agonist in normal men: an approach toward the development of a male contraceptive. *N Engl J Med* 305:663–667.

The Medical Research Council Prostate Working Party Investigators Group (1997) Immediate versus deferred treatment for advanced prostatic cancer: initial results of the Medical Research Council Trial. *Br J Urol* 79:235–246.

Naitoh J, Belldegrun A (1998) Gene therapy—the future is here: a guide to the practicing urologist. *Urology* 51:367–380.

Oliver RT, Williams G, Paris AM, et al. (1997) Intermittent androgen deprivation after PSA-complete response as a strategy to reduce induction of hormone-resistant prostate cancer. *Urology* 49:79–82.

Paulson DF (1994) Impact of radical prostatectomy in the management of clinically localized disease. *J Urol* 152:1826–1830.

Pfitzenmeyer P, Foucher P, Piard F, et al. (1992) Nilutamide pneumonitis: a report on eight patients. *Thorax* 47:622–627.

Pont A, Williams PL, Azhar S, et al. (1982) Ketoconazole blocks testosterone synthesis. *Arch Intern Med* 97:370–372.

Roach M Optimal use of various forms of radiotherapy with or without hormonal therapy for treatment of clinically localized prostate cancer, ASCO Educational Book.

Robinson MRG (1993) A further analysis of European Organization for Research and Treatment of Cancer Protocol 30805. *Cancer* 72:3855–3857.

Sato N, Gleave ME, Bruchowsky N, et al. (1996) Intermittent androgen suppression delays progression of androgen-independent regulation of prostate-specific antigen gene in the LNCaP prostate tumor model. *J Steroid Biochem Mol Biol* 58:139–146.

Schally AV, Arimurea A, Baba Y, et al. (1971) Isolation of properties of the FSH and LH-releasing hormone. *Biochem Biophys Res Commun* 43:393–399.

Scher HI (1999) Management of prostate cancer after prostatectomy: treating the patient, not the PSA. *JAMA* 281:1642–1645.

Sharifi R, Chodak G, Venner P, et al. (1993) Casodex versus castration in treatment of stage D2 prostate cancer: prostate specific antigen (PSA) as a measure of outcome. *Proc Am Soc Clin Oncol* 12:241.

Slovin SF, Kelly WK, Scher HI, et al. (1998) Immunological approaches for the treatment of prostate cancer. *Sem Urol Oncol* 16:53–59.

Small EJ, Vogelzang NJ (1997) Second-line hormonal therapy for advanced prostate cancer: a shifting paradigm. *J Clin Oncol* 15:382–388.

Solaway MS, Matzkin H (1993) Antiandrogenic agents as monotherapy in advanced prostatic carcinoma. *Cancer* 71:1083–1088.

Soloway MS, Sharifi R, Wajsman Z, et al. (1995) Randomized prospective study comparing radical prostatectomy alone versus radical prostatectomy preceded by androgen blockade in clinical stage B2 (T2bNxM0) prostate cancer. The Lupron Depot Neoadjuvant Cancer Study Group. *J Urol* 154:424–428.

Thompson IM, Zeidman EJ, Rodriguez FR (1990) Sudden death due to disease flare with luteinizing hormone-releasing agonist therapy for carcinoma of the prostate. *J Urol* 144:1479, 1480.

Tomic R, Bergman G (1987) Hormonal effects of cessation of estrogen treatment for prostatic carcinoma. *J Urol* 138:801–803.

# VIII Penile Disorders

## 24  Practical Dermatology for the Urologist

*Scott Podnos, MD
and Allison T. Vidimos, RPh, MD*

**CONTENTS**

    INTRODUCTION
    UNIQUE DERMATOSES
    INFLAMMATORY DERMATOSES
    DRUG REACTIONS
    PIGMENTED LESIONS
    BLISTERING DISORDERS
    ULCERATIVE CONDITIONS
    INFECTIONS
    INFESTATIONS
    BENIGN TUMORS
    MALIGNANT TUMORS
    SELECTED READING

## INTRODUCTION

Many diseases of the skin involve the penis and surrounding skin, making it important for the dermatologist to include the genitals in a full skin exam. Table 1 lists many of these conditions. In contrast, very few diseases involve only the skin of the penis. Therefore, the patient who presents to a urologist with a cutaneous disease should be examined for evidence of other skin diseases. This examination often reveals a diagnosis that would have been difficult otherwise. History—especially sexual—also plays an important role. Although not covered in this chapter, sexually transmitted diseases are a feature of virtually every differential diagnosis. Other important factors include systemic disorders, immune status, allergies, symptoms, travel history, and symptoms of sexual and close contacts. All medications should be documented, including parenteral, topical, herbal, and over-the-counter preparations.

Dermatological diagnosis is often based on clinical features, and a correct description is important. Lesions are described by their size, elevation, color, grouping, and any other clinical features, such as scale or crust. Laboratory studies are often needed to

From: *Current Clinical Urology: Office Urology: The Clinician's Guide*
Edited by: E. D. Kursh and J. C. Ulchaker © Humana Press Inc., Totowa, NJ

**Table 1**
**Dermatological Conditions of the Penis and Surrounding Skin**

**Unique Dermatoses**
  Pearly penile papules
  Cysts
    Apocrine hydrocystoma
    Median raphe cyst
    Epidermal inclusion cyst
  Sclerosing lymphangitis
  Angiokeratomas
    Angiokeratoma corporis diffusum
  Lichen sclerosis
**Inflammatory dermatoses**
  Balanoposthitis
  Allergic contact dermatitis
  Balanitis circinata
  Psoriasis
  Lichen planus
  Lichenoid dermatitis
  Lichen niditus
  Zoon's balanitis
  Seborrheic dermatitis
  Atopic dermatitis
  Pityriasis lichenoides
  Pityriasis rosea
  Glucagonoma syndrome
  Sarcoidosis
  Granuloma annulare
  Necrobiosis lipoidica diabeticorum
  Vasculitis
**Drug reactions**
  Fixed drug eruption
  Coumarin skin necrosis
  Foscarnet ulcers
**Pigmentary changes and lesions**
  Melanotic macules
  Lentigo
  Nevi
  Tattoos
  Postinflammatory changes
  Vitiligo
**Blistering disorders**
  Erythema multiforme
  Toxic epidermal necrolysis
  Bullous pemphigoid
  Cicatricial pemphigoid
  Pemphigus vulgaris, vegetans, and foliaceus
  Paraneoplastic pemphigus
  Epidermolysis bullosa
  Hailey-Hailey disease

**Ulcerative conditions**
  Aphthous ulcers
  Behçet's disease
  Pyoderma gangrenosum
  Crohn's disease
  Factitial ulcers
**Infections**
  Viral
    Herpes simplex[a]
    Molluscum contagiosum[a]
    Human papillomavirus[a]
    Varicella zoster virus
  Mycotic
    Candida
    Dermatophyte
    Histoplasma
    Blastomycosis
    Cryptococcus
    Penicillium
    Pityrosporum ovale
  Bacterial
    Infectious balanoposthitis
    Erysipelas
    Cellulitis
    Fournier's gangrene
    Erythrasma
    Trichomycosis
    Folliculitis
    Hidradenitis suppurativa
    Syphilis[a]
    Gonorrhea[a]
    Chancroid[a]
    Lymphogranuloma venereum[a]
    Granuloma inguinale[a]
    Tuberculosis
**Infestations**
  Filariasis
  Schistosomiasis
  Scabies
  Pubic lice
**Benign tumors**
  Vascular
    Capillary hemangiomas
    Varices
    Masson's tumor
    Lymphangioma circumscriptum
    Glomangioma
    Hemangioendothelioma
  Seborrheic keratosis
  Sebaceous hyperplasia

**Benign tumors** cont'd
  Dermatofibroma
  Xanthogranuloma
  Angiomyolipoma
  Dartoic leiomoma
  Syringomas
  Schawnnoma
**Malignant tumors**
  Squamous cell carcinoma
  Erythroplasia of Queyrat
  Verrucous carcinoma
  Bowenoid papulosis
  Pseudoepitheliomatous keratotic and micaceous balanitis of Civatte
  Basal cell carcinoma
  Melanoma
  Kaposi's sarcoma
  Extramammary Peget's disease
  Malignant schwannoma
  Histocytoma
  Lymphoma
  Leukemia cutis
  Langerhans cell histiocytosis
  Metastases
  Sarcomas
**Miscellaneous**
  Amyloidosis
  Angioid hyperplasia with eosinophilia
  Achrochordons
  Calcinosis cutis
  Ichthyosis
  Epidermal nevi
  Traumatic
    Fracture
    Bites
    Paraffinoma (factitial)
    Persistent fissure
    Gunshot wounds
    Burns
    Crush injuries
    Frostbite
    Zipper entrapment
    Iatrogenic

[a]Covered in Chapter 10.

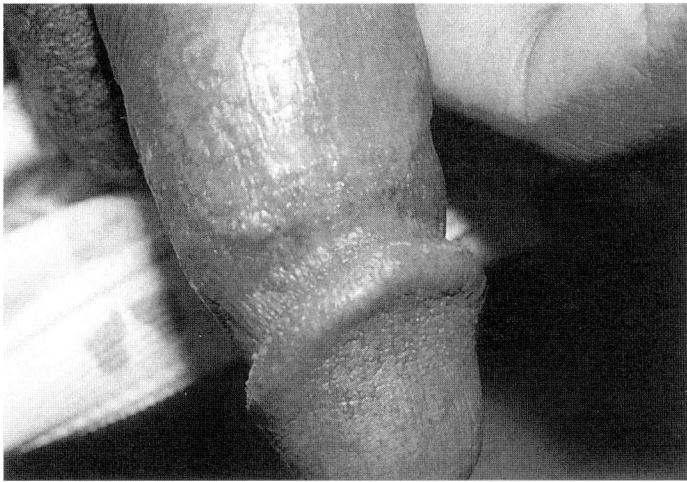

**Fig. 1.** Pearly penile papules. Flesh-colored tiny papules circumferentially around the corona. *See* color plate following p. 338.

aid in diagnosis. Potassium hydroxide preparations are useful for fungal and yeast infections. The skin can be cultured for bacterial, fungal, and viral infections when these are suspected. Biopsy for histology is often required for definitive diagnosis. Shave biopsies can be used for thin, noninflammatory lesions. More often, a full-thickness specimen is required, which is obtained with a circular punch biopsy or incisional technique. Solitary lesions may be cured if the diagnosis is obtained in this fashion.

Dermatologic therapy runs the gamut from reassurance to topical, systemic, and surgical modalities. In general, the least invasive therapy—or option with the least potential for harm—should be the first choice. Topical steroids deserve special emphasis because of their common use. The weakest effective preparation should be used on the thin skin of the genitals to avoid side effects, such as atrophy and striae. Over-the-counter 0.5% or 1.0% hydrocortisone may be all that is needed. Factors that increase the strength of a topical steroid include occlusion, the specific compound, and the vehicle (ointments are the most potent). Textbooks of dermatological therapy provide tables that rank steroids in order of potency. It is sometimes difficult to differentiate a benign inflammatory dermatosis from a lesion that requires histologic diagnosis. In practice, response to a short course of treatment with a mild topical steroid may obviate the need for more extensive evaluation. Topical steroids should generally be avoided if infection is suspected.

The following section lists several dermatologic entities that may involve the penis and scrotum. The most common diagnoses will be discussed in this chapter. Sexually transmitted diseases will be discussed in another chapter.

## UNIQUE DERMATOSES

*Pearly penile papules* (*see* Fig. 1) are a common condition that can be confused with warts if not in the usual location or typical pattern around the corona. They are

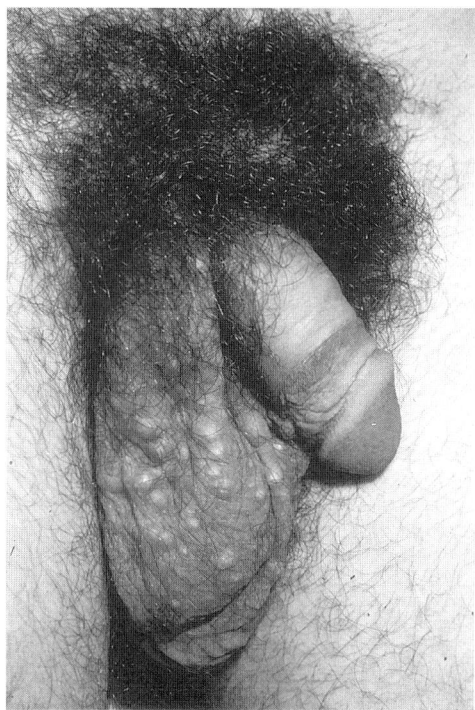

**Fig. 2.** Epidermal inclusion cysts of the scrotum. Whitish-yellow subcutaneous nodules.

actually angiofibromas, and are asymptomatic. If they are cosmetically disturbing to the patient, ablative laser treatment can be performed.

*Cysts* are common in many locations, and may occur on the penis. *Apocrine hydrocystomas* are benign cyst-like sweat-gland tumors that also occur on the penis. The most common cyst of the penis is the *median raphe cyst*. This embryologic abnormality lies on the midline ventral base of the penis. Benign in nature, it presents as a soft, compressible nodule. *Epidermal inclusion cysts* can occur on the shaft of the penis, but are more common on the scrotum (*see* Fig. 2). These yellow or flesh-colored cysts may lose their lining and calcify, forming several hard nodules called *idiopathic calcinosis* of the scrotum. Also benign, they can be excised if they are troubling.

*Sclerosing lymphangitis* (*see* Fig. 3) of the penis is a thrombosed or sclerotic lymphatic vessel found in young adults with a history of frequent sexual activity. It presents as a firm subcutaneous, cord-like nodule, which eventually resolves without treatment. *Angiokeratomas of Fordyce* (*see* Fig. 4) are firm, 1–2 mm violaceous or red papules on the shaft of the penis or the scrotum. Individual papules may be scaly or thrombosed, resembling a melanoma. Histologically, they are ectatic dermal blood vessels. Treatment is only for cosmesis or the rare episode of bleeding after trauma. Electrodesiccation, laser ablation, or topical coagulants are effective. *Fabry's disease (Angiokeratoma corporis diffusum)* is an X-linked storage disease caused by a deficiency of alpha-galactosidase-A. The accumulation of ceramide-trihexoside eventually causes death from renal failure, myocardial infarction, or stroke. Multiple angiokeratomas, especially around the waist, should alert the clinician to this or other rare storage diseases.

Chapter 24 / Practical Dermatology

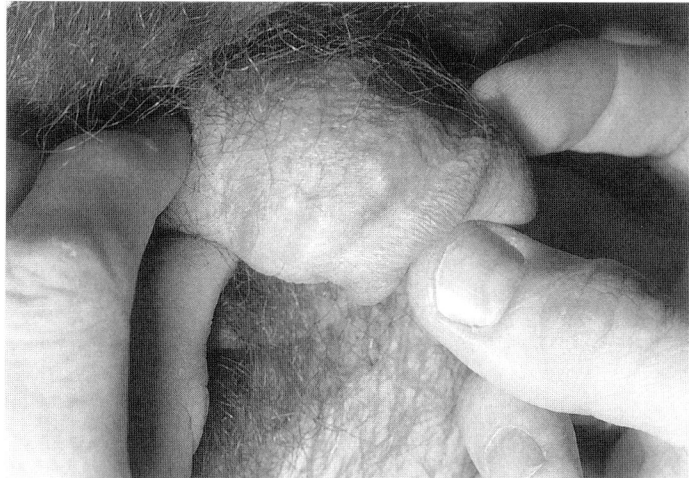

**Fig. 3.** Sclerosing lymphangitis. Firm subcutaneous nontender cord parallel to the corona on the distal penile shaft. *See* color plate following p. 338.

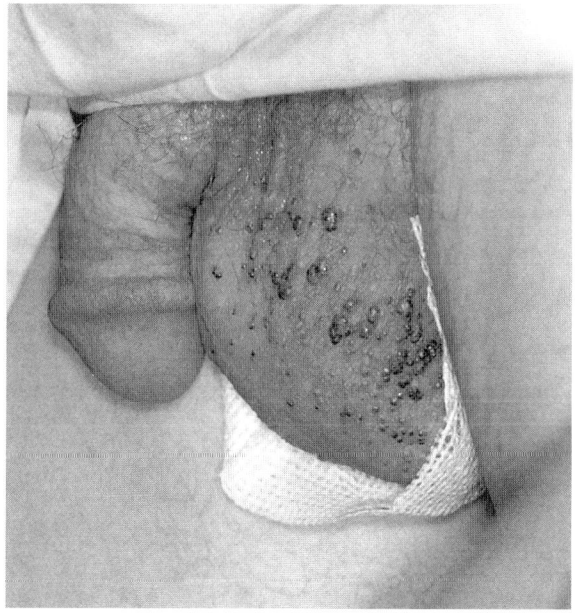

**Fig. 4.** Angiokeratomas of Fordyce. Variably-sized purple vascular papules of the scrotum. *See* color plate following p. 338.

*Lichen sclerosis,* or *lichen sclerosus et atrophicus* (LSA) (*see* Fig. 5), is a chronic, inflammatory dermatosis that may affect almost any skin site, but commonly involves the genitalia. It is common in middle-aged, uncircumcised males, but rarely occurs in circumcised men. *Balanitis xerotica obliterans* is used to describe the end stage of progressive LSA characterized by narrowing of the urethral meatus and phimosis. The

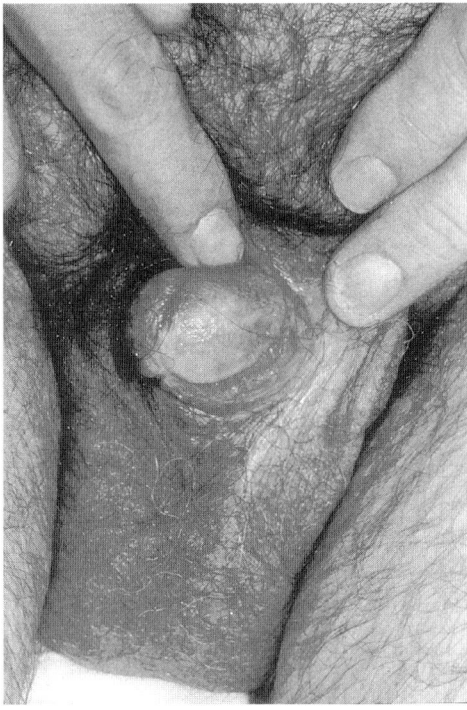

**Fig. 5.** Lichen sclerosis et atrophicus. Bluish-white atrophic plaque of the glans. *See* color plate following p. 338.

actual cause of LSA is unknown and is probably multifactorial. No infectious cause is known, but abnormal regulation of interleukin-1 may play a role. A recent report implicates alprostadil intracavernous injections, and hypothesizes that prostaglandin E1 may be an etiologic factor. Other postulated causes include late circumcision (after age 13), genetic and hormonal factors, and autoimmune disease.

Clinically, LSA begins as erythematous or white, atrophic papules or plaques that often coalesce into large atrophic patches or plaques. Bullae, erosions, fissures, and petechiae are rarely present. Lesions of the glans and prepuce greatly outnumber those of the frenulum, meatus, fossa navicularis, and shaft. As commonly seen in females, LSA may progress with obliteration of the normal anatomy, such as the coronal sulcus, the frenulum, and narrowing of the external meatus. If required for diagnosis, the histopathology is specific. Mild early complaints may progress to pruritus, phimosis, burning or hypoesthesia, and impaired sexual or urinary function. Treatment consists mainly of therapeutic circumcision. LSA is one of the rare penile dermatoses that requires potent topical steroids, such as clobetasol propionate. Topical steroids can reverse early disease in some cases. Carbon dioxide laser vaporization is useful, especially for meatal stenosis. Alternative treatments include other topical steroids, intralesional steroids, oral etretinate, or topical testosterone propionate cream, which is falling out of favor. Periodic examinations are needed, because chronic LSA can undergo malignant degeneration into squamous-cell carcinoma (SCC) (*see* Fig. 6), verrucous carcinoma, and adenosquamous-cell carcinoma.

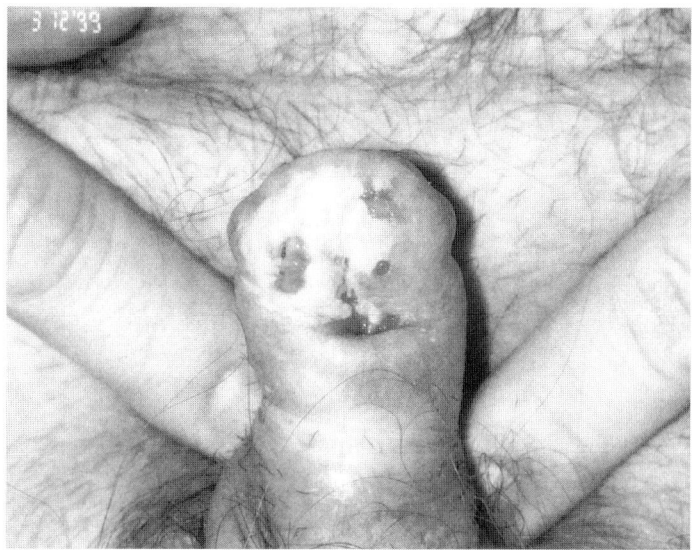

**Fig. 6.** Chronic lichen sclerosis et atrophicus with foci of invasive SCC in a patient who underwent urethral meatotomy, and later, distal ventral urethrectomy. *See* color plate following p. 338.

## INFLAMMATORY DERMATOSES

Although *dermatitis* of the penis is quite common, it is often difficult to pinpoint a diagnosis. Histological examination of these disorders may only confirm an inflammatory condition that requires clinical correlation. Common features include erythema, oozing, scaling, itching, and burning. There can be specific patterns of inflammation, or nonspecific disease. *Balanitis* and *posthitis* are inflammation of the glans and foreskin, respectively. *Balanoposthitis* (*see* Fig. 7) is usually idiopathic, and circumcision is curative. Symptomatic relief may require a topical mixture of steroid and antifungal treatments such as Vytone Cream (hydrocortisone and iodoquinol). Erosive balanitis rarely occurs, and responds to topical antibiotics, such as mupirocin ointment (Bactroban), or compresses of saline or dilute acetic acid (vinegar).

*Allergic contact dermatitis (ACD)* is a frequent cause of inflammation of the penis, as well as many other sites (*see* Figs. 8,9). The term "eczema" is sometimes used to describe this type of inflammation, and implies erythema, weeping, and intercellular edema. The clinical picture ranges from bright red, weeping skin that can be quite edematous or blistered, to a more chronic condition of dry, scaly, wrinkled skin with pigmentary changes. Chronic dermatitis is usually accompanied by changes secondary to scratching. The skin thickens, or lichenifies, in response to chronic manipulation. Skin markings are accentuated, with this change commonly seen on the scrotum (*see* Fig. 9). Severe inflammation can damage the melanocytes, often leaving hypopigmented patches when the process resolves. Certain rubber products may also cause both dermatitis and a bleaching reaction.

Allergens may directly contact the penis or be transferred by the hands or clothing. History is usually the best clue to direct exposure. Since ACD is an immune-mediated, type IV delayed hypersensitivity response, the reaction may not occur until several

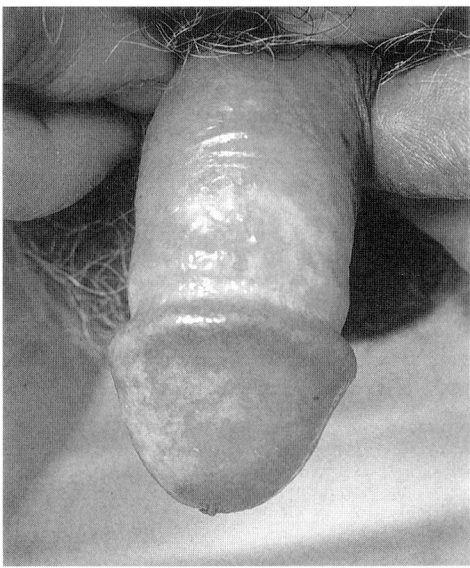

**Fig. 7.** Balanoposthitis. Inflammation of the glans and prepuce. *See* color plate following p. 338.

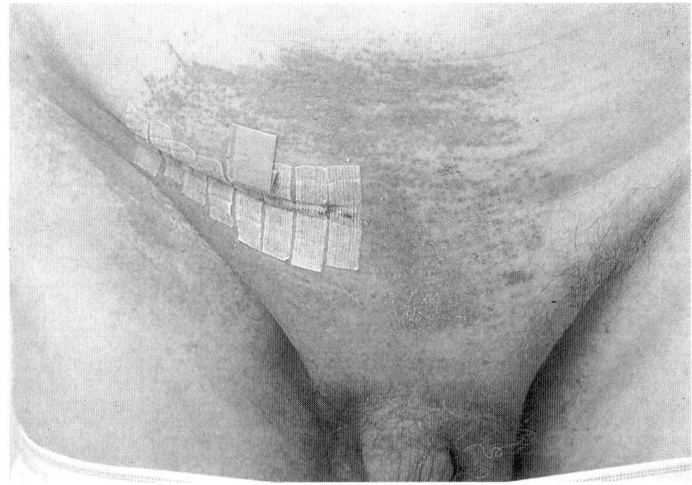

**Fig. 8.** Acute allergic contact dermatitis to Betadine surgical solution used at time of inguinal hernia repair.

days after the first or repeated exposure. Well-delineated dermatitis at the tip or base of the penis may be caused by contact with a diaphragm or condom. Patients with a type I, IgE-mediated latex allergy may experience contact urticaria (hives) during intercourse. This consists of local itching and swelling, potentially accompanied by severe systemic and respiratory symptoms. Less frequent allergens include condom additives, such as lubricants, spermicides, anesthetics (benzocaine), and preservatives. Feminine hygiene products may also be implicated, as well as clothing, metal (nickel),

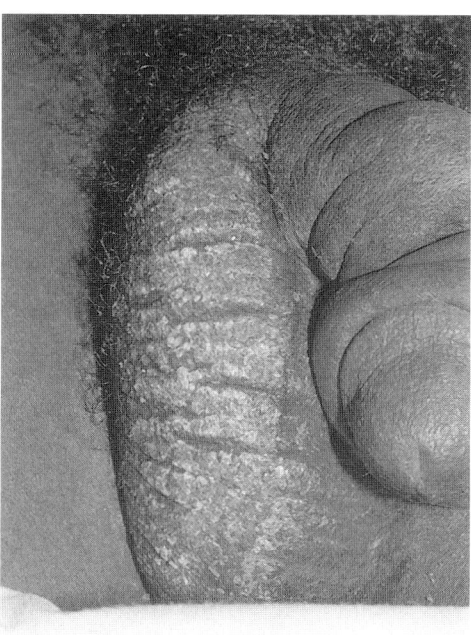

**Fig. 9.** Chronic allergic-contact dermatitis with edema and lichenification of the scrotal skin and penile edema.

perfumed sprays or lotions, and cleansers. Propylene glycol—which is found in KY jelly and many other products—can cause allergic contact dermatitis of the penis. Some patients even develop allergies to topical steroids and antibiotics. Allergens transferred from the hands include poison ivy (Rhus oleoresin) and creams intended for other areas of the body.

A diagnosis of ACD requires strong suspicion of an allergen, which may be confirmed by avoidance or rechallenge. A more precise identification may be achieved by patch testing with all suspected antigens. Irritant dermatitis and atopic dermatitis must also be included in the differential diagnosis. Atopic dermatitis has both genetic and immunologic components, and often accompanies a personal or family history of asthma, seasonal allergies, or eczema. Serum IgE levels are often elevated, but this is nonspecific. Involvement of the skin is usually not localized to one area. Patients with atopy are also more likely to suffer from irritant dermatitis.

Irritant dermatitis (*see* Fig. 10) is a nonimmune-mediated response that produces a similar picture without a true allergy. The dermatitis may occur immediately after exposure for this reason. Chronic exposure to urine, and the subsequent release of ammonia, is a common cause of irritation. Topical therapies for HPV infections, such as podophyllin, podophyllotoxin, imiquimod, 5-fluorouracil, and bi- or trichloroacetic acid, can cause irritant contact dermatitis. Frequent cleansing—as well as ingredients in the cleansers—are also causes. Occlusion of an allergen or irritant can intensify the response. Treatment requires removal of the inciting agent in either case. Symptomatic therapy is usually necessary. Short, tapering courses of oral steroids are appropriate in

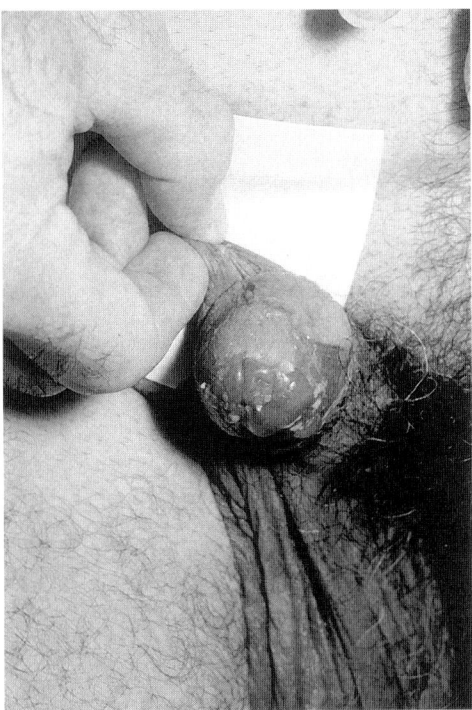

Fig. 10. Acute irritant dermatitis of glans with bullae formation secondary to ammonia burn.

severe cases. Often topical steroids are sufficient, again using the weakest preparation and shortest course possible. Weeping skin can be dried and soothed by normal saline or diluted Burow's compresses for 20 min two to three times a day. Atopic dermatitis, which is often diffuse, may require the use of antihistamines, such as hydroxyzine or doxepin hydrochloride, to control pruritus.

*Balanitis circinata* is the most common mucocutaneous lesion of Reiter's syndrome. The classic triad of asymmetric polyarthritis for at least 1 mo, conjunctivitis, and urethritis may be associated with mucocutaneous lesions that resemble psoriasis both clinically and histologically. Balanitis circinata in the circumcised male appears psoriasiform around the urethra and glans, often in an annular or circinate pattern. If the foreskin is intact, the affected area may consist of moist, erythematous plaques with a distinct border. There may be painless erosions. The histologic findings in balanitis circinata are very similar to psoriasis. Examination of the hands and feet may reveal hyperkeratotic plaques. Most common in young adult males, Reiter's syndrome appears to be a reactive disorder with both a strong genetic predisposition (HLA B27 positivity) and a previous venereal or gastrointestinal infection. These include *Chlamydia trachomatis* most commonly, as well as *Salmonella, Shigella, Yersinia, Campylobacter,* and *Mycoplasma.* Local treatment of balanitis circinata consists of weak topical steroids, which readily clear the lesions.

*Psoriasis* is a papulosquamous disorder of unknown etiology that frequently involves the penile skin. A complete skin exam may reveal similar scaly papules and plaques in a classic distribution involving the scalp, elbows, knees, and sacrum. Inverse-pattern psoriasis involves the occluded skin of the axilla, groin, intergluteal cleft, and preputial

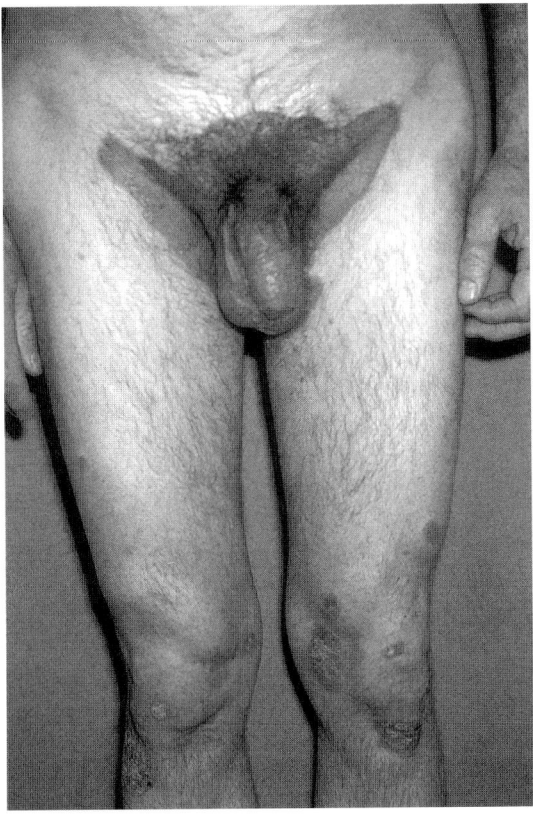

**Fig. 11.** Psoriasis. Scaly, erythematous plaques on thighs, knees, and legs, and well-demarcated red plaques with little to no scale in inguinal creases and on suprapubic skin.

sac, and is characterized by well-demarcated erythematous plaques with little-to-no scale (*see* Fig. 11). Characteristic nail changes of pitting, onycholysis, and oil spots may also aid in the diagnosis of psoriasis. A family history of psoriasis is often found. A punch biopsy of a penile lesion may be necessary to confirm the diagnosis in atypical cases. Treatment of penile plaques consists of low- to midpotency steroids and topical calcipotriol.

*Lichen planus* (*see* Fig. 12) is a T-cell mediated, inflammatory disease of the skin and mucosa. It is classically described as purple, polygonal papules that often display a white, lacy scale called Wickham's striae. On mucosal surfaces, the scale is obscured and the lesions may become erosive. The papules can coalesce to annular plaques and become pigmented. Diagnosis is aided by the identification of typical lichen planus lesions on the ventral wrists, lower back, and oral mucosa. Several of the papulosquamous diseases mentioned above, as well as secondary syphilis and SCC, must be excluded. The histopathology shows a band of inflammation at the epidermal-dermal junction with several other distinctive features. A lichenoid reaction to certain ingestants can mimic lichen planus, but should resolve after withdrawal of the offending agent.

*Lichen planus* lesions typically resolve spontaneously, and only require treatment if symptomatic. Patients should be reassured that the condition is not contagious. Intermittent treatment with topical or intralesional steroids may ease the pruritus, but may not

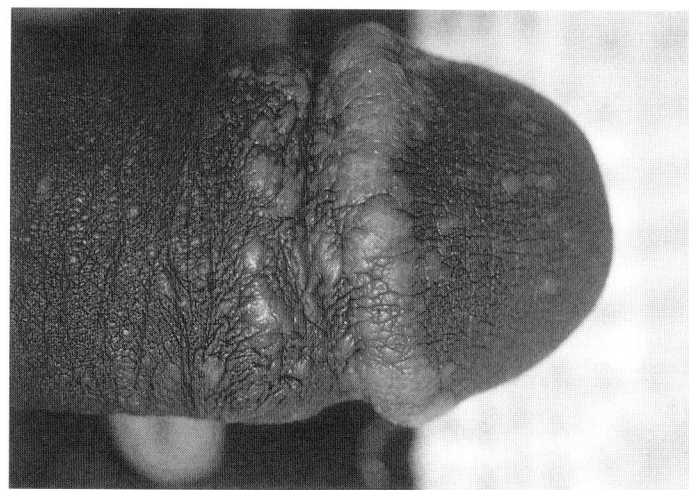

**Fig. 12.** Lichen planus. Purple polygonal papules and plaques on glans, corona, and distal shaft. *See* color plate following p. 338.

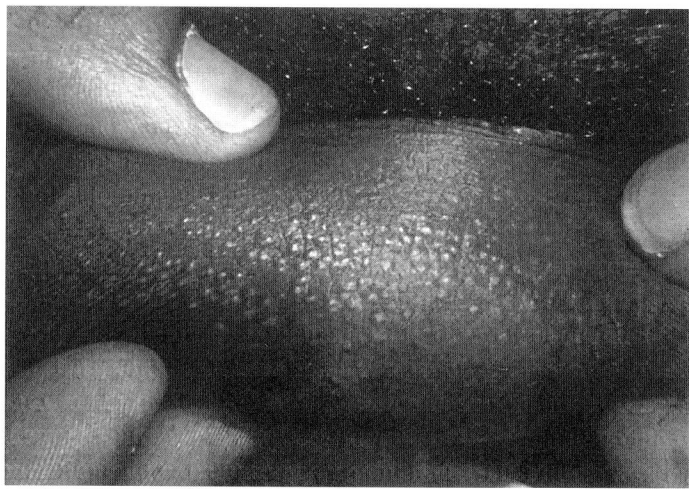

**Fig. 13.** Lichen niditus. Small, discrete, flesh-colored papules on penile shaft.

affect the course of the disease. Some patients experience disabling erosive oral lichen planus, requiring systemic immunosuppressive medications to control symptoms. Severe disease can also affect the gastrointestinal and vaginal mucosa. Squamous-cell carcinoma rarely occurs at sites of chronic lichen planus.

*Lichen nitidus* (*see* Fig. 13) may be a variant of lichen planus with distinctive clinical and histological features. This rare disorder presents as very tiny, flesh-colored papules on the penis, arms, and abdomen. There is a band of inflammation under a thinned epidermis, surrounded by a characteristic claw-like extension of the epidermis. Biopsy and treatment are not usually required once the benign and noncontagious nature of lichen nitidus is confirmed. Symptoms are rare, and lichen nitidus may be self-limited

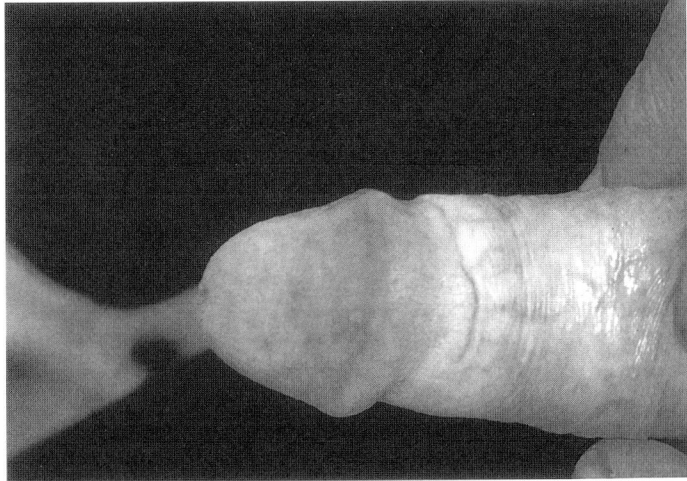

**Fig. 14.** Zoon's balanitis. Smooth, red-orange plaque on glans. *See* color plate following p. 338.

or persist chronically. If therapy is desired, topical steroids, ultraviolet light, and oral retinoids have been used with varying success.

*Zoon's balanitis (balanitis circumscripta plasmacellularis/plasma-cell balanitis)* is an unusual, benign condition of unknown etiology that occurs in uncircumcised, middle-aged and older men (*see* Fig. 14). The cause is unknown, but theories include chronic irritation or infection with *Mycobacterium smegmatis*. Analogous lesions have been described on other mucosal locations. Zoon's balanitis presents as a chronic, solitary, smooth, shiny, red-orange plaque on the glans, and may extend to the distal shaft. Variations in color include purpuric spotting, hyperpigmented macules, and yellowish coloration. Symptoms may include mild tenderness, and pruritus and erosions may occur. Biopsy is mandatory to rule out *in situ* SCC and melanoma in pigmented lesions. Histologically, a characteristic, dense plasma-cell infiltrate under a spongiotic or ulcerated epidermis is seen. The standard therapy is circumcision. If this is not curative, ablation with the carbon dioxide laser may be successful. Other reported therapies include topical antifungals, antibiotics, steroids, and fusidic 2% cream.

## DRUG REACTIONS

Several cutaneous reactions to medications may occur, including a nonspecific morbilliform eruption and the lichenoid reaction already mentioned. However, there are a few specific reactions to watch for. *Fixed drug eruptions (see* Fig. 15) are specific reactions to medications that occur on the glans and shaft. There is usually a sensitization period of a few weeks to a new medication, although fixed drug reactions can occur immediately after the first exposure to the offending agent. The usual presentation is a bright red patch or a plaque that may blister. In rare cases, it may become eroded or ulcerated. Other variations include multiple lesions and a number of symptoms, including burning, itching, or pain. The affected skin may become dusky or brown, and heals with discontinuation of the offending medication, often with residual hyperpigmentation. The most distinctive feature is the recurrence of the eruption—usually in the same location—if the medication is reintroduced. Common offending drugs include

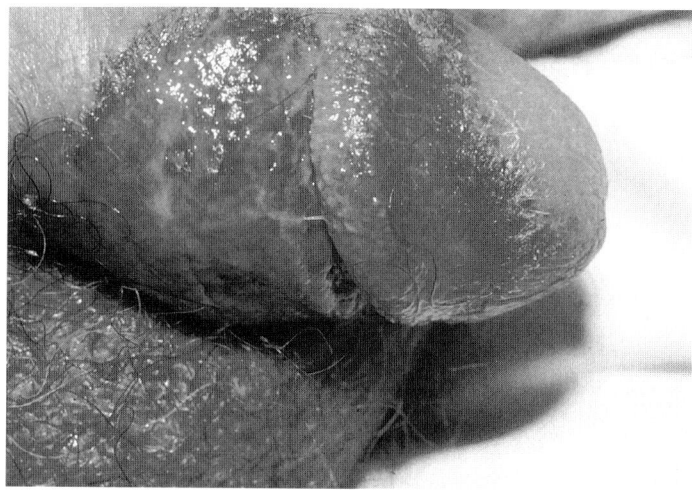

**Fig. 15.** Fixed drug eruption to Bactrim (sulfamethoxazole/trimethoprim). Erythematous eroded plaque on glans and distal shaft (photo courtesy of Kimberly Hollandsworth, MD).

tetracyclines, sulfonamides, barbiturates, phenolphthalein, salicylates, nonsteroidal anti-inflammatory agents, penicillins, carbamazepine, dapsone, griseofulvin, acetaminophen, and hydroxyzine. Diagnosis and treatment require only stopping and starting the suspected drug.

*Coumarin skin necrosis* may occur on the penis, but is more common on fat-rich areas on women. During the initial phase of anticoagulation, a hypercoagulable state may develop because of a deficiency of protein C. This results in thromboses and dermal hemorrhage, which may be seen on biopsy. Three to ten days after starting Coumarin therapy, pain and edema are followed by petechiae and ecchymoses. These areas progress to hemorrhagic bullae and necrosis. This condition may be associated with priapism. Therapy includes discontinuation of the warfarin analog, heparinization, and vitamin K. Severe necrosis requires debridement or amputation.

Foscarnet is a viral DNA- and RNA-polymerase inhibitor used to treat cytomegalovirus and acyclovir-resistant herpes infections. It can cause penile ulcerations up to 28% of the time in HIV-positive patients. It is probably a direct irritant effect, because the foscarnet is excreted unchanged in the urine. The ulcers are characteristically painful, and are more common in uncircumcised men. Although usually periurethral, they also occur on the shaft and scrotum. Rarely, oral ulcers are also present. Healing occurs with discontinuation of the foscarnet.

*Angioedema* is a deep urticarial reaction that occurs as a reaction to several medications. Rapid swelling of the penis and scrotum occurs, which subsides with discontinuation of the drug. The swelling may recur if the drug is reintroduced. Antihistamines speed up the recovery process.

## PIGMENTED LESIONS

Although not specific to the genital skin, many pigmented lesions can develop on the penis. *Melanotic macules* occur on the penis, and have an oral analog that is more common in women. These present as irregular, hyperpigmented macules that can be

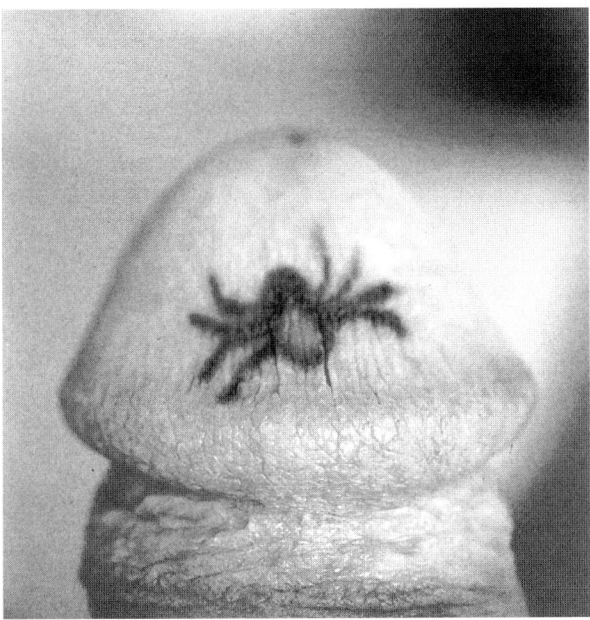

**Fig. 16.** Decorative tattoo of the glans (photograph courtesy of S. Teri McGillis, MD). *See* color plate following p. 338.

light brown to brown-black in color. Since they closely resemble a superficial melanoma, a biopsy is generally required for diagnosis. If the entire lesion cannot be practically removed, several small punch biopsies can be performed. The pathology shows only basal-layer hyperpigmentation and pigment incontinence, without cellular atypia.

*Lentigines* (singular, lentigo) generally look more benign in nature. These are light brown macules, unrelated to sun exposure. Although not usually performed, a biopsy will demonstrate hyperpigmentation, increased number of melanocytes, and elongation of the epidermal rete ridges. Treatment is unnecessary.

*Melanocytic nevi*, or common moles, may also appear on the penis. Nevi may be junctional, compound, or intradermal, depending on the depth of the nevus cells. The type does not affect the prognosis. The junctional type, which is flat, is most common on the glans. Excisional biopsy is often needed if severe atypia or a melanoma is suspected. Examination is guided by the *A, B, C,* and *D*s of any nevi. The patient should be instructed to look for changes of *a*symmetry, irregular *b*orders, variations in *c*olor, and large *d*iameter (> 5 mm).

Decorative *tattoos* (*see* Fig. 16) are occasionally placed on the penis. If desired, several nonablative lasers are available for removal with a very low risk of residual scarring. Foreign bodies can be traumatically introduced into the skin, forming tattoos. Black substances deep in the skin may look blue on the surface. The foreign body may also cause a granulomatous reaction. History of trauma is usually known, and treatment may involve excision or laser surgery to remove the foreign body.

*Postinflammatory pigment changes* are very common. Any cause of inflammation in the skin, especially a chronic process, can leave an area of hyperpigmentation. If left alone, the pigment slowly fades. *Hypopigmentation* may also follow inflammatory lesions, including contact dermatitis to rubber products. Certain treatment modalities—

such as cryosurgery to treat condyloma acuminata—may damage melanocytes, leaving hypopigmented macules.

*Vitiligo* is an acquired depigmentary disorder with the loss of melanocytes. Vitiligo is fairly common, and mild cases may go unnoticed by the patient. Generalized, segmental, and focal types exist, and the penis is frequently involved. Treatment is unsatisfactory. Topical steroids and Psoralen plus ultraviolet light A (PUVA) therapy are used in other locations but are unsuitable for treatment of vitiligo on the genitals. Screening for other autoimmune diseases may be indicated. Vitiligo is generally thought to have both genetic and autoimmune components, and is frequently associated with other autoimmune diseases, such as diabetes mellitus, thyroiditis, pernicious anemia, alopecia areata, Addison's disease, and multiglandular insufficiency. It has also been associated with malignancies and infection with the human immunodeficiency virus.

## BLISTERING DISORDERS

The skin diseases in this category generally involve the penis as part of a generalized eruption. Most are genetic or autoimmune in nature. One exception to both of these is *erythema multiforme (EM)*. As the name implies, EM has a myriad of presentations, although the classic is the "target" or "iris" lesion. An erythematous papulae with concentric color changes typically has a dusky center, with a surrounding pale ring. The central portion may blister. The lesions may occur in crops, and resolve in 2–4 wk. EM can occur almost anywhere, but is most common on the extensor extremities. The cause may not be identified, but EM is considered to be a reaction to infection or drugs. Common causes include herpes simplex virus, Epstein-Barr virus, and *Mycoplasma pneumoniae* infections, but almost every type of infectious agent has been implicated. Likewise, a number of drugs have been reported to be associated with EM. The most commonly reported medications are sulfonamides, penicillins, anticonvulsants, nonsteroidal antiinflammatory drugs, and allopurinol. In cases of recurrent EM, infections seem more likely. Although the classification system is frequently modified, EM can be thought of as the mildest end of a spectrum of disease that includes Stevens-Johnson syndrome and Toxic Epidermal Necrolysis (TEN).

*Stevens-Johnson syndrome* or *EM major* is generally a more severe but self-limited reaction that involves at least two mucosal surfaces. The cutaneous eruption is more widespread, with more frequent vesiculation and bullae formation. Epidermal necrosis and detachment may involve up to 10% of the skin surface. Balanitis may cause difficulty with urination. Systemic symptoms vary, and mortality is rare. The disease resolves within 6 wk. The workup may be directed, but typically includes a complete blood count, Mycoplasma titers, chest X-ray, and cultures from the skin and blood.

TEN is the most severe end of the spectrum, with at least 30% epidermal necrosis and detachment and widespread purpuric macules. Various prodromal symptoms are followed by a burning or painful rash that evolves into sheet-like loss of the epidermis. Large, flaccid bullae appear, which may be extended by lateral or direct pressure. Mucosal involvement is almost universal. Painful micturation may occur, and phimosis can result. High fever and systemic involvement usually requires hospitalization for many weeks, and the mortality rate is approx 30%. Drugs are the most common cause. Drugs started within 2–3 wk are the most likely cause, but the list of implicated agents is extensive. The same agents listed for EM are the most common culprits, but over

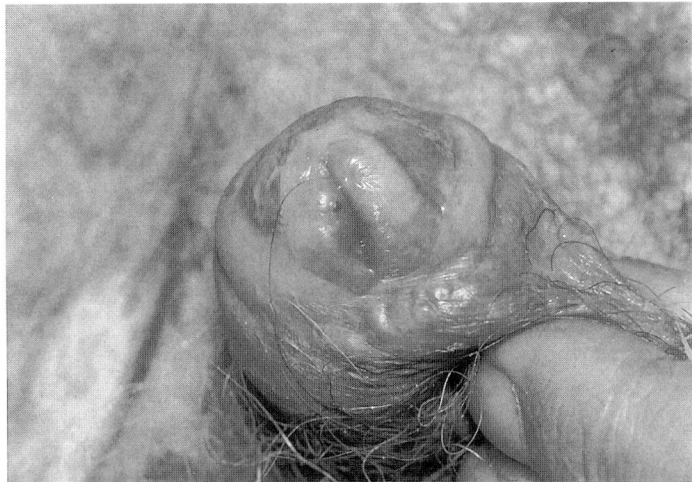

**Fig. 17.** Cicatricial pemphigoid. Large erosions on glans with underlying scarring.

100 drugs have been blamed. This list can include additives or fumigants not always considered in a drug history. Treatment involves discontinuation of any suspected agent, and intensive supportive care. A burn unit is ideal for treatment. The erosions typically heal without scarring, but pigment changes are frequent. Mucosal lesions may persist for months, and the penis is typically one of the last areas to heal. Phimosis may require corrective surgery after healing is complete.

Several autoimmune blistering diseases can affect the penile skin and mucosa. These are rare, and should be managed by a dermatologist who is familiar with their diagnosis and treatment. *Bullous pemphigoid* is mainly a disease of the elderly. Tense bullae form on normal or erythematous skin and generally do not expand. Symptoms are few, but occasionally the disease begins as an urticarial plaque that can produce burning or pruritus. This condition is difficult to diagnose, and may be confused with a drug reaction or other dermatitis. Biopsy is required for proper diagnosis, demonstrating a subepidermal split with many eosinophils. Direct immunofluorescence shows linear IgG deposition along the basement membrane. This illustrates the cause of the disease, since autoantibodies are produced against an integral protein in the lamina lucida. Treatment consists of high-dose prednisone, followed by a taper or switch to other immunosuppressive medications. The combination of tetracycline and niacinamide is an effective steroid-sparing regimen in some cases.

*Cicatricial pemphigoid* (*see* Fig. 17) is similar to bullous pemphigoid with a nearly identical histological picture. It is mainly a disease of the mucous membranes, and can cause severe scarring and morbidity. CP primarily affects the eyes and oral cavity, but may affect the skin of the penis, with vesicles, erosions, and scarring, and phimosis. Treatment consists of aggressive immunosuppression, and consultation with ophthalmology is essential.

*Pemphigus vulgaris* and its variants are autoimmune diseases in which IgG antibodies are directed against a protein on the surfaces of epidermal keratinocytes. This leads to separation of the epidermal cells, forming superficial, flaccid bullae and vesicles. Both of these findings are demonstrated with routine histology and immunofluorescence. As

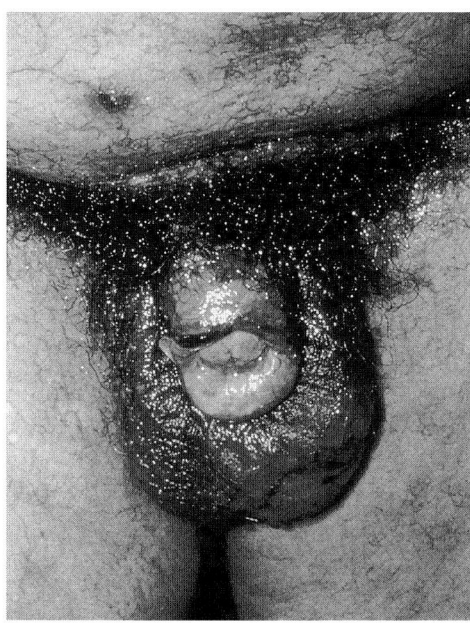

**Fig. 18.** Paraneoplastic pemphigus in patient with chronic lymphocytic leukemia. Ruptured bullae with erosions involving the lower abdomen, penis, and scrotum.

with other blisters on the penis, they often rupture and form erosions before they are noticed. This presentation is important, because erosions may be the only sign of a blistering disease. Herpes simplex infection—which is in the differential diagnosis—can present the same way. Pemphigus is most common in the oral cavity, but can affect any epithelialized surface. A full skin exam may reveal more characteristic flaccid bullae and erosions elsewhere. Pemphigus vulgaris should be considered a severe disease, and carried a high mortality rate before the advent of systemic steroids, which are still the mainstay of treatment. *Pemphigus foliaceus* is characterized by erosive plaques on the inguinal skin with seborrheic dermatitis or psoriasis-like lesions on the scalp, face, and upper trunk. *Pemphigus vegetans* can occur solely on the glans penis and is characterized by moist, verrucous plaques on intertriginous areas.

*Paraneoplastic pemphigus* (*see* Fig. 18) is a recently described entity that clinically resembles pemphigus vulgaris and is associated with an underlying neoplasm that is most frequently leukemia or lymphoma (especially non-Hodgkin's lymphoma). Clearing or improvement of the mucocutaneous blistering disease generally follows successful treatment of the underlying malignancy. Persistent pemphigus lesions may require treatment with immunosuppressive therapy of prednisone and cyclophosphamide. Response to therapy is somewhat less predictable than in patients with classic pemphigus vulgaris.

*Epidermolysis bullosa (EB)* and *Hailey-Hailey disease (benign familial pemphigus)* are genetic disorders that cause blistering and erosions of the penis. EB, which has one acquired form, is actually a large group of inherited defects in structural proteins that lead to blistering and erosions of the skin and mucosa. A family history is often present, but electron microscopy may be required to accurately delineate the specific type of EB. Treatment is only supportive, but there is active research in gene therapy

Chapter 24 / Practical Dermatology

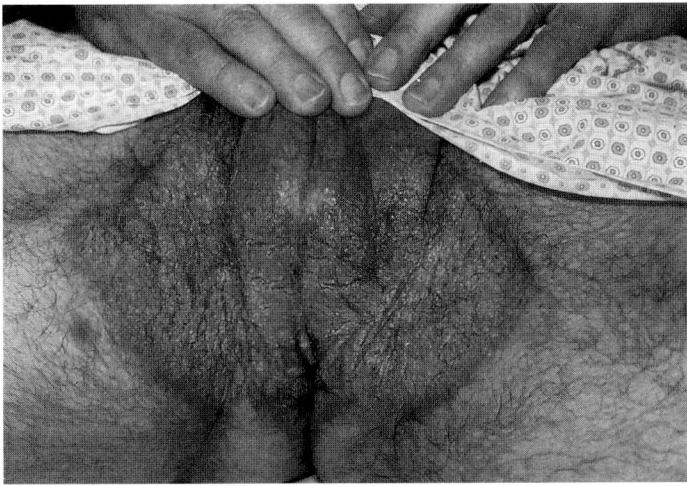

**Fig. 19.** Hailey-Hailey disease (benign familial pemphigus). Macerated, malodorous skin in inguinal folds, thighs, and scrotum with scattered erosions.

for these patients. Hailey-Hailey disease is an autosomal dominant, chronic condition that mostly affects intertriginous areas (*see* Fig. 19). The groin, neck, axillae, and trunk have sheets of small vesicles that rupture quickly with friction. These often become superinfected and crusted. Rarely, it may present as papules resembling condyloma acuminata. The cause is unknown, but there appears to be a defect in cellular adhesion demonstrated histologically by a form of epidermal separation called acantholysis. Treatment can be difficult and frustrating. Superinfection with bacteria, yeast, and herpes simplex are common and should be addressed. Chronic therapy with topical antibiotics, steroids, and drying agents or compresses are helpful. Localized areas can potentially be excised and grafted, or ablated with a laser.

## ULCERATIVE CONDITIONS

Ulcers are deeper than erosions, and extend at least to the dermis. The most common causes of genital ulcers are sexually transmitted diseases, which are included in the differential diagnosis of all other conditions. *Aphthous ulcers* are usually a diagnosis of exclusion. Similar to the common presentation in the mouth, these small, often painful ulcers may occur on the penis or scrotum. Some oral lesions have been linked to iron or vitamin deficiencies, but little is written about genital aphthous disease.

*Behçet's disease* is a rare disease that presents with aphthous-like ulcers on the genitalia as one of the secondary features, although this occurs with most patients. Diagnosis is based on the presence of recurrent oral ulcers along with two of the following: recurrent genital ulceration, eye lesions, skin lesions, and a positive pathergy test. Oral ulcerations are the main clinical feature and diagnostic requirement. Genital ulcers are generally fewer in number, deeper, more painful, and more likely to scar than their oral counterpart (*see* Fig. 20). Any organ system can be affected, and some patients exhibit uveitis and visual changes, cranial-nerve palsies, thrombophlebitis, arthritis, gastrointestinal disturbances, and psychiatric symptoms. The cause is unknown, but there appears to be a genetic predisposition, and it is more common in people of

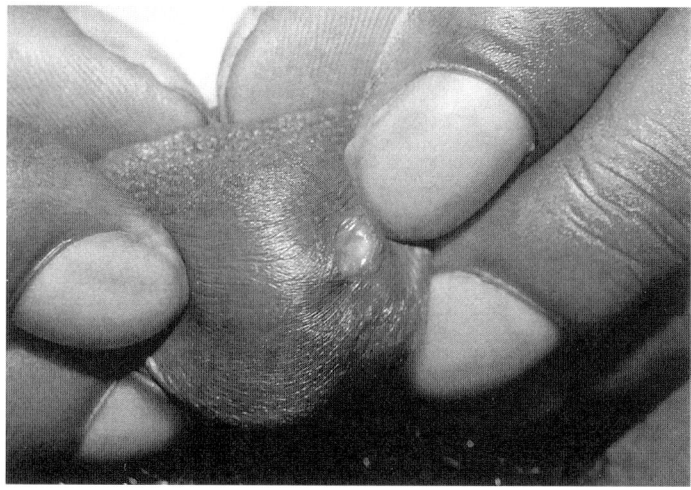

**Fig. 20.** Behcet's disease. Small, well-demarcated ulcer of glans.

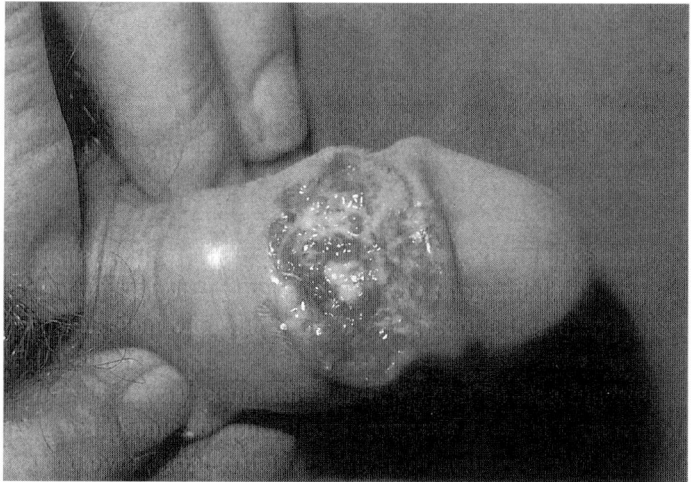

**Fig. 21.** Pyoderma gangrenosum. Large, undermined ulcer of distal shaft.

Japanese or Mediterranean descent. The pathology may not be specific, but should demonstrate a neutrophilic vascular reaction, often with subtle changes of vasculitis. The course is episodic, and treatment options vary with the degree of disease severity. Cutaneous ulcerations may respond to potent topical steroids or anesthetics. Systemic therapy is usually needed. The antineutrophilic drugs dapsone (100–200 mg/d) and colchicine (0.6 mg bid) are first-line therapy. More severe disease is treated with a variety of immunosuppressive and cytotoxic agents.

*Pyoderma gangrenosum* is a painful, chronic, ulcerative condition associated with a systemic disease in about 50% of patients (*see* Fig. 21). These diseases include inflammatory bowel disease (ulcerative colitis more often than Crohn's disease), arthritis, and lymphoproliferative diseases. The ulcers are most common on the legs, but

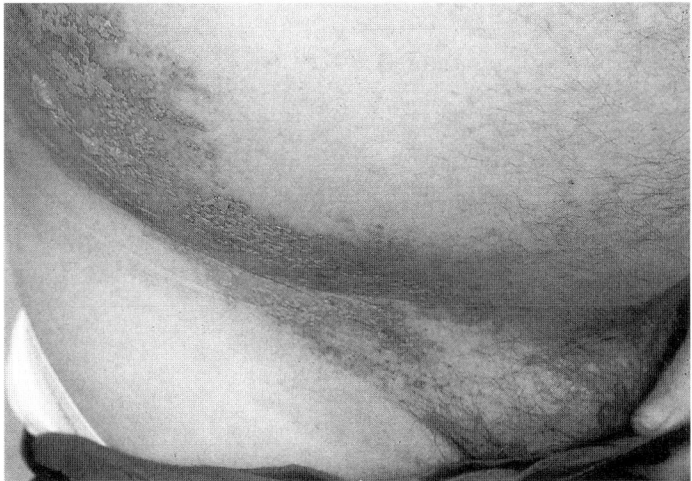

**Fig. 22.** Varicella zoster virus (shingles). Unilateral discrete and confluent vesicles and pustules with surrounding erythema on lower abdomen extending to suprapubic skin.

can rarely occur on the penis. A pustule forms and ulcerates with a violaceous, undermined border. Topical and intralesional steroids are the first lines of therapy, but any progression should be treated with aggressive immunosuppression. A rare destructive form of pyoderma gangrenosum can consume the entire penis if treatment fails. Inflammatory bowel disease may also extend to the perineal and genital skin. *Metastatic Crohn's disease* may produce the granulomatous lesions at distant sites, including the genitals. These vary from nodules to ulcers, and may require biopsy to differentiate from pyoderma gangrenosum. Treatment is directed at the bowel disease and local wound care. Cryoglobulinemia and end-stage renal disease secondary to diabetes can produce a dry necrosis of the penis, which may look similar to pyoderma gangrenosum. This is a harbinger of severe disease, and is frequently followed by death from the systemic disease.

*Factitial ulcers* are found in patients who chronically scratch the penis or scrotum. The patient may not be fully aware of his actions. Linear ulcers or excoriations are often present. Chronic rubbing of the skin produces thick, lichenified papules. Any secondary infection must be treated, and the underlying neurosis should be addressed.

## INFECTIONS

### Viral

Aside from the sexually transmitted diseases, a wide variety of infectious agents affect the genitals and surrounding skin. As the number of immunosuppressed patients increases, so does the potential for unusual pathogens. There are relatively few viral infections to consider. *Varicella zoster virus* typically causes chickenpox in children and young adults, and reactivates as herpes zoster (shingles) in older adults. The reactivation occurs in a unilateral, dermatomal pattern, which is often sudden and painful (*see* Fig. 22). The eruption may last several weeks, with crusting of the vesicles. Imvolvement of the penis is rare, but occurs when dermatomes S1–4 are involved. The

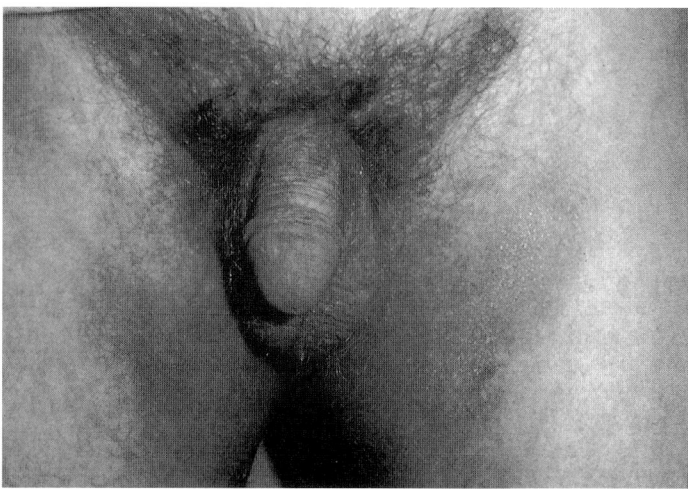

**Fig. 23.** Candida intertrigo. Erythematous patches of inguinal creases and medial proximal thighs with scattered pustules and erosions.

vesicles may extend to the pubic area, scrotum, and thigh. The distribution and course of varicella zoster vesicles aid in the diagnosis, since the individual vesicles are identical to herpes simplex infections. Culture and direct fluorescent antibodies differentiate between the two herpes virus types. Treatment for mild eruptions is mainly symptomatic, using normal saline or Burow's compresses twice a day and an antibacterial ointment applied to the crusted lesions. Cases in immunosuppressed patients, or severe cases, in general are improved with systemic antiviral therapy. Three effective agents are now available: acyclovir 800 mg five times a day for 7 d, famcyclovir 500 mg TID for 7 d, and valacyclovir 1000 mg BID for 7 d. Valacyclovir should not be used in immunosuppressed patients.

## Mycotic Infections

Mycotic infections of the genitals are common. The most common cause of infectious balanitis is *Candida spp*. The appearance is similar to other sites of infection, with erythema, tiny satellite pustules or erosions, and a white, curd-like accumulation. Patients may experience pruritus and mild burning, which may be accentuated by a superimposed bacterial infection with staphylococci or streptococci. Predisposing factors include treatment with antibiotics, exposure to an infected sexual partner, immunosuppression, and diabetes mellitus. Men with the last two conditions may progress to an ulcerative or severe edematous variant. The transmission rate from infected females to male sexual partners is about 10%, and hypersensitivity reactions to candida also occur. Diagnosis is confirmed by the recognition of pseudohyphae in a potassium hydroxide scraping. A wide range of topical antifungals, such as clotrimazole, produce high cure rates. An alternative treatment is a single 150-mg dose of fluconazole. If sexual transmission is suspected, the partner should be treated as well. *Candida intertrigo* (*see* Fig. 23) is also very common. In addition to antifungal therapy, absorptive clothing or powder, as well as aeration, are helpful.

*Tinea cruris (jock itch)* is a very common fungal infection of the groin, pubic area, and buttocks. Erythematous, pruritic, scaly plaques may spread in an annular fashion with a raised border. The scrotum is involved much more often than the penis. Dermatophytosis of the glans has been reported, but is exceedingly rare. It is most commonly caused by *Trichophyton rubrum,* although other species can be responsible. Most topical antifungals are quite effective. Widespread infections are better managed with oral griseofulvin. The newer agents itraconazole and terbinafine are also effective. The feet should also be examined for active dermatophyte infection, since they can infect the groin during clothing change. Other fungi or yeast that have been reported to rarely infect the penis include *Histoplasma capsulatum, Blastomycosis dermatitidis, Cryptococcus neoformans, Pityrosporum ovale (Malassezia furfur),* and penicillium.

## *Bacterial Infections*

Bacteria are the second most common cause of infectious balanitis. Streptococcus spp. are the most common bacterial pathogens, and may cause an infectious balanitis, erysipelas, or cellulitis. *Erysipelas* refers to a superficial infection that does not go deeper than the dermis. The erythematous, warm patches have borders that are sharp and may be raised. *Cellulitis* refers to a deeper infection that may extend to subcutaneous fat. Both conditions present as warm, erythematous, and swollen patches of skin that may be near a conspicuous break in the skin barrier. Both group A and group B beta-hemolytic streptococci cause skin infections of the penis. The former has been reported in prepubertal boys, and may follow autoinoculation from perianal cellulitis, or group A streptococcal pharyngitis. Group B hemolytic streptococcal balanoposthitis generally occurs in postpubertal men. The major reservoir for group B streptococci is the female genital tract, implicating sexual transmission. Treatment of streptococcal disease should be taken very seriously. The first line of therapy is penicillin, but effective alternatives include erythromycin, cephalexin, and ampicillin. The infection may become recurrent, leading to edema, scarring, and elephantiasis of the penis and scrotum, with permanent loss of sexual function. Some authors suggest the addition of prednisone tapers over several weeks, along with high-dose penicillin. These infections may also progress rapidly, with tissue necrosis that results in scarring.

*Staphylococcus aureus* can cause local infection or generalized disease. One strain produces an exotoxin that causes staphylococcal scaled-skin syndrome in infants and children. Although the infection is usually in the nasopharynx, it is a systemic disorder characterized by flaccid blisters and erosions that are frequently present on the genitals. The pattern of disease and biopsy differentiate this entity from toxic epidermal necrolysis, which is rare in children. Appropriate treatment is intravenous penicillinase-resistant antistaphylococcal antibiotics.

*Fournier's gangrene* refers to a necrotizing fasciitis of the male genitalia. It is typically a mixed flora infection, often including streptococci, gram-negative bacilli, and anaerobes, especially Bacteroides. In children, streptococcal and staphylococcal species are the most common isolates. Areas of erythema and warmth develop into malodorous, blue-brown, necrotic lesions. There may be a preceding trauma, and diabetes may be a predisposing factor. These patients become quite ill, and extreme pain is a characteristic symptom. There is a significant potential for morbidity and mortality, requiring early diagnosis and treatment. In addition to broad-spectrum antibi-

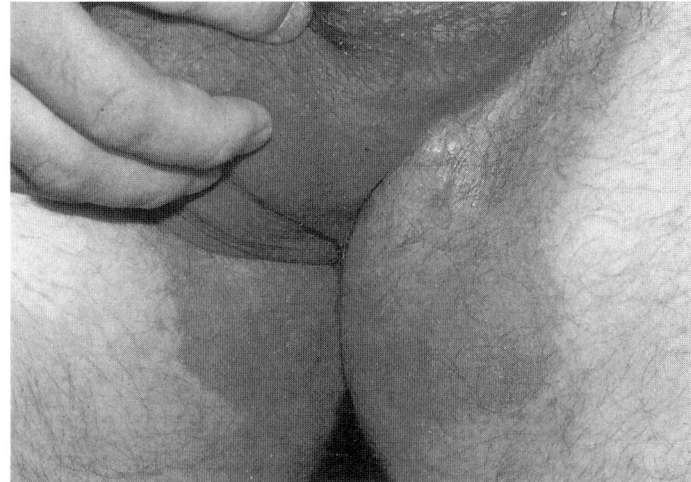

Fig. 24. Erythrasma. Symmetric, well-demarcated tan patches on medial thighs.

otics, surgical debridement is needed to halt extension to the perineum and abdominal wall.

*Ecthyma gangrenosum* is a gangrenous cellulitis caused by *Pseudomonas aeruginosa*, which frequently results in pseudomonal sepsis. The organism is present in tense vesicles on erythematous skin that become necrotic, gray ulcers. The groin and male genitalia are commonly affected sites. Treatment requires early use of antipseudomonal antibiotics, and debridement if indicated. The prognosis for *Ecthyma gangrenosum* with associated pseudomonal septicemia is grave, with a >50% mortality rate. *Ecthyma gangrenosum*-like lesions may also occur with *Staphylococcus aureus, Escherichia coli, Neisseria meningitidis, Aeromonas hydrophila, Serratia marcescens,* and fungi of Aspergillus and Rhizopus genera.

*Erythrasma* (*see* Fig. 24) is a chronic bacterial infection of the groin caused by *Corynebacterium minutissimum*. This eruption, which is usually between the scrotum and thighs, is often misdiagnosed as *tinea cruris* because of its similar appearance. Both conditions may be pruritic. Clinically, well-demarcated, tan-to-pink patches form symmetrically on the medial thighs. Examination with a Wood's lamp reveals a coral-red fluorescence caused by a porphyrin produced by the bacteria, and KOH preparation is negative unless a concomitant dermatophyte infection is present. Although it may improve with use of certain topical antifungals, the treatment of choice is topical or oral erythromycin. Topical clindamycin and benzoyl peroxide are also effective treatments.

*Trichomycosis* is an unusual infection caused by the diphtheroid bacteria *Corynebacterium tenuis*. It is associated with hyperhidrosis, and presents in the pubic area and axillae as hard concretions attached to the base of hairs. The concretions may be yellow, red, or black, and must be differentiated from the nits left by lice. Shaving the hair is the most effective treatment. Topical antibiotics, such as erythromycin and benzoyl peroxide, and a reduction in sweating may be effective, but recurrences are common.

*Balanoposthitis* is inflammation of the foreskin and glans. Occasionally, an infectious agent can be identified. A significant number of cases of the ulcerative form of balanoposthitis are caused by a mixed infection with nontreponemal spirochetes and anaerobic

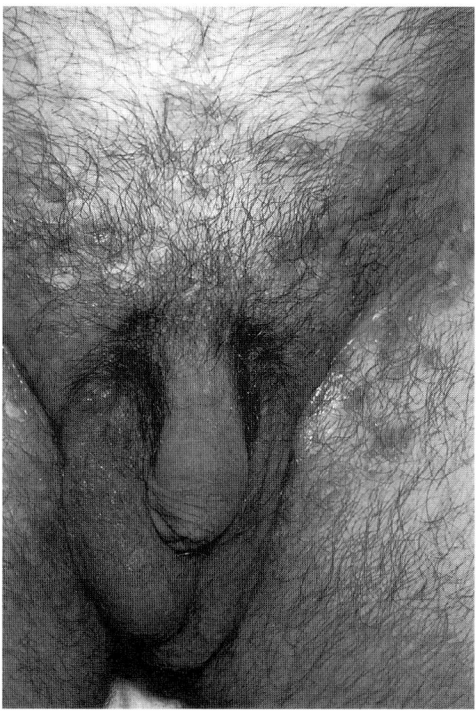

**Fig. 25.** Hidrandenitis suppurativa. Multiple, inflamed draining nodules, scarring, and sinus tracts of suprapubic skin, inguinal creases, thighs, and scrotum.

bacteria—usually Bacteroides. Poor hygiene and relative phimosis are predisposing factors. Transmission is thought to occur by orogenital contact, and less commonly by vaginal transmission. Metronidazole is an effective treatment. Circumcision is the most definitive treatment.

*Folliculitis* is a very common condition of hair-bearing skin, including the pubic area. Small, red papules or pustules are present at each affected follicle. This condition may be caused by external irritation, but is frequently a result of staphylococcal infection. Less frequently, pseudomonal, yeast, or herpes infections may cause folliculitis. Antibiotic treatment is dictated by the severity of the eruption and culture results. Irritation should be reduced, and using antibacterial cleansers may reduce future episodes. A *furuncle* is a perifollicular abscess that may be up to several centimeters in size. Pus may drain from a small opening spontaneously or with external pressure. An *abscess* is typically warm, swollen, and tender. *Staphylococcus aureus* is the most frequent pathogen. In immunosuppressed patients, unusual bacteria may be identified on culture. All patients are started on an antistaphylococcal antibiotic, such as dicloxacillin. Fluctuant lesions should be incised and drained.

Although not usually classified as an infectious disease, *hidradenitis suppurativa* is mentioned because of its similar appearance, and sometimes treatment, to furuncles or abscesses (*see* Fig. 25). This condition is part of the "follicular occlusion triad," which also includes acne conglobata and dissecting cellulitis of the scalp. All three entities are chronic, suppurative, inflammatory lesions of the pilosebaceous units or apocrine glands. Chronic inflammation and infection often lead to sinus-tract formation and scarring in all three conditions. Hidradenitis involves the groin, buttocks, axillae, and rarely a few other areas. Anogenital involvement is more common in males than axillary disease. It is usually found in postpubescent young adults, many of whom are obese or smoke. The first lesion may be a single, inflamed nodule in the groin. Solitary lesions may be drained or injected with corticosteroid. Hidradenitis usually requires chronic systemic treatment with antibiotics, such as tetracycline. A recent study suggests that topical clindamycin is just as effective. Topical antibacterial cleansers also help. Chronic disease may require surgical therapy, with excision of large areas of diseased tissue. Isotretinoin (Accutane), although effective in cystic acne, has been of little benefit in the treatment of hidradenitis. Rarely, aggressive squamous-cell carcinomas may develop in any chronic inflammatory focus.

There are reports of other types of bacteria that cause skin infection. These rare pathogens include *Haemophilus parainfluenzae, Klebsiella, Staphylococcus epidermidis, Enterococcus, Proteus, Morganella, Pseudomonas,* and *E. coli.* Mycobacterial disease of the male genitalia is very rare and most commonly reported outside of the United States.

## INFESTATIONS

Infestations frequently present in the genital area. *Scabies,* caused by the mite *Sarcoptes scabiei,* is fairly common in the general population. Transmission results from sexual or close contact, and even from fomites soon after contact with an infested individual. Scabies should be considered in the differential diagnosis of any intensely pruritic dermatosis, although this symptom is occasionally absent. The penis is one of the most commonly affected sites. The lesions can occur in any location below the head in immunocompetent individuals, especially in the finger webs or along the waist. Erythematous—sometimes scaly—papules, or nodules—are usually present in multiple locations (*see* Fig. 26). Linear burrows are pathognomonic. A rare variety—Norwegian scabies—presents as yellow-white scaly patches. This condition is most common in immunocompromised patients, and is caused by massive numbers of mites.

Diagnosis of scabies is by identification of the mite. Firm scrapings of the papules with a scalpel blade are viewed microscopically, revealing live mites, feces, or eggs. Patients are usually treated under strong suspicion, even when the search for mites is unsuccessful. Several effective treatments are available, including permethrin, lindane, precipitated sulfur, crotamiton cream, and oral ivermectin. Permethrin 5% cream (Elimite) is the usual choice, and is applied from the neck down for at least 12 h and washed off. The treatment may be repeated in 1 wk, and all household members and sexual contacts should be treated simultaneously. The papules or nodules may persist after effective treatment, but slowly resolve. Secondary bacterial infection may also occur with excoriation.

*Pediculosis pubis* is caused by the crab louse, *Phthirus pubis* (*see* Fig. 27). Small, dark brown or black lice and nits can be seen at the base of the hairs, and may be mobile. Small, blue macules (maculae ceruleae) representing dermal hemorrhage may be seen on the abdomen. Transmission requires close contact, usually of a sexual nature. Many patients will diagnose and treat themselves after noticing pruritus and a crawling sensation. Over-the-counter shampoos and lotions, such as permethrin (Nix) and pyre-

# Chapter 24 / Practical Dermatology

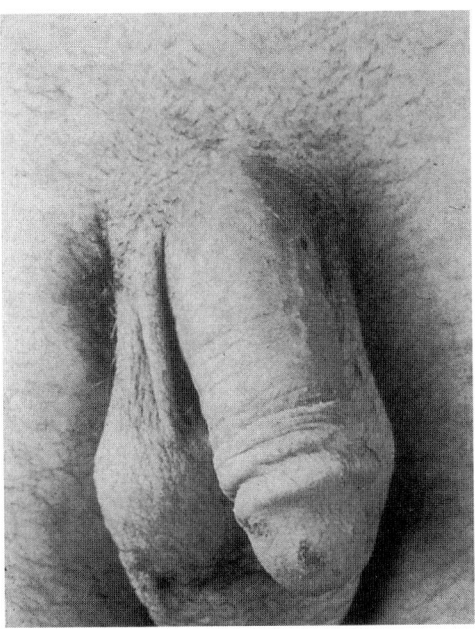

**Fig. 26.** Scabies. Linear burrows and excoriated papules of penile shaft and glans.

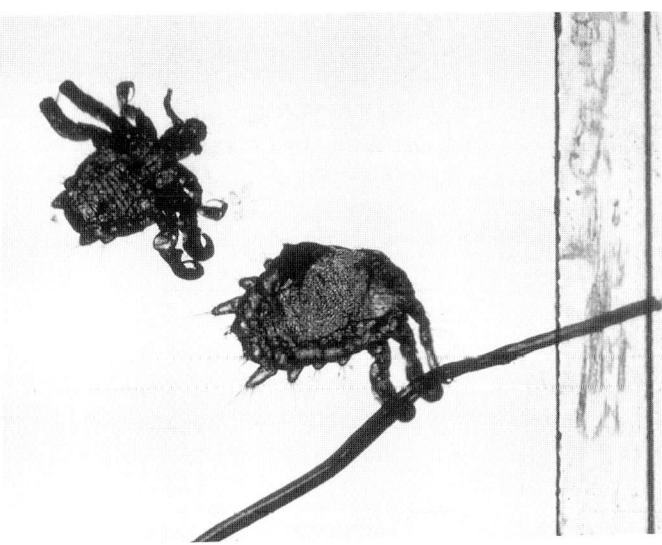

**Fig. 27.** Crab louse (*Phthirus pubis*).

thrins (RID), are usually effective. Because a single application may not be sufficient, the patient and any sexual contacts should repeat the treatment in 7–10 d.

## BENIGN TUMORS

Some of the more common benign growths have already been discussed. Other fairly common growths of vascular origin include *capillary hemangiomas*. These are red or

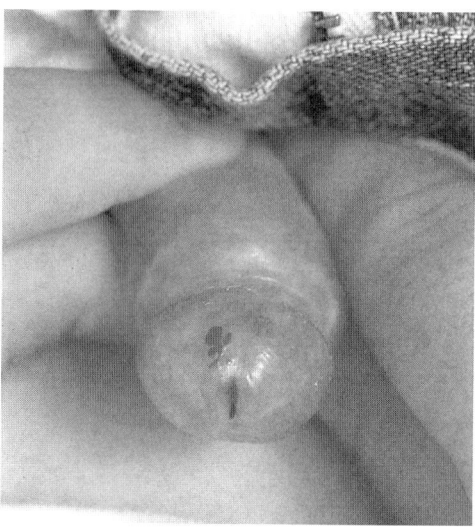

**Fig. 28.** Capillary hemangioma of glans in a child. Grouped, red vascular papules. *See* color plate following p. 338.

purple papules or depressed patches that are asymptomatic (*see* Figs. 28, 29). Treatment—which is only necessary if bleeding occurs—may be done with a vascular laser. *Varicose veins* occur rarely on the penis as a soft, blue nodule. In atypical or questionable cases, a biopsy can confirm the diagnosis. Another bluish, subcutaneous nodule on the shaft is *intravascular papillary endothelial hyperplasia,* or *Masson's tumor.* This is a rare condition diagnosed and cured by excisional biopsy. *Lymphangioma circumscriptum* (*see* Fig. 30) is a benign dilation of lymph vessels that can present as soft, compressible vesicles or blebs. Treatment is unnecessary, unless problems with lymphatic fluid leakage occur. Excision or carbon-dioxide laser ablation may be helpful in this scenario.

*Seborrheic keratoses* are brown, waxy growths with a "stuck on" appearance. They may fall off and grow back, and commonly occur on the rest of the body. They can be treated with liquid nitrogen or curettage if they become inflamed or painful. *Sebaceous hyperplasias* are small, yellow papules on the shaft that may be confused with warts. They are merely enlarged sebaceous glands, and treatment is unnecessary. *Verruciform xanthoma* is a rare condition with foam cells and verrucous epidermal hyperplasia seen on microscopic examination. Although usually found in the oral mucosa, it may occur on the scrotum or penis. The yellow, verrucous papules or plaques resemble a giant condyloma or squamous-cell carcinoma. A biopsy is needed for proper diagnosis.

## MALIGNANT TUMORS

*Penile carcinoma* is a significant problem worldwide, but is relatively rare in the United States. Nearly all occurrences are *squamous-cell carcinomas (SCC)* (*see* Fig. 31). Risk factors for penile carcinoma include smoking; history of genital warts; chronic irritation caused by poor hygiene, friction, smegma, inflammation, or trauma; late or no circumcision; and ultraviolet light treatment for other dermatoses. Chronic dermatoses that may cause squamous-cell carcinoma include lichen sclerosis et atrophicus (*see*

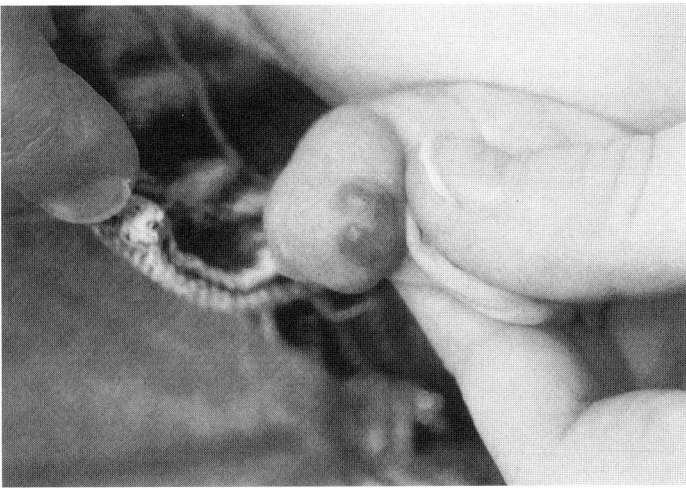

**Fig. 29.** Capillary hemangioma of glans. Purple, compressible blanchable soft nodule. *See* color plate following p. 338.

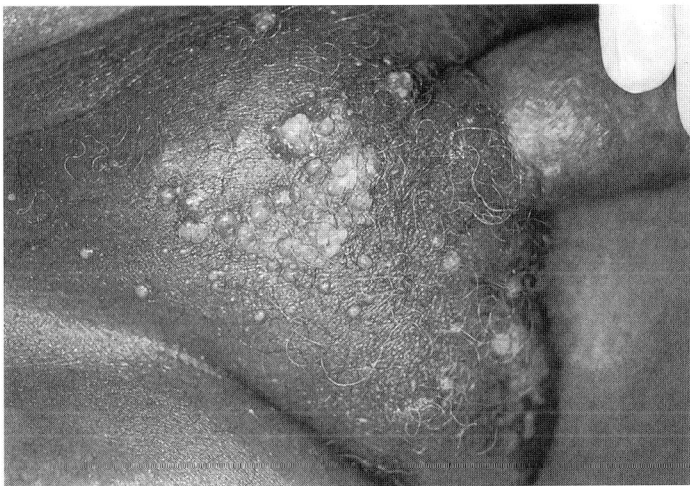

**Fig. 30.** Lymphangioma circumscriptum. Multiple discrete and confluent soft, compressible clear blebs on scrotum.

Fig. 6) and leukoplakia. The most commonly associated HPV type is HPV-16, followed by 18, 31, and 33. A pregnant woman with HPV-16 can transmit this virus to a newborn male, with subsequent development of intraepithelial atypia or *in situ*-SCC in the infant.

*Erythroplasia of Queyrat* (*see* Figs. 32, 33) refers to the *in situ* form of SCC on the mucous membranes of the glans penis or lining of the foreskin. It is the analog to Bowen's disease on keratinized skin. Both conditions can be confused with inflammatory dermatoses, but will not respond to treatment with topical steroids. Lesions on the penis are slow-growing, erythematous, shiny, well-demarcated patches or plaques. They may be velvety, scaly, or verrucous. There may be symptoms of pain or pruritus, bleeding, or difficulty in retracting the foreskin. Biopsy is needed to make the diagnosis

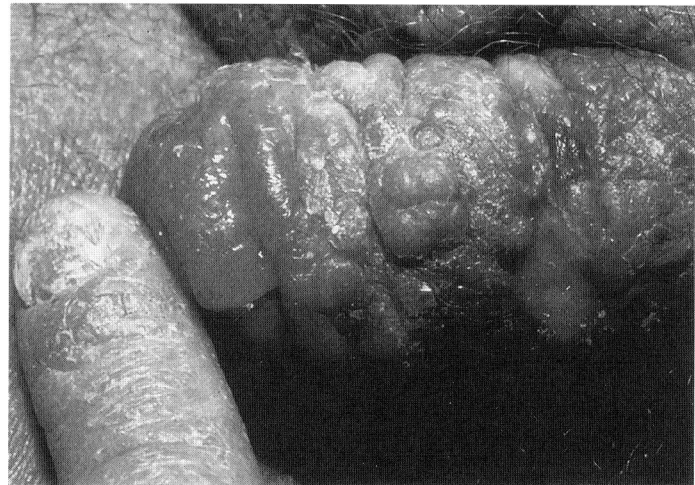

**Fig. 31.** Squamous-cell carcinoma in a patient with chronic dermatitis.

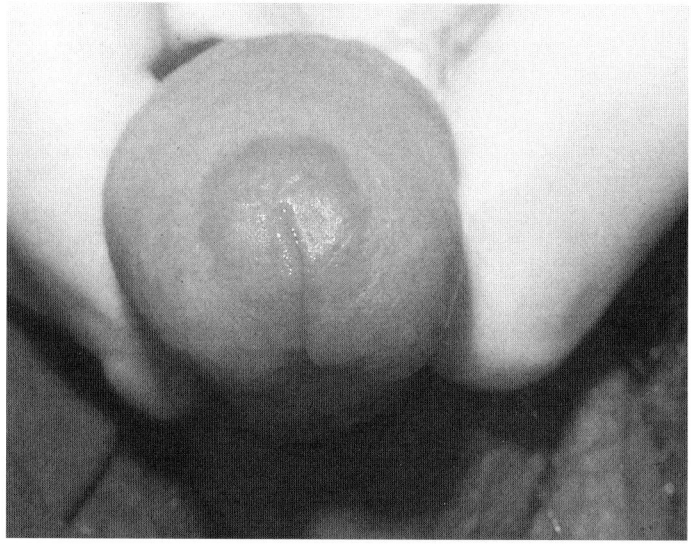

**Fig. 32.** Erythroplasia of Queyrat. *In situ* SCC presenting as velvety red plaque on glans and periurethral skin. The tumor extended proximally on the urethral mucosa (photograph courtesy of Kenneth Angermeier, MD). *See* color plate following p. 338.

and to rule out invasive SCC. Nonsurgical approaches to treatment are 5-fluorouracil cream or radiation. Other options include carbon-dioxide laser ablation, excision, circumcision, electrosurgery, and Moh's micrographic surgery. Lesions that recur after treatment should be biopsied, because an inflammatory dermatitis or invasive SCC can develop at the same site. Importantly, the recent application of podophyllin to condyloma acuminata may cause histologic changes similar to SCC *in situ.*

*Invasive SCC* on the penis may present as erythematous patches or plaques that ulcerate early or papillary tumors on the glans that slowly enlarge and eventually

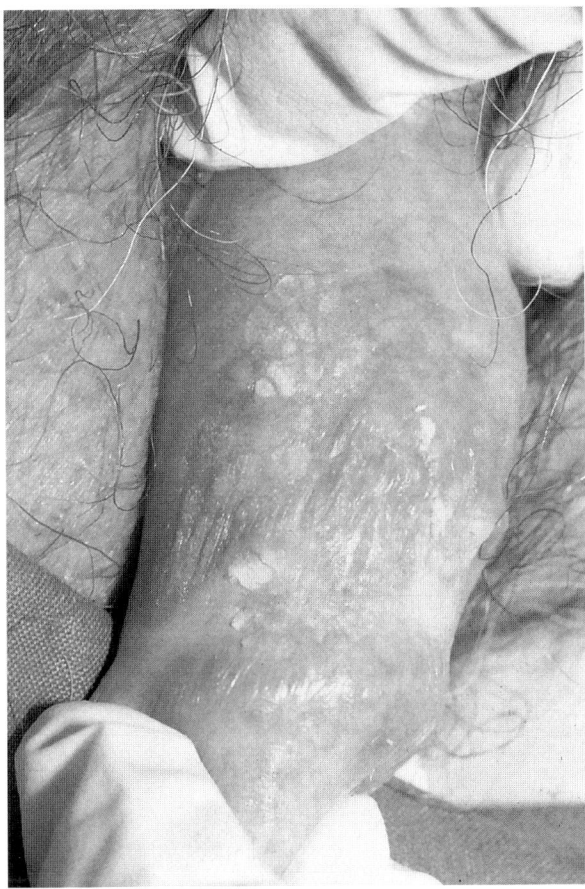

**Fig. 33.** Erythroplasia of Queyrat. *In situ* SCC of prepucial skin and glans presenting as chronically inflamed red plaque with verrucous foci. *See* color plate following p. 338.

ulcerate (*see* Fig. 31). Primary penile SCC most frequently arises on the glans, but may occur in any location on the penis. Early symptoms include pruritus or burning under the foreskin, which may be followed by pain, discharge, bleeding, voiding difficulties, and phimosis. Approximately one-half of penile SCC patients have palpable lymphadenopathy at the time of diagnosis, and 20% have nonpalpable nodal metastases. Treatment options for the primary tumor are the same as for *in situ* SCC, excluding topical therapy. Mohs micrographic surgery is the most tissue-sparing treatment for the invasive SCC, but still may be disfiguring. Lymphadenectomy is indicated for treatment of metastatic disease.

Squamous-cell carcinoma of the scrotum is far less common than SCC of the penis. Etiologic factors include exposure to inorganic arsenic, HPV, tar, paraffin, shale oil, and petroleum products. Clinically, patients present with a slow-growing, painless nodule that may ulcerate and become painful. The recommended treatment is wide excision and lymphadenectomy for proven metastatic disease.

*Verrucous carcinoma* (*see* Fig. 34), also named the Buschke-Löwenstein tumor, is a low-grade SCC of the glans penis that occurs predominantly in uncircumcised middle-

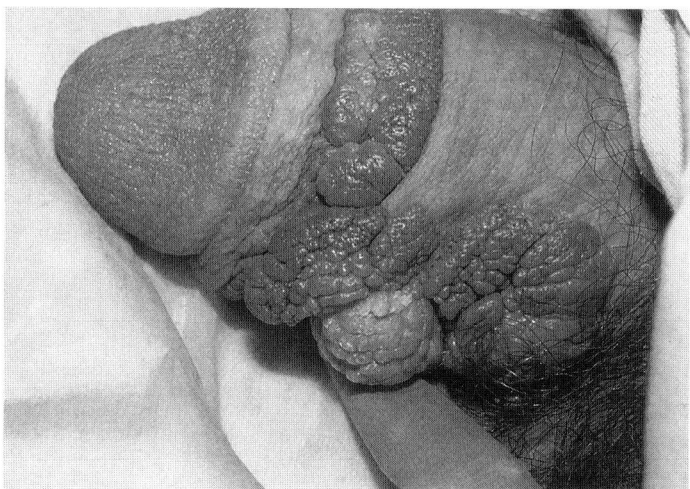

**Fig. 34.** Verrucous carcinoma (Buschke-Löwenstein tumor). Large, cauliflower-like tumor of penile shaft. *See* color plate following p. 338.

aged men. These are exophytic, cauliflower-like locally invasive tumors that occur on the glans or anogenital mucosa and may require a deep biopsy to differentiate them from a large condyloma. Patients frequently have a history of ulceration, balanitis, or phimosis. Human papilloma virus (HPV) types 6 and 11 may play a role in the pathogenesis of Buschke-Löwenstein tumors. Radiation therapy may predispose patients to metastatic disease, which is otherwise rare. These tumors can reach enormous sizes, and have a tendency to recur, even after extensive wide excision.

*Bowenoid papulosis* (*see* Fig. 35) is an HPV-related variant of SCC *in situ.* The pathology is similar, but with a more random pattern of atypical keratinocytes. The most commonly associated HPV types are 16, 18, 32, and 33. These papules may be flesh-colored, white, red, or hyperpigmented, and are typically found in young adults on the penis and scrotum. Differential diagnosis includes psoriasis, lichen planus, and warts. Most occurrences follow a benign course or regress without invasion. Treatment is similar to condyloma, including close follow-up and local destructive methods, such as liquid nitrogen, vesicants, or carbon-dioxide laser ablation. Treatment is required, because female sexual partners can develop cervical carcinoma.

*Pseudoepitheliomatous keratotic* and *micaceous balanitis (PKMB)* is a rare papulosquamous dermatitis of the glans in elderly men. It presents as a white-to-gold, scaly, well-demarcated plaque that may extend proximally on the corona and distal shaft as it slowly grows. Symptoms include pain, phimosis, and interference with sexual activity. Early excision is the recommended treatment because of the potential for malignant degeneration. Biopsy is needed for diagnosis, and shows variable degrees of epidermal atypia. PKMB is now considered a premalignant condition, and has been associated with SCC, verrucous carcinoma, and fibrosarcoma. Early excision is the recommended treatment.

*Basal-cell carcinomas* (*BCCs*) of the genitalia are exceedingly rare, with an unclear pathogenesis, although chronic inflammation and prior exposure to ionizing radiation have been implicated. To date, no link to HPV DNA has been found in genital BCCs.

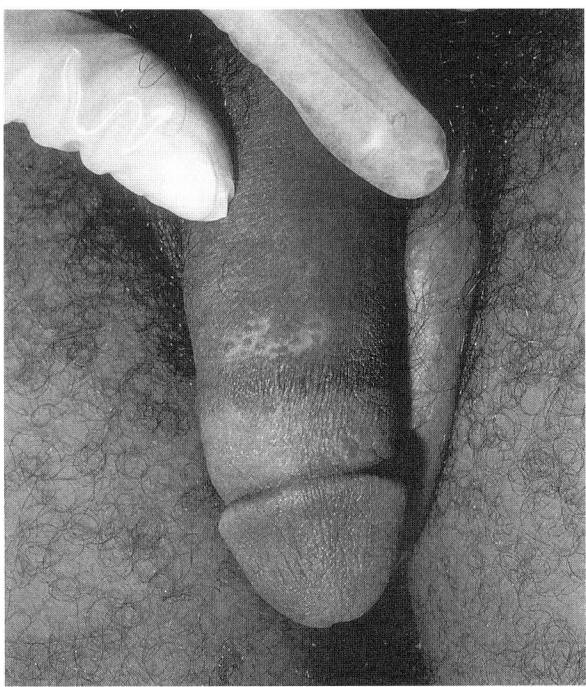

**Fig. 35.** Bowenoid papulosis. Recurrent flesh-colored papules in the area of previous liquid nitrogen cryotherapy (photograph courtesy of Charles Camisa, MD). *See* color plate following p. 338.

Genital BCCs present in similar clinical and pathologic forms as sun-exposed skin, and tend to be larger at the time of diagnosis. The most common site for penile BCC is the shaft, followed by the prepuce and the circumcised glans penis. Metastases have been reported from vulvar and scrotal BCCs. Treatment options include wide excision, Mohs micrographic surgery, and radiation therapy.

*Melanoma* of the penis is rare, and represents approx 1% of all penile cancers. It presents most commonly as an enlarging pigmented papule or nodule that may ulcerate. Patients are usually diagnosed in the sixth to seventh decades of life. Approximately 40–60% of patients have metastatic disease at the time of diagnosis and, therefore need a full metastatic workup as well as surgical excision. The most common histologic type of penile melanoma is acral-lentiginous melanoma. Distal amputation is usually performed for melanoma of the glans with a margin of 1–3 cm, depending on tumor thickness.

*Kaposi's sarcoma* (*see* Fig. 36) has become much more common since the HIV epidemic. Kaposi's sarcoma is a proliferation of vascular endothelial cells caused by human herpes virus 8. Lesions on the penis and scrotum are common, and are clinically violaceous or brown macules, papules, or plaques that can occasionally cause local edema or obstruction. Treatment may be cosmetic or functional, and includes cryosurgery, radiation, laser coagulation, electrocoagulation, or intralesional injection of vinblastine.

*Extramammary Paget's disease* (*see* Fig. 37) is a rare, slow-growing, epithelial neoplasm that classically involves the apocrine-gland-bearing skin of the perianal skin,

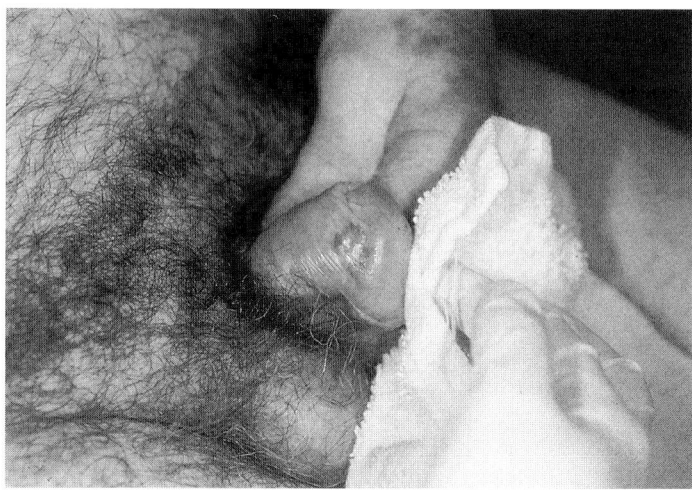

**Fig. 36.** Kaposi's sarcoma. Violaceous plaque on glans. *See* color plate following p. 338.

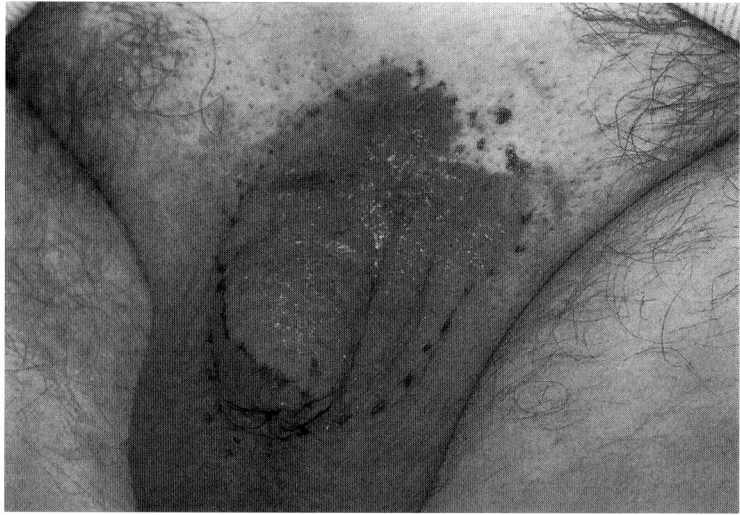

**Fig. 37.** Extramammary Paget's disease. Scaly, erythematous plaques with erosions on suprapubic skin, scrotum, and foreskin. *See* color plate following p. 338.

penis, axilla, or vulva. It is three times more prevalent in women. A few cases have been reported to occur on the glans, and each has been associated with an underlying genitourinary malignancy. Clinically, the well-demarcated brown or red scaly plaques can look eczematous or infectious. If these lesions are treated as such and do not respond, a biopsy is essential. Paget cells are seen scattered throughout the epidermis, and most stain with antisera to carcinoembryonic antigen. These cells are large, with abundant cytoplasm and large central nuclei. Moh's micrographic surgery has a lower recurrence rate than wide excision (23 vs 33%). Radiation therapy is an option if the

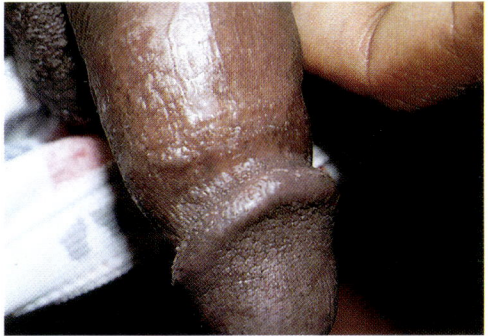

**Fig. 1.** Pearly penile papules. Flesh-colored tiny papules circumferentially around the corona.

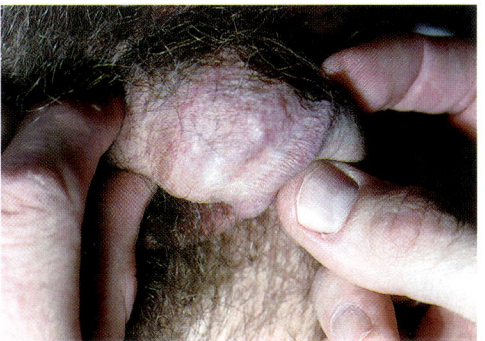

**Fig. 3.** Sclerosing lymphangitis. Firm subcutaneous nontender cord parallel to the corona on the distal penile shaft.

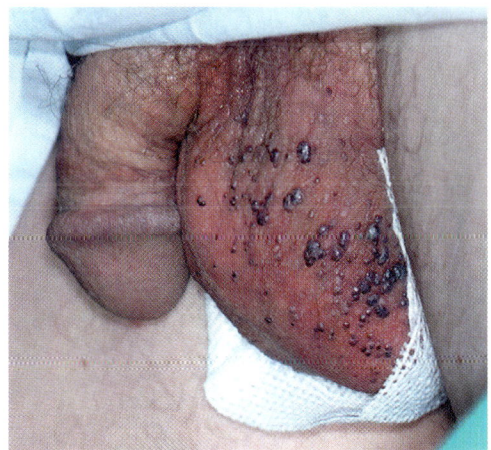

**Fig. 4.** Angiokeratomas of Fordyce. Variably-sized purple vascular papules of the scrotum.

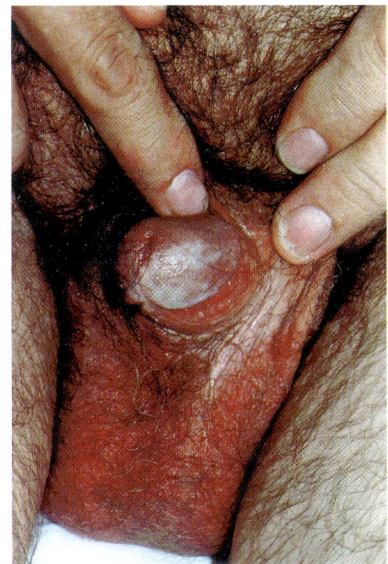

**Fig. 5.** Lichen sclerosis et atrophicus. Bluish-white atrophic plaque of the glans.

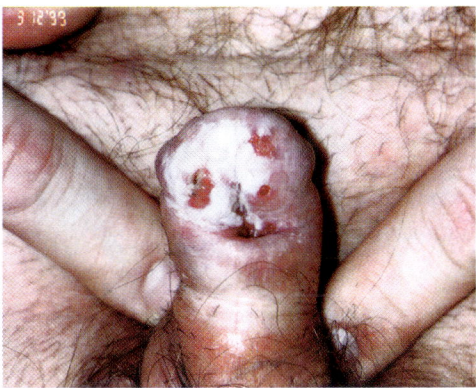

**Fig. 6.** Chronic lichen sclerosis et atrophicus with foci of invasive SCC, in a patient who underwent urethral meatotomy, and later, distal ventral urethrectomy.

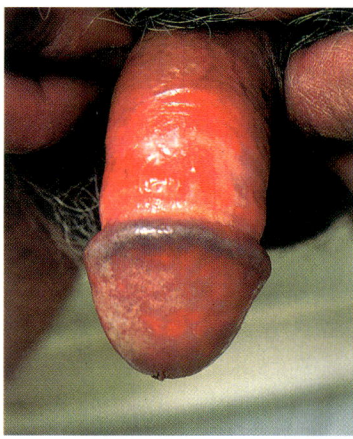

**Fig. 7.** Balanoposthitis. Inflammation of the glans and prepuce.

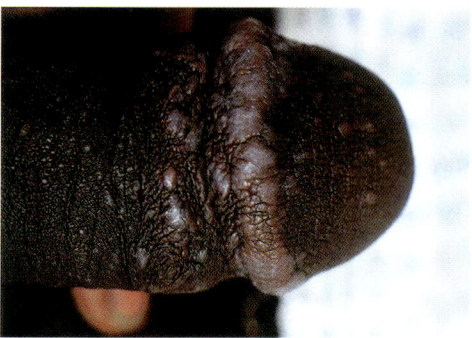

**Fig. 12.** Lichen planus. Purple polygonal papules and plaques on glans, corona, and distal shaft.

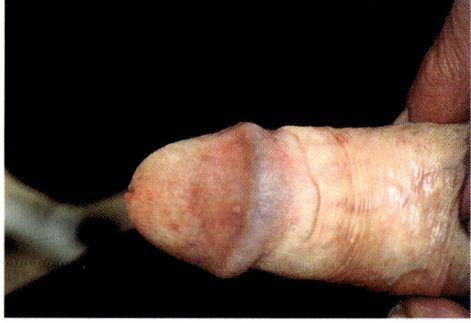

**Fig. 14.** Zoon's balanitis. Smooth, red-orange plaque on glans.

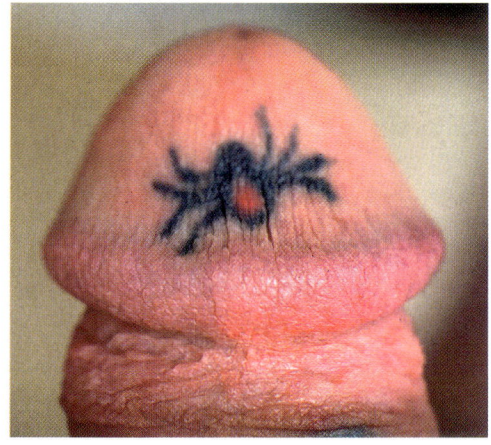

**Fig. 16.** Decorative tattoo of the glans (photograph courtesy of S. Teri McGillis, MD).

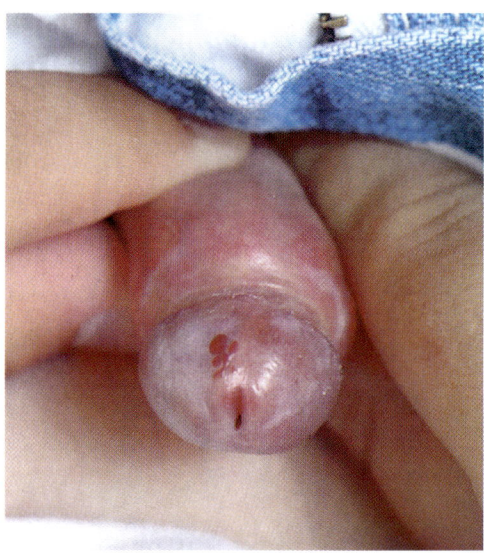

**Fig. 28.** Capillary hemangioma of glans in a child. Grouped, red vascular papules.

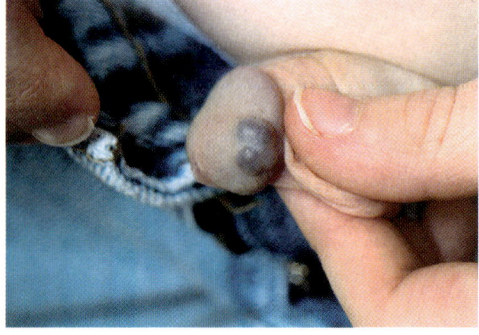

**Fig. 29.** Capillary hemangioma of glans. Purple, compressible blanchable soft nodule.

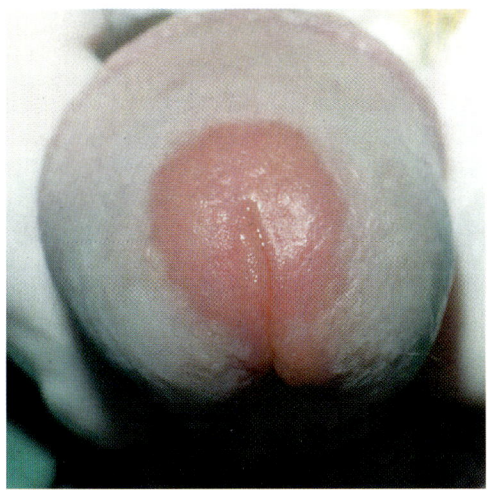

**Fig. 32.** Erythroplasia of Queyrat. *In situ* SCC presenting as velvety red plaque on glans and periurethral skin. The tumor extended proximally on the urethral mucosa (photograph courtesy of Kenneth Angermeier, MD).

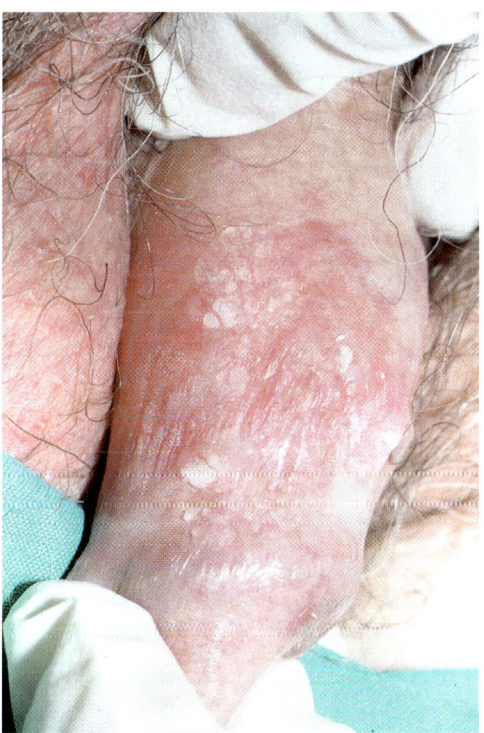

**Fig. 33.** Erythroplasia of Queyrat. *In situ* SCC of prepucial skin and glans presenting as chronically inflamed red plaque with verrucous foci.

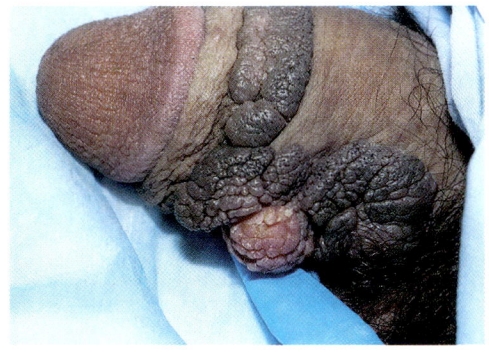

**Fig. 34.** Verrucous carcinoma (Buschke-Löwenstein tumor). Large, cauliflower-like tumor of penile shaft.

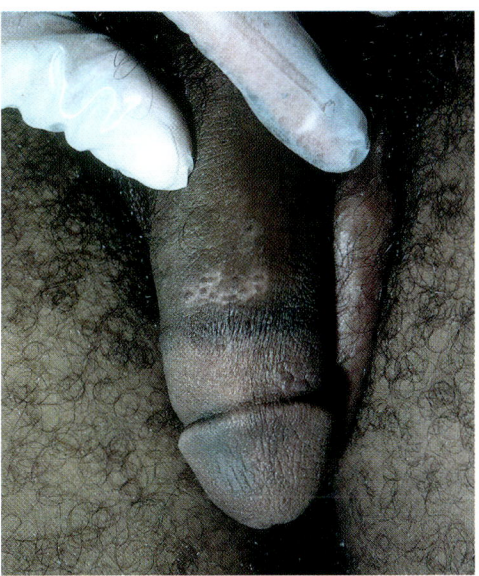

**Fig. 35.** Bowenoid papulosis. Recurrent flesh-colored papules in the area of previous liquid nitrogen cryotherapy (photograph courtesy of Charles Camisa, MD).

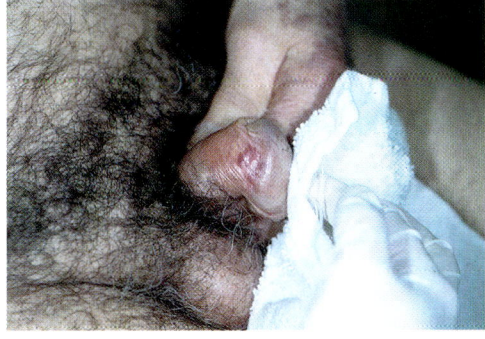

**Fig. 36.** Kaposi's sarcoma. Violaceous plaque on glans.

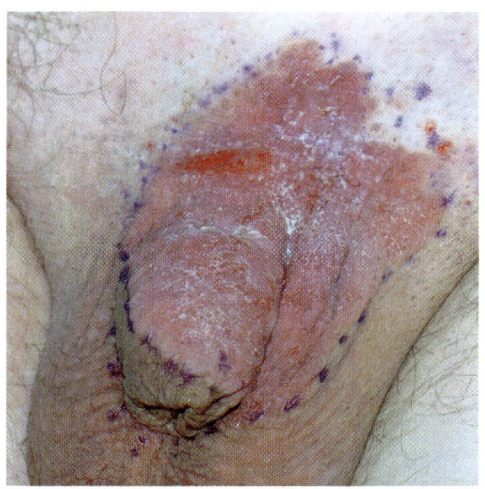

**Fig. 37.** Extramammary Paget's disease. Scaly, erythematous plaques with erosions on suprapubic skin, scrotum, and foreskin.

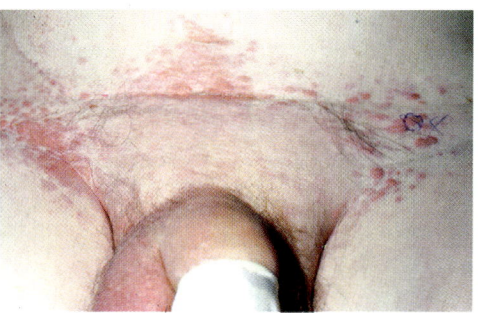

**Fig. 38.** Metastatic prostate carcinoma. Discrete and confluent pink papules and plaques of lower abdomen, suprapubic skin, and inguinal creases.

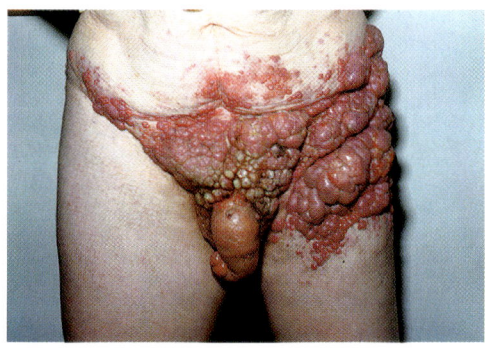

**Fig. 39.** Metastatic prostate carcinoma. Massive erythematous tumors and nodules of lower abdomen, genitalia, and thigh (photograph courtesy of Kenneth Tomecki, MD).

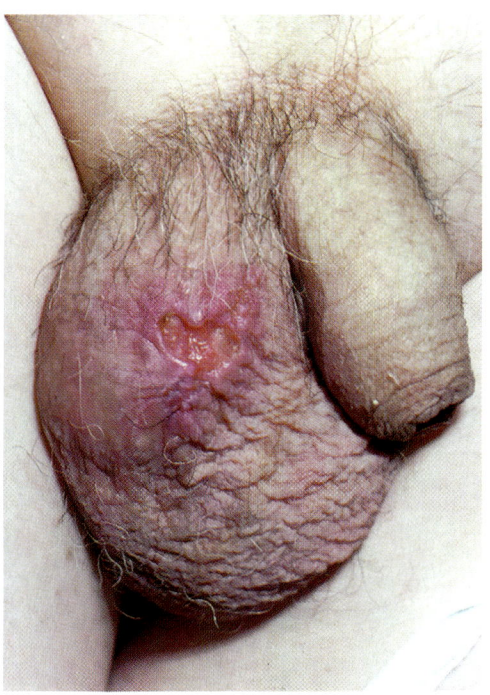

**Fig. 40.** Metastatic SCC of the lung to the scrotum. Ill-defined erythematous plaque with central, undertermined ulcer.

Chapter 24 / Practical Dermatology 339

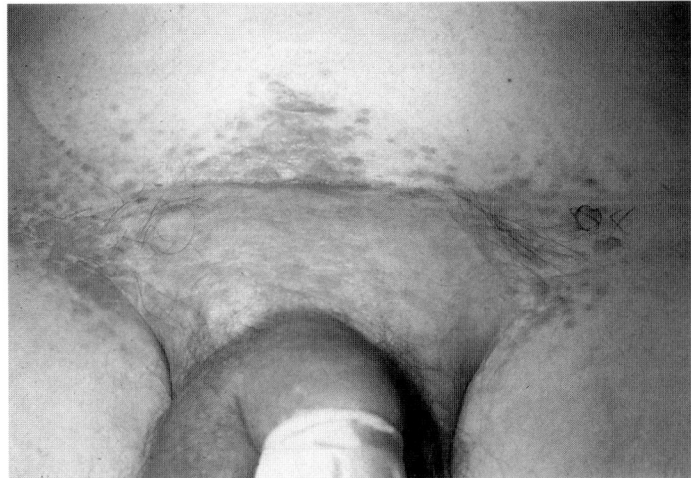

**Fig. 38.** Metastatic prostate carcinoma. Discrete and confluent pink papules and plaques of lower abdomen, suprapubic skin, and inguinal creases. *See* color plate following p. 338.

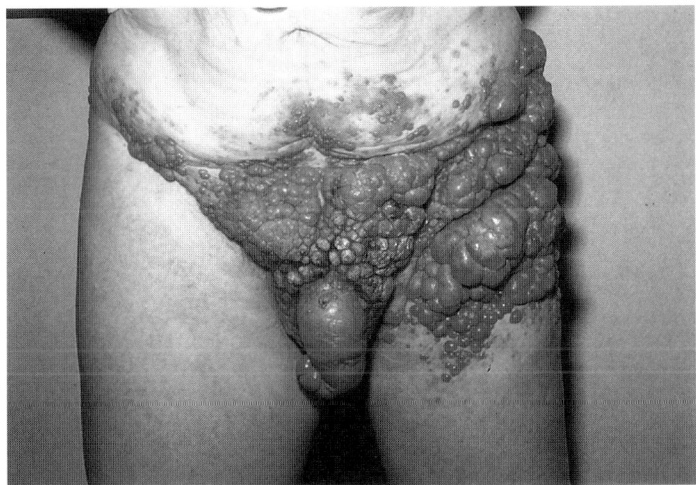

**Fig. 39.** Metastatic prostate carcinoma. Massive erythematous tumors and nodules of lower abdomen, genitalia, and thigh (photograph courtesy of Kenneth Tomecki, MD). *See* color plate following p. 338.

patient is not a surgical candidate. Metastases to regional lymph nodes occur late in the course of the disease. Identification and treatment of the associated underlying malignancy—which is present in up to 25% of cases—is essential.

*Metastatic tumors to the penis* are relatively rare. The most common primary sites are the genitourinary and gastrointestinal tracts. Clinical presentations include erythematous-to-violaceous papules or nodules (*see* Figs. 38, 39) or ulcers (*see* Fig. 40). Stasis and priaprism may occur secondary to metastases to the corpora cavernosum.

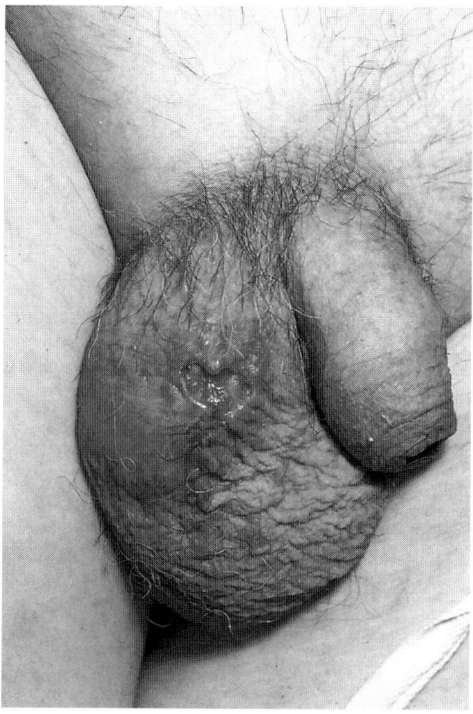

**Fig. 40.** Metastatic SCC of the lung to the scrotum. Ill-defined erythematous plaque with central, undermined ulcer. *See* color plate following p. 338.

## SELECTED READING

Arnt AA, LeBoit PE, Robinson JK, Wintroub BU, eds., (1996) *Cutaneous Medicine and Surgery*. Philadelphia: WB Saunders.

Bour J, Steinhart G (1984) Penile necrosis in patients with diabetes mellitus and end-stage renal disease. *J Urol* 132:560, 561.

Broughton G (1996) Management of the brown recluse spider bite to the glans penis. *Mil Med* 161(10):627–629.

Cohen HA, Barzilai A, Matalon A, Harel L, Gross S (1997) Fixed drug eruption of the penis due to hydroxyzine hydrochloride. *Ann Pharmacother* 31(3):327–329.

Coldiron BM, Goldsmith BA, Robinson JK (1991) Surgical treatment of extramammary Paget's disease. A report of six cases and a re-examination of Mohs micrographic surgery compared with conventional surgical excision. *Cancer* 67:933–938.

English JC III, Laws RA, Keough GC, Wilde JL, Foley JP, Elston DM (1997) Dermatoses of the glans penis and prepuce. *J Am Acad Dermatol* 37:1–24.

English JC, King DH, Foley JP (1998) Penile shaft hypopigmentation: lichen sclerosis occurring after the initiation of aloprostadil intracavernous injections for erectile dysfunction. *J Am Acad Dermatol* 39:801–803.

Fisher BK, Margesson LJ (1998) *Genital Skin Disorders. Diagnosis and Treatment*. St. Louis: Mosby, pp. 3–96.

Kato N, Matsue K, Sotodate A, Tomita Y (1996) Extramammary Paget's disease with distant skin metastasis. *J Dermatol* 23(6):408–414.

Konety BR, Cooper T, Flood HD, Futrell JW (1996) Scrotal elephantiasis associated with hidradenitis suppurativa. *Plast Reconstr Surg* 97(6):1243–1245.

Ladocsi LT, Siebert CF Jr, Rickert RR, Fletcher HS (1998) Basal cell carcinoma of the penis. *Cutis* 1(1):25–27.

Margolis DJ (1998) Cutaneous Diseases of the Male External Genitalia. In: PC Walsh, et al., eds., *Campbell's Urology*, Philadelphia: WB Saunders Co. pp. 717–732.

McKee PH (1996) *Pathology of the Skin with Clinical Correlations.* Barcelona: Times Mirror International Publishers, Ltd.

Mohsin SK, Lee MW, Amin MB, Stoler MH, Eyzaguirre E, Ma CK, Zarbo RJ (1998) Cutaneous verruciform xanthoma: a report of five cases investigating the etiology and nature of xanthomatous cells. *Am J Surg Pathol* 22(4):479–487.

Nagore E, Sanchez-Motilla JM, Febrer MI, Aliaga A (1997) Median raphe cysts of the penis: A report of five cases. *Pediatr Dermatol* 14(2):129, 130.

Nehal KS, Levine VJ, Ashinoff R (1998) Basal cell carcinoma of the genitalia. *Dermatol Surg* 24:1361–1363.

Schwartz RA (1995) Verrucous carcinoma of the skin and mucosa [published erratum appears in *J Am Acad Dermatol* May 1995; 32(5 Pt 1): 710] [see comments]. *J Am Acad Dermatol* 32(1):1–21.

Smith JH, von Lichtenburg F (1996) Parasitic diseases of the genitourinary system. In: Gillenwater JY et al., eds., *Adult and Pediatric Urology,* St. Louis: Mosby pp. 733–768.

Sanchez MH, Sanchez SR (1997) Pyoderma gangrenosum of penile skin. *Int J Dermatol* 36:634–639.

# 25 Erectile Dysfunction

*Drogo K. Montague, MD*
*and Milton M. Lakin, MD*

**CONTENTS**
    INTRODUCTION
    CLINICAL EVALUATION OF THE MAN WITH ED
    TREATMENT OF ASSOCIATED DISORDERS
    IDENTIFICATION OF ASSOCIATED DISORDERS
    TREATMENT OF ERECTILE DYSFUNCTION
    SELECTED READING

## INTRODUCTION

Erectile dysfunction (ED), the inability of a man to achieve and maintain an erection, is often classified as psychogenic, organic, or mixed. Although ED can exist for only psychogenic reasons, organic ED is almost always associated with some degree of psychogenic dysfunction; thus, nonpsychogenic ED is actually mixed. In the past, when the principal treatment for ED was penile prosthesis implantation, the distinction between psychogenic and organic or mixed ED was of considerable importance. Since many of today's treatment options are nonsurgical, this distinction is less critical. For men who are contemplating surgical treatment, such as penile prosthesis implantation, however, it is still desirable to exclude temporary or potentially reversible forms of erectile impairment, such as psychogenic ED. Erectile dysfunction must also be distinguished from other sexual disorders, such as decreased libido, premature or retarded ejaculation, painful erections or orgasm, and erectile deformity. Of course, any of these disorders may coexist.

The Massachusetts male aging study (MMAS) was a community-based survey of 1290 men ages 40–70. In this survey, ED was classified as mild, moderate, or complete. There was a 52% probability of the presence of some degree of ED across all age categories. The overall incidence of any degree of ED at age 40 was 39%, and it increased with each decade to reach 67% at age 70. Extrapolating these data, there are an estimated 30 million men in the United States who experience some degree of erectile impairment.

ED clearly increases with age, but is it an inevitable consequence of aging? Since normal erectile function is known to persist in healthy men well into advanced age,

From: *Current Clinical Urology: Office Urology: The Clinician's Guide*
Edited by: E. D. Kursh and J. C. Ulchaker © Humana Press Inc., Totowa, NJ

Table 1
Treatment Options for ED

| 1970s | 1990s |
|---|---|
| Sex therapy | Sex therapy |
| Penile prostheses | Systemic therapy |
|  | Vacuum constriction devices |
|  | Intraurethral pharmacotherapy |
|  | Penile injections |
|  | Penile prostheses |
|  | Vascular surgery |

Table 2
Diagnostic Testing for ED

| 1970s | 1990s |
|---|---|
| NPT testing | NPT testing |
|  | Diagnostic penile injections |
|  | Duplex ultrasonography |
|  | Cavernosometry |
|  | Cavernosography |
|  | Arteriography |

the increase in ED seen with aging is considered to be the result of age-related diseases, such as atherosclerosis, diabetes, and other poorly understood factors. Although erectile function persists in healthy men of all ages, the clinician should be aware of some age-related changes in male sexual function. As men age, there is usually a decrease in libido. Erections require more direct stimulation of the external genitalia. The force and volume of ejaculation decrease with age, and the latency period—defined as the time from an orgasm to the time at which the man can achieve another erection—increases with age. With aging, difficulty in reaching orgasm is also sometimes experienced.

The selection of a treatment for ED in the 1970s was relatively simple. Sex therapy was the treatment of choice for psychogenic ED, and penile prosthesis implantation was the only reasonable treatment option for organic or mixed ED. Today, a variety of treatment choices are available, including sex therapy, systemic therapy, vacuum constriction devices, intraurethral pharmacotherapy, penile injections, penile prosthesis implantation, and vascular surgery (see Table 1). Likewise, diagnostic testing has evolved from nocturnal penile tumescence (NPT) testing in the 1970s to testing in the 1990s, which includes: NPT testing, diagnostic intracavernous injections, duplex ultrasonography, cavernosometry, cavernosography, and penile arteriography (see Table 2).

We will address the following questions: What is the purpose of the diagnostic evaluation for ED? How much evaluation is necessary? Which specialized tests, if any, should be performed? We will also discuss the indications, risks, and benefits of the various treatment options for ED.

| Table 3 |
| --- |
| Rationale for ED Evaluation |
| Verify chief complaint |
| Uncover underlying disorders |
| Exclude reversible ED in surgical candidate |
| Satisfy some patients' need to know |

## CLINICAL EVALUATION OF THE MAN WITH ED

Many of the treatment options for ED work regardless of etiology, thereby fostering the concept of "the patient's goal-directed approach to therapy." The purpose of the evaluation of ED (*see* Table 3) therefore is not primarily for treatment selection, but instead to verify the chief complaint (for example, some men presenting with apparent ED actually have premature ejaculation), to identify significant underlying diseases or risk factors, and to exclude temporary or reversible disorders in men who are candidates for surgical therapy. An additional reason for the ED evaluation is that some men need to know what might be causing their problem.

### *Sexual History*

The evaluation should begin with the patient's chief complaint and sexual history. Immediately addressing the problem in a straightforward manner helps put the patient at ease. If the chief complaint is a problem with erections, when did it begin? Was the onset sudden or gradual? The sudden onset of ED in the absence of a precipitating cause (eg, surgery or trauma) suggests a psychogenic etiology. Does the patient have a problem achieving or maintaining erections, or both? Is the ED global, or does it vary with different partners or in different circumstances (for example, in masturbation vs in sex with a partner)? Erections that vary in different situations suggest a psychogenic cause. In terms of firmness on a scale of 0–10, how does the man rate his best erection? What percentage of coital attempts are successful? The history should proceed to a sexual review of symptoms, including libido, orgasm, and ejaculation (normal, premature, or retarded), pain with erection or at orgasm, and erectile deformity.

The man's relationship with his partner or partners, if any, should be explored. Other than the sexual dysfunction, are there any significant relationship conflicts? Are there any other significant sources of stress in the man's life? When possible, the above information should be confirmed by an interview with the partner. Finally, any previous evaluation or treatment should be explored.

### *Medical History*

A complete medical history should be taken, including past and present illnesses, operations, radiation treatment, and injuries. In addition to a review of systems, a list of medications, illicit drugs, smoking habits, and alcohol use is made.

### *Physical Examination*

A physical examination is performed, with particular attention to secondary sex characteristics, blood pressure, cardiovascular and peripheral pulses, the abdomen, external genitalia, prostate, bulbocavernosus reflex, and lower-extremity motor and sensory exams.

## *Laboratory Studies*

Laboratory tests complete the initial evaluation, and are conducted to help screen for risk factors that may contribute to the ED. A complete blood count, SMA profile, serum testosterone and prolactin, and urinalysis are done. Depending on the results of the history and physical examination, the following additional studies may be ordered: lipid profile, EKG, glucose tolerance test, or hemoglobin A1C, PSA, and thyroid studies. If the screening serum testosterone is low, a repeat total testosterone and a free testosterone and luteinizing hormone (LH) are obtained.

## TREATMENT OF ASSOCIATED DISORDERS

### *Relationship Conflict and Depression*

After the evaluation, the patient—and, whenever possible, his partner—should meet with the urologist to discuss the results of the initial evaluation and to choose a treatment option. If a conflict in the patient–partner relationship is present, focusing exclusively on ED treatment is unlikely to be successful. We would refer this couple for marital therapy. If the ED is associated with signs of depression, which include loss of libido, sleep disturbances, unexplained weight gain or loss, fatigue, and loss of interest in usual activities, referral to a psychiatrist may be indicated.

### *Hypogonadism*

Signs and symptoms of hypogonadism include decreased libido, low ejaculate volume, difficulty achieving and maintaining erections, decreased testicular size, and decreased secondary sex characteristics. Hypogonadism can be suspected when one or more of these factors are present; however, unless hypogonadism is long-standing, a diagnosis based on clinical signs and symptoms is often difficult. For this reason, we believe that most men with erectile dysfunction should have a serum testosterone determination as part of the initial screening evaluation.

Since serum testosterone varies significantly throughout the day, a low serum testosterone should be confirmed by repeat determination. At the time that the repeat total testosterone is ordered, a free serum testosterone and LH should also be ordered. A low total and free serum testosterone together with high values for serum LH suggests that the problem is testicular failure (primary or hypergonadotropic hypogonadism). A low serum testosterone together with low or normal values for serum LH suggests that the hypogonadism is caused by pituitary disease (secondary or hypogonadotropic hypogonadism). In this case, an MRI or sector CT scan of the sella turcica should be obtained to see if a pituitary mass is present.

When present, hypogonadism is treated by parenteral testosterone or by testosterone skin patches. The patches have the advantage of providing a more uniform level of hormone replacement, but they are often associated with skin rashes and irritation. We give testosterone enanthate im either every 2 wk (200 mg) or every 3 wk (300 mg). Oral forms of testosterone are either not reliably absorbed or are potentially hepatotoxic. Testosterone replacement in the hypogonadal male generally results in increased libido, better erections, and increased ejaculatory volume. We find that hypogonadism is associated with erectile dysfunction in only 3–5% of our cases.

### *Hyperprolactinemia*

Hyperprolactinemia in men is associated with low sexual desire and/or erectile dysfunction; gynecomastia and galactorrhea are rare. Men with hyperprolactinemia usually have low levels of serum testosterone; however, serum testosterone sometimes will be within the normal range. For this reason, we usually obtain both serum testosterone and serum prolactin as part of the initial screening evaluation. Pituitary micro- and occasionally macro adenomas are frequent etiologic factors as are medication, hypothyroidism, renal disease, and other systemic illnesses. Hyperprolactinemia may also be associated with hypothyroidism. The prevalence of hyperprolactinemia in men is still unknown; however, this disorder occurs much less frequently than hypogonadism.

Normal male levels of serum prolactin are below 20 ng/mL. Levels between 20 and 50 ng/mL are indeterminate, whereas levels above 50 ng/mL suggest excessive prolactin release. Serum prolactin levels above 100 ng/mL are usually associated with pituitary adenomas.

Testosterone replacement therapy in men with ED who have hyperprolactinemia is usually not effective. Bromocriptine, a dopaminergic agonist, given in doses of 7.5–25 mg daily, usually corrects prolactin hypersecretion, reduces pituitary size, and restores normal sexual function. When hyperprolactinemia is associated with use of certain medications, withdrawal of the drug(s) will treat the disorder. Hyperprolactinemia associated with hypothyroidism is usually effectively treated by thyroid replacement.

### *Sleep Disorders*

Sleep disorders in men can also be associated with ED. The probability of a sleep disorder being present increases if the man is obese, hypertensive, or if he has a history of loud snoring, excessive daytime sleepiness, or morning headaches. When a sleep disorder is suspected, referral to a sleep-disorder clinic is indicated. Successful treatment may improve the patient's quality of life and reduce the chance of motor vehicle accidents, and it may also may relieve the ED.

### *Prescription Medications, Alcohol Abuse, Smoking, and Illicit Drug Use*

Erectile Dysfunction is sometimes associated with the onset of a new medication. Many medications have been known to be associated with ED; and it is usually prudent, if possible, to change the medication to see if the ED resolves. In our experience, ED in this setting often persists, and then treatment of the ED *per se* should be considered. Alcohol abuse, smoking, and illicit drug use may also be associated with ED, and these issues should be addressed.

### *Psychogenic ED*

Sex therapy may be selected as the initial treatment option if the cause of the sexual dysfunction is believed to be primarily psychogenic. For psychogenic erectile dysfunction, the therapist teaches the couple sensate focus and other exercises designed to reduce performance anxiety and to restore pleasure to the sexual act by focusing attention on pleasurable sensations and not on whether an erection is present. Sex therapy can be particularly helpful in the treatment of premature ejaculation. The therapist teaches the man or the couple either the squeeze or the stop-start technique. Using this method, the man learns to recognize the point of ejaculatory inevitability, thus gaining control over ejaculation.

Sex therapists also evaluate the quality of the couple relationship. Sexual dysfunction may be a manifestation of an underlying relationship disturbance. Sex therapy will not be helpful under these circumstances, and the sex therapist will recommend couple therapy. When depression or other psychiatric disorders are present, the sex therapist will recommend psychiatric consultation for appropriate treatment.

The sex therapist should work with the urologist as a team. Treatment options for sexual dysfunction are not mutually exclusive, and they should more often be combined. When penile prosthesis implantation is planned, for example, the couple may benefit from a preoperative evaluation and counseling session with the sex therapist as well as one or two postoperative counseling sessions. This helps to ensure that the couple has realistic expectations regarding outcomes, and it helps them resume sexual activity using a prosthesis.

## IDENTIFICATION OF ASSOCIATED DISORDERS

The initial ED evaluation should also reveal significant underlying disorders that are frequently associated with ED. Examples of these include hypertension, coronary artery disease, peripheral vascular disease, and diabetes mellitus. Although treatment of these disorders is unlikely to help resolve the ED, it is still important to help prevent other complications.

## TREATMENT OF ERECTILE DYSFUNCTION

After the initial evaluation and treatment of any of the associated disorders identified here, the algorithm in Fig. 1 may be followed. For the man who wishes to learn more about the etiology of his ED, nocturnal penile tumescence (NPT) testing and duplex ultrasound (DUS) examination are often indicated. For the man who is willing to accept empiric treatment, the use of the oral agent sildenafil citrate is considered. The sequence of treatment options is shown in Table 4.

### *Sildenafil Citrate*

Nitric oxide (NO) released by sexual stimulation results in the formation of cyclic guanosine monophosphate (cGMP), which causes the arterial dilation and cavernosal smooth-muscle relaxation needed for erection. Sildenafil citrate (Viagra; Pfizer, Inc., New York, NY), is an oral type-5 phosphodiesterase inhibitor that acts primarily in the corpus cavernosum to block the breakdown of cGMP. Because of its effects on the NO/cGMP pathway, sildenafil citrate can help many men with ED to achieve and maintain a better erection in response to sexual stimulation. Although sildenafil is effective for ED of diverse etiologies, it is less effective in severe vascular insufficiency, diabetes mellitus, and after nonnerve-sparing radical prostatectomy.

Because sildenafil citrate potentiates the hypotensive effects of nitrates, its use in men who take any form of nitrates is strictly contraindicated. Sildenafil citrate is available in 25-, 50-, and 100-mg tablets. The usual starting dose is 50 mg, taken 1–2 h before coitus. If this is not effective, the dose may be increased to 100 mg. Use more than once daily is not advised. A starting dose of 25 mg is recommended for the elderly,

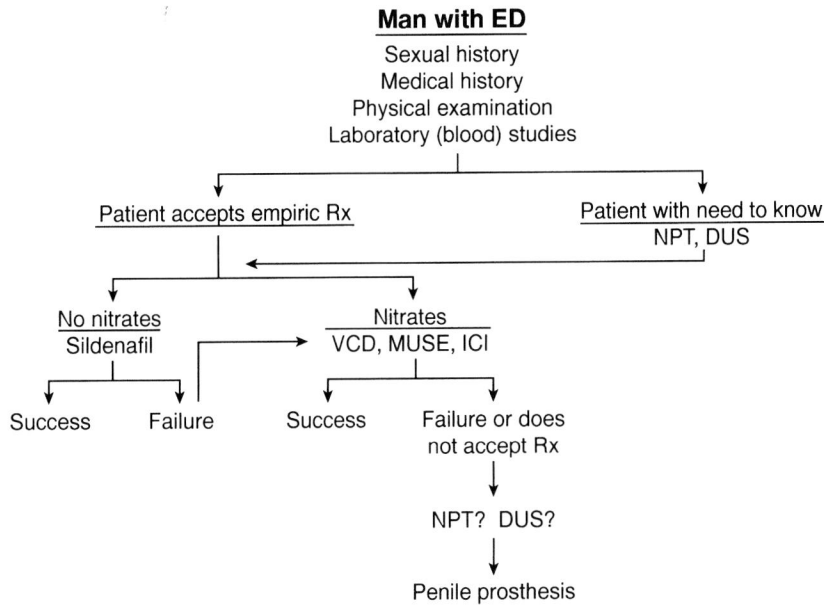

**Fig. 1.** Management of erectile dysfunction.

Table 4
Treatment Options for ED

Treatment of associated disorders
    Relationship conflict, depression
    Hypogonadism, hyperprolactinemia
    Sleep disorders
    Prescription medicines, alcohol, smoking, illicit drugs
    Psychogenic ED (sex therapy)
First-line therapies for ED
    Oral sildenafil citrate
    Oral or sublingual phentolamine (investigational)
    Oral apomorphine (investigational)
Second-line therapies for ED
    Vacuum constriction devices
    Intraurethral pharmacotherapy
    Intracavernous injection therapy
Third-line therapies for ED
    Penile prosthesis implantation
    Vascular surgery

for men with renal or hepatic insufficiency, or for men taking erythromycin, cimetidine, ketoconazole, or itraconazole. Side effects include headaches (16%), flushing (11%), dyspepsia (7%), and visual disturbances (3%).

### *Investigational Systemic Agents*

Other systemic agents currently in phase III clinical trials include an alpha-adrenergic blocker (oral or sublingual phentolamine) and a centrally acting agent (oral apomorphine). Because sildenafil, phentolamine, and apomorphine all have different mechanisms of action, future directions for ED treatment may include combination systemic drug therapy.

## Vacuum Constriction Devices

In men who cannot use sildenafil citrate because they are taking nitrates, or who reject or fail treatment with sildenafil, the use of second-line treatment options should be considered. The first of these are vacuum constriction devices (VCDs). Several vacuum constriction devices are currently available. Some are manually operated, and some are battery operated.

With vacuum constriction, a plastic chamber is placed over the penis, and the pump is used to create a vacuum, producing an erection-like state that is maintained by a tension band applied to the base of the penis. It is recommended that the tension band be left on no longer than 30 min. The most frequent complaints relating to the use of these devices include lack of spontaneity, insufficient rigidity, pivoting erection, discomfort from the constriction band, blocked ejaculation, and bruising.

## Intraurethral Pharmacotherapy

Drugs introduced into the distal urethra are partially absorbed into the overlying corpora cavernosa. Alprostadil—a form of prostaglandin E1—is formulated as a urethral suppository delivered by a plastic applicator in a product known as MUSE (Vivus, Inc., Menlo Park, CA). Dosage forms include 125, 250, 500, and 1000 µg. Side effects include pain and hypotension. Although the primary advantage of this method of drug delivery to the corporeal bodies is that it avoids the needles associated with intracavernous injection (ICI) therapy, the response rate is considerably less than it is for ICI. Other drugs and drug combinations for intraurethral use are currently under development.

## Intracavernous Injection Therapy (ICI)

Vasoactive drugs injected directly into the corpora, intracavernous injection therapy, and ICI have been used since the mid-1980s. ICI is effective in the treatment of ED of diverse etiologies, and prior to the introduction of sildenafil, ICI was the most widely used ED treatment option. ICI may be useful in situations in which treatment with sildenafil citrate is less successful, such as ED associated with diabetes mellitus or following nonnerve-sparing radical prostatectomy. The drugs most frequently used in ICI are papaverine hydrochloride, phentolamine, mesylate, and prostaglandin E1. These drugs may be used alone or in combination. Side effects include pain, prolonged erection, and fibrosis.

## Penile Prosthesis Implantation

In men who fail treatment with VCDs, MUSE, and ICI, or in men who find these treatment options unacceptable, third-line treatment options should be considered. The first of these is penile prosthesis implantation. Penile prostheses are available in semirigid rod or mechanical devices and in hydraulic or inflatable devices. These devices can be implanted under local anesthesia, but they are most often implanted under spinal or general anesthesia. Outpatient surgery or overnight surgery requiring less than a 24-h stay are most commonly used. Complications include infection, erosion, and mechanical failure. Most complications require additional operative procedures.

## Vascular Surgery

Because of poor long-term results, penile venous ligation surgery is seldom performed today. Likewise, arterial revascularization for older men with atherosclerotic disease has not been proven to be generally effective. However, young men with arteriogenic ED following pelvic or perineal trauma may be suitable candidates for penile arterial revascularization.

## SELECTED READING

Arver S, Dobs AS, Meikle AW, Allen RP, Sanders SW, Mazer NA (1996) Improvement of sexual function in tesetosterone deficient men treated for 1 year with a permeation enhanced testosterone transdermal system. *J Urol* 155:1604–1608.
Buffum J (1992) Prescription drugs and sexual function. *Psychiatr Med* 10:181–198.
Carter JN, Tyson JE, Tolis G, Van Vliet S, Faiman C, Friesen HG (1978) Prolactin-secreting tumors and hypogonadism in 22 men. *N Engl J Med* 299:847–852.
Feldman HA, Goldstein I, Hatzichristou DG, Krane RJ, McKinlay JB (1994) Impotence and its medical and psychosocial correlates: results of the Massachusetts male aging study. *J Urol* 151:54–61.
Goldstein I, Lue TF, Padma-Nathan H, Rosen RC, Steers WD, Wicker P (1998) Oral sildenafil in the treatment of erectile dysfunction. *N Engl J Med* 338:1397–1404.
Kolettis PN, Lakin MM, Montague DK, Ingleright BJ, Ausmundson S (1995) Efficacy of the vacuum constriction device in patients with corporeal venous occlusive dysfunction. *Urology* 46:856–858.
Lakin MM, Montague DK, Mendendorp SV, Tesar L, Schover LR (1990) Intracavernous injection therapy: analysis of results and complications. *J Urol* 143:1138–1141.
Lue TF (1990) Impotence: a patient's goal-directed approach to treatment. *World J Urol* 8:67–74.
McClure RD (1998) Endocrine evaluation and therapy of erectile dysfunction. *Urol Clin N Am* 15:53–64.
Mohr DC, Beutler LE (1990) Erectile dysfunction: a review of diagnostic and treatment procedures. *Clin Psychol Rev* 10:123–150.
Montague DK (1989) Penile prostheses: an overview. *Urol Clin N Am* 16:7–12.
Montague DK, Barada JH, Belker AM, Levine LA, Nadig PW, Roehrborn CG, Sharlip ID, Bennett AH (1996) Clinical guidelines panel on erectile dysfunction: summary report on the treatment of organic erectile dysfunction. *J Urol* 156:2007–2011.
Nadig PJ, Ware JC, Blumoff R (1986) Noninvasive device to produce and maintain an erection-like state. *Urology* 27:126.
Padma-Nathan H, Hellstrom WJG, Kaiser FE, Labasky RF, Lue TF, Nolten WE, Norwood PC, Peterson GA, Shabsigh R, Tam PY, Place VA, Gesundheit N (1997) Treatment of men with erectile dysfunction with transurethral alprostadil. *N Engl J Med* 336:1–7.
Peterson CA, Bennett AH, Hellstrom WJG, Kaiser FE, Morley JE, Nemo KJ, Padma-Nathan H, Place VA, Prendergast JJ, Tam PY, Tanagho EA, Todd LK, Varady JC, Gesundheit N (1998) Erectile response to transurethral alprostadil, prazosin and alprostadil-prazosin combinations. *J Urol* 159:1523–1528.
Schiavi R, Schreiner-Engel P, Mandeli J, et al. (1990) Healthy aging and male sexual function. *Am J Psychiatry* 147:766–771.
Schover LR (1989) Sex therapy for the penile prosthesis recipient. *Urol Clin N Am* 16:91–98.
Schover LR, von Eschenbach AC (1985) Sex therapy and the penile prosthesis: a synthesis. *J Sex Marital Ther* 11:57–66.
Sheeler LR, Lakin MM (1988) Hypogonadism and hyperprolactinemia. In: Montague, DK, ed., *Disorders of Male Sexual Function*, Chicago: Yearbook Medical Publishers, Inc., pp. 120–127.
Spark RF, Baker R, Bienfang DC, Bergland R (1982) Bromocriptine reduces pituitary size: requiem for pituitary surgery. *JAMA* 247:311–316.
Anonymous (1996) Testosterone patches for hypogonadism. *The Medical Letter,* 38:49–50.

# IX THE SCROTAL CONTENTS

# 26 Evaluation and Management of the Scrotal Mass and Acute Scrotum

*Edward E. Cherullo, MD
and James C. Ulchaker, MD*

**Contents**
INTRODUCTION
DIAGNOSIS
DIFFERENTIAL DIAGNOSIS
SELECTED READING

## INTRODUCTION

There are many causes of acute and chronic scrotal pathology. Some of these require emergency medical or surgical treatment, but others do not require immediate intervention. Appropriate evaluation of the patient with any scrotal abnormality is crucial, as a delay in recognition of the offending process or administration of treatment may result in testicular loss, infertility, or significant morbidity. Careful history, physical examination, and prudent radiologic and laboratory testing define the physician's armamentarium to establish the correct diagnosis. When this diagnosis is reached in a timely fashion, appropriate therapy can be instituted, thus minimizing any associated complications.

## DIAGNOSIS

Diagnosis of an acute or swollen scrotum is largely dependent on a detailed history and careful examination. Often, the use of ancillary radiologic or laboratory tests only confirms or refutes a working diagnosis determined by history and physical examination. In contrast, the scrotal mass often requires radiographic and laboratory evaluation for accurate diagnosis.

### History

Although patients often present to the emergency department with atypical medical histories, frequently the physician may accurately identify the offending pathology through appropriate and thorough questioning. The following section serves to highlight

From: *Current Clinical Urology: Office Urology: The Clinician's Guide*
Edited by: E. D. Kursh and J. C. Ulchaker © Humana Press Inc., Totowa, NJ

the most important historical components of the patient with acute scrotal swelling or scrotal mass.

1. Onset of pain or swelling: Did the patient notice the mass or discomfort acutely? Was the abnormality associated with trauma or exercise? Was the patient awakened from sleep? Has the pain or swelling been present in the past with interval improvement? The answers to these questions often help to distinguish a patient with potential testicular torsion, who requires immediate surgical intervention, from a patient with a more insidious disease process.
2. Duration of symptoms: Defined by the amount of time in minutes, hours, or days since the onset of symptoms. When torsion occurs, testicular loss is likely within 8–12 h if not surgically corrected. This information will help in diagnosis, and also aids in treatment planning.
3. Evolution of pain or mass: Did the pain begin sharply and suddenly, or become more intense in a gradual manner? Is the pain colicky in nature? Is the mass or swelling increasing in size, becoming more tender, or changing in a significant manner?
4. Associated information: Is the process associated with nausea? Does the pain radiate? Is the scrotal process unilateral or bilateral? The presence of fever or associated abdominal or flank discomfort are also important pieces of a patient's history that help to narrow the differential diagnosis. Additionally, a thorough urologic review of systems is important, including: urgency, frequency, dysuria, hematuria, history of stone disease, sexual activity, and previous surgical procedures.

Again, an accurate and thorough patient history helps to narrow the differential diagnosis of acute scrotal pain or mass and to define the few surgical emergencies—such as testicular torsion or strangulated inguinal hernia—that may present with scrotal pain or a mass as a chief complaint.

## *Physical Examination*

Thorough physical examination of the scrotum and its contents—including a careful abdominal exam—is essential in any patient who presents with scrotal pain, swelling, mass. Inspection, palpation, and auscultation are integral components of the abdominal and scrotal examination. Additionally, transillumination of the scrotal contents is indicated if there is any suspected scrotal pathology on exam.

1. Age and developmental stage: During the initial examination, the patient's age and pubertal development should be determined. Testicular torsion is much more common than epididymitis or testicular-appendage torsion in the prepubescent patient. Conversely, testicular tumors most often present after puberty in young men, and epididymitis usually presents after the onset of sexual activity.
2. Surgical scars: Has the patient undergone previous scrotal or inguinal surgery? Was this bilateral? Previous orchiopexy scars in a patient with a scrotal mass are an important finding, because cryptorchid testis—even when fixed to the scrotal wall—have an increased incidence of tumor development. Previous surgery for inguinal hernia, hydrocele, or varicocele should also be determined.
3. Other cutaneous findings: Warmth, swelling, pain, and erythema are findings suggestive of an underlying inflammatory process. Gynecomastia can be associated with certain testicular tumors. A large hemiscrotum with an impalpable testis is often suggestive of a primary or secondary hydrocele. Fixation of the scrotal skin over the testis suggests necrosis.

4. Testicular palpation and position: Is the testis palpable? What is its location in the scrotum? A testis positioned high in the scrotum, with associated inflammation and tenderness, is suggestive of testicular torsion. The relationship of the testicle to the epididymis and any scrotal masses should be assessed. Is the testicle tender? Are there any associated masses? Is the scrotum tender? The size and consistency of the testicle should also be determined. Is the testicle firm, soft, nodular, or enlarged? All findings should be compared to the contralateral side. Is the cremasteric reflex present? The absence of this reflex is notable in cases of testicular torsion. An attempt to reduce inguinal masses should be made.
5. Other findings: Flank pain and renal colic may suggest a calculus as the etiology of the patient's scrotal pain. Ileus and abdominal tenderness may suggest an incarcerated inguinal hernia. The examiner should always entertain other abdominal pathology in the differential diagnosis of scrotal pain, because this pain may be referred.

## *Laboratory Evaluation*

Laboratory information needed for a complete evaluation of the acute or swollen scrotum includes a urinalysis, urine culture, complete blood count, and evaluation of meatal secretions or discharge. If the patient is sexually active, gonorrhea and Chlamydia tests are mandatory. In the evaluation of the nontender testicular mass, a urinalysis and alpha-fetoprotein and beta human chorionic gonadotropin are the minimal laboratory tests necessary to diagnose testicular tumors.

## *Radiologic Evaluation*

It is important to emphasize that testicular torsion is a clinical diagnosis. If the examining physician has a high suspicion for testicular torsion in a young patient, prompt surgical exploration of the scrotum is necessary. No laboratory or imaging studies need to be obtained. It has been demonstrated, however, that only approx 30% of young males presenting with acute scrotal pain and/or swelling require surgical intervention. Therefore, a careful history and physical examination, combined with selective imaging studies, should help identify the appropriate patient population for surgical operation. Testicular loss usually occurs within 8–12 h after the onset of vascular compromise.

## *Ultrasound*

Color Doppler ultrasound is perhaps the most common study currently obtained for the evaluation of the acute scrotum or the scrotal mass. It allows for the evaluation of the testicular tissue and can demonstrate organ blood flow and return, making it very useful for the evaluation of both the testicular mass and the acute scrotum.

Doppler ultrasound has been found to be 90–95% accurate in establishing or refuting the diagnosis of testicular torsion. This radiographic test is relatively easy to perform, and the contralateral testicle can be used for comparison. There have been no reports of false-positive results (demonstration of blood flow when in fact it is absent) in patients who present <12 h since the onset of scrotal pain. False-positive results can occur if the patient presents >12 h after the onset of pain. In these cases, the inflammation and increased blood flow in the tunics of the testis are the causes of the false-positive finding. Scrotal inflammation secondary to testicular torsion or infarction has been reported to produce this false-positive result. Because any inflammatory condition of the scrotum can lead to a false-positive reading, color Doppler ultrasound becomes an unreliable study in the presence of significant scrotal edema or inflammation.

Doppler ultrasound is also compromised as a diagnostic tool in the prepubescent age group. Because the prepubertal testicle is small, it can be difficult to reliably demonstrate a pulse. This information does not preclude use of Doppler ultrasound in the evaluation of the prepubescent-age testicle, but rather suggests cautious interpretation of the results.

Ultrasound is an excellent ancillary test for the evaluation of other potential causes of the acute scrotum or the scrotal mass. Epididymo-orchitis has demonstrated reproducible ultrasound findings, including increased flow. Testicular tumors often appear as hypo-echoic areas that arise from the testicular parenchyma. Testicular evaluation in the presence of a hydrocele is also possible. This is important for surgical planning, because the testicle is often not palpable and the hydrocele may be secondary to tumor or trauma. Determination of the integrity of the testicular tunics is also possible with ultrasound after blunt testicular trauma. When this testicular "capsule" has been ruptured or violated, surgical correction is indicated.

### *Nuclear Orchiogram*

This nuclear scan performed with $^{99m}$Tc-pertechnetate may be used to evaluate many acute and chronic scrotal conditions. It has been shown to be most useful in the diagnosis and management of testicular torsion and acute epididymo-orchitis. This study, like Doppler ultrasound, has its limitations. It is often unavailable in a timely fashion during late or weekend hours, and it allows for more variation in interpretation than Doppler ultrasound. The study is also of limited value in the prepubertal testicle, because of small size. It is often difficult to obtain an adequate study when evaluating children because of the length of the exam and the inability of the sick child to keep still for the necessary length of time.

Testicular torsion appears on the nuclear ochiogram as a spot of nucleotide deficiency caused by compromised blood flow. This is referred to as a "cold spot." Alternatively, inflammatory conditions of the scrotum—including epididymo-orchitis and torsion appendix testis—demonstrate increased uptake of $^{99m}$Tc on this nuclear scan secondary to the resultant inflammation and hyperemia. Accuracy rates of this study have been reported to be as high as 90–95%—yet this is very variable, as many false-negatives and false-positives may result. False-negatives (torsion present but scan read as normal) result in cases of prolonged torsion where resultant scrotal-wall inflammation and hyperemia are interpreted as normal flow to the testicle. If the testicle has been torsed for >48 h, a rim of increased nucleotide uptake may surround a "cold spot." This is commonly called the "vascular rim." False-positives (incorrect interpretation as compromised vascular flow) can occur in the presence of a hernia, hydrocele, spermato-cele, or any nonvascular lesion of the testis. This is secondary to decreased concentration of nucleotide counts caused by the offending process. If the testicle is torsed <360°, the scan may appear as normal flow.

Again, it should be made clear that ancillary tests can not substitute for sound clinical judgment. Radiographic and laboratory tests should only be used when acute, emergency scrotal pathology is not clearly suggested by the history and physical exam. Prudent use of Doppler ultrasound and nuclear orchiogram can help reduce the number of unnecessary operations, and ultimately aid in providing optimal, appropriate therapy in cases of acute or chronic scrotal pathology.

## DIFFERENTIAL DIAGNOSIS

### *Testicular Torsion*

Testicular torsion refers specifically to a rotation of the spermatic cord and testicle that results in venous obstruction and congestion, progressive swelling, arterial compromise, and ultimately, gonadal loss secondary to infarction. Torsion of the spermatic cord must be considered in the differential diagnosis of any scrotal process, because the testicle can be salvaged with emergent surgical exploration. Previous orchiopexy does not obviate recurrent torsion. Testicular torsion occurs in several clinical settings.

**Extravaginal Torsion (Perinatal)**

Extravaginal testicular torsion can occur in the perinatal period (either in utero or up to 30 d after birth). In neonates, the testicular tunics and the gubernaculum have not yet become firmly attached to the scrotal wall, which secures the testicle in its correct anatomic position. This allows the testicle, epididymis, testicular tunics, and spermatic cord to rotate freely within the scrotum, and may lead to torsion of the spermatic cord. Because the testicular tunics rotate freely within the scrotum and twist with the testicle on the vascular pedicle, this type of torsion is termed "extravaginal". Extravaginal torsion accounts for <10% of all cases of testicular torsion, and clinically this process may present in one of two manners. First, on routine neonatal physical examination, the examiner may notice a hard nodule in the scrotum and a contralateral normal testicle. This scrotal lesion does not transilluminate, and the ipsilateral hemiscrotum may be ecchymotic. The spermatic cord on the suspect side can occasionally be palpated, and the atrophic testis is nontender with no associated inflammation. This scenario most likely represents an intrauterine torsion with resultant testicular loss. Upon examination, the hard nodule has been found to represent a gangrenous testicle. The testicular salvage rate is very poor when torsion presents in this manner, as ischemia has often been present for much greater than 24 h. Treatment of intrauterine torsion is controversial, and some authors advocate conservative management. This includes serial examination of the testicle and no intervention if the tissue is gradually reabsorbed. The possibility of clinical infertility later in adulthood has been raised secondary to a potential autoimmune reaction to the testicle or sperm because of reabsorption of the necrotic tissue. For this reason, some authors advocate early surgical exploration and removal of the gangrenous testis. Alternatively, neonatal torsion may present with the discovery of a tender, swollen hemiscrotum at or shortly after birth. This scenario represents an acute torsion of the spermatic cord, and immediate surgical exploration is mandatory, as salvage of the testicle in this instance is possible. Orchiopexy of the contralateral testis at this time is also indicated, because it may be at risk for torsion in the future.

**Intravaginal Torsion**

Intravaginal torsion can occur at any age, but is most common between the ages of 12 and 20. This process differs anatomically from extravaginal torsion. In this case, the testicular tunics and gubernaculum are fused to the scrotal wall and the testicle rotates on its blood supply between the visceral and parietal tunica vaginalis. An anatomic abnormality referred to as "the bell clapper deformity" has been described to explain the likelihood of testicular torsion in some testicles. This deformity occurs when the tunica vaginalis inserts in a high position on the testicle. The result is that the tunica vaginalis completely surrounds the testicle and epididymis. The testicle is often found in a transverse position on palpation, and a narrowed vascular mesentery is found to insert at the lateral edge of the testis. These anatomic abnormalities predispose the testicle to twist on its blood supply and the subsequent resultant ischemia.

Patients with intravaginal testicular torsion present with an acute onset of testicular pain, which may be associated with testicular and scrotal swelling. This pain may be associated with minor trauma or exercise, or may awaken the patient from sleep, but often there is no precipitating history. Patients may also describe a history of a similar discomfort in the past, with spontaneous resolution—suggestive of spontaneous torsion and detorsion of a susceptible testicle in the past. Other associated symptoms include lower abdominal pain and cramping, nausea, vomiting, and contralateral scrotal discomfort. On examination, the testicle will be acutely tender and enlarged. It may be located in a high scrotal position secondary to the torsed and subsequently shortened spermatic cord. A transverse lie and anteriorly positioned epididymis may also be appreciated. Elevation of the scrotum will not alleviate the patient's discomfort, sometimes referred to as a negative Prehn's sign. Swelling and erythema of the scrotum occur with prolonged ischemia. At times, the swelling and edema can become so severe that they preclude palpation of the epididymis or spermatic cord. Fixation of the overlying scrotal skin is an indication of testicular necrosis, and urinalysis is often negative.

It should be made clear that testicular torsion is a clinical diagnosis and when the physician has a high index of suspicion, immediate surgical exploration is mandatory. However, if the examining physician feels that torsion is unlikely, a nuclear orchiogram or testicular Doppler ultrasound can be performed to confirm the presence of testicular blood flow.

When the diagnosis of testicular torsion is made, manual detorsion of the testicle may be attempted after appropriate analgesia for the patient is administered. Cord block should be avoided, because it confuses the clinical picture. Detorsion is accomplished either by raising the scrotum or rotating the testicle and untwisting the spermatic cord. Often the epididymis is in an anterior position, and its rotation to a lateral and subsequently posterior position may successfully detorse the testicle. Manual detorsion has been likened to the opening of a book—the testicle is rotated in the direction of the ipsilateral thigh. Successful detorsion is confirmed by palpation of the testicle in a lower scrotal position and resolution of pain. If manual detorsion is successful, surgical exploration may be delayed for a short time. However, orchiopexy is mandatory, because the testicle may retorse in the future. If manual detorsion is unsuccessful, immediate surgical exploration and orchiopexy is mandatory.

Detorsion of the testicle within 4 h results in a salvage rate of near 100%, and after 12 h of ischemia the testicular salvage rate is near 20%. Between 12 and 24 h of ischemia time, recovery is possible and orchiopexy should be performed. In cases where the testicle may not appear viable, but is not grossly necrotic, orchiopexy may be performed. Although the tubular cells are not likely to recover, it is possible that the interstitial Leydig's cells—which are much more resistant to an ischemic insult—

will continue to produce testosterone. If the testicle is grossly necrotic or has been torsed for more than 48 h, the testicle should be removed. Orchiopexy is performed by fixing the testicle to the scrotal wall with three nonabsorbable sutures. Because of the risk of torsion to the contralateral testicle it should undergo orchiopexy regardless of the fate of the torsed testicle.

## *Epididymitis and Orchitis*

Acute epididymitis is an infection of the epididymis that results most commonly from the retrograde migration of bacteria down the vas deferens from the urethra. This process is most common in adolescent and elderly men, and is rare in the prepubertal age group. When epididymitis occurs in a prepubescent child, anatomic abnormalities must be considered. These include neurogenic bladder, ectopic ureter, meatal stenosis, urethral obstruction secondary to strictures, or valves. Risk factors in the adult population include unprotected intercourse, severe physical strain, chronic indwelling Foley catheter, and urethral stricture disease or instrumentation, including transurethral resection of the prostate (TURP).

The most common pathogens that cause epididymitis in men younger than 35 yr are *Chlamydia trachomatis* and *Neisseria gonorrhoeae*. In children and men older than 35 yr, *Escherichia coli* and *Pseudomonas* species are the most common offending organisms.

Patients with acute epididymitis often present with a heavy, dull ache in the ipsilateral hemiscrotum, and this discomfort may radiate to the ipsilateral flank. The patient may have fever and chills. If examination is performed early in the course of the infection, the epididymitis is palpable, and tenderness at the tail can be appreciated. As the inflammatory process progresses, the physical exam often demonstrates an epididymitis that is markedly swollen and exquisitely tender. If the infection is present for a prolonged period, the inflammatory process may spread to the testicle—termed epididymo-orchitis. In this instance, the hemiscrotum may become warm, erythematous, and edematous, and on physical exam the testicle and epididymis will become clinically indistinguishable. A reactive hydrocele may develop within a few days of onset of infection secondary to a reaction by the tunica albuginea to the severe inflammation. The spermatic cord may be tender upon palpation. If an abscess is present, the overlying skin may be thinned, dry, and shiny. In sexually active men, a urethral discharge often accompanies this clinical scenario. Elevation of the scrotum over the symphysis may relieve the symptoms—termed a positive Prehn's sign. Urinalysis often demonstrates pyuria and or bacteruria, and the patient frequently has an elevated white blood-cell count. Urine culture results play a critical role in the appropriate treatment of epididymitis.

When evaluating this clinical entity, testicular torsion must always be ruled out. Torsion most commonly occurs in the adolescent age group, and is uncommon in older patients. Epididymitis also occurs more commonly than torsion in men older than 30 yr. A positive Prehn's sign is suggestive of epididymitis instead of torsion, but is not a perfect differentiating tool. It is clinically appropriate for the examining physician to formulate a working diagnosis based on history and physical exam alone. If the diagnosis of torsion is reached, surgical exploration is indicated. False-positive surgical exploration for torsion is considered clinically appropriate in approx 10% of patients. However, if the examiner feels that epididymitis is likely, Doppler ultrasound or nuclear orchiogram can confirm this diagnosis. As previously discussed, Doppler ultrasound and nuclear orchiogram demonstrate increased flow to the affected testicle in cases of severe inflammation secondary to infection.

Treatment of epididymitis is achieved by first providing broad-spectrum antibiotic coverage until the culture results return. Antibiotic coverage is then tailored to the specific offending organism(s), based on the culture and sensitivity report. Around-the-clock nonsteroidal analgesia in addition to scrotal elevation helps to reduce the associated inflammation and subsequent scrotal pain. It may take several weeks or months, and long-term antibiotic therapy, for the patient to experience complete resolution of symptoms.

Acute epididymitis can be a severe infectious process, and complications from late diagnosis or misdiagnosis do occur. Testicular abscess can occur following severe epididymitis. Clinically, the examiner may notice that the overlying scrotal skin is fixed to the testicle. Constitutional symptoms, including fever, chills and malaise, may be present. Ultrasound confirms the presence of an abscess, and orchiectomy may be necessary as definitive treatment if antibiotics and drainage do not result in clinical improvement.

Testicular ischemia and necrosis may occur secondary to abscess or severe inflammation. This results when the spermatic cord becomes involved in the inflammatory process. The resultant swelling and the relative inelastic nature of the cremasteric muscle fibers cause venous outflow obstruction, and eventually, arterial compromise. Testicular loss can follow if treatment is not instituted in a timely fashion.

Chronic epididymitis can result from recurrent acute episodes secondary to particularly virulent strains of bacteria in addition to inappropriate antibiotic selection or short duration of treatment. The recurrent episodes of acute epididymitis eventually lead to chronic induration, swelling, and tenderness. Treatment is with long-term antibiotic therapy, anti-inflammatory agents, and scrotal support. Rarely, epididymectomy is needed to provide relief from chronic pain and discomfort.

Orchitis results from an involvement of the testicle with the inflammatory or infective process affecting the epididymis. The treatment of orchitis is essentially the same as that for epididymitis (support, NSAID analgesia, possible bed rest, antibiotics when appropriate) unless abscess or necrosis develops. In these instances, orchiectomy may be necessary. Mumps orchitis occasionally presents to the urologist. The development of testicular involvement occurs 4–7 d following the onset of parotitis. Up to one-third of patients who experience mumps orchitis have, as a result, at least some degree of testicular atrophy. The treatment of this viral entity is supportive care.

## *Torsion of Testicular Appendages*

Torsion of the testicular or epididymal appendages usually occurs between the ages of 2 and 12 y old. Less commonly, it occurs in adolescents or adults. The testicular appendage is a remnant of the mullerian ductal system, and is anatomically located at the upper pole of the testis. These appendages can be long and pendulous, and may twist at their base, causing ischemia and eventual infarction of the appendage.

Patients can present with the acute or gradual onset of unilateral scrotal pain, similar to that seen with true testicular torsion. The onset of the discomfort may be associated with exercise or injury. Patients may suffer from referred pain to the lower abdomen, nausea, or vomiting, but constitutional symptoms are usually less severe than those seen with true testicular torsion. Examination is important for an edematous, erythematous scrotum and a mildly tender testicle. A tender "nodule" may be palpable at the superior aspect of the testicle. The torsed testicular appendage may be visible through the thin scrotal skin as a "blue dot" over this tender palpable area. Torsion of the appendix testis should not be a clinical diagnosis unless the offending appendages can be palpated at the superior pole of the testis and confirmation can be provided that this is the source of the patient's pain.

Doppler ultrasound or nuclear orchiogram demonstrates normal or slightly increased blood flow to the testicle when torsion of the appendix testis has occurred. This finding confirms that the testicle is not in ischemic danger, and allows the examining physician to reassure both the patient and the family that the testicle is not in jeopardy. Treatment of a torsed testicular appendage consists of alleviation of symptoms and patient reassurance. Patients are encouraged to take nonsteroidal anti-inflammatory medications around the clock and wear supportive undergarments until symptoms improve. Complete resolution of symptoms usually occurs after appendage necrosis and resolution of the surrounding inflammation—typically between 10 and 14 d.

The testicular appendages can torse and untorse intermittently. This process may cause the patient to re-present to the physician several times with acute scrotal pain that occasionally complicates diagnosis and management. The knowledge of this possibility and the exclusion of vascular compromise to the testicle by Doppler ultrasound or nuclear orchiogram can help the physician arrive at the correct diagnosis.

### *Inguinal Hernia and Hydrocele*

An abdominal hernia is defined as a defect in the layers of the abdominal fascia that allow protrusion of the intra-abdominal contents into a sac or diverticulum. Herniation of the abdominal contents can and does occur in the inguinal region, and this process may result in significant scrotal swelling. The pathophysiology of inguinal hernia is different in pediatric and adult patients, and will be discussed separately.

Embryologically, the testicles develop retroperitoneally within the abdominal cavity. They usually descend into their anatomic position within the scrotum at or around the time of birth. As they migrate, the testicles bring with them some of investing layers of the abdominal cavity. It is these layers that contribute to the internal and external spermatic fascia, cremasteric fibers, and the tunica vaginalis. The processus vaginalis is an extension of the abdominal peritoneum that lies anatomically in a superior and medial location in relation to the spermatic cord and testis within the inguinal canal and scrotum. This extension of peritoneum is patent while the testis descend, and fuses into a flat testicular covering at or shortly after birth.

In the pediatric population, a communicating hydrocele occurs when the processus vaginalis fails to close and intra-abdominal fluid passes freely into and out of the scrotum through this anatomic connection. A hernia results from intra-abdominal fat or bowel segments passing through the patent process vaginalis from the abdominal cavity into the inguinal canal or scrotum. A communicating hydrocele often presents as painless unilateral or bilateral scrotal swelling. The testicles are often palpable, and most communicating hydroceles resolve spontaneously by 1 yr of age. However, if the communicating hydrocele is still present at that time, surgical correction is advised. A hydrocele of the spermatic cord (an encysted hydrocele) and a hydrocele of the tunica vaginalis occur much more rarely. In these instances, the fluid collection is either present in a segment of processes vaginalis associated with the spermatic cord, or solely within the tunica vaginalis surrounding the testicle. In both instances these is no communication between the fluid collection and the abdominal cavity. Because it can be difficult to clinically distinguish a communicating hydrocele from a hydrocele of the cord or tunica vaginalis, the true diagnosis is often made at the time of surgical exploration.

Hernia occurs when bowel segments or other abdominal contents are able to pass from the abdominal cavity into the inguinal canal or scrotum through the patent processus vaginalis. The clinical presentation differs slightly from that of communicating hydrocele because an inguinal bulge may be palpated and the parents may claim that this bulge is only present when the child is upset. If a hernia is present, an attempt at reduction should be made. If this is not clinically possible, the hernia is incarcerated, and surgical correction should occur in a timely fashion. If the child suffers from abdominal pain, nausea, emesis, or extreme tenderness over the inguinal bulge, a strangulated hernia is likely, which constitutes a surgical emergency. Surgical exploration should take place immediately.

In the older child and adult, a hydrocele is rarely secondary to a patent processus vaginalis. The most common causes of hydrocele in the adult population include idiopathic, inflammatory, traumatic, and malignant processes. These hydroceles result secondary to fluid accumulation between the visceral and parietal layers of the tunica vaginalis. Presentation usually consists of painless unilateral scrotal swelling, and the patient is often unable to give any history of trauma, infection, or other precipitating event. Occasionally, the patient may complain of a dull scrotal ache or heaviness. The scrotal swelling should be nontender and transilluminate. If the hydrocele is large enough to preclude examination of the testicle, scrotal ultrasound should be performed to evaluate for testicular pathology, including testicular tumor. In the absence of a testicular abnormality, a hydrocele carries little risk of complications if clinically observed. The two most common complications include testicular atrophy secondary to vascular compromise and trauma. This occurs when a large hydrocele compresses the spermatic cord and subsequently restricts blood flow to the testicle. Secondly, trauma may result in hemorrhage into the hydrocele sac and development of a large hematoma. Therefore, surgical repair of a hydrocele is indicated when the patient experiences discomfort or other symptoms, or the hydrocele is large enough to cause concern regarding testicular blood supply or scrotal hemorrhage.

Indirect or direct inguinal hernias may present as a large scrotal mass. In this instance, a substantial amount of omentum or bowel protrudes within a hernia sac into the scrotum. The testicle may not be palpable, and this process may be clinically indistinguishable from a large hydrocele. The distinction can be made if the patient is relaxed and the hernia is reducible; however, this is not always possible. Scrotal ultrasound can aid diagnosis when necessary by distinguishing between these two entities. A CT scan with oral contrast can help delineate the extent of the hernia when present. Hernias of this size rarely present with strangulation; however, surgical repair is appropriate.

### *Spermatocele*

A spermatocele clinically presents as a unilateral scrotal mass usually discovered incidentally by an examining physician. On examination the spermatocele is a nontender, cystic mass lying in a position superior and posterior to the testicle. They are usually <1 cm in size, but may become large enough to clinically resemble a hydrocele. Both spermatoceles and hydroceles can transilluminate. Differentiation is possible, as a hydrocele should cover the entire anterior aspect of the testicle and the testicle may not be palpable. Additionally, spermatoceles are often tense, and may feel solid. Differentiation from a testicular tumor or mesothelioma (spermatic-cord tumor) is possible, because these lesions are separate from the testicle, do not contain fluid, and should not transilluminate.

The etiology of this lesion is not entirely clear, but spermatoceles are likely to arise from tubules or cystic structures in the superior pole of the testis or head of the epididymis. When aspirated, microscopic examination of the contents often reveals murky fluid and sperm. Ultrasound may be useful in evaluating the lesion if the diagnosis is clinically difficult. Treatment consists of surgical spermatocelectomy or epididymectomy. Aspiration as a treatment option yields poor long-term results, because these lesions may recur. Sclerosing agents should be avoided because of the potential for chemical epididymitis. In young men concerned with fertility, therapy should be avoided altogether.

## *Trauma*

Blunt testicular trauma can occur at any age. Patients typically give a history consistent with an insult to one or both testicles, and the resultant discomfort is significant enough to cause concern. The presentations of testicular trauma include testicular contusion, hematocele, rupture of the testicular tunics, and torsion of the testis or its appendix. Additionally, scrotal trauma—if significant enough—can cause disruption of the blood–sperm barrier and the subsequent development of antisperm antibodies.

The physical exam in patients who present with a traumatic hematocele or rupture of the scrotal tunics is significant for severe, painful scrotal-wall ecchymosis and edema. The testicle often cannot be palpated. In most cases, scrotal ultrasound is an essential diagnostic tool. With ultrasound, the integrity of the testicle and its vascular supply may be assessed.

Occasionally, a patient may present to the physician with severe scrotal pain and swelling following strenuous activity or minor injury. These cases should be treated as testicular torsion until proven otherwise. In susceptible individuals, minor testicular trauma may precipitate torsion. Doppler ultrasound and nuclear orchiogram are particularly useful in these cases.

The treatment of traumatic hematoma or testicular disruption is surgical. The goals of intervention include control of bleeding, hematoma evacuation, and repair of testicular rupture. It has been argued that the use of ancillary radiologic examination in this patient group is unnecessary. Prompt surgical exploration is advocated for salvage of the testis and the prevention of antisperm antibodies.

## *Varicocele*

A varicocele is an abnormal dilation of the pampiniform plexus of veins within the spermatic cord. This abnormality of testicular venous drainage occurs primarily on the left, and there are several proposed etiologies for the formation of these varicies. Anatomic factors—including lack of venous valves in the pampiniform plexus and pressure differences in venous drainage—most likely explain the formation of a varicocele and the clinically apparent left-sided predominance.

This phenomenon is rarely diagnosed before puberty. The patient may present to the physician with concern about a scrotal "mass" that was not previously present.

Occasionally, the patient may also complain of a "dull ache" or "heaviness" in the ipsilateral testicle, often after strenuous activity or prolonged standing. Additionally, varicocele may be identified in patients who undergo routine physical exam or an infertility evaluation.

Diagnosis rests on clinical findings. Examination of the scrotum while the patient is standing upright usually allows for identification of the characteristic mass of veins usually located above and behind the testicle. During examination, smaller varicoceles may be made more clinically apparent by asking the patient to perform a Valsalva maneuver. Ancillary tests are not usually necessary for confirmation of the diagnosis; however, use of a Doppler stethoscope over the suspected area may help diagnosis. Identifying the audible, characteristic rush of blood while the patient performs a Valsalva maneuver is diagnostic evidence for the presence of the varicocele. The varicocele and any associated discomfort, when present, should be significantly reduced when the patient is supine.

The need for the surgical treatment of varicoceles is presently controversial. Correction is currently advocated in certain clinical settings. Varicoceles have been associated with infertility, and improved sperm quality has been demonstrated after repair. If a varicocele is diagnosed during adolescence and is associated with a smaller-volume testicle as compared to the contralateral gland, the current practice of most urologists is to offer the patient repair. Repair is also advocated in the setting of pain that can reliably attributed to the varicocele. Large varicoceles may be cosmetically significant, and cause the patient appreciable distress. In this setting, repair is appropriate.

Surgical correction of the varicocele consists of ligation or occlusion of the dilated testicular veins. This can be accomplished by radiologic techniques, microsurgical methods, or conventional surgery. Complications of treatment include wound infection, hematoma, hydrocele, recurrence of the varicocele, or testicular atrophy. All of these may be avoided through appropriate surgical techniques.

### *Testicular Tumor*

Although testicular tumors usually present in men in their third or fourth decades, they may present at any age. Most tumors are incidentally discovered by the patient during palpation, or by the physician during a routine physical examination. The usual presentation is a painless lump, nodule, or hardness associated with the testicle. The patient may complain of concomitant lower-abdominal or inguinal discomfort and heaviness, and may present with acute pain secondary to tumor growth and resultant necrosis or hemorrhage. Approximately 10% of patients will have clinical epididymitis associated with the testicular tumor. When a testicular tumor is present, laboratory evaluation includes serum beta-human chorionic gonadotropin and alpha-fetoprotein levels. Treatment for testicular tumors includes radical orchiectomy, and radiation with or without systemic chemotherapy (depending on the tumor's histologic composition, size, and staging).

### *Henoch-Schönlein Purpura*

This systemic vasculitic syndrome occurs primarily in male children aged 2–11 yr, and is manifested by nonthrombocytopenic purpura, colicky abdominal pain, joint pain and swelling, and glomerulonephritis. Acute swelling of the scrotum and spermatic cord can occur. Testicular involvement has been reported in up to one-third of affected patients. Diagnosis of this disorder rests on clinical observations.

Classic presentation consists of a maculopapular rash on the lower extremities and buttocks. This rash may spread to the scrotum. Testicular involvement consists of moderate swelling and tenderness of the testicles. Differentiation of this syndrome from a patient with testicular torsion may be made by careful history. The temporal association between the onset of the rash and scrotal swelling is very important. Testicular torsion has been reported in children with Henoch-Schönlein Purpura, and therefore, ancillary radiologic assessment should be obtained if any uncertainty regarding the diagnosis exists. In the absence of vascular compromise to the testicle, urologic treatment of this phenomenon is limited to symptom improvement.

## *Fournier's Gangrene*

Fournier's gangrene—a urologic emergency—is a form of necrotizing fascitis that originates in the perineum, and can be widespread and life-threatening. This process can affect any age group; however, presentation often occurs in older diabetics. Patients typically present with the sudden onset of scrotal edema, pain, and areas of black or bluish skin. Crepitus of the tissues may or may not be present. Sources of infection may include periurethral, perirectal, or ischiorectal abscesses, but often no definitive source can be determined.

Treatment must take place immediately after diagnosis, and includes aggressive antibiotic coverage of possible offending microbes—including aerobic and anaerobic organisms—in addition to wide debridement of all involved tissues. This may include large portions of the anterior abdominal wall when necessary. Salvage of the testicle is possible if the deep tissues are uninvolved with the infective process. Treatment then involves placement of the testicle into an ectopic subcutaneous pouch. A scrotal pouch can be reconstructed after resolution of the infectious process.

## SELECTED READING

Altaffer LF III, Steele SM, Jr (1980) Torsion of testicular appendages in men. *J Urol* 124:56.
Barada JH, Weingarten JL, Cromie WJ (1989) Testicular salvage and age-related delay in the presentation of testicular torsion. *J Urol* 142:746.
Bickerstaffe KI, Sethia K, Muric JA (1988) Doppler ultrasonography in the diagnosis of acute scrotal pain. *Br J Surg* 75:238.
Clark WR, Kramer SA (1986) Henoch-Schönlein purpura and the acute scrotum. *J Pediatr Surg* 21:991.
Dandapat MC, Padhi NC, Patra AP (1990) Effect of hydrocele on testis and spermatogenesis. *Br J Surg* 77:1293.
Dresner ML (1973) Torsed appendage diagnosis and management: Blue Dot Sign. *Urology* 1:63.
Eshghi M, Silver L, Smith AD (1987) Technetium 99m scan in acute scrotal lesions. *Urology* 30:586.
Gartman E (1964) Torsion of the spermatic cord and testicular appendage in adult scrotal testes. *Am J Surg* 108:802.
Golimbu M, Florio FE, Al-Askari S, Morales PA, Passalaqua A (1985) Value of scrotal scanning. *Urology* 25:92.
Holder LE, Meloul M, Chen D (1981) Current status of radionucleotide scrotal imaging. *Semin Nucl Med* 11:232.
Holland JM, Graham JB, Ignatoff JM (1981) Conservative management of twisted testicular appendages. *J Urol* 125:213.
Kass EJ, Stone KT, Cacciarelli AA, Mitchell B (1993) Do all children with acute scrotum require exploration? *J Urol* 150:667.

Krarup T (1978) The testis after torsion. *Br J Urol* 50:43.

Lutzker LG (1982) The fine points of scrotal scintigraphy *Semin Nucl Med* 12:387.

Nadel NS, Gitter MH, Han LC (1973) Preoperative diagnosis of testicular torsion. *Urology* 1:478.

Nagler HM, White RD (1982) The effect of testicular torsion on the contralateral testis. *J Urol* 128:1343.

Perri AJ, Morales JO, Feldman AE, Kendal AR, Karafin L (1976) Necrotic testicle with increased blood flow on Doppler ultrasound monitoring. *Urology* 8:265.

Perri AJ, Slachta GA, Feldman AE, Kendall AR, Karafin L (1976) The Doppler stethoscope and the diagnosis of the acute scrotum. *J Urol* 116:598.

Puri P, Guiney EJ, O'Donnell B (1984) Inguinal hernia in infants: the fate of the testis following incarceration. *J Pediatr Surg* 19:44.

Ransler CW, Allen TD (1982) Torsion of the spermatic cord. *Urol Clin N Am* 9:245.

Rodriguez WC, Rodriguez DD, Fortuo RF (1981) The operative treatment of hydrocele: a comparison of 4 basic techniques. *J Urol* 125:804.

Ryken TC, Turner JW, Hayes T (1990) Bilateral testicular torsion in a pre-term neonate. *J Urol* 143:102.

Sayfan J, Soffer Y, Orda R (1992) Varicocele treatment: prospective randomized trial of 3 methods. *J Urol* 148:1447.

Schulsinger D, Glassberg K, Strashun A (1991) Intermittent torsion: association with horizontal lie of the testicle. *J Urol* 145:1053.

Siegel A, Synder H, Duckett JW (1987) Epididymitis in infants and boys: underlying urogenital anomalies and efficacy of imaging modalities. *J Urol* 138:1100.

Skogland RW, McRoberts JW, Ragde H (1970) Torsion of testicular appendages: presentation of 43 new cases and a collective review. *J Urol* 104:598.

Stadalnik RC (1981) Bullseye sign in scrotal imaging. *Semin Nucl Med* 11:316.

Thomas AJ, Geisinger MA (1990) Current management of varicoceles. *Urol Clin N Am* 17:893.

Thomas WEG, Cooke ER, Davies ER, Jackson PC, Williamson RCN (1981) Dynamic radionucleotide scanning of the testis in acute scrotal conditions. *Br J Surg* 68:621.

Thurston A, Whitaker R (1982) Torsion of testis after previous testicular surgery. *Br J Surg* 70:217.

Vordermark JS, Buck AS, Brow SR, Tuttle WK (1981) The testicular scan: use in diagnosis and management of acute epididymitis. *JAMA* 245:2512.

Williamson RCN (1976) Torsion of the testis and allied conditions. *Br J Surg* 63:465.

# 27 Genital Pain

*Elroy D. Kursh, MD*

**CONTENTS**
- INTRODUCTION
- CAUSES OF GENITAL PAIN
- DEFINITION OF CHRONIC GENITAL PAIN
- INNERVATION OF THE TESTICLES AND SCROTUM
- EVALUATION
- MEDICAL THERAPY
- LOCAL ANESTHETIC BLOCKS
- SURGICAL INTERVENTION
- PSYCHOLOGICAL FACTORS
- NEUROMUSCULAR PELVIC-FLOOR DYSFUNCTION
- MULTIDISCIPLINARY APPROACH TO THE MANAGEMENT OF CHRONIC GENITAL PAIN
- SELECTED READING

## INTRODUCTION

Recurrent or chronic genital pain is a frequent problem in a urologic practice. Most urologists cringe at the thought of seeing these patients. Despite the frequency of the problem, very little has been written about this condition. Frequently, no physical cause for the man's symptoms can be found. The pain has an obscure etiology, or is ascribed to vague entities, such as prostatitis or prostatodynia, with little or no objective diagnostic evidence. Treatment is generally ineffective.

Most patients become indignant and incredulous at the suggestion that their pain is psychosomatic, and are reluctant to accept a referral to a mental health professional. Therefore, a variety of treatments, such as antibiotics, are usually prescribed, even when the urine cultures and prostate-fluid cultures are negative. Other treatment—such as sitz baths, pain medication, anti-inflammatory drugs, and reassurance—may be prescribed to little or no avail. When all else fails, some clinicians even recommend orchiectomy.

In the absence of organic findings, some investigators have suggested that men with genital pain have a high incidence of life stress and psychological disturbance. Their observations primarily concern patients who complain of pain in the testis, groin, perineum, suprapubic area, and flank, often accompanied by urinary urgency and frequency, and pain during ejaculation.

Men with chronic genital pain are often diagnosed as having chronic prostatitis. Despite the frequency of establishing a diagnosis of chronic prostatitis according to reviews of coding records, I believe that this is a rare disease. Since so little is understood about the disease, some investigators are starting to classify it as chronic prostatitis/chronic pelvic pain syndrome. Recent data suggests that an autoimmune component may play a role in some men. Frankly, I have serious doubts that a diagnosis of chronic prostatitis even exists or—to be more precise—I doubt that the prostate is the source of pain in men with chronic genital pain ascribed to nonbacterial prostatitis or prostatodynia. There is no doubt that the prostate may be the seat of infection, as evidenced in patients with acute prostatitis or recurrent acute prostatitis, which could be correctly classified as chronic prostatitis. Over the years, I have treated many men who present to the office during a routine follow-up visit with an asymptomatic urinary-tract infection. Their expressed prostatic secretion or urine voided after prostatic massage (VB3) reveal many WBCs. Cultures confirm the diagnosis of a urinary-tract infection with the common pathogens, and the infection clearly resides in the prostate. What has intrigued me is the fact that these men have no symptoms linked to the urinary tract and no genital discomfort whatsoever, despite the apparent infection in the prostate.

In our experience, men with nonorganic genital pain are psychologically similar, regardless of the site of discomfort. We have adopted a novel new approach to the management of these patients. It is clear that dealing with patients with chronic genital pain is difficult and time-consuming. We believe a unified multidisciplinary approach is crucial to achieving a successful outcome.

## CAUSES OF GENITAL PAIN

The causes of acute genital pain have been well-described, and include a variety of problems, such as acute epididymitis, testicular torsion, torsion of the appendix testis, acute urethritis, and testicular or scrotal abscess.

The causes of chronic genital pain are more subtle and less well-defined. Some of the described causative factors include infections (such as chronic prostatitis or urethritis), tumors (such as a testicular tumor), inguinal hernia, intermittent testicular torsion, hydrocele, spermatocele, and varicocele. In our experience, hydrocele and spermatocele are rarely, if ever, associated with pain. Any described discomfort with these entities is most likely the result of the large size of the mass, which may cause a dragging or heavy sensation. Similarly, even large varicoceles are rarely associated with pain, and it is my opinion that surgical correction for pain alone is rarely, if ever, indicated. Trauma, such as recurrent testicular trauma, and referred pain may also be responsible for chronic genital discomfort.

Finally, chronic genital pain may be caused by a previous operation. Vasectomy represents the most common operation reported to be responsible for chronic genital pain, but other scrotal and inguinal procedures, such as inguinal herniorrhaphy, may play an etiological factor. In a review of 172 patients, 4 yr following vasectomy, McMahon and colleagues reported the surprisingly high incidence of chronic genital pain of 33%, with 15% considering the pain to be troublesome. Despite this high incidence of chronic pain, only three patients regretted having the vasectomy.

## DEFINITION OF CHRONIC GENITAL PAIN

Chronic genital pain is defined as pain without an identified organic cause, that includes at least one of the following sites: the perineum, testicles, scrotum, penis, or urethra. Dysuria or suprapubic pain alone are excluded from the definition, but may be reported with the other types of pain. Additionally, non genital pain syndromes may coexist with genital pain.

## INNERVATION OF THE TESTICLES AND SCROTUM

The innervation of the scrotal wall and the scrotal contents is complex, because it contains the testis with a distant splanchnic supply (T10–12) surrounded by somatic nerves of widely separated segments (L1–2 and S2–3) that also supply other viscera with autonomic nerves. Therefore, the potential for referred sensations in both directions is substantial. The sensory innervation of the testis and epididymis or pain originating in either of these structures is mediated by both autonomic and somatic fibers that accompany the internal spermatic vessels.

The somatic fibers from the parietal and visceral layers of the tunica vaginalis and cremaster are carried by the genital branch of the genitofemoral nerve to L1, 2. Other somatic nerve endings are apparently carried from the tunica vaginalis and scrotal skin by the posterior scrotal nerves (S2,3).

The testes bring their sympathetic nerve supply with them on their descent from the T10–12 segments. These nerves accompany the internal spermatic vessels. After penetrating the tunica albuginea, they are distributed to the interior of the testis between the seminiferous tubules. The main function of these nerves appears to be supplying arteries and stimulating the smooth muscle of the tunica albuginea, but afferent nociceptive fibers from the testicles travel in the sympathetic plexus to invest the testicular artery and vein and terminate in thoracolumbar segments. Acute distention of the testis by injecting saline after anesthetizing the skin and tunica vaginalis produces pain that is felt not in the scrotum, but instead low in the ileac fossa—presumably caused by reference to the corresponding somatic segments.

The sympathetic fibers to the vas deferens and epididymis are distinct from those that supply the testis. They arise from the sympathetic outflow of T10–L1 and pass down the sympathetic chains into the pelvic plexus, and then extend along the vas deferens to the epididymis. These fibers supply the smooth muscles of the vas deferens and epididymis, but afferent nociceptive fibers also travel in them. There is no description of sensory nerve endings in these sites, but the pain sometimes produced by acute distention of the epididymis after vasectomy produces pain vaguely felt in the inguinal area and scrotum, presumably because of reference to the ilioinguinal and genitofemoral nerves (L1).

Referred pain to the scrotum or its contents is a well-known phenomenon. Pain may be referred to superficial somatic segments from either viscera or deep somatic structures with the same segmental nerve supply. By far, the most common cause of referred pain to the scrotum is a stone in the mid or lower part of the ureter. The pain may be referred to the testis alone—which actually represents the tunica vaginalis—but usually there is associated referred pain to the groin and sometimes to the skin over the femoral triangle. This pain emanates from splanchnic (L1,2) ureteric stimulation to the same somatic segments via the genital branch of the genitofemoral nerve. In other words, the ureteral automonic afferent fibers cross over to the testis-afferent fibers in the autonomic ganglia, thus "referring" the perception of pain to the testis. Alternatively, direct irritation of the genitofemoral nerve as the ureter lies on it may occasionally cause a similar pattern of referred pain.

## EVALUATION

Patients who present with chronic genital pain are typically tense, anxious, confused, and convinced that they have a serious problem. Invariably, the men have consulted multiple physicians regarding their genital pain, and have received a variety of treatments, such as antibiotics and anti-inflammatory drugs, for various diagnoses, such as prostatitis or epididymitis. Multiple courses of treatment rarely—if ever—offer more than temporary relief. A variety of costly tests may also have been performed, such as scrotal ultrasound, computerized tomography of the abdomen and pelvis, and even cystoscopy, without revealing an apparent abnormality. Therefore, obtaining a thorough and accurate history is a critical part of the evaluation for these patients, but it is often a difficult and time-consuming task that requires a great deal of patience. These men are too often scheduled in the course of a busy day in the office, when finding time to deal with them is almost impossible.

Patients are questioned about the onset, location, duration, and activities that trigger the pain, such as exercise, sexual intercourse, or ejaculation. Previous treatments, evaluations, and results are recorded. It is important to obtain a history of the patient's social support and satisfaction with marital and dating relationships; assessment of current stresses; stressors coinciding with the onset of pain; assessment of sexual function, including sources of sex guilt, such as paraphilic fantasies; extramarital sexual activity; very strong religious views about sexual issues; and assessment of mood and anxiety.

Physical examination includes examination of the penis, scrotum testis, epididymides, and spermatic cords, and assessment of the inguinal areas for the presence of an inguinal hernia. The prostate and rectum are evaluated through a digital rectal examination. In these patients, the physical examination very rarely reveals a discernible abnormality.

At the time of the initial examination, routine laboratory tests include urinalysis and microscopic examination of the expressed prostatic secretion or the urine voided after prostatic massage (VB3). When indicated, culture and sensitivities of the urine or VB3 are obtained.

A variety of more specific diagnostic studies have been obtained to attempt to define the cause of chronic genital pain, including scrotal ultrasound, excretory urography, cystoscopy, urodynamics, and computerized tomography of the abdomen and pelvis. In a review of 48 predominantly young, active servicemen with chronic genital pain, Costabile and colleagues reported that 221 diagnostic procedures were performed, for an average of 4.7 diagnostic procedures per patient. Four of the patients in their series had significant voiding symptoms, such as dysuria, frequency, and urgency, in addition to scrotal discomfort, and they accounted for the majority of significant abnormal findings on the diagnostic studies. Table 1 provides an analysis of the results of the diagnostic procedures performed on men with orchialgia, including the four patients with voiding dysfunction. A significant finding was considered to be an abnormality found in the study that would require intervention even in the absence of pain. An

## Table 1
### Results of Diagnostic Procedures Performed on Patients with Orchialgia

| Study | No. | Normal no. (%) | Significant abnormality no. (%) | Incidental no. (%) |
|---|---|---|---|---|
| Excretory urography | 22 | 20 (91) | 0 | 2 (9) |
| Cystoscopy | 16 | 16 (100) | 0 | 0 |
| Urinalysis | 38 | 38 (100) | 0 | 0 |
| Culture | 31 | 31 (100) | 0 | 0 |
| Scrotal ultrasound | 30 | 22 (73) | 0 | 8 (27)[a] |
| Other uroradiology | 21 | 20 (95) | 1 (5) | 0 |
| Urodynamics | 10 | 10 (100) | 0 | 0 |
| Computerized tomography | 13 | 12 (92) | 1 (8) | 0 |
| Other | 28 | 27 (96) | 0 | 1 (4) |
| Totals | 209 | 196 (94) | 2 (1) | 1 (4) |

[a] Subclinical hydroceles and varicoceles

From Costabile RA et al (1991) Chronic orchialgia in the pain-prone patient: the clinical perspective. J Urol 146: 1571–1574, with permission.

incidental finding was an anatomical genital abnormality that normally would not require surgical intervention, but would be observed. Excluding the patients with voiding dysfunction, only 2 of 209 studies (<1%) showed significant abnormalities. Based on these data, the examiners concluded that streamlining of the process in patients with chronic orchialgia is not only needed to decrease medical costs, but is necessary to decrease the risk of complications brought on by invasive testing. We believe that in the absence of clinical findings, extensive diagnostic testing is not indicated and may even be detrimental—it may increase the patient's concern about the etiology of the pain or intensify their focus on their genitals. In some instances, it is reasonable to perform a scrotal ultrasound, because the underlying fear of the physician (and occasionally, the patient) is the possibility of missing an occult neoplasm. Scrotal ultrasound is valuable in excluding a testicular tumor.

## MEDICAL THERAPY

Despite little or no objective evidence of a specific problem that is responsible for the pain in an overwhelming majority of instances, a variety of medications have been prescribed. Initially, various antibiotics are often administered, but these are rarely, if ever, beneficial. The same situation applies to nonsteroidal anti-inflammatory drugs.

Some investigators recommend the administration of alpha-adrenergic blocking agents in patients with so-called prostatodynia or nonbacterial prostatitis. This recommendation is based on clinical and video urodynamic studies of prostatodynia patients which demonstrate that some have "spastic" dysfunction of the bladder neck and prostatic urethra (the internal urinary sphincter). Principle findings are depressed urinary-flow rates, incomplete relaxation of the bladder neck, and prostatic urethra to a point just proximal to the external urinary sphincter. It is suggested that these men have an acquired functional disorder—a type of bladder-internal sphincter dyssynergia that has been called bladder-neck/urethral spasm syndrome. The postulated basis for symptoms is that smooth-muscle spasm of the bladder neck and prostatic urethra causes elevated prostatic urethral pressures, resulting in intraprostatic and ejaculatory-duct urinary reflux. This leads to chemical prostatitis, seminal vesiculitis, and even epididymitis. In our experience, alpha-adrenergic blocking agents are seldom successful in relieving chronic unexplained genital pain, including patients with so-called prostatodynia and nonbacterial prostatitis.

## LOCAL ANESTHETIC BLOCKS

Nerve blocks have been used with limited success in some men with chronic, unrelenting genital pain, but long-lasting success is rarely achieved. The most common attempted blocks have been ilioinguinal, genitofemoral, and spermatic-cord blocks, generally with a long-acting local anesthetic such as bupivacaine, which sometimes includes steroids. Other nerve blocks that have been employed are paravertebral nerve-root blocks at the T10 to L1 level, and even injection of the pelvic plexus via a transrectal route using transrectal ultrasound guidance.

## SURGICAL INTERVENTION

Testicular denervation has been described for the treatment of intractable testicular pain. The procedure is performed through an inguinal incision after the external oblique aponeurosis is incised. The spermatic cord is mobilized and skeletonized, leaving behind the testicular artery and one vein with or without the vas deferens. A Doppler probe is helpful in identifying the testicular artery, which is quite small and often goes into spasm after handling. Using bipolar diathermy, the periadventitial layers of the artery are stripped over a length of 2–3 cm, thus interrupting the afferent nociceptive sympathetic fibers from the testicles to the T10–L1 level. The ilioinguinal nerve is left undisturbed, but the cremaster fibers are divided completely, resulting in transection of the genital branch of the genitofemoral nerve. One investigator described the use of this technique in four patients with chronic testicular pain, resulting in immediate and lasting relief.

More recently, Brooks and colleagues reported the use of laparoscopic resection of both spermatic cords to denervate the testicles in a patient with chronic orchialgia. Complete pain relief was achieved in this single patient, but the authors imply that relief may have resulted from complete removal of a significantly inflamed area of spermatic cord related to the use of Gianturco coils used to treat bilateral varicoceles that were considered responsible for the pain.

Epididymectomy has been attempted to resolve the chronic pain thought to be caused by this structure, but almost never affords pain resolution. In the series reported by Davis and colleagues, 9 of 10 patients who underwent epididymectomy required subsequent orchiectomy for definitive treatment. Epididymectomy was initially selected because the pain seemed to be localized to that region and the patients preferred a testis-sparing procedure. The average interval between epididymectomy and orchiectomy was 15 mo.

Other surgical approaches have included bilateral orchiectomy for an apparent diagnosis of intermittent testicular torsion, hydrocelectomy, spermatocelectomy, and varicocele repair with variable results. I do not share the assertion that varicocele causes chronic orchialgia of any consequence. Varicocele is an extremely common finding, occurring in approx 15% of the general population of men. It is well known to experienced urologists that varicoceles, even very large varicoceles, are rarely, if ever, symptomatic. The one possible exception to this is the rare patient with a thrombus in the pampiniform plexus, which resolves with conservative management. Therefore, I strongly discourage surgical intervention for relief of pain secondary to varicocele. If varicocele repair is planned as a last resort, it is essential that the patient have a clear understanding that the overwhelming odds are that the pain is not likely to be relieved.

Orchiectomy has been the most commonly recommended procedure for chronic genital pain. Davis and colleagues concluded that inguinal orchiectomy was the procedure of choice for the management of chronic testicular pain when conservative measures were unsuccessful. Of the 15 patients in their series who underwent inguinal orchiectomy, 11 (73%) reported complete relief of pain and four had partial relief. Alternatively, of the nine patients who underwent scrotal orchiectomy, 5 (55%) reported complete relief of pain; three had partial relief, and one denied any improvement. The recommendation for inguinal orchiectomy was made despite the fact that the difference between the two approaches was not statistically significant.

Costabile and colleagues reported that surgery offered no benefit following a large variety of surgical procedures performed to relieve testicular pain. These authors performed 74 different surgical procedures in 48 men with chronic orchialgia. Of the patients who underwent orchiectomy, 80% continued to complain of pain. It is interesting to observe that the pathological findings of the testicles following removal was benign, and the primary diagnosis was normal tissue with no pathological diagnosis in 80%. Only 2 of the 10 specimens who underwent orchiectomy revealed a minor abnormality, minimal focal tubular atrophy—a diagnosis not indicative of a chronic pain etiology. Other surgical procedures included epididymectomy, varicocele ligation, scrotal inguinal exploration, vasectomy, hernia repair, transurethral resection of the prostate or bladder neck, and a variety of other procedures. Each patient had an average of 1.6 operations, and some underwent as many as five or six operations in an attempt to resolve the complaint. For the most part, surgery offered no benefit. The authors reported that the common sequence observed after surgical intervention was a brief period of improvement followed by subsequent recurrence of the pain. They concluded that surgical intervention should be limited to cases in which a clear indication is present. We wholeheartedly agree with this approach.

The literature clearly shows variable and generally poor results following a variety of surgical procedures for chronic genital pain. Despite multiple surgical procedures, the patients usually continue to experience unrelenting pain. It is our firm belief that with rare exception, invasive surgical procedures should be avoided.

## PSYCHOLOGICAL FACTORS

There is increasing data to indicate that men with genital pain and no organic findings have a high incidence of life stress and psychological disturbance. Schover reported that among 48 men with genital pain and no organic findings psychological disorders were diagnosed frequently, including somatization disorder (56%), nongenital chronic-pain syndrome (50%), major depression (27%), and chemical dependency (27%) (Table 2). About one-third of the men were socially isolated, and 18% had an important emotional loss at the time of pain onset. Despite their mean age of 41 yr, only one-half of the men were married. Additionally, sexual anxiety and dysfunction were quite

Table 2
Stresses at Pain Onset (48 Men)[a]

| Stresses | N (%) |
|---|---|
| History of significant loss | 23 (48) |
| Recent breakup of relationship | 17 (35) |
| Job stress | 16 (33) |
| Social isolation | 15 (31) |
| Financial problems | 13 (27) |
| Pressure to commit to a new partner | 13 (27) |
| Illness of spouse or partner | 4 (8) |
| Infertility | 3 (6) |

[a]From Schover LR (1990) Psychological factors in men with genital pain. *Clevel Clin J Med* 57: 697–700, with permission.

common. These data suggested that genital pain without organic findings is often related to psychological disorders, life stress, and poor social support.

Costabile and colleagues concluded that chronic testicular pain is a fairly common manifestation of chronic pain syndrome associated with a high incidence of clinical depression. They believed that treatment of these patients is best managed by a multidisciplinary approach involving the urologist and a pain-clinic environment. Others have also indicated that some of these patients have chronic pain syndrome.

Increasing evidence suggests that psychological factors play an important role in genital pain that has no identifiable organic cause. Various studies indicate that features of patients with chronic genital pain are similar to those of patients with chronic pain syndromes. The most consistent psychological features in these men are somatization disorder, major depression, anxiety, and a constellation of difficulty establishing relationships, sexual anxiety, and sexual dysfunction. These factors must be addressed when managing patients with chronic genital pain.

## NEUROMUSCULAR PELVIC-FLOOR DYSFUNCTION

Some investigators have described a condition involving the pelvic-floor muscles or areas of attachment that may be responsible for the discomfort observed in some patients with chronic genital pain. We have coined the term "neuromuscular pelvic-floor dysfunction" to encompass these patients. There is support for this disorder in the literature, which is familiar to specialists in physical medicine and rehabilitation, but not generally familiar to the overwhelming number of practicing urologists.

Sinaki and colleagues described a condition called pelvic-floor tension myalgia, which is characterized by continuous habitual contraction of the muscles of the pelvic floor (levator ani and short external rotators of the hip). The syndrome occurs in both men and women, and may be secondary to some local, painful, inflammatory condition, or there may be no such local factors. These patients complain of perineal or genital pain that is aggravated by sitting or automobile riding and is accompanied by suprapubic pressure or pain and variable urinary symptoms. The pain is often ascribed to and the patient often managed for a diagnosis of chronic prostatitis or prostatosis despite the absence of physical findings or objective criteria to establish this diagnosis. Some men also report difficulty urinating in public restrooms. Affected patients are usually tense, impulsive individuals, and appear to be somewhat neurotic. Segura and colleagues have discussed the diagnosis and treatment of this disorder. Patients often complain of perineal discomfort or pain, usually within a short time after sitting down. The discomfort may be accompanied by testicular ache and a feeling of heaviness or aching in the area of the pelvis. Frequency and urgency are common. After sitting or riding for a short time, patients become uncomfortable because of pain resulting from compression or painfully contracting, fatigued, and sore pelvic muscles. As the pain increases, the tension and contraction of the pelvic muscles also increases in a vicious cycle. Objective findings are limited to pain or tenderness of the muscles of the pelvic floor during rectal examination. Palpation of the levator ani on either side, and of the short external rotators, may be painful. The prostate is not usually tender. Because the primary pathological process is probably habitual contraction and spasm of the pelvic-floor muscles, therapy is directed at reduction of pain and relaxation of the affected muscles. Tenderness is decreased when the patient is urged to relax those muscle groups. A counterpart of the above-described syndrome of chronic genital pain in men has also been observed in women with vulvar vestibulitis syndrome marked by a significant history of long-term moderate to severe chronic introital dyspareunia and tenderness of the vulvar vestibule.

Although it is unclear what impact physical therapy has in the management of patients with chronic unexplained genital pain, we feel it is an important facet of the approach to treatment. Physical therapy may have a significant therapeutic benefit in men with definitive neuromuscular pelvic-floor dysfunction. The use of physical therapy has the added important advantage of meeting the patient's expectation for a medical rather than psychological intervention. We do not feel it is productive to emphasize to the patient that the problem is psychogenic. Rather, we present the problem as one of stress-related chronic pelvic-muscle tension.

## MULTIDISCIPLINARY APPROACH TO THE MANAGEMENT OF CHRONIC GENITAL PAIN

The treatment of patients with chronic genital pain is difficult and time-consuming. Patients are typically tense, anxious, and concerned that they have a dreaded condition. Generally, they have a history of consulting a number of other physicians and have experienced a variety of tests and treatments. When all else fails, the hapless man may have been advised to undergo surgery or is told that the problem is "all in his head." In order for the urologist or other physician to achieve any degree of success in dealing with such a patient, it is critical to approach them with compassion, and convey an interest in helping them.

We have adopted a systematic multidisciplinary approach for patients with chronic genital pain, intended for those who have had chronic genital pain for several months or longer—not those with relatively new, unexplained genital pain that can often be managed by reassurance alone. The initial evaluation is done by a urologist. A careful history is taken, and a physical examination is conducted. It is essential to rule out any possible organic cause of the pain. Basic laboratory tests are done as previously outlined. Any additional diagnostic studies that the urologist wishes to obtain, such as scrotal ultrasound, are arranged. The urologist usually introduces the diagnosis of neuromuscular pelvic-floor dysfunction to the patient and advises him that we have a special program to help men with their particular disorder. Rather than focus on the psychological aspects of the disorder, the urologist relates that the pain is often attributed to stress-related chronic muscle tension, and informs the patient of the program that we have available to help manage this disorder. The patient is asked to read a specific patient information sheet describing the details of the program. The urologist arranges referrals to a mental health professional and a physical therapist who has a specific interest and knowledge in managing this disorder. The urologist will usually see the patient in follow-up visits at variable periods to monitor his progress. The role of the urologist, therefore, is to rule out an organic explanation for the patient's pain, to introduce the patient to our specialized neuromuscular pelvic-floor dysfunction program, and to monitor the patient's progress.

The mental health professional conducts a psychological evaluation interview. This structured interview includes a brief developmental history, current and lifetime major disorders of mood, anxiety, somatization, chemical dependency, current social support, past and current sexual function, history of sexual trauma or paraphilia, and recent life stresses, especially emotional losses. Written psychological testing is also performed. Patients are requested to complete a Brief Symptom Inventory, in which the man relates the degree he is distressed in relation to 53 problems. The patient also completes a male pain questionnaire covering a variety of questions on sexual function and the degree of genital or pelvic pain experienced during various sexual and nonsexual activities. Depending on the outcome of the testing, ongoing psychotherapy is provided as indicated, often focusing on stress management and treating sexual problems. In some instances, antidepressants may be prescribed.

An initial physical therapy evaluation is performed. The therapist takes a history and examines the patient. Initial values for pelvic-muscle strength are recorded, and the patient is introduced to pelvic-muscle biofeedback, which is performed using appropriately placed pads. Homework exercises are prescribed to increase pelvic-muscle strength and voluntary control over pelvic-floor muscle contraction. The theory behind increasing muscle strength is that a maximal contraction is followed by maximal relaxation. Therefore, the patient not only increases pelvic-muscle strength but also learns how to relax the pelvic muscles and control pelvic-floor muscle instability. Ongoing physical therapy is provided, and progress is monitored. After 6 mo of treatment, ending values for pelvic-muscle strength are recorded, and the therapist provides an outcome evaluation.

It is too early to determine the outcome of this multidisciplinary approach for the management of chronic genital pain, but initial experience with this program is promising. A majority of patients appear to receive some benefit and return to a more productive lifestyle. As already emphasized, many types of treatments for patients with this disorder have almost always been unsuccessful. We believe that our multidisciplinary program for men with so-called "neuromuscular pelvic-floor dysfunction" is a rational means of dealing with and understanding this chronic, unrelenting pain disorder. We recommend that others adopt a similar approach for patients with this extremely difficult form of chronic pain. Not only does this program provide a compassionate attempt to resolve the problem, but it represents a cost-effective approach in a rapidly changing period of health-care delivery. The ultimate goal for the management of these men may not be to completely resolve the pain, but to provide better coping mechanisms for dealing with it.

## SELECTED READING

Brooks JD, Moore RG, Kavoussi LR (1994) Laparoscopic management of testicular pain after embolotherapy of varicocele. *J Endourol* 8:361–363.
Choa RG, Swami KS (1992) Testicular denervation. A new surgical procedure for intractable testicular pain. *Br J Urol* 70:417–419.
Costabile RA, Hahn M, McLeod DG (1991) Chronic orchialgia in the pain prone patients: the clinical perspective. *J Urol* 146:1571–1574.
Davis BE, Noble MJ, Weigel JW, et al. (1990) Analysis and management of chronic testicular pain. *J Urol* 143:936–939.
Egan KJ, Krieger JN (1994) Psychological problems in chronic prostatitis patients with pain. *Clin J Pain* 10:218–226.
Glazer HI, Rodke G, Swencionis C, et al. (1995) Treatment of vulvar vestibulitis syndrome with electromyographic biofeedback of pelvic floor musculature. *J Reprod Med* 40:283–290.
Holland JM, Feldman JL, Gilbert HC (1994) Phantom orchialgia. *J Urol* 152:2291–2293.
Keltikangus-Jarvinen L, Jarvinen H, Lehtonen T (1981) Psychic disturbances in patients with chronic prostatitis. *Ann Clin Res* 13:45–49.
Kursh ED, Schover LR (1997) the dilemma of chronic genital pain. *AUA Update Series* 16(37):290–296.
McMahon AJ, Buckley A, Taylor SN, et al. (1992) Chronic testicular pain following vasectomy. *Br J Urol* 69:188–191.
Meares EM, Jr (1986) Prostatodynia: clinical findings and rationale for treatment. In: Weidner W, Brunner, Krause W, Ruthauge CF, eds., *Therapy of Prostatitis*. Munich: W Zuckswerdt Verlag, pp. 207–212.
Miller HC (1988) Stress prostatitis. *Urology* 32:507–510.
Schover LR (1990) Psychological factors in men with genital pain. *Clevel Clin J Med* 697–700.
Segura JW, Opitz JL, Green LF (1979) Prostatosis, prostatitis, or pelvic floor tension myalgia? *J Urol* 122:168–169.
Sinaki M, Merritt JL, Stillwell GK (1997) Tension myalgia of the pelvic floor. *Mayo Clin Proc* 52:717–722.
Yeates WK (1985) Pain in the scrotum. *Br J Hosp Med* 101–104.

# 28 A Practical Approach to Male Infertility

*James A. Daitch, MD
and Anthony J. Thomas, Jr., MD*

**CONTENTS**

    INTRODUCTION
    HISTORY
    GONADOTOXINS
    REVIEW OF SYSTEMS
    PHYSICAL EXAMINATION
    VARICOCELE
    ABSENCE OF THE VAS DEFERENS
    SEMEN ANALYSIS
    TESTS OF SPERM FUNCTION
    SUMMARY
    SELECTED READING

## INTRODUCTION

Approximately 50% of couples who are actively attempting to conceive a child will achieve conception within 6 mo. Eighty to 85% will conceive within 1 yr. Infertility, therefore, is defined as the failure to establish a pregnancy after 1 yr of frequent, unprotected intercourse. The term "primary infertility" refers to couples who have never had children, whereas "secondary infertility" refers to those who have had children in the past but subsequently cannot initiate another pregnancy. A significant number of the 15–20% who do not easily conceive will seek professional help in their quest to have children. As more people defer parenthood until later in life, the number of infertile couples will continue to increase. The growing numbers of affected couples combined with the exciting and well-publicized advances in assisted reproductive techniques (ART) have led to an increase in the requests for infertility evaluations by over 200% just in the last 10 yr. This chapter outlines some of the more important aspects of the outpatient evaluation, as well as some of the treatment options available to the infertile male.

From: *Current Clinical Urology: Office Urology: The Clinician's Guide*
Edited by: E. D. Kursh and J. C. Ulchaker © Humana Press Inc., Totowa, NJ

Of the estimated 4.5 million infertile American couples, a male factor alone is identified in approx 20–30% of cases. A combination of problems involving both the man and the woman accounts for an additional 20%.

An early and thorough evaluation of the male patient may identify a significant problem causing the infertility, thereby avoiding unnecessary and inappropriate testing and treatment for his partner. Occasionally, the examination may uncover a more serious health problem linked to the patient's fertility status, such as testis or pituitary tumors, an endocrine disorder, or generally poor health habits, such as smoking, use of inappropriate drugs, or excessive alcohol consumption.

The initial fertility investigation of the male patient includes a well-directed history, a careful physical examination, and at least two properly performed semen analyses. Further testing—including hormonal assessment, functional sperm testing, and sonographic imaging—may subsequently be indicated based on the initial assessment.

## HISTORY

A thorough history with emphasis on past medical problems related to reproductive function may identify a potential cause for the couple's infertility. It is important to know if the patient or his partner has ever initiated a pregnancy, either between them or with another partner. If they have, are there or have there been any problems that may have altered one or the other's fertility potential? Knowing how long the couple has been trying to achieve a pregnancy, as well as what prior contraceptive techniques were used, puts their past efforts into a temporal perspective. Since the natural pregnancy rate is approx 25–30% per menstrual cycle, if they have been trying for less than a year or have been having intercourse infrequently, there may not have been adequate time or exposure for them to establish a conception. The couple's sexual frequency and timing should be assessed to determine whether intercourse is taking place at the right time of the cycle and often enough to allow for a pregnancy to occur. All too often, working couples complain of being too tired to have intercourse during the week, and play "catch up" on the weekends. Couples who are actively trying to conceive need to make a concerted effort to have intercourse every day or every other day during the days prior to and the day of ovulation. Waiting for these days to have intercourse— the so-called "saving up technique"—should be discouraged, as any prolonged abstinence may lessen sperm motility. When discussing the frequency of intercourse, it is also important to assess whether there are any sexual difficulties, such as erectile dysfunction or premature or retarded ejaculation. Some couples may be using artificial vaginal lubricants for intercourse. Most of these substances (including water-soluble surgical gel) can adversely affect sperm motility, and should be strictly avoided.

## GONADOTOXINS

It is estimated that as many as 20 million American workers are exposed to potentially harmful substances in the workplace. Pesticides, fumigants, herbicides and fungicides, organic solvents, and heavy metals are just some of the toxins that may affect a man's fertility (see Table 1). These effects may be transitory or permanent, depending on the type of toxin and duration of exposure.

Of the more common self-inflicted potential toxins, tobacco and marijuana can contribute to a decreased sperm concentration and diminish motility and normal mor-

## Table 1
### Gonadotoxins/Sperm Function Inhibitors

**Industrial**
- Fumigants
- Heavy metals
  - Cobalt
  - Lead
  - Manganese
- Herbicides/fungicides
- Organic solvents
  - Benzene
  - Ethylene glycol
  - Toluene
- Pesticides
  - Carbamates
  - Organochlorines
  - Organophosphates

**Drugs**
- Anaboloic steroids
- Cigarettes
- Cocaine

**Drugs** cont'd
- Heroin
- Marijuana
- Methadone
- Nitrous oxide

**Medications**
- Allopurinol
- Calcium-channel blockers
- Chemotherapy
- Cimetidine
- Colchicine
- Cyclosporine
- Ketoconazole
- Minocycline
- Nitrofurantoin
- Radiation therapy
- Spironolactone
- Sulfasalazine
- Valproic acid

phology. Excessive alcohol and various illicit narcotics can directly affect testicular function by causing alterations in the hypothalamic-pituitary-testicular axis.

Anabolic steroids, taken to enhance muscle mass and strength, are becoming more commonplace in sports, even at the high-school level. This class of androgenic drugs is often taken in very large, nonphysiologic quantities without medical supervision. The reproductive consequences include a halt in sperm production and the occurrence of testicular atrophy and rarely, gynecomastia. These changes—like those of many of the other drugs mentioned—can be reversed in most—but not all—cases if the offending drug is withdrawn.

Certain medically prescribed drugs can also lead to impaired spermatogenesis or sperm function. Sulfasalazine, commonly used by patients with inflammatory bowel disease, adversely affects sperm production. Similarly, nitrofurantoins and some of the tetracycline-like drugs can lead to decreased sperm concentration when taken for an extended period of time. Calcium-channel blockers have been implicated in the inhibition of the acrosome reaction, thereby decreasing sperm–egg interaction. All drugs should be suspect until carefully studied. Chemotherapeutic agents and radiation therapy may severely and sometimes permanently interfere with spermatogenesis. Azoospermia occurs in 20–40% of men treated with chemotherapy for testicular cancer, and in 70% of men after MOPP (a regimen of mechlorethamine, Oncovin, procarbazine, and prednisone) combination therapy for Hodgkin's disease.

A history of prior medical or surgical problems and procedures may reveal a possible cause for impaired fertility. Cryptorchidism, even with early orchidopexy, is associated with decreased spermatogenesis. Oligospermia may be found in 30% of unilateral cryptorchid patients and in 50% of men with a history of bilateral cryptorchidism. Past testicular trauma, such as torsion or direct injury, may impair spermatogenesis. Mumps orchitis is almost unheard of today because of immunization practices, but in the past could affect the postpubertal male and cause unilateral or more rarely, bilateral testicular atrophy. Some sexually transmitted diseases can cause ductal obstruction in the vasa or epididymides, resulting in azoospermia or severe oligospermia. Other medical illnesses, such as multiple sclerosis or diabetes mellitus, can alter fertility potential by affecting erectile and ejaculatory ability.

A history of a recent significant febrile illness, such as pneumonia, influenza, mononucleosis, or hepatitis, may temporarily disturb spermatogenesis for 3–6 mo before the sperm concentration returns to baseline.

If the patient has a history of a hernia repair, particularly as a child, it is possible that he could have an inguinal vasal obstruction. It has been estimated that injury to the vas occurs in 2–3% of children and 0.5% of adults who undergo inguinal hernia repair. A unilateral injury may never be noticed if the contralateral testis is normal. If the contralateral testis is poorly functioning but has an intact vas deferens, the patient may be oligospermic or azoospermic, depending on the degree of sperm production from that unobstructed side.

A surgical procedure performed on some boys in the past, but rarely done today, is a YV-plasty of the bladder neck. This procedure can result in an open bladder neck and retrograde ejaculation.

Retroperitoneal lymph-node dissection for testicular cancer may interrupt the sympathetic nerve chain and cause either retrograde ejaculation or anejaculation. Currently, nerve-sparing techniques, when possible, are allowing these young men to preserve their ejaculatory capacity.

Total colectomy for ulcerative colitis, pull-through operations for an imperforate anus, or surgery for rectal cancers can also lead to ejaculatory problems caused by either nerve disruption or injury to the vas deferens and seminal vesicles.

## REVIEW OF SYSTEMS

A directed review of systems may reveal problems that the patient considers unrelated to infertility. Recurrent respiratory infections can be associated with nonmotile sperm, or even azoospermia. Depending on their severity and chronicity, they may suggest conditions such as Kartagener's syndrome (a primary ciliary dyskinesia causing chronic sinusitis, bronchiectasis, situs inversus, and immotile sperm), Young's syndrome (chronic bronchitis associated with obstructive azoospermia), or cystic fibrosis coupled with congenital absence of the vas deferens. Congenital anosmia may be associated with hypogonadotropic hypogonadism (Kallmann's syndrome). Galactorrhea, decreased libido, or impaired visual fields are symptoms that can be associated with a prolactin-producing pituitary tumor. Excessive thirst and urinary frequency, combined with a small or absent semen volume, may be an early manifestation of diabetes mellitus with partial or complete retrograde ejaculation.

## PHYSICAL EXAMINATION

A thorough examination should be performed, with particular attention to the genital area.

The presence of normal virilization is easily assessed through an observation of the patient's body and hair, muscle, and genital development. Failure to develop full masculine features along with small testicles might lead to a diagnosis of hypo- or hypergonadotropic hypogonadism. Most of the testicular parenchyma is composed of sperm-producing cells. Therefore, testicular size correlates somewhat with histology to the extent that the smaller the testicles, the less sperm-forming function they may possess. Normal testicular size is approximately equal to or larger than $4 \times 3 \times 2.5$ cm—or by volume, more than 20 cm$^3$. The consistency of a normal testis is firm and pliant, but not hard. The epididymides and vasa deferentia should be palpated and characterized for their presence or absence as well as their consistency. Thickening or induration of the epididymides or vasa suggests an obstructive problem. A digital rectal examination is performed if indicated by the patient's age (>40 yr) or if clinical signs warrant it (leukocytospermia, low semen volume, or absence of seminal emission).

## VARICOCELE

Examination of the spermatic cords with the patient standing upright in a warm, well-lit room is the best method to identify a varicocele. These dilated veins of the pampinaform plexus are present in approx 15% of the general male population, but may be found in 30–40% of men who present with primary infertility. They are most commonly found on the left side, but may be bilateral and rarely on the right side only. Varicoceles are graded according to size, with Grade I being palpable only when the patient performs a Valsalva maneuver. Grade II varicoceles can be palpated at rest and during Valsalva. Grade III varicoceles can be easily visualized through the scrotal skin. A Doppler stethoscope may aid in varicocele detection. Reflux of blood can be heard during Valsalva. Color Doppler ultrasonography can also assist in confirming the diagnosis.

The precise pathophysiology of varicoceles and their effect on fertility has not been fully elucidated or agreed on, although most evidence points toward a decrease in semen quality associated with an increase intratesticular temperature. This may be caused by an increased arterial inflow combined with the effect of the dilated veins as they impair the countercurrent heat exchange necessary for normal spermatogenesis. Improvement in semen parameters has been reported by some in approximately two-thirds of men who undergo varicocele ablation, with associated pregnancy rates averaging about 40%.

## ABSENCE OF THE VAS DEFERENS

Absence of the vas deferens should be readily diagnosed by physical examination alone, and does not generally require surgical exploration. Men with either unilateral or bilateral vasal absence comprise 1–2% of all infertile men and approx 10% of all azoospermic men. When there is unilateral vasal absence, there may be associated congenital renal abnormalities, such as absence of the ipsilateral kidney. Those with bilateral vasal absence may have varying anatomic abnormalities of the seminal vesicles, most commonly absence or hypoplasia. The caput epididymis is usually present when there is vasal absence, but the remainder of the epididymis is often absent, since it—

Table 2
Normal Semen Parameters

Volume: 1.5–5.0 mL
pH: 7.2–7.6
Concentration: >20 million/mL
Total count: >40 million
Motility: >50%
Forward progression: >2 (scale 0–4)
Morphology: ≥30% normal forms WHO criteria
>14% normal forms Kruger criteria
White blood cells: <1 million/mL
No evidence of sperm agglutination or red blood cells

like the vas—is derived from the mesonephric duct. The testicles are usually normal in size and function with regard to spermatogenesis and testosterone production.

The association between both unilateral and bilateral congenital absence of the vas (CAVD) and the cystic fibrosis transmembrane conduction gene mutation is undisputed. Nearly 80% of men with congenital bilateral absence of the vas (CBAVD) will harbor at least one known CF gene mutation. Men with CAVD and their spouses should be offered genetic testing for CF mutations, since these mutations can also be found in approx 4% of the healthy, unaffected spouses. The absence of a positive test does not mean there is no mutation, since not all mutations have been identified, and not all can be tested for. These couples should receive genetic counseling to inform them of their risk for having a child with cystic fibrosis or of passing on the CF mutation gene(s) to their child. These couples will require sperm extraction from the testis or epididymis combined with intracytoplasmic sperm injection (ICSI) if they wish to have their own biologic child.

## SEMEN ANALYSIS

The semen analysis is the cornerstone of the laboratory evaluation for male infertility. At least two analyses should be obtained, separated by a period of several weeks. Two or three days of sexual abstinence are requested prior to each collection. Masturbation is the preferred collection method, although special silicone condoms are commercially available for men who are unable to obtain a semen sample by manual stimulation. The specimen containers used should be made of a material that will not affect sperm viability or motility. The criteria most commonly used for normal values have been established by the World Health Organization (see Table 2). Although it is rare to have only a single abnormal parameter, each will be discussed separately to put into perspective what problems can be found and how they may best be addressed with the infertile male.

### Semen Volume

The normal volume of ejaculate is 1.5–5 mL. Some men have a higher volume, which is not generally a problem unless it is associated with a low sperm concentration. This may cause a relative dilutional effect on the sperm as it comes into contact with the cervix. Low semen volume—particularly volumes of <1 mL—can be a significant causative factor in infertility in and of itself, because it may be insufficient to allow the sperm to contact the cervical mucus. It may also be a sign or symptom indicating a more serious problem.

A low ejaculatory volume may be reported as the result of either an incomplete semen collection or a short abstinence period prior to collection. If these causes are ruled out and the volume is repeatedly <1.5 mL, further evaluation should be carried out to determine if the patient has ejaculatory-duct obstruction, congenital absence of the vasa and ejaculatory ducts, seminal vesicle hypoplasia, retrograde ejaculation, or anejaculation. Some men who have had urethral reconstructive surgery for strictures or hypospadius may have irregular scarring or diverticula within the urethra that prevents efficient expulsion of the semen. They will report that the semen does not come out with force, but rather dribbles out during and after the sensation of ejaculation occurs. Other men ejaculate in a retrograde fashion when there is incompetence of the bladder neck caused by anatomic or neurologic causes. When the semen volume is low or absent, a urine sample obtained within minutes after ejaculation should be examined for sperm to confirm retrograde ejaculation. If sperm are present in the urine and there is no urethral obstruction that needs to be addressed, sympathomimetic medications, such as Ephedrine sulfate, pseudoephedrine, or Phenylpropanolamine hydrochloride, may stimulate the sympathetic nerves sufficiently to cause an antegrade ejaculation to occur. If this fails, the urine can be alkalinized using oral sodium bicarbonate (600 mg every 6 h the day before sperm collection and 1200 mg every 4 h on the day of collection) and the postejaculatory urine can be collected and the sperm separated to be used for insemination or another assisted reproductive procedure. If there is no sperm in the postejaculatory urine, there may be a complete failure of seminal emission. The most common causes for this are spinal cord injury and prior non-nerve sparing retroperitoneal node dissection. Ejaculatory-duct obstruction and absence of the ejaculatory ducts have similar semen parameters. The volume of fluid is usually <1 mL and of thin consistency. No sperm are present in the semen, and its pH is acidic (<6.5) because it is composed mostly of prostatic secretions. When the ejaculatory ducts are obstructed, the epididymides and vasa are often palpably thickened. Transrectal ultrasonography will confirm ejaculatory-duct obstruction. The seminal vesicles are generally enlarged, measuring more than 1.5 cm in antero-posterior diameter. Some authors advocate aspirating the obstructed seminal vesicles transrectally, using ultrasound guidance prior to attempting resection of the ejaculatory ducts. If sperm are found, spermatogenesis is confirmed, as is the absence of a secondary epididymal obstruction.

Some men with spinal cord injuries cannot ejaculate because of the level and completeness of their injury. Some can be stimulated to ejaculate with the use of a high-frequency, hand-held vibrator applied to the ventral aspect of the glans penis. Others may need more intense electrical stimulation to the vasal ampulla and seminal vesicles by means of a transrectal electrical probe. With both methods of stimulation, the most significant risk for men with a high-level spinal cord lesion is the occurrence of autonomic dysreflexia. Careful monitoring, pretreatment with nifedipine, and stopping the stimulation if the blood pressure begins to rise too high or too fast will minimize the risk, but one must be well-prepared to treat the symptoms of dysreflexia if they do occur, as this can pose a life-threatening situation.

## Sperm Concentration

The minimum concentration of 20 million sperm per milliliter of semen is not an absolute number required for pregnancy to occur. If the volume is high, a lower count may still indicate a satisfactory sperm concentration. Even when the concentration is low, if the overall quality is good with regard to motility and percent of normal morphology, pregnancies may readily occur. Deficiencies in the number of sperm, however, are the single factor that most concerns patients.

If a semen sample is found to be totally devoid of sperm on routine analysis, the sample should be centrifuged at 1500–3000 rpm for 10 min and the pellet reexamined for sperm. Sperm may be found in up to 20% of such cases. The remaining patients are truly azoospermic, and although the evaluation of these two groups of men is similar, the ultimate prognosis may be better for those with at least some sperm present in the semen. Azoospermia can be the result of either hormonal abnormalities (pretesticular), primary spermatogenic failure (testicular), or excurrent ductal obstruction (posttesticular).

## Hormonal Evaluation

Testicular function is regulated by the pulsatile release of gonadotropin-releasing hormone (GnRH) from the hypothalamus, which in turn stimulates the release of follicle stimulating hormone (FSH) and luteinizing hormone (LH) from the anterior pituitary gland. FSH facilitates the later stages of spermatogenesis and supports Sertoli cell function. Sertoli cells, in turn, secrete inhibin that serves as a feedback inhibitor for FSH release. LH stimulates the Leydig cells to produce testosterone (T). Testosterone—along with its aromatized metabolite, estradiol—serves as a feedback inhibitor for both hypothalamic GnRH release and the pituitary release of LH. Any defect in this hypothalamic-pituitary-gonadal axis (HPG axis) can result in abnormal or absent spermatogenesis.

Azoospermic men should have a serum FSH and T level obtained to help determine if they have spermatogenic failure, deficiencies in sperm maturation, or obstructive azoospermia (*see* Fig. 1).

When both FSH and T are low, serum LH and prolactin levels should be obtained. If an individual is found to have hypogonadotropic hypogonadism, treatment is directed at hormonal replacement. If the serum prolactin is elevated, imaging of the pituitary gland by MR or CT should be done to determine if the patient has a prolactin-producing pituitary tumor, which may require medical or surgical treatment. Most of these tumors are small, and almost all are benign. Treatment with a dopamine agonist, such as bromocriptine, can be highly effective in lowering the prolactin level and restoring spermatogenesis.

If the FSH and T levels are normal and the testicles >20 cm$^3$ with palpably normal vasa, a testis biopsy is appropriate to determine if the patient is obstructed or has a maturation arrest. If active spermatogenesis is found, further surgery to correct an obstruction or sperm aspiration can be carried out, depending on what is most appropriate for the couple. If the biopsy reveals maturation arrest and there is a varicocele present, consideration should be given to correcting the varicocele, because complete spermatogenesis will sometimes occur. Otherwise, these individuals are left with the options of trying to find sperm somewhere in the testicles by performing multiple biopsies com-

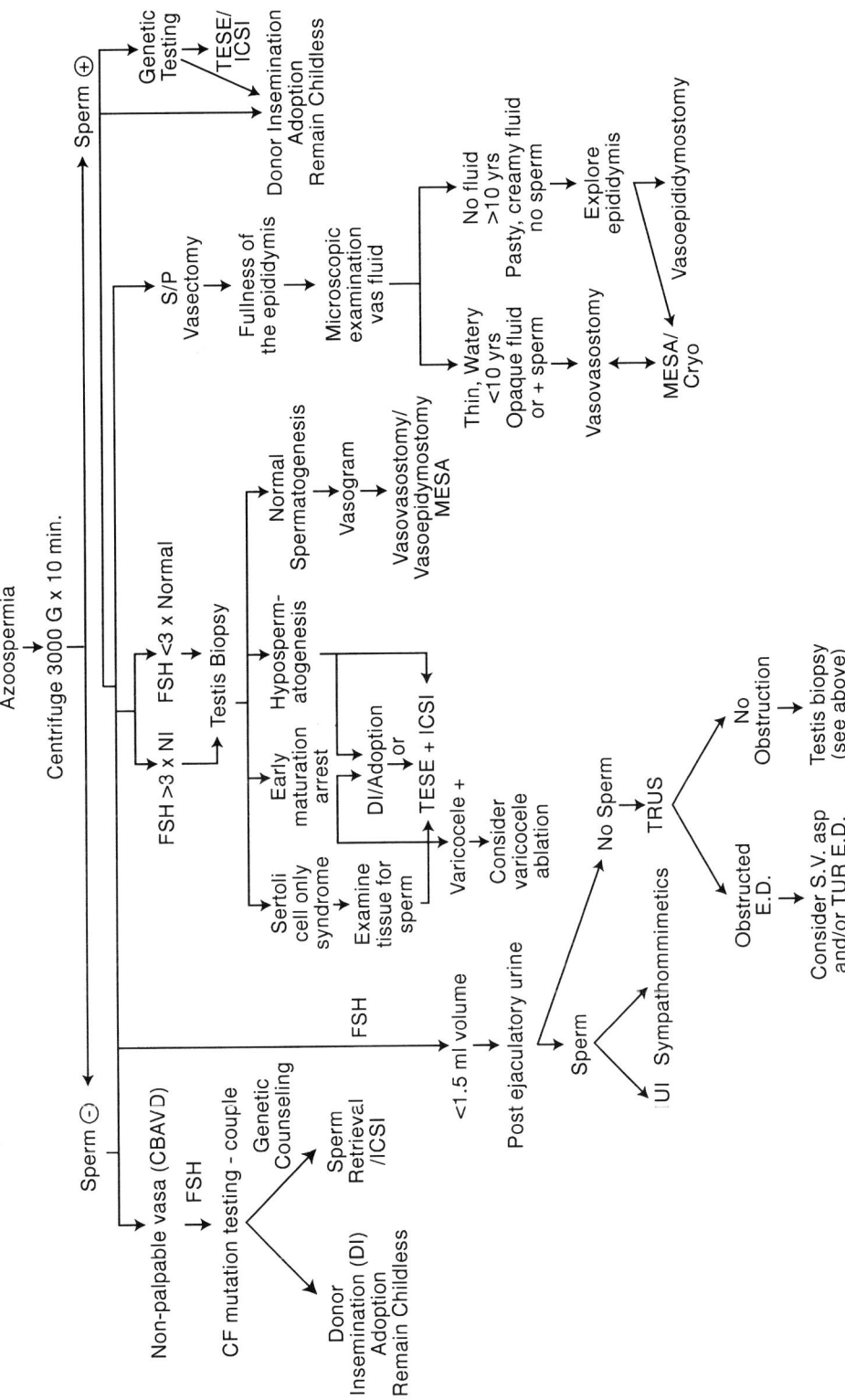

**Fig. 1.** Flowchart of treatment options for azoospermia.

bined with in vitro fertilization (IVF) and intracytoplasmic sperm injection (ICSI) or choosing adoption, donor insemination, or remaining childless.

Patients with azoospermia or severe oligospermia and elevated FSH levels (>3 × normal) have primary spermatogenic failure. A testis biopsy is not needed to confirm the diagnosis. No specific medical treatment is available for these patients to improve sperm production. Some recent reports of such patients have showed improved sperm production if a varicocele is found and is corrected. Although very occasional spontaneous pregnancies were reported in these men after varicocele ligation, most of those who had sperm appear in their semen still required IVF-ICSI, but with ejaculated sperm rather than testicular sperm extraction.

Regardless of whether the man has nonobstructive azoospermia or severe oligospermia, if the couple is going to pursue the possibility of having their own biologic child with assisted reproductive techniques using sperm from his semen or extracted from his testicles, it is appropriate to recommend genetic testing. A simple karyotype may identify a patient with Klinefelter's syndrome, the most common (10–13%) sex-chromosome abnormality found in azoospermic men or one of the other, less common sex-chromosome anomalies. Some men have autosomal abnormalities—such as a chromosomal translocation, inversion, or ring chromosome—that may limit the chance of fathering a viable conceptus, or have significant developmental implications for the child.

Gene deletions on the long arm of the Y chromosome were first described in azoospermic men in the mid 1970s. Since that time, more sophisticated testing has identified microdeletions on the long arm of the Y chromosome in 10–12% of azoospermic men and 3–10% of oligospermic men. These individuals have a normal karyotype. Using special techniques, the Y chromosome has been examined, and at least three regions have been identified (termed AZFa, AZFb, and AZFc) as having the genes needed for spermatogenesis to occur. With microdeletions, spermatogenesis is impaired or absent. As expected, when sperm are found from some of these men and IVF with intracytoplasmic sperm injection (ICSI) is used to establish a pregnancy, the male offspring will also have the Y-chromosome microdeletion and will inherit the father's infertility problem. Couples should be counseled regarding the availability of these tests. They can be done anywhere, in any office in the country, by drawing the patient's blood, with special test tubes, or obtaining a buccal smear with prepackaged kits supplied by the laboratories and sending the sample in to the laboratory by overnight mail. Genetic testing is often not enough, and counseling should be made available for these couples to help them understand the implications of their choices.

## *Oligospermia*

If the sperm concentration is $<10 \times 10^6$/mL, serum FSH and T levels should be obtained to identify a primary endocrine abnormality or to determine if the testis is being maximally stimulated as evidenced by a normal testosterone and a high-normal or elevated serum FSH level. Hormonal deficiencies should be treated appropriately. Men with normal FSH levels and low or normal T levels with normal genital examinations are more difficult to treat, because there may be little other than empirical treatment or ART to fall back on. Most empirical treatment has generally been unsuccessful. Commonly recommended drugs are the antiestrogenic clomiphene citrate and tamoxifen citrate. These agents may act by decreasing the negative feedback on the anterior pituitary, thereby increasing FSH and LH release. The increased FSH and LH are hoped to stimulate increased sperm production. Although controlled studies have failed to show any beneficial results with these drugs, in our experience a small subpopulation of patients (perhaps <10%) appear to respond to these drugs. Our experience has led us to try stimulation for 1 mo, and then to recheck FSH and T levels. If the FSH is >1.5 times the upper limits of normal, or the testosterone is higher than the laboratory's upper normal limits, the drug is withdrawn because it will not be effective. If the values are still within the above parameters, the drug is continued for 6–9 mo, and the patient is examined and semen analysis obtained at 3-mo intervals.

### *Sperm Motility*

Motility is defined as any sperm-tail movement, regardless of whether there is any forward progression. Subjectively, examining a slide containing motile sperm, the technologist determines the percent motile and the quality of the motility by grading the progressive movement of 200 consecutively viewed sperm, divided into two groups of 100 each and averaged. The grade of motility is listed a–d. Grade a) is rapid, progressive motility; b) slow or sluggish but still progressive movement; c) is nonprogressive motility but still with tail twitching; and d) is immotile sperm. When the analysis is performed in a laboratory using a computer assist, the actual velocity of the sperm is averaged, but the percent of slow vs fast-moving sperm is not distinguished.

Asthenospermia (poor sperm motility) is uncommon, but not unheard of, as an isolated deficiency in the semen analysis. It usually coexists with other poor-quality sperm parameters, such as a low count and poor morphology. When it is the sole abnormality, first consider if it was a collection or transport problem. Was the container in which the sample was collected free of sperm toxins? Did the specimen get cold during transit to the laboratory? If it was not a collection problem, some specific testing may identify the cause of the low motility.

It is often helpful for the treating physician to directly view the patient's semen sample to have some idea of the quality of the sperm—particularly the concentration and degree of forward progressive motility. Even the inexperienced eye can determine lack of progressive motility, with sperm shaking with great fervor yet going nowhere. This type of tail movement may indicate the presence of sperm antibodies. Clumping or agglutination of sperm may also be present associated with this type of useless movement.

Testing for antibodies bound to sperm can be done with a variety of commercial kits. One of the most common is the Immunobead Assay. Small beads composed of polyacrylamide bound with antihuman immunoglobulin G (IgG) and A (IgA) are mixed with the patient's washed sperm. If antibody is present on the sperm surface, the beads will bind to the sperm. The test is positive if more than 20% of the sperm exhibit the antibody, but only of clinical significance if there is >50% binding. Therapy in general, and immunosuppressive therapy in particular, have been disappointing and can have significant and lasting side effects. Sperm washing with a buffering solution, such as human tubal fluid (HTF), may sometimes provide enough unbound sperm to attempt intrauterine inseminations. If pregnancy is not achieved, these couples may best be advised to consider IVF/ICSI. The resulting pregnancy rates have been reported to be similar to rates found in couples without antibodies.

Various sperm tail defects have been described that could severely affect the motility of the sperm. Whenever there is consistently <20% motile sperm on a fresh, properly collected semen sample, ultrastructural tail defects must be considered. These defects may also be associated with similar defects in ciliary movement in the respiratory system (immotile cilia syndrome) caused by the congenital absence of dynein arms in the sperm tail and cilia. These and other defects are identifiable by examining the sperm by transmission electron microscopy.

### *Teratozoospermia*

Identifying the morphologic variations of sperm (teratozoospermia) requires a well-trained eye and patience to carefully evaluate 100–200 stained sperm under oil immersion at 600–1000 × magnification. Sperm are currently evaluated for morphologic abnormalities using one of two methods—that defined by the World Health Organization and the more strictly defined criteria described by Kruger et al. By these latter criteria, the percent of normal shape sperm heads has been correlated with the ability to fertilize an egg under laboratory conditions. According to standards set forth by the World Health Organization, more than 30% of examined sperm should be classified as morphologically normal. Using the more strict criteria, 14% or more should be judged as normal. This does not mean that less than the lower limits of normal relegates a couple to ICSI or remaining infertile, but it is likely that morphologically abnormal sperm are much less likely to fertilize the egg.

### *Leukocytospermia*

Round cells reported to be present in the semen deserve special mention. To the inexperienced technologist performing the analysis, some round cells—which are actually immature sperm cells—can be misread as while blood cells (WBCs). Since more than $1 \times 10^6$ white cells/mL are considered abnormal, whenever there are this many or more round cells, a test to differentiate immature sperm from white cells should be performed. Staining of the cells on a dry, fixed slide will allow an experienced person to identify the different types of cells. Other more objective methods are available that enable the observer to identify and quantify granulocytes (PMNs)—the most common excess white cells found in the semen—by using a peroxidase straining technique. All types of white blood cells present in the semen can be identified using monoclonal antibody (MAb) staining methods specific for each cell type.

Excessive granulocytes in the semen may indicate an infective or inflammatory condition, generally emanating from the prostate and almost always without clinical symptoms. These white cells may adversely affect sperm function by increasing the free radicals (reactive oxygen species—ROS) and overwhelming the naturally occurring antioxidants within the semen. Treatment has been somewhat empirical, because antibiotics are given along with antioxidants (vitamins E and C) and instructions to ejaculate frequently to clear the white cells from the prostate. Semen or prostatic fluid cultures can be performed, but generally are obtained if the patient is symptomatic or fails to clear the white cells after the regimen outlined here is conducted.

## TESTS OF SPERM FUNCTION

The semen analysis is the first and most important test to be requested when a male patient is being evaluated for infertility. Depending on the results, other tests would be requested to more clearly identify where the problem lies and what possible solutions

## Table 3
## Tests of Sperm Function

| Test | What is done | What is measured |
| --- | --- | --- |
| Bovine mucus penetration test | A open capillary tube filled with bovine cervical mucus (CM) is placed in a container with some of patient's semen. The distance that the sperm swim in the tube is measured after 60 min. It should be > 30 mm. | This test may identify problems with excessive viscosity (inability of sperm to transfer from semen to CM), poor quality motility, and the possibility of sperm antibodies if penetration is poor. |
| Eosin-Y viability stain | Eosin-Y stain is taken up only by dead sperm. | Determines if sperm are nonmotile or nonviable. |
| Hypoosmotic swelling test | Sperm are exposed to hypoosmotic environment. | Live sperm in a hypoosmotic environment can absorb fluid that is manifested by swelling and curling of the tail. Can be used to differentiate nonmotile live from dead sperm for IVF/ICSI. |
| Sperm penetration assay | Hamster oocytes, stripped of their zona pellucida, are incubated with human sperm. Number of sperm penetrating and decondensing in oocytes are determined. | Indirectly measures ability of sperm to undergo some of the changes necessary to carry out the fertilization process, namely capacitation and the acrosome reaction. |
| Acrosome reaction assay | Variety of assays available to determine the percent of sperm that can undergo the physical and biochemical changes necessary for sperm–egg fusion and penetration. | The acrosome covers more than half of the sperm head and contains the acrosin and hyaluronidase needed for oocyte penetration after capacitation takes place. Test determines ability of sperm to penetrate the zona pellucida. |
| Reactive oxygen species | Measures potentially toxic oxygen radicals present in the semen and derived from spermatozoa and white-blood cells. | High levels of ROS have been correlated with decreased fertility. |

exist. Some of the more useful tests used to determine the functional integrity of the sperm are listed in Table 3.

## SUMMARY

Recent advances in the field of male reproduction—particularly the ability to use very few sperm to establish a pregnancy through IVF/ICSI—have expanded our knowledge of human reproduction. These developments have allowed physicians to offer patients assistance when previously there was no hope. Most infertile men do not require the use of advanced reproductive techniques. An evaluation can be carried out that is both cost-effective and efficient. It is necessary to have a thorough understanding of the various laboratory tests available for these men and when each should be ordered. The physician must be aware of the various problems that can affect the male reproductive system and how best to identify a cause and a possible solution.

## SELECTED READING

Carbone DJ, Jr (1999) Male reproductive physiology and assisted reproductive technology. *AUA Update Series* 18(21):162.

Hallak J, Hendin BN, Thomas AJ, Jr, Agarwal A (1998) Investigation of fertilizing capacity of cryopreserved spermatozoa from patients with cancer. *J Urol* 159:1217.

Howards SS (1995) Treatment of male infertility. *N Engl J Med* 332(5):312.

Jarow JP, Sigman M (1999) Office evaluation of the subfertile male. *AUA Update Series* 18(23):178.

Kim ED, Leibman BB, Grinblat DM, Lipshultz LI (1999) Varicocele repair improves semen parameters in azoospermic men with spermatogenic failure. *J Urol* 162(3 Pt 1):737–740.

Kruger TF, Menkveld R, Stander FS, Lombard CJ, Van der Merwe JP, van Zyl JA, Smith K (1986) Sperm morphologic features as a prognostic factor in *in vitro* fertilization. *Fertil Steril* 46:1118.

Lipshultz LI, Howards SS, eds., (1997) *Infertility in the Male.* St. Louis: Mosby-Year Book, Inc.

Mathews GJ, Matthews ED, Goldstein M (1998) Induction of spermatogenesis and achievement of pregnancy after microsurgical varicocelectomy in men with azoospermia and severe oligoasthenospermia. *Fertil Steril* 70(1):71.

Schlegel PN (1997) Is assisted reproduction the optimal treatment for varicocele-associated male infertility? A cost effectiveness analysis. *Urol* 49:83.

Schlesinger M, Ilene FW, Nagler H (1994) Treatment outcome after varicocelectomy. *Ur Clin N Am* 21:517.

Vine MF, Margolin BH, Morrison HI, Hulka BS (1994) Cigarette smoking and sperm density: a meta-analysis. *Fertil Steril* 61:35.

Wilcox AJ, Weinberg CR, Baird DD (1995) Timing of sexual intercourse in relation to ovulation. Effects on the probability of conception, survival of the pregnancy, and sex of the baby. *N Engl J Med* 333(23):1517.

World Health Organization (1992) The influence of varicocele on parameters of fertility in a large group of men presenting to infertility clinics. *Fertil Steril* 57:1289.

*WHO Laboratory Manual for the Examination of Human Semen and Sperm-Cervical Mucous Interaction* (1992) New York: Cambridge University Press, (3rd ed.).

# 29 Elective Sterilization

*Roy A. Brandell, MD*
*and Marc Goldstein, MD*

**CONTENTS**
    INTRODUCTION
    PREOPERATIVE CONSIDERATIONS
    TECHNIQUE
    COMPLICATIONS
    CONCLUSION
    SELECTED READING

## INTRODUCTION

Approximately 500,000 men undergo vasectomy in the United States each year. Although it is generally considered a safe and effective method of contraception, over 30% of paid malpractice claims against urologists involve vasectomy-related complications. Thus, it is imperative that urologists be well-versed in the management of men seeking permanent sterilization. The key to avoiding problems is thorough preoperative counseling of the patient, with appropriate documentation and consent. Meticulous operative technique and follow-up will also help to minimize unfortunate outcomes.

## PREOPERATIVE CONSIDERATIONS

### Patient Selection

It is entirely appropriate for urologists to refuse vasectomy if they believe it is not in the patient's best interest. Permanent sterilization may not be appropriate for young, unmarried men with no children. Recently divorced men should be cautioned that divorce with subsequent remarriage to a woman who desires children is the most common reason for requesting vasectomy reversal. Although not required, involvement of the spouse or partner in the decision-making and in witnessing the consent is highly recommended.

From: *Current Clinical Urology: Office Urology: The Clinician's Guide*
Edited by: E. D. Kursh and J. C. Ulchaker © Humana Press Inc., Totowa, NJ

## *Evaluation*

A brief history and physical are appropriate, focusing on those areas relevant to the procedure. The patient should be questioned regarding medications, drug allergies, and any history of bleeding disorders. Prior scrotal surgery, such as orchidopexy or hydrocelectomy, should be noted, because this may make the procedure more difficult. Any history of testicular or scrotal pain should also be clearly documented.

Physical examination of the genitalia should be performed in a warm room to allow for relaxation of the scrotum and detection of any anatomic abnormalities or unusual tenderness. Since men who request vasectomy usually have no specific complaints, it is tempting to perform a cursory exam to simply document the presence of two vasa. This temptation must be resisted. Many men requesting vasectomy are in the age group for which the incidence of testicular cancer is highest. Furthermore, hernias, hydroceles, or symptomatic varicoceles that need repair should be diagnosed, so that treatment can be offered concurrently with the vasectomy. Any abnormalities on scrotal examination or unexplained testicular symptoms should be evaluated with a scrotal ultrasound.

If one of the vasa is congenitally absent, an abdominal ultrasound should be obtained, because these patients have a high incidence of renal agenesis. A vas that is difficult to palpate may require performance of the vasectomy in the operating room. In our experience, this is fairly unusual. Penile or scrotal infections should be diagnosed and treated prior to the vasectomy. Routine laboratory testing is unnecessary in most cases, and should only be obtained for specific indications.

## *Counseling*

It is extremely important for the patient to understand how the procedure is done and all potential complications, both short-term and long-term. They should be reassured that vasectomy does not change semen volume or appearance, erectile function, libido, or quality of orgasm. The role of vasectomy as a *permanent* form of sterilization must be emphasized. Patients need to be aware that vasectomy reversal is possible, but success is not guaranteed and the procedure is costly, lengthy, and rarely covered by insurance. They should also be counseled that cryopreservation of sperm is a service widely available in most metropolitan areas. However, men should not count on cryopreserved semen as a guarantee of future fertility.

Some urologists perform all patient education themselves, whereas others make use of videotapes or nursing personnel as a time-saving measure. Preprinted instructions outlining what to expect before, during, and after the vasectomy are highly recommended. The consent form should clearly indicate that patient education has been provided and seems to be understood, and that all questions have been answered.

## TECHNIQUE

A myriad of techniques for vasectomy have been described over the years. Most urologists who perform the procedure have made their own personal modifications to the reported techniques based on their individual experience and preferences. We will describe the "No-scalpel" vasectomy in detail, and briefly summarize some of the other options available.

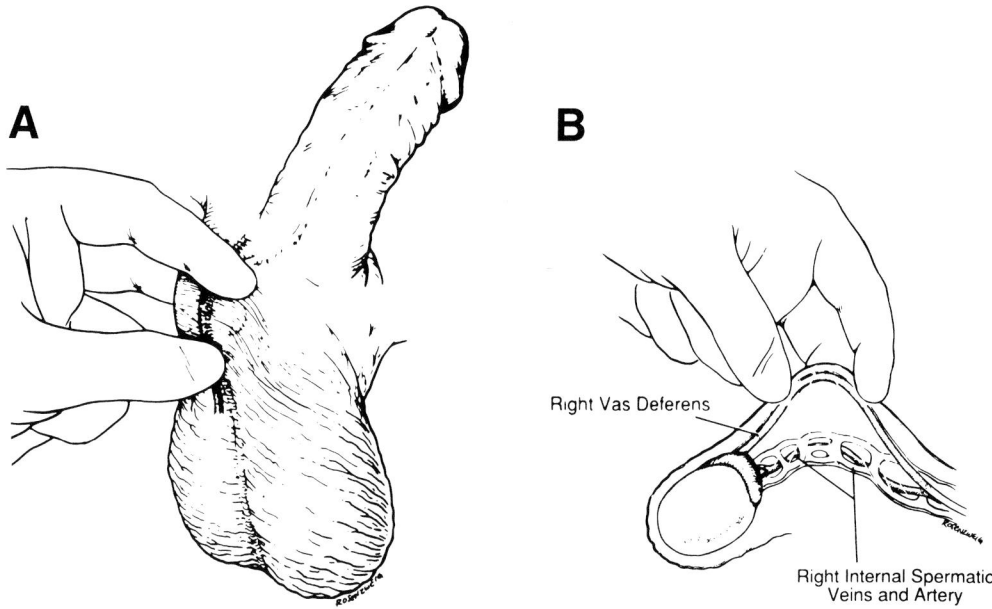

Fig. 1. (A,B) Three-finger technique for isolation of the vas deferens just below the scrotal skin near the median raphe. (From Schlegel, PN, Goldstein, M (1995) Vasectomy. In: Goldstein, M, ed., *Surgery of Male Infertility*, Philadelphia: WB Saunders Co., p. 36, with permission.)

## *Preparation and Local Anesthesia*

The procedure is greatly facilitated by having a relaxed patient with a relaxed scrotum. This is accomplished by giving the patient 10 mg of oral diazepam after arrival to the office. A warm room and warm antiseptic solutions for prepping help to relax the scrotum for easier identification of the vas deferens.

Local anesthesia is obtained by isolating the vas below the median raphe, using the three-finger technique depicted in Fig. 1. One percent plain lidocaine buffered with sodium bicarbonate to prevent burning is injected via a 25-gauge, 1.5-in. needle, raising a superficial skin wheal. The needle is then advanced its full length immediately adjacent and parallel to the vas. Five cubic centimeters of lidocaine is injected within the external spermatic sheath as the needle is withdrawn. The vas deferens is released, and the opposite vas is anesthetized using the same technique. Most of the anesthetic is injected away from the vasectomy site, toward the external inguinal ring. This effects a vassal block while avoiding edema immediately around the vasectomy site, thus facilitating isolation of the vas.

## *Delivery and Occlusion of the Vas*

The vas should again be fixed beneath the previously formed skin wheal using the nondominant hand (*see* Fig. 1). A specially designed extracutaneous fixation clamp is used to stabilize the vas (*see* Fig. 2), and a sharpened, curved hemostat (*see* Fig. 3) is used to puncture the scrotal skin. The vas deferens is punctured and delivered from the scrotum using a rotational motion (*see* Fig. 4). The fixation clamp is removed from

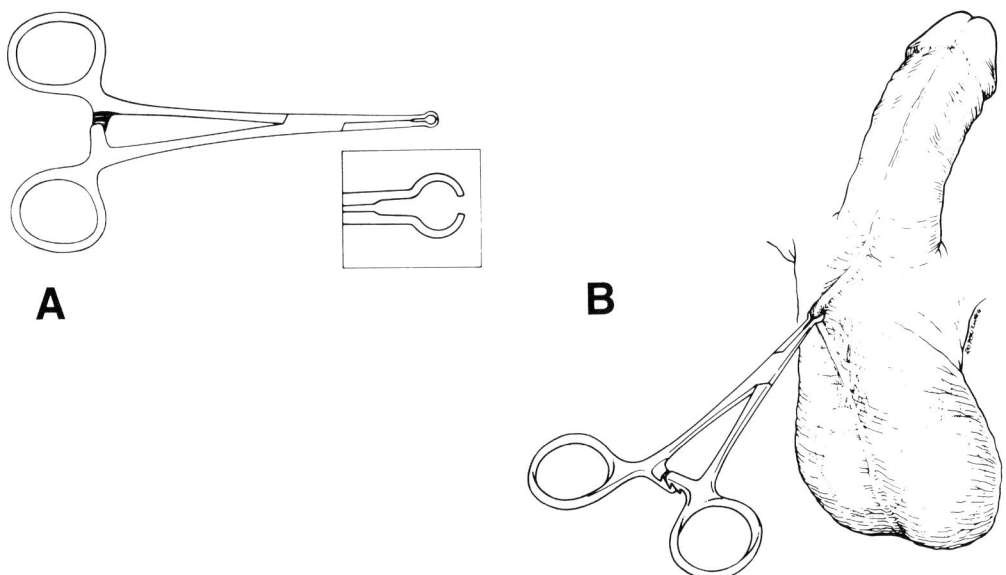

**Fig. 2.** Extracutaneous ring fixation clamp (**A**) used to isolate the vas deferens (**B**) for vasectomy. (From Schlegel, PN, Goldstein, M (1995) Vasectomy. In: Goldstein, M, ed., *Surgery of Male Infertility*, Philadelphia: WB Saunders Co., p. 37, with permission.)

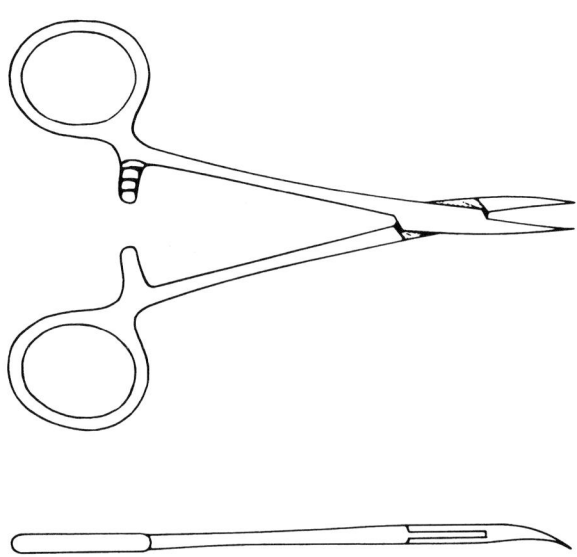

**Fig. 3.** A sharpened curved hemostat-dissecting clamp is used to puncture and deliver the vas deferens. (From Schlegel, PN, Goldstein, M (1995) Vasectomy. In: Goldstein, M, ed., *Surgery of Male Infertility*, Philadelphia: WB Saunders Co., p. 37, with permission.)

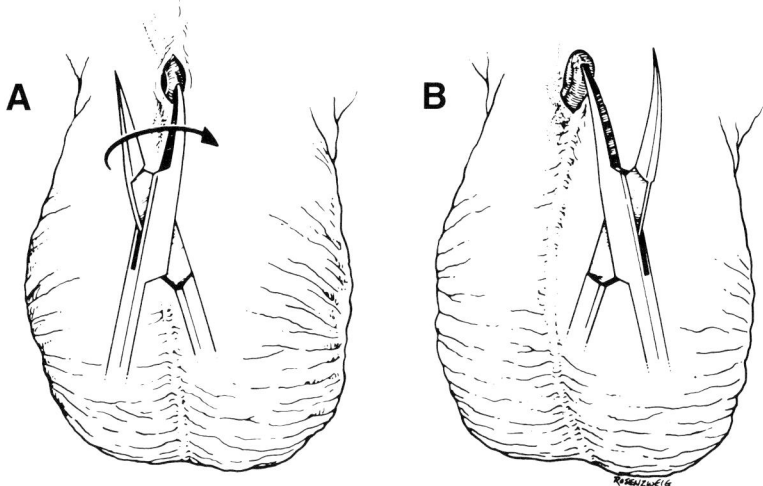

**Fig. 4.** The vas deferens is punctured and, with a rotational motion, delivered (**A**) through the small puncture site (**B**) using the sharp curved hemostat. (From Schlegel, PN, Goldstein, M (1995) Vasectomy. In: Goldstein, M, ed., *Surgery of Male Infertility*, Philadelphia: WB Saunders Co., p. 38, with permission.)

the skin and used to grasp the vas directly. The vasal vessels should then be separated from the vas deferens itself and excluded from the vasectomy site (*see* Fig. 5).

A 1-cm segment of vas is excised. Removing larger segments is unnecessary, and may make future attempts at vasectomy reversal more difficult. Sending the segment for pathologic identification is probably unnecessary for the experienced vasectomist, and is of no proven value from a medico-legal standpoint. A battery-operated cautery needle is placed 1 cm into both lumen of the vas, and then slowly withdrawn while rotating the needle as current is applied. The goal is to cause fibrosis and obliteration of the vasal lumen. Full-thickness burns of the vasal wall should be avoided, because necrosis may result in an increased risk of recanalization. Medium metal clips are then applied to both ends of the vasa in the middle of the cauterized segment. Again, care is taken not to apply the clips so tightly that vasal necrosis ensues. The vassal ends are released and allowed to retract into the scrotum. The opposite side is then performed through the same puncture hole in an identical fashion. Hemostasis should be carefully maintained throughout the procedure, because even minimal bleeding can lead to a large scrotal hematoma.

The skin puncture wound does not require closure with sutures. In fact, leaving a small entry site open may help to prevent hematoma formation. The wound will seal itself within 24 h and is virtually invisible within 1 wk. Antibiotic ointment and a gauze dressing are applied and held in place with a scrotal support.

There are numerous alternatives to the no-scalpel approach. The procedure can certainly be accomplished through one or two small incisions. The incision may be made over the vas prior to applying any clamps. The vas is then secured through the incision with an Allis clamp or towel clip. Rather than clips, the vasal ends can be occluded using absorbable or nonabsorbable suture. Recanalization and subsequent vasectomy failure rate are higher with pure ligature techniques. Alternatively, cautery

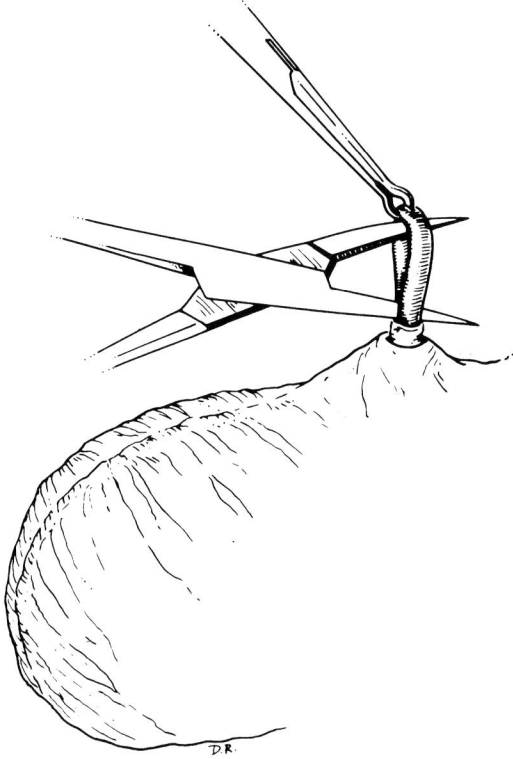

**Fig. 5.** The vasal vessels are dissected off the vas deferens using the hemostat. Sparing these vessels is preferred, but meticulous hemostasis is essential. (From Schlegel, PN, Goldstein, M (1995) Vasectomy. In: Goldstein, M, ed., *Surgery of Male Infertility*, Philadelphia: WB Saunders Co., p. 38, with permission.)

alone may be used, or an "open-ended" vasectomy performed. If the testicular end of the vas is left open, a sperm granuloma is likely to develop. Although this makes future attempts at vasectomy reversal easier (by diminishing epididymal pressure and decreasing the incidence of eipdidymal "blowouts"), it also leads to higher recanalization rates. If an open-ended vasectomy is to be performed, it is wise to bury the vasal ends in different fascial layers to decrease the failure rate. Some urologists perform this maneuver even if the vasal ends have been occluded.

Another practice that has received attention over the years is the irrigation of the abdominal vas with normal saline or unused local anesthetic. Although easily accomplished, a recent study revealed that this practice does not decrease the time or number of ejaculations needed to achieve azoospermia. It also has not been found to decrease the number of postoperative semen analyses required.

## *Postoperative Care*

The patient should be instructed to limit physical activity and lie supine as much as possible during the first 24 h. Intermittent application of an ice pack during the first 12 h helps to decrease pain and swelling. Patients may return to desk work the next day, but heavy lifting, vigorous activity, and sexual intercourse should be avoided for

1 wk. Most patients require only over-the-counter medications for pain control, but occasionally acetaminophen with codeine or a similar-strength analgesic is necessary.

Patients must understand that other forms of contraception should be continued until two separate semen analyses document azoospermia. The disappearance of sperm from the ejaculate correlates more with the number of ejaculates than with the time interval after vasectomy. Approximately 90% of men will be azoospermic after 15 ejaculations. About 80% of men will be azoospermic 6 wk after vasectomy, regardless of ejaculatory frequency. If early failure from recanalization occurs, it will usually do so within the first 12 wk. Based on these observations, we recommend an initial semen analysis 6 wk postoperatively followed by a confirmatory test 4–6 wk later. Only after two consecutive centrifuged semen specimens document azoospermia can the patient be told it is safe to discontinue other forms of contraception. However, he also needs to understand that no procedure is 100% successful, including vasectomy. Late recanalization, even many years after the vasectomy, can occur. We have observed that 10% of men who present for vasectomy reversal will be found to have sperm in their centrifuged semen specimen. Fortunately, the sperm are usually nonmotile and of insufficient quantity to initiate a natural pregnancy. We inform couples that the chance of failure after our no-scalpel vasectomy is about 0.1%.

If the first postoperative semen analysis shows sperm—especially if they are motile—we ask the patient to continue contraception and provide another specimen in 6–8 wk. The presence of motile sperm persisting 3 mo after the vasectomy is a clear sign of failure, and in these cases the procedure should be repeated. Some patients will have rare, nonmotile sperm in their ejaculate for many months. Although the exact risk of pregnancy in this population cannot be determined, it is estimated to be below 1%. Couples should be counseled in this regard and offered a repeat procedure if they desire.

## COMPLICATIONS

### *Short-Term*

Hematoma is the most common early complication of vasectomy, occurring in 0.1–3% of patients. The incidence of hematomas diminishes considerably as the urologist becomes more experienced. Hematomas can grow to a large size, potentially requiring surgical evacuation and hospitalization. Smaller hematomas can be managed with restricted activity, pain medication, and warm compresses. Patients should be instructed to avoid aspirin and nonsteroidal anti-inflammatory drugs (NSAIDs) for 10 d before the vasectomy to further reduce the chances of bleeding complications.

Sperm granulomas result from leakage of sperm at the testicular end of the vasectomy site. Sperm granulomas occur in 1–30% of patients, and can usually be managed conservatively, most are asymptomatic. However, urologists should be aware that sperm granulomas do predispose the patient to recanalization.

Wound infections and epididymitis are rare complications of vasectomy, occurring in 1–3 of every 500 cases. Local wound care and oral antibiotics should be administered as needed.

### *Long-term*

Scrotal discomfort occurring weeks or months after vasectomy is fairly common, occurring in up to 30% of patients. However, it is usually self-limited, and only about

5% ever seek medical attention for their symptoms. The pain is most likely secondary to congestion of the epididymal tubules. Most patients respond to NSAIDs but referral to a pain clinic is occasionally warranted. Even more rare—occurring in perhaps 1 in 1000 cases—is severe, debilitating pain requiring surgical intervention. Options include conversion into an open-ended vasectomy, vasectomy reversal, total epididymovasectomy, and denervation of the spermatic cord. Although these complications are rare, patients should be warned of this potential outcome preoperatively.

No adverse systemic effects have been proven to be associated with vasectomy. Possible antisperm antibody-mediated effects have been hypothesized. Sperm are shielded from the immune system by the blood–testis barrier and by virtue of the fact that they do not appear until puberty. Vasectomy traumatizes the blood–testis barrier, leading to antisperm antibody formation in most men. Antisperm antibodies are only of concern if the patient later desires vasectomy reversal. High levels of sperm-bound antibodies in the semen decrease the chances of successful natural conception, intrauterine insemination, and in vitro fertilization. Despite these observations, pregnancy rates following vasovasostomy for vasectomy reversal remain in the 40–60% range, with patency rates over 90% when microsurgical techniques are used.

Patients should be informed that many large, well-controlled studies have been conducted analyzing the long-term systemic effects of vasectomy. Vasectomized men demonstrate no evidence of a significant increase in any systemic disease, including atherosclerotic cardiovascular disease, prostate cancer, or testis cancer. Early reports suggesting an association between vasectomy and these conditions were severely flawed. In 1993, a panel assembled by the National Institute of Health, the Association for Voluntary Surgical Contraception, and the National Cancer Institute reaffirmed the conclusion of most medical experts that vasectomy is a safe and effective means of permanent birth control.

## CONCLUSION

Vasectomy is a simple and effective method for providing permanent contraception. Newer techniques, such as the "no-scalpel" vasectomy, have decreased the incidence of local complications and have enhanced the popularity of vasectomy as a means of birth control. Careful counseling of patients is required to prevent misunderstandings and all patient education should be clearly documented in the medical record. The overwhelming evidence to date indicates that vasectomy is safe and is not associated with any serious, long-term, adverse sequelae.

## SELECTED READING

Benger JR, Swami SK, Gingell JC (1995) Persistent spermatozoa after vasectomy: a survey of British urologists. *Br J Urol* 76:376, 379.

Bernal-Delgado E, Latour-Perez J, Pradas-Arnal F, Gomez-Lopez LI (1998) The association between vasectomy and prostate cancer: a systematic review of the literature. *Fertil Steril* 40:191–200.

Haws JM, Morgan GT, Pollack AE, Koonin LM, Magnani RJ, Gargiullo PM (1998) Clinical aspects of vasectomies performed in the United States in 1995. *Urology* 52:685–691.

Jarow JP, Budin R, Dym J, el al. (1985) Quantitative pathological changes in the human testis after vasectomy: a controlled study. *N Engl J Med* 313:1252–1256.

Kendrick JS, Gonzales B, Huber DH, Grubb GS, Rubin GL (1987) Complications of vasectomy in the United States. *J Fam Pract* 25:245–248.

Li S, Goldstein M, Zhu J, Huber D (1991) The No-scalpel vasectomy. *J Urol* 1455:341–344.

Li PS, Li S, Schlegel PN, Goldstein M (1992) External spermatic sheath injection for vasal nerve block. *Urology* 39:173–176.

Linnet L (1983) Clinical immunology of vasectomy and vasovasostomy. *Urology* 22:101–114.

McMahon AJ, Buckley J, Taylor A, Lloyd SN, Deane RF, Kirk D (1992) Chronic testicular pain following vasectomy. *Br J Urol* 69:188–191.

Philliber SG, Philliber WW (1985) Social and psychological perspectives on volutary sterilization: a review. *Stud Fam Plann* 16:1–12.

Schlegel PN, Goldstein M (1985) Vasectomy. In: Goldstein M, ed., *Surgery of Male Infertility*. Philadelphia: WB Saunders Co., pp. 35–45.

West PJ, Bartelt RC (1980) Medicolegal aspects of urology. *Urol Clin NA* 7:153–163.

Zhu K, Stanford JL, Daling JR, et al. (1996) Vasectomy and prostate cancer: a case-control study in a health maintenance organization. *Am J Epidemiol* 144:717–722.

# X VOIDING DYSFUNCTION

# 30 Office Urodynamics

*John P. Lavelle,* MB, BCH, FRCSI,
*Michael W. Phelan,* MD,
*Seamus Teahan,* MB,
*and Michael B. Chancellor,* MD

**CONTENTS**

INTRODUCTION
URODYNAMIC TERMINOLOGY
URODYNAMIC LABORATORY
ASSESSMENT
TESTING
TECHNIQUE OF CYSTOMETRY
SELECTED READING

## INTRODUCTION

In this chapter, we present the basis of office urodynamics and provide guidance on the administration and interpretation of the office urodynamic test. This includes the indications, pitfalls, and interpretation of urodynamic evaluation. The importance of the history and physical findings combined with the objective but simple urodynamic findings cannot be overemphasized. It is also important that all the diagnostic findings be integrated into a cohesive unit without omitting pertinent data.

## URODYNAMIC TERMINOLOGY

The purpose of a urodynamic study is to reproduce the patient's symptoms in the office. The primary problems of the bladder are failure to store urine correctly (incontinence), or failure to empty the bladder (retention), or a combination of both. Table 1 provides the Wein classification of voiding dysfunction, which is a functional classification. Many other classification systems are available for the description of urodynamic problems. The terminology in urodynamics is also important. In past years, the actual definitions used by various individuals have varied. A clarification of the current terminology used for urodynamics has been defined by the International Continence Society. Advances in urodynamics and video-urodynamics have improved

## Table 1
### Classification of Voiding Dysfunction

| Failure to store: | Failure to empty: |
|---|---|
| Caused by bladder | Caused by bladder |
|   Detrusor hyperactivity |   Detrusor dreflexia |
|     Involuntary contractions |   Impaired detrusor contractility |
|     Suprasacral neurologic disease |   Psychogenic learned behavior |
|     Bladder-outlet obstruction | Caused by outlet |
|     Idiopathic |   Anatomic obstruction |
|   Decreased compliance |   Detrusor sphincter dyssynergia |
|     Fibrosis |   Psychogenic learned behavior |
|     Idiopathic | |
|   Sensory urgency | |
|     Inflammatory | |
|     Infectious | |
|     Neurologic | |
|     Psychological | |
|     Idiopathic | |
| Caused by outlet | |
|   Urethral hypermobility | |
|   Intrinsic sphincter deficiency | |

the understanding of the normal and abnormal function of the bladder and sphincter. The testing allows us to prospectively identify patients at risk for upper-tract deterioration, and has improved therapeutic selection in relation to the underlying pathophysiology.

## URODYNAMIC LABORATORY

The area of the urologist's office dedicated to urodynamic assessment is important. Attention to detail is essential to the proper performance and interpretation of the tests. The area should allow privacy for the patients to change (preferably in an adjacent room) and to be examined without disturbance from other activities of the office. The area should also include an examination room where the patient is examined and the testing is performed. A history and physical exam may also be performed in the room. A bathroom with uroflow equipment should be adjacent to the room to allow the patient to void in privacy, and to assess the patient's voiding pattern. The urodynamic equipment should be maintained and operated by personnel who are dedicated to and competent in the equipment's maintenance and performance of the various tests. This setting allows a smooth setup and performance of testing between the physician and patient with minimum disruption, stress, or disturbance to the patient. The staff used for urodynamic assessment should have a thorough understanding of the nature and theory of each test, a sound understanding of the equipment required for each test, and the ability to circumvent or quickly adapt in the event of equipment malfunction. Since all modern urodynamic equipment is based on digital technology, a knowledge of computer software and hardware is also strongly advisable.

Table 2
Segmental Innervation of the Genitourinary System

| Level | Organ |
|---|---|
| T8–T12 | Abdominal-wall sensation |
| T8 | Testis |
| S2 | Penile sensations and reflex erections |
| S3–4 | Rectal and anal contractions |
| S2–4 | Bladder |
| S2–3 | External sphincter |
| S2–3 | Bulbocavernosus reflex |
| S3 | Anal reflex |

## ASSESSMENT

The initial assessment should include a comprehensive history and physical examination. Routine laboratory tests, including a urinalysis and culture (if required), and serum creatinine, should be obtained. An elevated creatinine may indicate significant upper-tract deterioration in an otherwise asymptomatic patient.

### Clinical Assessment

The general history includes questions relevant to neurological and congenital abnormalities and details of prior urinary-tract infections and surgery. History of prior medications, and a sexual, menstrual, bowel function, and obstetrical history must also be obtained. The complete description of each symptom regarding time course, onset, and aggravating and relieving factors should be obtained. Attempts to define and separate symptoms of obstruction from other bladder dysfunctions have been unsuccessful. Symptoms classified as obstructive or irritative are extremely unreliable indicators of the actual micturitional disorder. Yet the symptoms cannot be ignored. They must fit in with the final diagnosis. When dealing with incontinent patients, some assessment of the severity and quantity of lost urine should be made.

### Physical Examination

The physical examination should include a general urological—and, if appropriate, a gynecological examination—as well as an assessment of perineal sensation, the perineal reflexes supplied by the sacral segments S2–4, and anal-sphincter tone and control. Sensory dermatomes are summarized in Table 2. Spinal-cord lesions produce varied loss of neurological function, depending on the nature of the lesion (complete or incomplete) and the areas affected if incomplete. Most complete spinal-cord lesions interfere with the micturition reflex with detrusor hyperreflexia and external-sphincter dyssynergia. Sensory neurogenic bladders may present with urinary retention, because the patients lack the sensation of bladder fullness. The cremasteric reflex is elicited by striking the inner thigh, and results in an ipsilateral elevation of the testicle. The anal reflex is elicited by lightly stroking the perianal skin, and results in anal contraction. The bulbocavernosus reflex in men is elicited by squeezing the glans penis (not the body of the penis), and monitoring the external anal-sphincter contractions. For women, the clitoris is pressed. Decreased anal tone also suggests laxity of the urinary sphincters. The spinal-cord segments for anal tone are primarily S2–4. An IVP or renal ultrasound to exclude upper-tract deterioration and hydronephrosis should also be performed.

Incomplete bladder emptying results from impaired detrusor contractility which may be neurologic, myogenic, or learned. The reflexes associated with micturation may be disrupted by sensory problems with diabetes mellitus and peripheral neuropathy, or by cauda equina or conus medullaris lesions. Patients with neurological lesions and long-standing neurogenic bladder dysfunctions are usually unaware that their voiding habits are abnormal. Long-term acontractile bladder and straining to void often present with urgency and urge incontinence, and incomplete bladder emptying.

## *Bladder Diary*

A simple record of the voiding pattern, with the amount voided and time together with intake and a rough guide to any incontinence episodes, is an invaluable tool in the evaluation of patients. The diary should be kept for a full 24-h period. The record also provides information on the number of voidings, the distribution of voidings, and the volume voided. Records of urgency and leakage with the number of incontinence pads used may be also kept.

If the patient complains of incontinence, a pad test may be performed. Generally this is performed over a 1-h period, although this time is not universally set. The subject drinks 500 mL of a sodium-free drink and performs certain activities over the course of 1 h. The pad is weighed prior to and after the 1-h period, and the amount of incontinence is recorded. If it is a satisfactory test (one that produces incontinence) the patient voids and the volume is recorded.

Residual urine is the integral result of bladder contractility and urethral resistance. Generally, if the volume is large, this is considered undesirable. If the volume is low, this is indicative of a normal lower urinary tract. However, the volume may be low when the bladder contraction can overcome increased urethral resistance with obstruction. A high residual volume (RV) may be a warning of contractile failure in response to urethral resistance increases. This test has poor test–retest reliability, and currently there is no defined abnormal RV. The actual measurement of the postvoid residual urine is best performed with a catheter; however, a number of ultrasound devices are now available for the purpose of residual urine measurement.

## TESTING

In patients at risk, a serum creatinine can be obtained to determine if there is any renal function impairment. This should be particularly important for patients with neurological injury (with a small, noncompliant bladder), or patients with detrusor-sphincter dyssynergia caused by the risk of renal impairment from vesicoureteric reflux from a high-pressure bladder.

A plain abdominal film can also be performed to exclude any spinal disease or stone disease. An ultrasound of the kidneys is also useful as a screening tool, particularly in children, to exclude hydronephrosis and check the kidney size and any gross renal deformities (such as ectopy, cysts, evidence for scarring, tumors).

The primary tests for urodynamic evaluation are cystometry and uroflowmetry. Video-urodynamics, sphincter electromyography, and urethral pressure profilometry are not discussed here because these are rather specialized test that present more technical challenges and pitfalls, and are not generally required in the general office setting.

## *Cystometry*

For cystometry, any catheter that is comfortable for the patient may be used (generally, a 12–14-F catheter). However, if uroflowmetry is attempted with cystometry, the size of the catheter is important, and generally an 8–10-Fr catheter with multiple ports is used. The problem is that the larger catheters tend to artifactually obstruct the urethra, leading to an erroneous diagnosis of obstruction. Some systems use two catheters—a small 4-Fr measuring catheter and a larger 10-Fr filling catheter. The filling catheter is removed after the filling phase of the cytometry. In a complete cystometry to assess both the filling phase and voiding phase, liquid is used as a filling agent. A number of machines use gas (usually $CO_2$)—however, this leads to lower pressures recorded and an assessment of the voiding phase cannot be performed.

The decision to use a multichannel or a single-channel cystometer depends on the budget and expertise of the individual urologist. The technical challenges of the single-channel machines are greater, because determinations must be made about intraabdominal pressure, which are additive to the single-channel cystometrogram (CMG). This process may be difficult, and is much easier on a multichannel machine. However, these are more expensive, and more difficult to set up and maintain.

## TECHNIQUE OF CYSTOMETRY

Cystometry measures the pressure/volume relationship of the bladder. It is an interactive process that permits examination of motor and sensory function, and is used to assess detrusor activity, sensation, capacity, compliance, and control of micturition process. After a detailed explanation to the patient, the examination is begun by passing a catheter into the bladder, measuring residual urine, and filling the bladder. Close verbal contact is maintained between the patient and the examiner as predefined motor and sensory landmarks are observed and annotated.

A number of definitions are shown in Table 3 to cystometry. Commonly used terms used to describe sensory phenomena include:

1. First sensation of bladder filling.
2. First desire to void.
3. Normal desire to void (this is defined as the feeling that leads the patient to pass urine at the next convenient moment, but voiding can be delayed if necessary).
4. Strong desire to void (this is defined as a persistent desire to void without the fear of leakage).
5. Urgency (this is defined as a strong desire to void accompanied by fear of leakage or fear of pain).
6. Pain (site and character of pain should be specified). Pain during bladder filling or micturition is abnormal.

These are the usual markers of progress during the filling phase of the CMG.

Bladder contractions can be voluntary or involuntary. In the presence of neurological disease, involuntary contractions are defined as detrusor hyperreflexia. Otherwise, in the normal bladder, involuntary contractions are caused by detrusor hyperactivity (*see*

## Table 3
### Definitions Relating to Cystometry

| | |
|---|---|
| Vesical pressure | The pressure within the bladder |
| Abdominal pressure | Pressure surrounding the bladder. Estimated from rectal-pressure measurement |
| Detrusor pressure | The component of the vesical pressure that is created by forces in the bladder wall (passive and active). Estimated by subtracting abdominal pressure from vesical pressure |
| Bladder capacity | Maximum cystometric capacity in patients with normal sensation in the volume at which the patient feels he/she can no longer delay micturition. Otherwise it is when the patient voids involuntarily. If the bladder capacity is >1L the examiner may stop the examination. |
| Detrusor leak-point pressure | This is the pressure at which the bladder leaks during filling cystometry |
| Abdominal or Valsalva leak-point pressure | The pressure that the bladder leaks in response to coughing, straining, or Valsalva maneuver. |

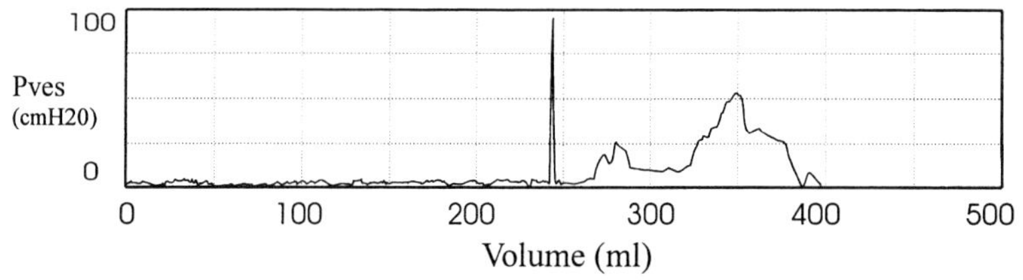

**Fig. 1.** A 54-yr-old woman with symptoms of urgency, frequency, urge incontinence, and stress incontinence, who underwent a CMG study. At 240 mL she was asked to cough, and generated a abdominal pressure of nearly 100 cm $H_2O$ without leakage. However, she developed two involuntary bladder contractions at 280 mL and 350 mL. The patient was successfully treated with an anticholinergic drugs, time voiding, and moderate fluid restriction.

Fig. 1). It is important to determine whether the patient's symptoms are caused by involuntary contractions or whether the involuntary contractions are just present and asymptomatic. The International Continence Society has restricted the term "unstable bladder" to indicate an involuntary phasic increase in detrusor pressure >15 cm $H_2O$, but in practice, contractions are often of lesser magnitude.

One of the primary functions of the bladder is storage of urine. The bladder should distend and store urine at low intravesical pressure. It is accepted that if the bladder has a sustained high intravesical pressure, the patient has an increased risk of developing vesicoureteral reflux, hydronephrosis, stones, and urosepsis. The method of measuring the resistance of the bladder to distension is to measure the bladder compliance.

Compliance is defined as the change in volume over the change in pressure, and is the inverse of elastance. Compliance is a measure of the distensibility of the bladder in relation to the intravesical pressures. Initially the cutoff point for unacceptably high sustained pressure was 40 cm $H_2O$, but this may be lower depending on the compliance of the bladder. Bladder compliance should be measured with the bladder neck occluded (e.g., with a Foley balloon) for accuracy, or the compliance may be overestimated.

The detrusor leak-point pressure is the pressure point during filling cystometry that the bladder leaks. This is different than the abdominal leak-point pressure, which measures sphincteric function.

## *Methods of Cystometry*

The purpose of cystometry is to reproduce the patient's symptoms if possible, and to determine the underlying pathophysiology. The examination is explained to the patient, and is then begun by having the patient void and gown. A catheter is placed in the bladder, and the residual urine is measured. Large residual-urine volumes may alter detrusor function, especially in neuropathic disorders. All the systems are zeroed at atmospheric pressure, and the reference point is the level of the superior edge of the symphysis pubis. For catheter transducers, the reference point is the transducer itself. The patient should be awake and alert, with no anesthesia, and should not have taken any drugs that alter bladder function. The patient should be instructed to report what they feel to the examiner without instruction on voiding. Changes in observed pressure should be correlated with symptoms (if any), malfunction, or change in position of the catheter(s). The vessical pressure is the sum of the intra-abdominal pressure and the detrusor pressure. To determine artifact from the abdominal musculature, the abdominal pressure should be measured and subtracted from the vesical pressure to determine the true detrusor pressure.

Problems with cystometry include the calibration and maintenance of the transducers and electronic equipment. The fill rates—whether slow, medium, or fast—should be constant for a particular office to allow easy comparison of results over time. If gravity fill is performed, the time of infusion and infusion volume should be accurately measured to obtain the fill rate. Changes in position of the patient, or measurement in different positions, can change the pressure recordings. The normal recording position is supine, but CMGs may be performed in sitting or standing positions to reproduce the symptoms. If the patient has a perivesical mass, is very anxious, or is undergoing a significant diuresis, this may influence the quality of the cystometrogram. Other patient-compliance issues include a patient who is crying, uncooperative, moving around too much, or coughing. All these factors may decrease the quality of the recordings. Artifacts from coughing or moving should be annotated on the recording to make interpretation easier.

If the patient is difficult to catheterize, cystometry may be performed with a flexible cystoscope to introduce the fluid into the bladder. The pressures may be measured using the biopsy channel, and direct or fluoroscopic visualization of the bladder may be easily performed during the study. This technique may be useful in patients with spinal-cord injuries.

Occasionally a simple "eyeball" CMG may be performed, using an 18-F urethral catheter with an open 60-$cm^3$ syringe attached. The bladder is filled through the syringe barrel, and the pressure is recorded by watching the level in the syringe. The height of the meniscus of the fluid above the symphysis pubis is the intravesical pressure.

### Uroflowmetry

Uroflowmetry measures the expelled urethral urine rate per unit time (usually mL/s). There are many types of uroflowmeter, each with their own advantages and disadvantages. The primary types are shown in Table 4. These machines should have their calibration checked on a regular basis to maintain performance. The performance of

## Table 4
### Primary Types of Uroflowmeters

| Method | Mechanism | Advantage | Disadvantage |
|---|---|---|---|
| Weight | Measuring the weight of the collected fluid | Accurate regardless of site of stream impact | Sensitive to mechanical disturbances; density must be set |
| Electronic Dipstick | The electrical capacitance of a dipstick mounted in the collecting chamber changes as volume changes | Least expensive; no mechanical parts | Relatively large variation in volume and flow-rate calibration |
| Rotating Disk | The voided urine is directed onto a rotating disk. The power required to keep a rotating disk rotating at a constant rate is measured and is proportional to the mass flow rate of the fluid | Accurate and reliable, insensitive to mechanical disturbances | Density must be set. Affected by site of stream impact. |

uroflowmetry also requires a reporting of the pattern of the urinary flow, to help in the differential diagnosis and to sort out any technical problems with the performance of the test.

For proper uroflow interpretation, the following information must be provided about the test performance: the voided volume, the patient environment, the nature of the filling (by diuresis or catheterization), the type of voided fluid, the type of measuring equipment, whether other procedures were associated with the test, and whether the voiding pattern was typical of the patient's usual voiding patterns. It is currently theorized that the voided volume should exceed 150 mL, and that corrections or adjustments to the maximum flow rate are unnecessary for volumes in excess of this figure.

The other parameters that may be measured during uroflowmetry are shown in Table 5. The normal pattern of voiding is a single void with a bell-shaped curve. However, because of the variations in intra-abdominal pressure and sphincteric activity, this ideal pattern is rarely seen.

Significant pattern changes may be observed in patients with abnormal voiding processes. The classic example is the patient with outlet obstruction or a poorly contractile bladder who uses increased abdominal pressure to void. This produces a characteristic flow in spurts, with complete interruption between activity. Occasionally a patient may have a dramatic outflow of urine in a short period of time ($Q_{max} > 40$ mL/s). This is usually seen in women who are normal or have intrinsic sphincter deficiency with normal bladder contractility.

The diagnosis of lower urinary-tract obstruction may not made on the sole basis of the maximum flow rate ($Q_{max}$); however, the $Q_{max}$ may be used to help determine that the patient is obstructed in conjunction with the patient's symptoms and other findings. The usual pattern for the obstructed bladder is that of a low flow rate, sufficient voided volume, and prolonged flow time. However, this may also be found in patients with

Table 5
Parameters Measured During Uroflowmetry

| | |
|---|---|
| Voided volume | The total volume of urine expelled from the bladder |
| Residual urine volume | The total volume of urine remaining in the bladder after voiding |
| Flow time | The time over which measurable flow actually occurs |
| Maximum flow rate ($Q_{max}$) | The maximum measured value of the flow rate |
| Time to minimum flow | The elapsed time from the onset of flow to the point of minimum flow |
| Time to maximum flow | The elapsed time from the onset of flow to the point of maximum flow |
| Continuous urinary flow | A constant urinary stream without interruption |
| Mean flow rate | Volume voided divided by flow time. The average flow rate is only interpretable if flow is continuous and without anomaly at the start and end of voiding |

decreased bladder contractility because of overstretching (overly full following catheterized filling of the bladder) of the bladder, or neurological impairment of the micturition reflex (diabetes or neurological injury). Therefore, the uroflowmetry findings should always be interpreted with caution.

## *Diagnosis*

The actual diagnosis in the urodynamic laboratory/office setting is often difficult, as the findings may often be explained by more than one answer. Thus, it is imperative that the other symptoms and physical findings be taken into account.

## *Normal*

Normal urodynamic studies are relatively rare in patients with symptoms and physical findings. The common exception to this is in trying to make the diagnosis of unstable bladder, because 50% of the time a CMG is normal.

## *Spinal-Cord Injury*

The primary symptom to watch for here is increased intravesical pressure, which may lead to renal damage if vesicoureteric reflux occurs. The diagnosis of detrusor-sphincter dyssynergia should be considered in all patients with spinal-cord injuries. Care should be taken to make sure the bladder is monitored regularly to detect any subtle changes in bladder dynamics.

## *Cerebrovascular Accident and Parkinson's Disease*

Bladder instability and incontinence are the primary problems here, as suprapontine control of the bladder is lost. In elderly men, procedures to relieve obstruction (TURP or bladder-neck incision) should be used with caution, because the bladder instability may make matters worse. Generally, TURP is not indicated in Parkinson's disease, as the patient's obstructive symptoms are related to the bradykinesia of Parkinson's disease.

It is worth noting that elderly patients may experience vascular accidents that cause subtle neurological changes that are relatively asymptomatic but have profound urological effects.

### Multiple Sclerosis and Diabetic Neurogenic Bladder

In multiple sclerosis, the demyelination injury may affect any part of the micturition reflex, and thus the symptoms, signs, and urodynamic findings may be varied and separate. Treatment should be related to the findings and symptoms. Bladder instability is the most common problem. In diabetic cystopathy, the bladder is often insensate, and overflow incontinence may occur. The bladder may also become unstable, and should be treated symptomatically.

### Stress Incontinence

This is a common problem, which often affects women after childbirth or difficult deliveries. The patient coughs and loses urine. The patient may have also an unstable bladder, a condition that may be revealed following treatment of stress incontinence. The Valsalva leak-point pressure is low (<60 cm $H_2O$). There may be associated cystocele, rectocele, and enterocele.

### BPH and Bladder-Neck Obstruction

The diagnosis of lower urinary-tract obstruction should be combined with the diagnosis of an adequate bladder contraction. A low uroflow, which is often associated with an obstructed lower urinary tract, is also found in patients who have inadequate bladder contractions—usually caused by diabetes or prolonged obstruction. In the latter case, about 50% of these patients recover adequate (although not necessarily normal) bladder function to allow adequate voiding.

### Postprostatectomy Incontinence

Severe post-radical-prostatectomy incontinence is relatively rare (<5%); however, the development of bladder instability can occur. This may be diagnosed with the aid of the CMG and symptoms. The treatment is symptomatic and is based on the clinical findings.

## SELECTED READING

Abrams P, Blaivas JG, Stanton SL, Andersen JT (1988) Standardization of terminology of lower urinary tract function. *Neurourol & Urodynam.* 7:403–426.

Blaivas JG, Chancellor MB, eds., (1996) *Atlas of Urodynamics.* Philadelphia: Williams & Wilkins.

Blaivas JG, Olsson CA (1988) Stress incontinence: classification and surgical approach. *J Urol* 139:727–731.

Chancellor MB, Blaivas JG, eds., (1995) *Practical Neuro-Urology. Geritourinary Complications in Neurologic Disease.* Stoneham, MA: Butterworth Heinemann.

Kaplan SA, Te AE, Blaivas JG (1995) Urodynamic findings in patients with diabetic cystopathy. *J Urol* 153:342, 343.

McGuire EJ, Woodside JR, Borden TA, Weiss RM (1981) Prognostic value of urodynamic testing in myelodysplastic patients. *J Urol* 126:205–209.

# 31 Assessment of the Incontinent Woman

*Edward J. McGuire, MD*

**CONTENTS**
    BACKGROUND
    SYMPTOMS
    URGE INCONTINENCE AND URODYNAMICS
    URODYNAMICS OF STRESS INCONTINENCE
    TREATMENT OF MOTOR-URGE INCONTINENCE
    ASSESSMENT
    CHARACTERIZATION OF STRESS INCONTINENCE AND
        PROLAPSE CONDITIONS
    PLANNING APPROPRIATE SURGICAL MANAGEMENT
    SELECTED READING

## BACKGROUND

Urinary incontinence is a very common condition which seems to be more common in women than men. Epidemiologic studies suggest that as many as 15% of adult women have some degree of incontinence, and a recent study of college women athletes found that a substantial percentage had incontinence associated with effort. If the degree of "bother" is considered, the percentage of women with "troublesome" incontinence at the time of the survey ranges from 3 to 5%. The *prevalence* of incontinence, which means the cumulative incidence of the problem over time, is much higher than 15%. As a population ages, the incidence of incontinence gradually rises, and as many as 30% or more of the elderly to very elderly are incontinent on a daily basis. A recent English study suggests that approx 11% of women in a rural area undergo surgery for vaginal prolapse and incontinence during their lifetime. A similar study from Hong Kong found that 25% of all gynecologic admissions to hospitals were related to vaginal prolapse and incontinence. Incontinence associated with surgery for prolapse is most often stress incontinence related to urethral dysfunction, but the most common cause of urinary incontinence in women in the industrialized world is uncontrolled detrusor contractility. These figures suggest that incontinence of all kinds is a problem for a substantial number of women during their lifetime. Other data indicates that many—

From: *Current Clinical Urology: Office Urology: The Clinician's Guide*
Edited by: E. D. Kursh and J. C. Ulchaker © Humana Press Inc., Totowa, NJ

and perhaps most—people with incontinence do not seek medical help for the problem. A German study found that although a substantial number of general practitioners' patients admitted they had a problem with incontinence, most had never told their doctor about the problem. More surprising, an even higher percentage of urologists' patients were incontinent, but most had never mentioned it and had not been asked about the problem. Perhaps this explains the large areas in drugstores and grocery stores devoted to adult protective padding diapers and protective undergarments.

## SYMPTOMS

Symptoms of urinary incontinence are often grouped into two categories: those that suggest stress incontinence, and those that suggest a lack of bladder contractile control. These are, respectively, "stress" and "urge" incontinence. A third category—"mixed" incontinence—refers to symptoms of both stress and urge incontinence present in the same patient. In most studies, the latter is the largest group. When a tentative diagnosis based on symptoms is "validated" with a full clinical evaluation and conventional urodynamics, a problem arises. Most of the published work in this area suggests that a tentative diagnosis based on symptoms leads to an overestimation of the incidence of urge and mixed incontinence and an underestimation of the incidence of stress incontinence, when compared to diagnoses based on clinical and urodynamic evaluation. Although the initial conclusion drawn from these findings was that symptoms are unreliable as a guide to the actual cause of incontinence, the problem may actually lie in the urodynamics.

## URGE INCONTINENCE AND URODYNAMICS

Motor-urge incontinence is a condition characterized by urinary loss related to uncontrolled or uncontrollable detrusor contractility. Urinary urgency usually accompanies the sudden, unanticipated bladder contractile activity. Uncontrolled detrusor contractility occurs commonly in neurogenic conditions, but in that circumstance the problem is termed *detrusor hyperreflexia*. This is considered a different condition than "idiopathic detrusor overactivity," where uncontrolled detrusor contractility seems to occur in the absence of a definite neural deficit, although this situation seems unlikely. Indeed, detrusor hyperreflexia related to a stroke appears to be the same problem as ideopathic motor-urge incontinence or nocturnal eneuresis—only worse. Detrusor instability is an observation during a cystometrogram (CMG): the bladder contracts without the subject's permission (the subject of the CMG). In the past this finding on urodynamic testing was thought to be required for the diagnosis of "motor-urge incontinence." More recently, it became obvious that the CMG is insensitive and not specific for motor-urge incontinence. At least 50% of adults with motor-urge incontinence have "a normal or stable bladder" by cystometry. The information regarding a lack of sensitivity of the CMG resulted from data derived from continuous ambulatory monitoring of detrusor contractile activity and other clinical data. A CMG cannot screen for the presence of motor-urge incontinence in any population. There are very high false-negative rates with the test, and lower but substantial false-positive rates as well. Artibani recently suggested that the International Continence Society should revise its terminology on detrusor overactivity, since it is still based on CMG findings, and Griffiths wrote in a recent paper in *European Urology* that "detrusor instability" was a urodynamic observation only, not a diagnosis or a condition. The inaccuracy and high false-negative rate for the CMG is a major reason why symptoms do not correlate with urodynamics, and the former "gold standard," which was the CMG, is now probably symptoms, since we have nothing more definitive. The false-positive rate for the CMG approaches 15% in the elderly, and no one knows what that might mean. Continuous ambulatory monitoring of bladder pressure while the subject goes about daily activities (CAM) was the test that destroyed the CMG. CAM testing of persons with urge-incontinence symptoms and a normal CMG picked up very high rates of detrusor contractility. Unfortunately, the test has a 60% false-positive rate in normal volunteers, and is rarely used now. The CMG is no longer considered the standard method to make the diagnosis of motor-urge incontinence, or to "rule out" detrusor contractility as a potential cause of incontinence in a given patient.

Currently, symptoms are a better guide to detrusor contractility as a cause of incontinence that urodynamics. Patients usually describe a random pattern of sudden short warning, or no warning, before detrusor contractility where urgency occurs just before or at the same time as actual wetting. It is the lack of warning that leads to the problem. These patients almost always have a normal response to filling on a CMG. There are often associations with the syndrome of incontinence, which include running water, returning home, and other situations, such as arising in the morning or getting up from a chair. The syndrome could be described as a sensory problem as well as a motor problem, and agents that inhibit detrusor contractility do not improve subjective sensation or the person's ability to sense what the bladder might do and thus control it. The incontinence episodes are not associated with any particular urine volume, and they occur in an almost completely random pattern, first described by Pat D. O'Donnell based on the study of incontinence patterns in the elderly. The random pattern seems to be partly responsible for the lack of a response to treatment with anticholinergic agents. The bladder is basically normal, but occasionally the control mechanism fails.

## URODYNAMICS OF STRESS INCONTINENCE

Stress incontinence is characterized by urinary leakage, and the force for expulsion is abdominal pressure and not detrusor pressure. This condition is associated with abnormal urethral function, and can be objectively identified on physical examination, by urodynamics, and more precisely by video urodynamics. There is no definitive information on how precise and sensitive these methods are, but most experts would agree that the methods are much more sensitive than those that exist for the identification of urge incontinence. This is, in part, the reason why symptoms seem to underestimate the incidence of stress incontinence, since stress incontinence is easily detected even if there are no symptoms, which suggest that it is a problem. There is also a clear, if imperfect, linkage between stress and motor-urge incontinence. In the past, detrusor overactivity was regarded as a problem that would result in a poor outcome for the concomitant surgical treatment of stress incontinence. Conventional wisdom held that motor-urge incontinence should be ruled out with a CMG, and only then was the diagnosis of "genuine stress incontinence" possible. In effect, the diagnosis of stress incontinence was clinical and based on the exclusion of motor-urge incontinence with CMG—which could not be done. There are excellent methods to establish the diagnosis of stress incontinence (leakage of urine driven by abdominal pressure). Stress incontinence is not one condition, but several—and proper characterization of the exact condition present and treatment based on that characterization improve outcomes dramatically. Surprisingly, objective cure of stress incontinence is usually associated with resolution of urge-incontinence symptoms. This finding, which is consistent in virtually all prospective studies, suggests that SUI and motor-urge incontinence are associated with cause-and-effect in as many as 70–75% of individuals with both conditions. As many as 60–65% of patients with video-urodynamically identified stress incontinence also have urge-incontinence symptoms. These symptoms cannot be better characterized by cystometry, and as many as 70% will no longer have urge-incontinence symptoms after successful treatment of their stress incontinence. Thus, our efforts should properly be directed toward the precise characterization of the stress incontinence to ensure the best possible result of treatment of that condition. Based on late-outcome assessment, it is clear that no single procedure can provide good results when applied to large numbers of women with generic "stress incontinence" not otherwise characterized. The problem with this data is the lack of certainty regarding who should have the procedure. Thus, we conclude that the procedure studied does not work, and we then develop a new one with the same results.

## TREATMENT OF MOTOR-URGE INCONTINENCE

When a tentative diagnosis of motor-urge incontinence is established based on historical detail and physical assessment, the next step is a search for conditions that might produce the overactive bladder. These include stress incontinence; vaginal prolapse; cerebral vascular disease; occasionally diabetes; certain medications, including antihypertensive medication, diuretics, sedatives, and hypnotics; obstructive uropathy after prior stress-incontinence surgery; and occult neurological disease or injury. In the elderly, and sometimes the nonelderly, a lack of mobility and/or toilet access can make a mild problem into a major one.

## ASSESSMENT

A pelvic examination in the supine—and upright position if possible—is essential (*see* Fig. 1). One looks for any prolapse condition, urethral mobility, and the position of the urethra at rest after any prior stress-incontinence surgery (*see* Fig. 2). An assessment of perineal sensation and of the contractility and strength of the pelvic-floor musculature and anal sphincter provides useful information. A urine analysis and determination of residual urine by an accurate method are also helpful. If a patient claims to have a prolapse condition, an upright exam may be required to diagnose it. At this point a CMG helps to define the condition to be treated. If the CMG is normal and no contraction is elicited—even if the study makes the patient uncomfortable—a reasonably solid diagnosis of ideopathic motor-urge incontinence is established. Treatment must take into account the fact that this bladder, when watched (as during the CMG) behaves normally. A method that focuses the patient's attention on the bladder is essential here. This can be timed voiding, a diary, behavioral therapy, or biofeedback, but some effort in this direction is essential. Anticholinergic agents alone will not work in these cases. If the CMG is positive and an uninhibited contraction is elicited, ideopathic instability may be present, but a search for another underlying cause of the bladder overactivity is worthwhile. Although anticholinergic agents will delay the bladder response, they alone cannot ensure that the patient will be dry. A method to

## Chapter 31 / Assessing the Incontinent Woman

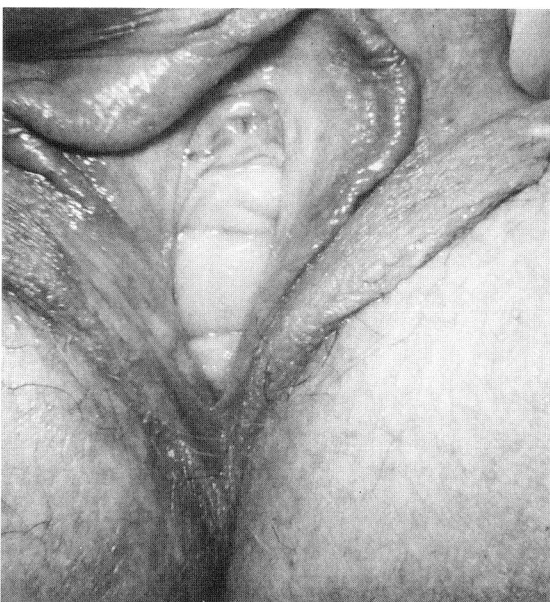

**Fig. 1.** Standard position for a pelvic examination. On careful assessment there was prolapse of the anterior, apical, and posterior vaginal segments, and there is a deficient perineal body, which is obvious on inspection. That abnormality is in the midline posteriorly.

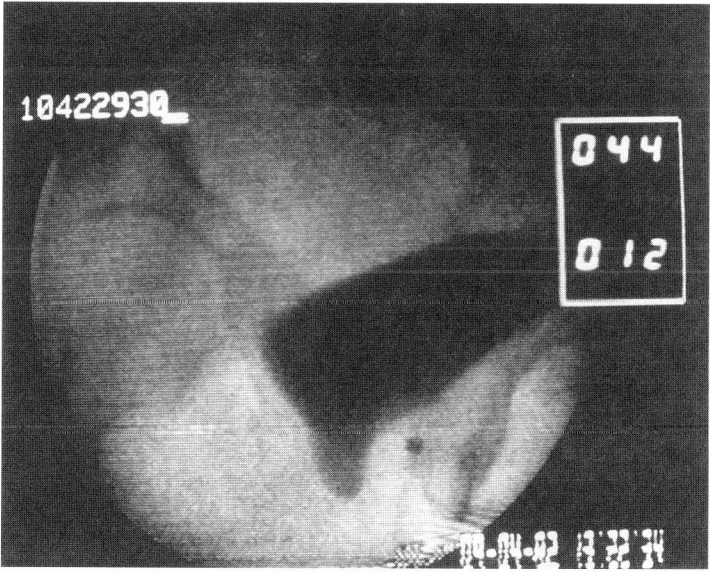

**Fig. 2.** Lateral video urodynamic image. A 65-yr-old woman with a grade 2 or 3 cystocele, and difficulty voiding, intermittent retention, and urge incontinence. The urethra is in a relatively high, fixed position with the cystocele just behind it. This is obstructive uropathy, but it is complicated, and both the cystocele and the urethral position contribute to the problem. Her urethral suspension was a sling. This kind of cystocele, in conjunction with the urethral hypersuspension, can have two long-term effects, both negative: retention or altered voiding dynamics, and perhaps worse, traction forces operating on the sling and the attachments of that structure to the arcus tendineus, can break the sling, leading to more prolapse and recurrent stress incontinence.

empty the bladder on a regular basis must be combined with the drug therapy, just as would be done in a patient with a spinal-cord injury treated with intermittent catheterization. In nonneuropathic conditions, timed regular voiding works quite well.

These conservative methods do fail, but the frequency is unclear because there is no certain way to identify the overactive bladder. More complex but effective treatments exist, but they carry higher risks and they may not be applicable to all patients. These include the Ingleman-Sundberg transvaginal partial bladder dennervation, which can be considered if a subtrigonal injection of a local anesthetic is associated with a transient but dramatic and complete resolution of all symptoms. Bladder augmentation with bowel is effective, but usually requires intermittent catheterization on a lifelong basis, and is associated with a theoretical risk of neoplasia in the bowel segment used and the long-term problems associated with bowel resection. Autoaugmentation, first used in pediatric patients, is a reasonable alternative method. It does not require intermittent catheterization, and in the short-term, results are equivalent to bowel augmentation.

### *Other Conditions Associated with Involuntary Urinary Loss*

Much more subtle and dangerous than stress or urge incontinence is incontinence associated with poor bladder compliance. Altered storage activity of the bladder with volume increments are associated with a progressive rise in pressure can result from injury related to radiation therapy or chemotherapy, chronic catheter drainage, peripheral neural injury, such as that occasionally incurred during abdominoperineal resection for rectal carcinoma, or radical hysterectomy. The abnormal pressure gain with volume results—at some point—in an isobaric bladder and proximal urethra (*see* Fig. 3). In this condition, minimal effort will induce leakage and the symptoms are very much like stress incontinence, although the expulsive force is detrusor pressure and not abdominal pressure. Further filling and pressure gain leads to continuous steady-state incontinence, where leakage basically occurs as the ureters deliver urine into the bladder. If the pressure of leakage in this circumstance is 40 or more, a serious and culmulative risk to upper-tract function exists, and renal failure may be the result. These states are associated with moderate residual urine volumes. As compared with overflow incontinence, which occurs at a very large volume when the limits of bladder viscoelastic distensibility are reached, in altered compliance the driving force is pressure exerted on a relatively small volume of urine by active muscular contractility or a fibrotic nondistensible bladder. A CMG is accurate and sensitive in the diagnosis of this condition. Any patient who has had radiotherapy or chemotherapy for various malignant conditions—especially for cervical and endometrial carcinoma and myeloproliferative or lymphatic malignancies—should be examined for this condition. Treatment is directed at bladder enlargement and regular emptying, and usually consists of intermittent catheterization and two or more anticholinergic agents. If this treatment is not successful, the surgical methods described in this section to enlarge the bladder can be used.

## CHARACTERIZATION OF STRESS INCONTINENCE AND PROLAPSE CONDITIONS

Stress incontinence occurs when the urethra cannot resist abdominal prseure as an expulsive force. This can be associated with posterior rotational descent of the urethra

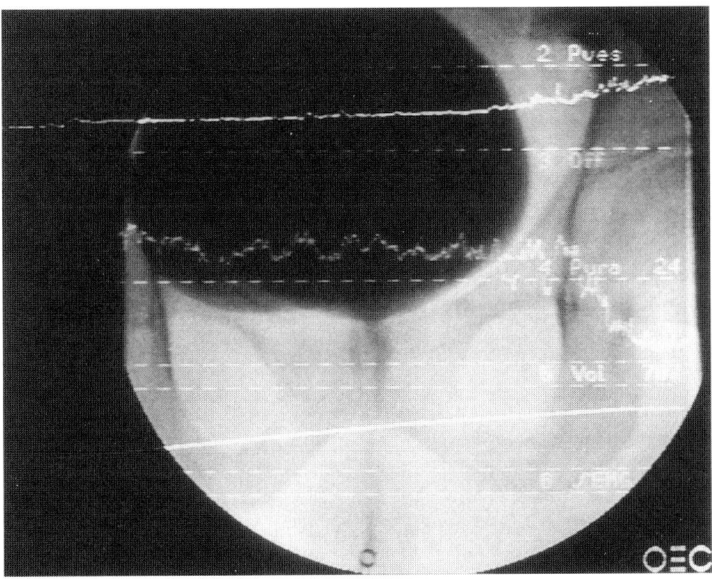

Fig. 3. A bad bladder. There is a progressive elevation in bladder pressure with filling (upper tracing). That finally results in an isobaric bladder and proximal urethra. The video image was made at that point. This situation is associated with a stress incontinence-like syndrome, in that any effort induces leakage, but the actual expulsive force is detrusor pressure generated by volume. Leakage is a bad problem here, but there is also a risk of ureteral functional impairment and renal failure if the pressure of leakage is high enough.

into the potential space of the vagina, or with poor closure of the proximal urethra, with poor coaptation and/or loss of the seal effect that is a property of the mucosal layer of the urethra. Abnormal closure leading to leakage need only involve the proximal mechanism from the bladder neck to the distal zone. The latter is partly under volitional control, whereas the proximal zone is not.

Urethral tissue loss resulting from prior surgery, stress incontinence, or a diverticulum can be associated with severe stress incontinence that prevents effective closure of the urethra. These conditions involve full-thickness injury, such as might be incurred with a urethrotomy or a transurethral resection, or loss of part of the periurethral fascial envelope that surrounds and supports the urethra. The latter injury leads to pseudodiverticular formation and stress incontinence. One mechanism for this injury is tearing of the fascia related to periurethral suture placement for needle suspension, necrosis related to Kelly-type plication sutures, or inadvertent injury related to excision of a urethral diverticulum.

### *Prolapse Conditions*

These can involve any vaginal segment: anterior, with prolapse of the urethra, bladder base, trigone, bladder and peritoneum and contents; superior (apical), with prolapse of the cervix and uterus, the peritoneum and occasionally the bladder, posterior, involving the peritoneum, the rectum, and the perineal body and the levator complex, which

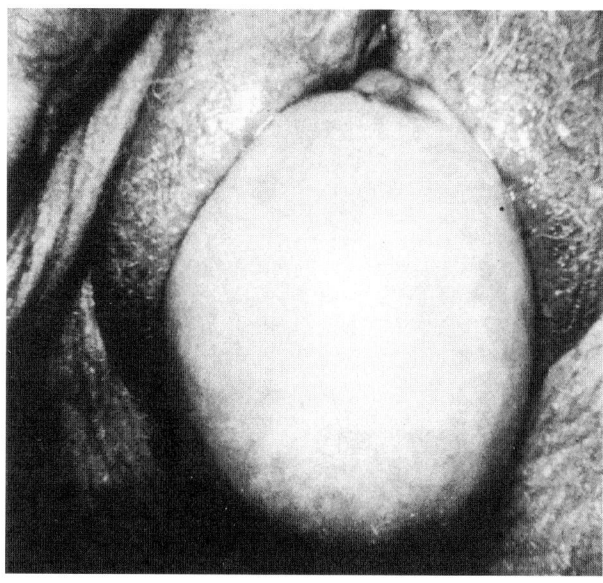

Fig. 4. Complete eversion of the vagina, with total vaginal prolapse.

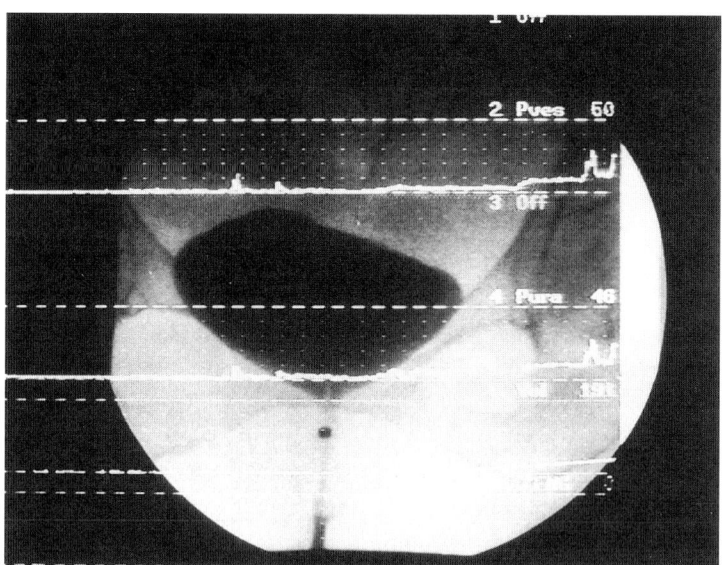

Fig. 5. A grade-one cystocele associated with severe low-pressure leakage related to intrinsic sphincter dysfunction. The cystocele will be reduced completely by the sling procedure, which is the most appropriate procedure.

supports everything. In addition, complete prolapse—where the vagina is completely everted—can also occur (see Fig. 4).

Precise diagnosis depends on a careful pelvic examination in the supine and upright position, if possible. The classic pelvic examination position may lead to an underestima-

# Chapter 31 / Assessing the Incontinent Woman

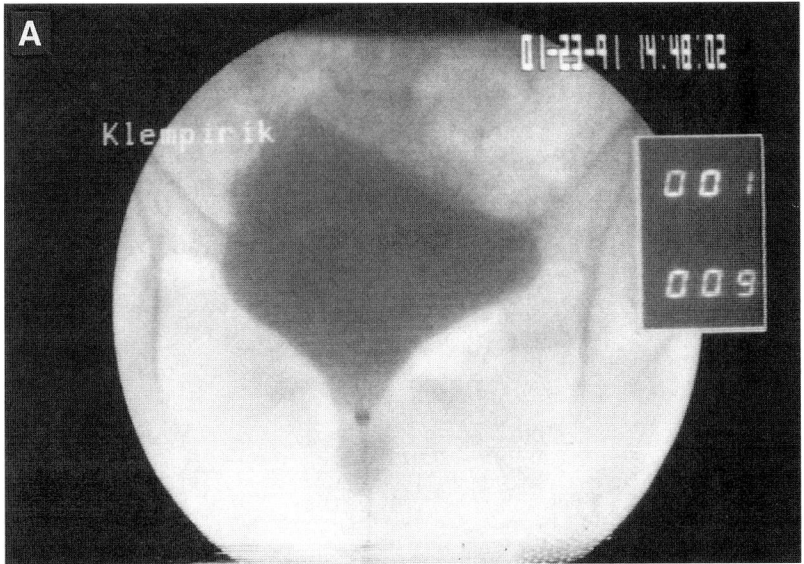

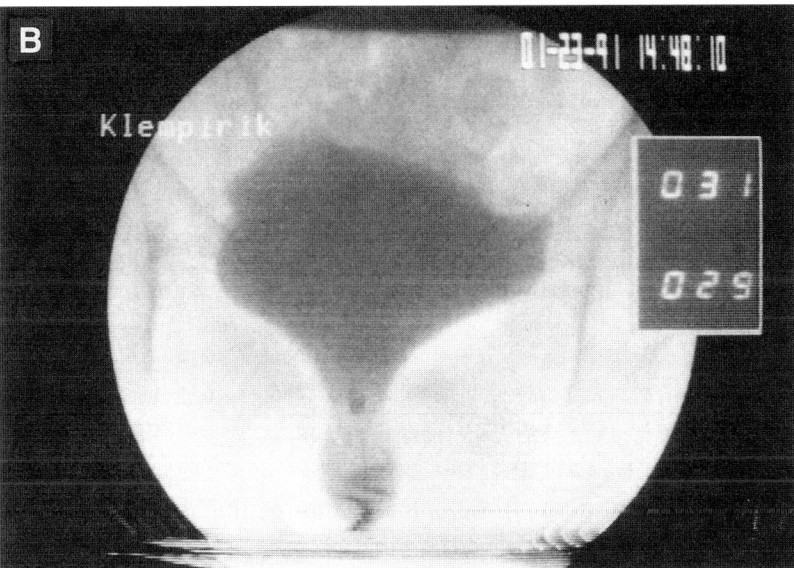

**Fig. 6.** (**A**) A central cystocele—there is a defect in the pelvic floor through which the bladder herniates. There defect is small and very central. (**B**) The cystocele is a little more prominent and larger, with an increase in abdominal pressure, but the defect is the same, small and very central. (**C**) A different patient with a somewhat larger defect in the pelvic floor seen in the lateral projection. The urethra (outlined by the urodynamic catheter) is also out of position, and although it does not leak, it should be suspended with a sling at the time of cystocele repair.

tion of the degree of prolapse and the extent of the defect through which the prolapse herniates. Failure to appreciate the extent of the prolapse can lead to an inadequate repair and recurrence. For example, a potent cause of failure of a rectus fascial sling is prolapse of a cystocele, or enterocele above and behind the sling. Even if the sling appears to be in good position, repair of a cystocele or enterocele often interferes with

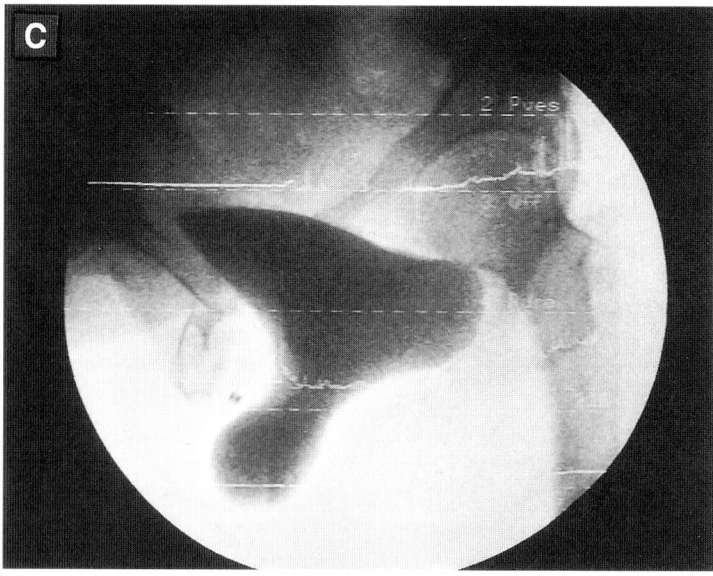

**Fig. 6.** Continued

the attachments of the sling at the arcus tendineus, and leads to failure with recurrent stress incontinence postoperatively.

## Cystoceles

These occur in 30% or more of women with primary-stress incontinence. Grade I and II cystoceles, which are anterior and do not herniate from the introitus, do not need a separate repair and are reduced more or less in conjunction with a urethral suspension (*see* Fig. 5). Higher-grade prolapse of a cystocele, where the mass extends beyond the introitus, usually requires a dedicated repair. Lasting repair of a cystocele depends on analysis of its component parts. A central cystocele herniates through a central defect in the pelvic floor (*see* Fig. 6A,B,C). The neck of the cystocele seen radiographically is relatively narrow, although presenting part of the cystocele may be large and spherical. This kind of cystocele may—when fully prolapsed—contain three-quarters or more of the bladder. The repair must concentrate on the defect through which the bladder herniates. One good way to do this is to use a rectus fascia patch or other fascial patch and fix it to the arcus on both sides the cervix or sacrouterine complex posteriorly and superiorly, and to a suburethral sling anteriorly.

Lateral detachment refers to loss of the normal vaginal support at the arcus tendineus on one or both sides (*see* Fig. 7A,B). This can be associated with loss or damage or dennervation of the levator complex, but not in all cases. This condition produces a broad-based descent of the anterior vaginal segment, and sometimes includes the vaginal cuff. On radiographic evaluation, the cystocele is very broad-based and deep in lateral projection, and usually requires some kind of vault suspension for adequate repair. Combined defects involve central herniation and lateral detachment. These require closure of the central defect and vault suspension to restore normal vaginal depth and axis. Repair of a central defect using tissue adjacent to the defect may induce a lateral

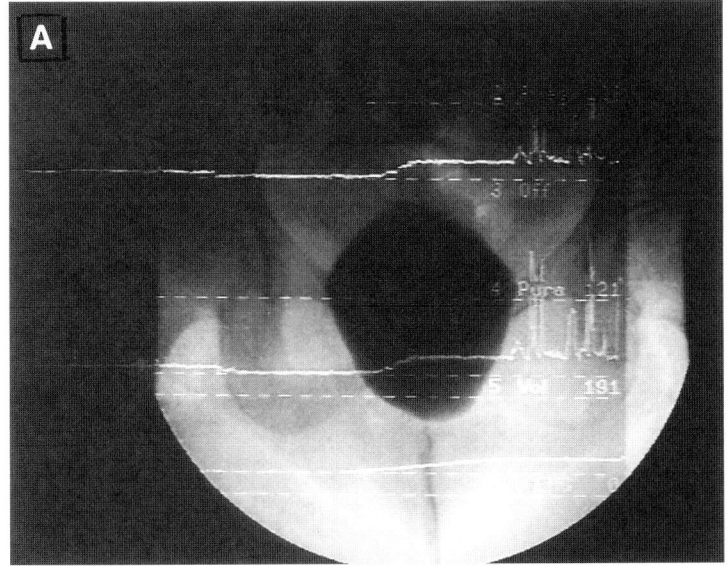

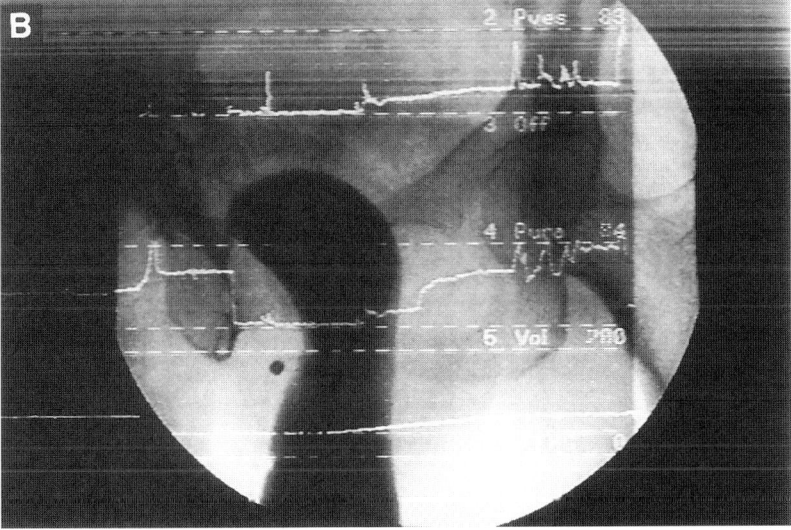

**Fig. 7. (A)** Lateral detachment. The prolapse has a broad base and descends as a unit. Often, the degree of descent is less with this kind of cystocele, although the repair may be more difficult. **(B)** Combined lateral and central cystocele, which requires separate repairs, although they are done through the same incision.

detachment, and a paravaginal repair to restore a lateral detachment may induce a central defect.

## PLANNING APPROPRIATE SURGICAL MANAGEMENT

### *Stress Incontinence*

The outcome data available for retropubic suspensions and needle suspensions suggests that most women of childbearing age with significant stress incontinence that

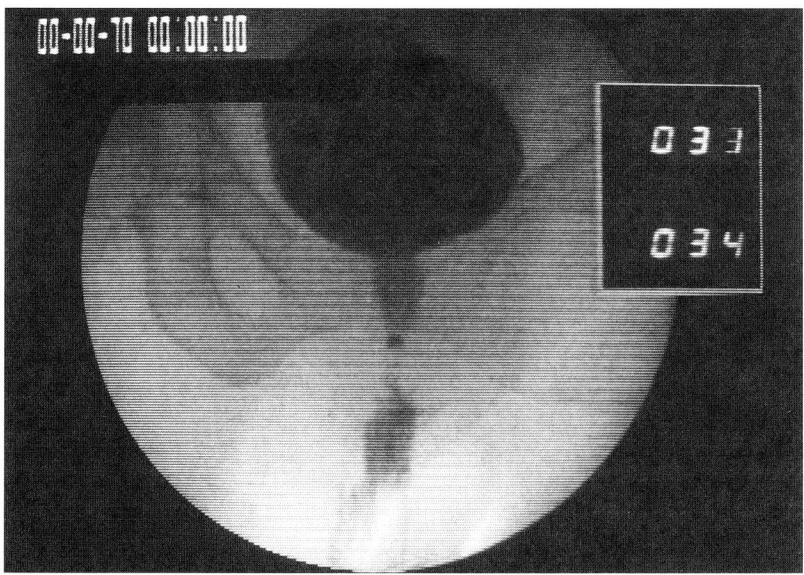

**Fig. 8.** Stress leakage at very low pressure. There is no motion of the urethra at all—it simply cannot resist abdominal pressure.

develops in association with labor and delivery should be treated with a sling—for both immediate and long-term outcome. Women who develop stress incontinence in the perimenopausal years are probably also best treated with some variety of sling, although retropubic suspension procedures in this group are also acceptable. Patients with gross violent urethral hypermobility should probably not be treated with a needle suspension. At present, the conditions suitably treated by a sling only are as follows: pure ISD with a low Valsalva leak-point pressure, leakage with little or no urethral mobility (although collagen could also be used here, it is not a permanent solution) (*see* Fig. 8). Other relative indications for a sling are: recurrent stress incontinence after a retropubic suspension; a needle suspension or sling; when a synthetic sling has eroded, or when a synthetic sling requires removal for one reason or another and stress incontinence redevelops; and in patients with hypermobility but a low Valsalva leak-point pressure. In this context, a low leak-point pressure ranges from 0–70, a high leak-point pressure is above 120, and the rest fall in the middle.

Slings are effective but problematic for the elderly patient, since detrusor strength is not normal and primary urge incontinence is also common. A good result with respect to urethral continence function can be overshadowed by prolonged retention and severe motor-urge incontinence. In the case of elderly and very elderly patients, a needle suspension and anterior repair or collagen are often better choices than a sling, but sometimes only a sling is strong enough to effect good urethral function.

### *Collagen*

This treatment, done transurethrally, produces continence in as many as 70% of carefully selected patients. The best candidates are elderly women with type I stress incontinence, with little or no mobility of the urethra but not a completely nonfunctional proximal mechanism. If there is no change after three injections, further injections are probably futile.

## SELECTED READING

### Urinary Incontinence Symptoms

Artibani W (1997) Diagnosis and significance of ideopathic overactive bladder. *Urology* 50:25.
Cross C, Manhot L, English S, et al. (1998) Urinary incontinence questionaires: do they correlate with urodynamic findings. *J Urol* 159: Abst. #829.
Cundiff GW, Harris RL, Coates KW, et al. (1997) Clinical predictors of urinary incontinence in women. *Am J Obstet Gynecol* 177:262.
Griffith DK (1998) Clinical aspects of detrusor instability and the value of urodynamics: a review of the literature. *European Urol* 34:13.
McGrother C, Resnick M, Yalla SV, et al. (1998) Epidemiology and etiology of urinary incontinence in the elderly. *World J Urol* 16:3.
Sandvik H, Hunskaar S, Vanvik A, Bratt H, et al. (1995) Diagnostic classification of female urinary incontinence: an epidemiologic study corrected for validity. *J Clin Epidemiol* 48:339.

### Continuous Ambulatory Monitoring

Brown K, Hilton P (1997) Ambulatory monitoring. *Int Urogynaecol J Pelvic Floor Dysfunction* 8:369.
Heslington K, Hilton P (1996) Ambulatory monitoring and conventional cystometry in asymtomatic female volunteers. *Br J Urol* 103:434.

### Urodynamics of Stress Incontinence

Nitti V, Combs AJ (1996) Correlation of Valsalva leak point pressure with subjective degree of stress incontinence. *Urology* 155:281.
Roamnzi LJ, Chaikin DC, Blaivas JG (1999) The effect of genital prolapse on voiding. *J Urol* 161:581.
Versi E, Lyell DJ, Griffiths DJ (1998) Video urodynamic diagnosis of occult genuine stress incontinence in patients with anterior wall relaxation. *J Soc Gynecol Invest* 5:327. (diagnosis of the condition SUI in patients without SUI symptoms).
Wan J, McGuire E, Bloom DA, et al. (1993) Stress leak point pressure. *J Urol* 150:700.

### Stress and Urge Incontinence

Alcalay M, Monga A, Stanton SL (1995) Burch culposuspension: a 10 to 20 year follow up. *Br J Obstet Gynaecol* 102:740. There was no effect on outcome of detrusor instability determined to be present preoperatively.
McGuire EJ (1992) The unstable bladder: clinical relevance of a urodynamic diagnosis. *Advances in Urology.* 5:107.
McGuire EJ, Cross CR (1998) Pubovaginal slings in patients with stress urinary incontinence. *J Urol* 159:1195. The same outcome with a high rate of resolution of DI symptoms, identical to the earlier series from the University of Michigan, and the Duke and Cornell series.
Morgan T, Westney OL, McGuire EJ (1999) Pubovaginal sling: 4 year outcome analysis and quality of life assessment. *J Urol* 161 abst # 394. There was a 75% resolution rate of urge incontinence symptoms in these 240 patients.

### Conditions Associated with Motor-Urge Incontinence

Cross CA, Cespedes RD, English S, et al. (1998) Transvaginal urethrolysis for urethral obstruction after antiincontinence surgery. *J Urol* 159:1199. Motor urge incontinence is very common in this setting—usually associated with residual urine, but not always.
McGuire EJ (1995) Urodynamic evaluation of stress incontinence. *Urol Clin NA* 23:551. Background on video urodynamics and the meaning of the findings in a large, diverse group of women.
Neri-Mendez C, Salas-Gonzales F, Rodriguez-Colorado C, et al. (1996) Incidence of pelvic genital static disorders in patients with urinary incontinence. *Gynecologica y Obstet de Mexico* 64:193. They looked at the problem from another angle and found 45% of the incontinent population had a significant prolapse.

Olsen AL, Smith VJ, Bergstrom JO, et al. (1997) Epidemiology of surgically managed pelvic organ prolapse and urinary incontinence. *Obstet Gynecol* 89:501. An interesting study detailing an 11% cumulative risk for American women for surgery for prolapse and incontinence—the same numbers as reported in an English study.

## *Assessment*

Montella JM, Ewing S, Cater J (1997) Visual assessment of urethrovesical junction mobility. *Int J Urogynaecol Pel Floor Dys* 8:13. They did not find this to be an effective method.

Neuman M, Lavie D, Gdansky E, et al. (1995) Early uterine prolapse following culponeedle suspension. Aust NZ J Obstet Gynaecol 35:339. Rapid development of prolapse after needle suspension, which suggests the condition was potentially there to begin with.

## *But LOOK Here*

Swift SE, Herring M (1998) Comparison of pelvic organ prolapse in the dorsal lithotomy position compared with the standing position. *Obstet Gynecol* 91:661. They did as well on exam with the patient supine as when she was standing, i.e., they found no difference. That has not been my experience when pelvic exam is compared to upright video urodynamics, but this is an interesting study suggesting that due care and expertise during an exam is rewarded with accurate findings.

## *Treatment of Motor Urge Incontinence*

Burgio KL, Whitehead WE, Engel BT (1985) Urinary incontinence in the elderly: bladder sphincter training and biofeedback and toileting skills training. *Ann Int Med* 103:507.

Cespedes RD, Cross CA, et al. (1996) Ingleman-Sundberg bladder dennervation for intractable urge incontinence. *J Urol* 156:1744.

Leng WW, Blalock J, Frederickson W, et al. (1999) Enterocystoplasty or detrusor mymectomy: a comparison of indications and outcomes for bladder augmentation. *J Urol* 161:758. Mymectomy was as effective as augmentation cystoplasty, is easier for patient and surgeon, and did not require intermittent catheterization.

## *Surgical Therapy of Incontinence and Prolapse*

Barrington JW, Calvert JP (1998) Vaginal vault suspension for prolapse after hysterectomy using an autologous fascial sling of rectus fascia. *Br J Obstet Gynaecol* 105:83.

Carr LK, Walsh PJ, Abraham VE (1997) Favorable outcome of pubovaginal slings for geriatric women with stress incontinence. *J Urol* 157:125.

Cross CA, Cespedes RD, McGuire EJ (1997) Treatment results using pubovaginal slings in patients with large cystoceles. *J Urol* 158:431.

Fisher-Rasmussen W (1998) Transvaginal needle bladder neck suspension: practical methods but non optimal results. *Obstet Gynecol Scand Suppl* 168:38.

Harris WJ, Jarvis RR (1999) Use of autologous rectus fascia graft for repair of cystocele. *Pelvic Surgery* 5:146.

Pelosi MA III, Pelosi MA (1998) Transvaginal needle suspension with Le Fort culpocleisis for stress incontinence and advanced utero vaginal prolapse in high risk patients. *J Am Asso Gynecol Laparoscopists* 5:7.

Trockman BA, Leach GE (1996) Needle suspension procedures past present and future. *Endourol* 10:217.

# 32 Selection, Treatment, and Counseling for Women with Urinary Incontinence

*Kathleen C. Kobashi, MD*
*and Gary E. Leach, MD*

**CONTENTS**
INTRODUCTION
TYPES OF URINARY INCONTINENCE
TREATMENT OPTIONS
CONCLUSIONS
SELECTED READING

## INTRODUCTION

The International Continence Society (ICS) defines urinary incontinence (UI) as the "involuntary loss of urine that represents a hygienic or social problem to the individual and which is objectively demonstrable." Estimates of the prevalence of urinary incontinence vary with the profile of the groups studied. Urinary incontinence is estimated to affect 13 million Americans, and costs approx $16 billion in health-care each year. A recent review of the societal cost of care of urinary incontinence in patients >65 yr of age by Wagner and Hu estimated a cost of $26.3 billion, or $3565 per patient. An approximated 10–20% of women aged 15–64 yr, 40% of women >60 yr, and >50% of institutionalized patients (including both sexes) are affected.

In this chapter, we discuss the types of urinary incontinence and provide a detailed discussion of treatment options and the risks and benefits associated with each option.

## TYPES OF URINARY INCONTINENCE

*Stress urinary incontinence* (SUI) is defined as leakage of urine with a sudden increased intra-abdominal pressure—such as seen with laughing, coughing, lifting, walking, or changing position—without a concomitant rise in intravesical pressure. The proposed mechanism is that the increased pressure is transmitted to the bladder, causing the intravesical pressure to rise above the urethral pressure. Under normal circumstances, the urethral pressure not only rises approx 250 ms before any increase

From: *Current Clinical Urology: Office Urology: The Clinician's Guide*
Edited by: E. D. Kursh and J. C. Ulchaker © Humana Press Inc., Totowa, NJ

Table 1
Possible Etiologies for Three Major Types of Incontinence

| Stress urinary incontinence | Urge incontinence | Overflow incontinence |
|---|---|---|
| Trauma<br>  Childbirth<br>  Pelvic surgery<br><br>Physiologic<br>  Atrophic vaginitis<br>    (hormonal)<br>  Pelvic prolapse<br><br>Medication side effects<br>  α-Blockers<br>    (for hypertension)<br>  β-Antagonists<br>  Benzodiazepines<br>    (muscle relaxants) | Neurologic<br>  Spinal-cord injury/back<br>    surgery<br>  Multiple sclerosis<br>  Cerebrovascular accident<br>  Parkinson's disease<br>  Aging<br><br>Obstruction<br>  Uncommon in females<br>    without prior pelvic<br>    surgery<br>  Cystocele/vault prolapse<br>  Previous pelvic surgery<br>  Malignancy<br><br>Fibrosis<br>  Aging<br>  Iatrogenic<br>    Long-term indwelling<br>      catheter<br><br>"Other"<br>  Infection<br>  Tumor/carcinoma *in situ*<br>  Stones<br>  Interstitial cystitis<br>  Idiopathic | Trauma<br>  Myogenic damage<br>    (2° to overdistension)<br><br>Neurologic<br>  Diabetes mellitus (70%<br>    decreased sensation;<br>    15% acontractile)<br>  Multiple sclerosis<br>    (5–10% acontractile)<br><br>Obstruction<br>  Previous antiincontinence<br>    surgery<br>  Malignancy<br><br>Medication side effects<br>  Drugs with anticholinergic<br>    side effects |

in the intravesical pressure, but the rise is sufficient to prevent urinary leakage from occurring (ie, protective mechanism). Etiologies are shown in Table 1. Patients with *urge incontinence* describe the sudden insuppressible sensation to void, resulting in variable leakage of urine. *Mixed incontinence*, as the name implies, includes components of both SUI and urge incontinence. *Overflow incontinence* may occur in cases in which the bladder is full to capacity, and any further urine production results in frequent low-volume loss of urine, ie "overflow." The clinician should be aware that patients who actually suffer from overflow incontinence may describe symptoms of urgency or stress incontinence. A patient's ability to empty the bladder must be evaluated to ensure that overflow incontinence is not being overlooked.

## TREATMENT OPTIONS

### *Stress Urinary Incontinence*

#### Nonsurgical Options

When counseling patients about treatment alternatives for SUI, all options must be considered. Most patients wish to try noninvasive therapy before surgery. The goal—

## Table 2
### Alpha-Agonists for SUI and Their Dosage[a]

| Medication | Dosage |
|---|---|
| Ephedrine sulfate | 25–50 mg QID |
| Pseudoephedrine (Sudafed®) | 30–60 mg TID |
| Phenylpropanolamine | 50–75 mg BID or TID |
| Chlorpheniramine maleate (Ornade®) | 1 tab BID |
| Guaifenesin (Entex La®) | 50 mg QD or BID |

[a]This group of medications may be used to increase bladder-outlet resistance.

regardless of treatment choice—is to improve the incontinence and improve the patient's quality of life.

### Medications

*Alpha-Agonists.* Alpha-agonists stimulate the alpha receptors at the bladder neck and proximal urethra, resulting in smooth-muscle stimulation and increased bladder-neck and proximal urethral resistance. Alpha stimulators are useful in the treatment of mild to moderate SUI, but are usually not sufficient to treat severe SUI. For maximal results, alpha-agonists should be used in conjunction with pelvic-floor exercises (PFEs) and estrogens.

Pharmacologic agents in this category are listed in Table 2. Alpha-stimulants should be used with caution in the elderly patient population, and it is prudent to consult the primary care physician prior to prescribing these medications. This especially applies to those patients with cardiac disease, hypertension, or hyperthyroidism, because alpha-agonists can cause drowsiness, anxiety, weakness, insomnia, headache, tremor, palpitations, cardiac dysrrhythmias, respiratory difficulty, and blood-pressure elevation. Tachyphylaxis may be seen. Ephedrine and pseudoephedrine are stereoisomers of each other and stimulate both alpha and beta receptors in addition to inducing the release of norepinephrine. Phenylpropanolamine is a pure alpha agonist that produces less central stimulation than ephedrine and pseudoephedrine. Therefore the adverse effects of anxiety, insomnia, and headache tend to be minimized.

*Tricyclic Antidepressants.* Tricyclic antidepressants (TCAs) increase bladder-outlet resistance through inhibition of peripheral reuptake of norepinephrine. This in turn increases stimulation of the alpha-receptors in the smooth muscle of the bladder neck and proximal urethra. TCAs also have anticholinergic and musculotropic effects, as well as a strong direct inhibitory effect on the detrusor, which is not anticholinergic or adrenergic. These effects make TCAs ideal for treatment of mild SUI, urge incontinence, and mixed stress and urge incontinence. The primary agent in this category is imipramine (Tofranil®), which is administered at a dosage of 10–25 mg BID to TID, and may be increased up to 150 mg total per day. Higher doses are used for treatment of depression.

Adverse effects of TCAs can be divided into alpha-adrenergic and anticholinergic effects. The medication is generally well-tolerated, but is contraindicated in patients with cardiac arrhythmia or heart block. Adrenergic side effects include tachycardia, restlessness, blood-pressure elevation, and exacerbation of heart block. Anticholinergic effects include orthostatic hypotension, dry mouth, ataxia, tachycardia, restlessness, hallucinations, and mental status changes. The latter effects are typically seen only at the higher doses used for antidepressive therapy.

*Estrogen.* The exact mechanism of action of estrogen in the treatment of incontinence is speculative. Theoretically, estrogen enhances the effects of alpha-agonists, perhaps by increasing the density of alpha-receptors. Estrogen also promotes mucosal proliferation, and increases submucosal blood flow, thereby enhancing the "mucosal seal" effect. Estrogen is indicated in patients noted to have changes in the vagina. Intravaginal use at a dose of one-third applicator three times per week amplifies the local effect of the estrogen over the effect of oral estrogen on the urethral and vaginal epithelium. Estrogen is usually used in combination with other medications, pelvic-floor exercises, and behavioral modification to achieve maximal benefit.

Oral estrogen supplementation has been implicated in increasing the risk of endometrial cancer when unopposed by progestins, and an association between estrogens and breast cancer has been shown with long-term use (>15 yr). However, this effect has not been definitively demonstrated with the use of vaginal hormone creams. Numerous studies have examined the effect of vaginally administered estrogens on the endometrium, and have shown minimal or no proliferation with varying doses. A vaginal estrogen ring (Estring®), which is maintained in the vagina for 90 d and releases 8 µm of estrogen per 24 h, has recently been introduced, and shows promising early results and satisfaction rates. Transdermal and vaginal administration of estrogens avoids the first-pass effect through the liver seen with oral dosage, and therefore, the risks of alteration in clotting factors and plasma renin substrate do not occur.

**Behavioral Therapy.** All patients considered mentally and physically fit for active participation are candidates for behavioral modification. However, it is important to remember that the candidates who appear to benefit the most are those who suffer from only mild SUI. Patients must also be dedicated to compliance in the program to benefit maximally.

Patients are encouraged to limit fluid intake to <40 oz/d and to avoid consumption of caffeine or alcohol. The use of Kegel exercises and vaginal weights have had variable success in the literature. Kato, et al reported on 77 patients with SUI who were treated with weighted vaginal cones. Nineteen of twenty-seven (70%) of the patients with mild SUI had complete or >50% improvement. Conversely, only 7 of 50 patients with severe SUI had similar success. Wilson and Borland studied 34 women with genuine stress-urinary incontinence treated with vaginal weight training for 6 wk. Subjective improvement was reported in 23 (47%). At a mean follow-up of 15.8 mo (range 12–24 mo), 14 (41%) still reported continued improvement.

Cammu et al showed that the cure/improved rates in two groups of 30 women who used either PFEs with weighted vaginal cones or PFEs alone were similar. However, patients in the cone group either dropped out of the study or discontinued cone therapy after completion of the 12-wk study. Use of the vaginal cones can decrease the number of visits to the physical therapist without affecting therapeutic outcome. However, poor patient compliance limits the usefulness of this treatment option.

**Biofeedback.** Biofeedback (BFB) is an excellent treatment option for those patients who can benefit from a nonsurgical approach to their incontinence based on either individual preference or clinical situation. It also enables the patient to take an active role in the management of her health-care issues. BFB employs monitoring equipment to facilitate the development of conscious control of various body functions of which the patient is unaware. A vaginal probe is inserted to measure the activity of the levator ani musculature and surface electrodes detect contractions of the abdominal or gluteal muscles that might otherwise be mistaken by the patient as contraction of the pelvic-floor musculature. Patients are taught to tighten the sphincter muscle without increasing abdominal pressure, and the BFB equipment relays auditory or visual feedback to patients regarding measurements of the physiologic activity.

Moderate success was noted in a study by Stein et al in which 5 of 14 (36%) patients showed a significant decrease in stress-urinary incontinence symptoms following 6 BFB sessions over a 3-wk period. The response was maintained over the period of follow-up, although the length of follow-up was not specified. It is important for the clinician to understand and explain to patients that long-term success with PFEs is only possible if the patient continues with the exercises following completion of their course of biofeedback.

**Injection Therapy.** Various materials, including collagen, Teflon, and fat, have been used in periurethral injection therapy for treatment of ISD. Only collagen is approved for use in the United States (*see* Fig. 1A, B). Complications with collagen injection are rare, but include tissue necrosis at the injection site, urethral prolapse, delayed hypersensitivity with systemic arthralgia, bladder-outlet obstruction, pseudocyst formation, and sterile abscess formation. Complications with autologous fat injection, although rare, have included fat reabsorption, persistent urinary incontinence, and one reported case of pulmonary embolism. Autologous fat is obtained by aspiration (liposuction) of the subcutaneous fat of the abdomen, and may therefore result in complications related to the fat harvest site. Haab et al. compared the efficacy of injection therapy using fat vs collagen, and found a significantly higher failure rate with fat injection.

In a review of 139 patients who underwent periurethral collagen injection therapy (median follow-up 18 mo, range 6–36 mo), Cross et al. showed that 103 (74%) had substantial improvement, 29 (20%) had improvement, and 7 (5%) had no change. The average duration since the last collagen injection was 18 mo. Thirty-nine patients (28%) developed *de novo* urgency, and 29 (20.8%) had persistent urgency. A total of 11.6% required a "booster injection" more than 6 mo after the first injection. Cross suggests that too superficial an injection risks tearing of the mucosa and leakage of the collagen, whereas too deep a placement requires a higher volume of collagen to achieve any effect.

Herschorn et al. advocate the use of collagen injection therapy for treatment of SUI, even in patients with urethral hypermobility. In a review of 187 patients treated with collagen injection therapy for SUI with a mean follow-up of 22 mo (range 4–69 mo), they found 43 (23%) patients cured, 97 (52%) improved, and 47 (25%) failed. There was no difference in outcome between patients with or without urethral hypermobility.

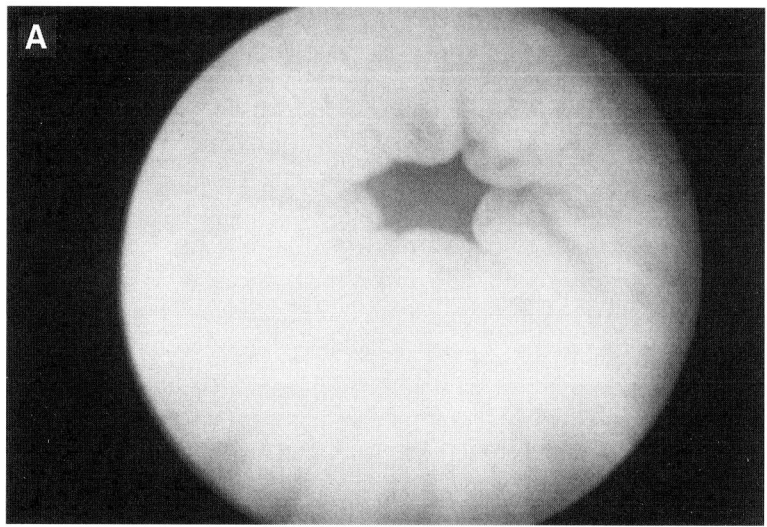
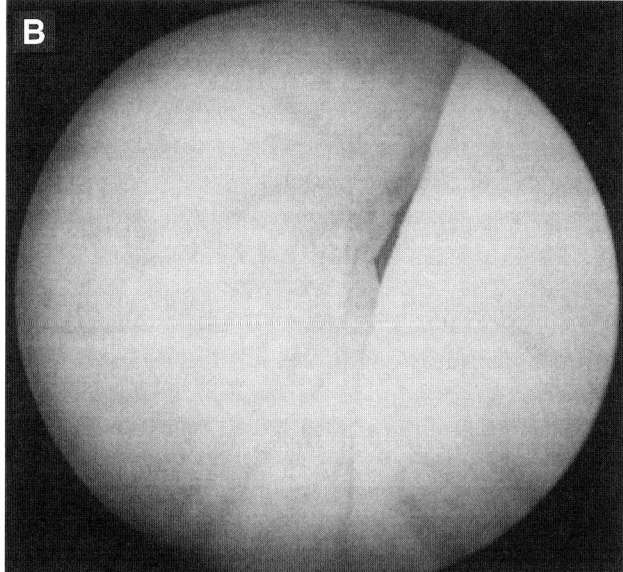

**Fig. 1.** Endoscopic view of the urethra of a patient with intrinsic sphincter deficiency before (**A**) and after (**B**) periurethral collagen injection.

**Urethral Plugs.** Instruments that physically occlude the urethral meatus have been introduced as treatment options for SUI. Results have been disappointing overall. Fuertes et al. reviewed the efficacy of a urethral plug in 20 patients with 4-wk follow-up. Ten (50%) patients refused to complete the study secondary to infection, difficulty with use, or urethral irritation. Of the remaining 10 patients, eight (40%) had a subjective decrease in incontinence; however, after completion of the study, only five patients wished to continue using the plug. In a similar study by Nielsen, et al., only 18 of 40 patients completed the study, which continued over a 3-mo period. Seven of eighteen

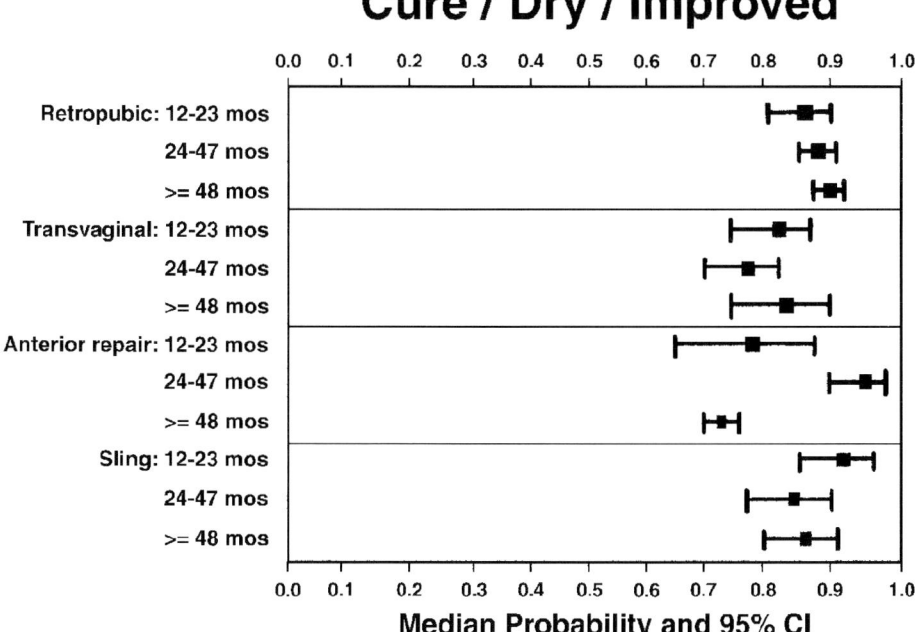

Fig. 2. The AUA Clinical Guidelines panel for treatment of female stress-urinary incontinence concluded that, based on the literature, slings and retropubic suspensions have the best long-term results (84–84% at 48 mo).

(42.5%) patients showed both subjective and objective improvement of their incontinence.

**Surgical Options**

The authors prefer to use pubovaginal slings for all female patients with SUI who opt for surgical therapy. Candidates for pubovaginal slings include those patients who have objectively demonstrated SUI, empty their bladders completely preoperatively, have no other bladder pathology such as tumors or stones, and do not have predominant symptoms of urgency that are not controlled by medications. Exceptions include those patients who only have urodynamically proven detrusor instability at high volumes, or patients in whom such instability does not correlate with their symptoms.

In their comprehensive review of the literature regarding surgical treatment for female stress-urinary incontinence, the AUA Clinical Guidelines panel categorized treatment options into four groups: retropubic suspensions, needle suspensions, anterior repair, and slings. The Panel found that all surgical techniques for treatment of SUI have similar outcomes up to 48 mo. Only beyond 48 mo do the differences in cure and dry rate become significant (*see* Fig. 2). Slings and retropubic suspensions maintain an 83–84% success rate beyond 48 mo, as compared to the needle suspensions, which decrease to 67% success at that point. It is important to consider that when the majority of the articles that were reviewed by the panel were written, slings were primarily used only for the more difficult cases of SUI, and were nonetheless able to stand up to the other popular surgical techniques. Slings clearly appear to be the most efficacious treatment over time, and the current trend is moving toward slings for treatment of all types of SUI for patients who choose operative therapy and are good surgical candidates.

**Retropubic Suspension.** Retropubic suspensions provide support of the bladder neck and proximal urethra by anchoring the perivesical and periurethral tissues to the pelvic wall, Cooper's ligament, or the pubic bone. Innumerable variations have been developed with an overall cure/dry rate comparable to that of the sling, both short-term and at >48 mo of 80–90%. The Marshall-Marchetti-Krantz (MMK) procedure utilizes bilateral bladder-neck sutures that are anchored to the symphysis pubis. The Burch retropubic suspension involves placement of four paravesical/perivaginal sutures that are secured to Cooper's ligament. Complications of retropubic suspensions include urinary retention, urethral obstruction, new-onset pelvic prolapse, persistent or *de novo* urgency or urge incontinence, osteitis pubis, and injury to the urethra, bladder, or bowel.

Gilja et al. reported an 89.3% continence rate in 44 patients who underwent a Burch retropubic suspension with 3 yr follow-up.

Clemens et al compared the results of the Stamey needle bladder-neck suspension (mean follow-up 15.2 yr, range 9.4–19.9 yr) with those of the MMK (mean follow-up 17.0 yr, range 13.2–21.9 yr). They found that both the dry-rate and long-term morbidity were higher for the Stamey procedure than the MMK. Dry-rate was 44 vs 33%, local pain was 9 vs 0%, and postoperative urgency was 70 vs 23%.

**Needle Suspension.** Needle suspension procedures involve suspension of the bladder neck and proximal urethra via placement of sutures through the periurethral and perivaginal tissues and suspending them from the rectus fascia or pubic symphysis. The long-term results are poor, with failures most likely secondary to tearing-through of the vaginal sutures.

Trockman, et al. reviewed the long-term success rate of the modified Pereyra bladder-neck suspension with a mean follow-up of 9.8 yr. They found that the length of follow-up had a significant impact on the reported success rates. There were no identified preoperative predictors of long-term outcome. Of this group, 51% of patients reported SUI with or without urgency at 5-yr follow-up, and only 20% reported no incontinence at 10 yr. Improvement in symptoms was reported by 71%, and 73% reported satisfaction with their results.

Although the Guidelines panel found no significant difference in the results of procedures within a given category of treatment, some authors describe differences in success of needle suspension techniques. Nonetheless the results have generally been relatively poor. Kondo et al. reviewed the results of Stamey ($n = 342$) vs Gittes ($n = 40$) needle BNS, and found that the Stamey procedure had a much higher continence rate than the Gittes (71.3% at 14 yr vs 31% at 6 yr). Elkabir et al reported on 52 patients (mean follow-up 53 mo, range 24–103 mo) who underwent a Gittes BNS and also showed a high failure rate with the Gittes. Twelve (23.1%) patients were dry, and 14 (26.9%) others were improved. Within 2 yr of surgery, 40 (80%) failed.

**Pubovaginal Sling.** Pubovaginal slings have been created from a variety of materials, including synthetics and autologous, allogenic, and xenogenic tissues. Slings are placed beneath the proximal urethra/bladder neck to provide a hammock effect with some degree of direct compression of the urethra. Slings have traditionally been used in the

Table 3
Comparison of Complications with Synthetic
vs Autologous Materials

| Complications | No. of autologous materials (%) n = 1715 | No. of synthetic materials (%) n = 1515 |
|---|---|---|
| Vaginal erosion | 1 (0.0001) | 10 (0.007) |
| Urethral erosion | 5 (0.003) | 27 (0.02) |
| Fistula | 6 (0.003) | 4 (0.002) |

Synthetic materials used for creation of pubovaginal slings have a greater tendency to erode into the vagina and/or urethra as compared to autologous materials. From AUA Clinical Guidelines panel on treatment of stress urinary incontinence.

treatment of intrinsic sphincter deficiency or in those patients who have failed previous anti-incontinence surgery. However, slings are now being advocated to treat all types of SUI. Although some surgeons may consider slings to have a higher complication rate and to be more technically complicated than retropubic and needle suspensions, the long-term success rate has proven to be superior to that of the other techniques.

Two main approaches to sling placement are widely used—the combined abdominal-transvaginal and the transvaginal approaches. The transvaginal approach—particularly with cadaveric fascia—has a significantly shorter operative time and hospital stay and recovery period. The cadaveric transvaginal sling (CaTS) technique also results in less postoperative pain, typically requiring no more than acetaminophen in our the experience, and achieves better cosmesis than the combined approach or when harvesting of fascia is necessary.

The general risks of slings include persistent or *de novo* urgency, which occurs in 20–40% and 10–12% of patients, respectively. Temporary urinary retention occurs in approx 50–60% of patients and is permanent in only 1–2% of patients who receive slings.

## Outcomes According to Type of Sling

*Synthetic Slings.* Review of the literature reveals that synthetic materials tend to have a higher complication rate than autologous tissues or allografts (*see* Table 3). The vaginal and urethral erosion rate of synthetic slings ranges from 0–14%, depending on the synthetic material used (*see* Table 4). Thus, the authors do not use synthetic sling material.

*Autologous Slings.* The biggest disadvantage of using fascia lata is pain at the harvest site. Sixty-seven percent of patients experience lateral thigh pain with walking. Cosmetic results are also a consideration. In Wheatcroft's series, 38% of patients complained about the appearance of the scar, and Naugle reported the complication of herniation of the muscle belly.

Use of rectus fascia provides the same excellent long-term results as fascia lata. The fascia is harvested through the abdominal incision used in the combined abdominal/transvaginal approach for sling placement. There is no proven risk of "rejection" or transmission of infectious disease with autologous fascia. Disadvantages of rectus fascia

Table 4
Comparison of Erosion Rates of Various Synthetic Materials[a]

| Reference | N | Sling material | Vaginal erosion, n (% total) | Urethral erosion, n (% total) | Number removed, n (% total) | Follow-up (range) | Interval–insertion to removal |
|---|---|---|---|---|---|---|---|
| Barbalias et al. | 16 | Gore-tex | 0 (0) | 2 (0.125) | 2 (0.125) | 30–38 mo | [c] |
| Stanton et al. | 30 | Silastic | — | 1 (0.03)[b] | 1 (0.03) | [c] | [c] |
| Hom et al. | 35 | Polypropylene | 0 (0) | 0 (0) | 0 (0) | 2–18 mo | N/A |
| Bryans et al. | 69 | Marlex | 5 (0.07) | 0 (0) | 2 (0.03) | 6 mo–8 yr | 7 yr |
| Chin et al. | 88 | Silastic | 5 (5.5) | 5 (5.5) | 10 (11) | 2 mo–5 yr | 16.6 mo (mean) |
| Staskin et al. | 122 | Gore-tex | 5 (4) | 0 (0) | | 24.4 mo (mean) | N/A |
| Morgan et al. | 274 | Marlex | 0 (0) | 2 (0.01) | 2 (0.01) | 1–5+ yr | 1–3 yr |

[a] This table summarizes the results of numerous studies that evaluated various materials used for creation of pubovaginal slings for their erosion into the vagina or urethra.
[b] Urethrovaginal fistula.
[c] Data not presented.

include the development of an abdominal hernia, inherent weakness of the patient's fascia—especially following multiple abdominal surgeries or radiation therapy, and a "pulling" sensation or pain radiating to the groin. This sensation is presumably secondary to the tension of the suspension sutures on the rectus fascia or nerve entrapment.

Cross et al. reviewed their results in 150 patients with type II, type III, or ISD with urethral hypermobility, who underwent rectus PVSs (mean follow-up 22 mo, range 6–42 mo). Of this group, 140 (93%) patients were cured. All failures presented within 3 mo (7/10 within 1 mo and 10/10 within 3 mo). Complications included urinary retention requiring further surgery in (2.8%), de novo UI in (19%), and persistent UI in (3%).

Chaikin et al. studied 251 patients who underwent autologous rectus fascia pubovaginal sling with a mean follow-up of 3.1 yr (range 1–15 yr). Ninety-two percent (231) of patients were cured or improved after surgery, 3% (7) of patients had de novo urge incontinence, 23% (58) had persistent urge incontinence, and 2% (4) experienced permanent urinary retention.

Govier et al. reported their experience with 32 patients with ISD who underwent placement of $2 \times 24$–28-cm fascia lata slings with a median follow-up of 14 mo (range 3–33 mo). Outcome analysis was based on a retrospective chart review and evaluation of the same patients by survey. Eighty percent of patients responded that they would undergo the same procedure again. In the chart review group, 87% (28) of patients wore no pads, 9% (3) were improved, and 3% (1) showed no improvement. The same group was evaluated by anonymous survey. Of this group, 70% (21) of patients required no pads, 20% (6) wore 1–3 small pads, and 10% (3) required >3 pads/d.

Carr et al. reported excellent results with rectus fascia slings in the geriatric patient population. They compared their outcomes in 96 patients with SUI treated with rectus slings, 19 of whom were >70 yr of age, and 77 of whom were <70 yr old. Mean follow-up was 22 mo (range 3–43 mo). The symptoms of SUI resolved in 100% of the geriatric patients and 97% of the patients <70 yr of age. Urgency symptoms in patients who had had preoperative detrusor instability improved postoperatively in >50% of patients in both groups. *De novo* urgency occurred in 10% of patients in both groups, but was controlled adequately in all patients with anticholinergic medications.

*Cadaveric Fascia Lata.* The risk of transmission of infection by transplanted cadaveric fascia has been shown to be minimal. The risk of acquiring HIV-infected tissue from a properly screened donor is reported to be 1/1,667,600, and the risk of transmission of HIV from banked cadaveric fascia is 1/8,000,000. The Tutoplast® has been used extensively in Europe with no reported cases of transmission of HIV. Wound infection or "rejection" has not been seen in the authors' experience to date. Handa reported that 2 of 16 (12%) patients developed abdominal-wound infections following placement of cadaveric slings, which is comparable to the incidence reported by Beck with autologous fascial slings.

Wright et al. evaluated their results in 92 patients with a mean age of 60 yr and mean follow-up of 11.5 mo. They compared autograft ($n = 33$) versus allograft ($n = 59$) fascia lata slings. The groups were similar with regard to preoperative SEAPI scores, number of previous antiincontinence procedures, and leak-point pressure. The procedures were equally well-tolerated, with marked improvement in both groups and no patients with infection or erosion of the sling. Mean operative time and hospital stay were significantly lower in the allograft patients.

Thus far, the authors have performed 95 *ca*daveric *t*ransvaginal *s*lings (CaTS) using a transvaginal bone anchoring system (*see* Fig. 3A, B). Patients have been admitted to the hospital for 23 h for intravenous antibiotics. Because there is no abdominal or leg incision for harvesting of the fascia or placement of the sling, analgesic requirements have been minimal, and the majority of patients who require pain medication are adequately controlled on acetaminophen alone. All patients have been evaluated with a preoperative and postoperative SEAPI score. The decrease in the mean score postoperatively has been statistically significant (5.36 vs 1.27, $p < 0.001$). Less than 50% of patients require temporary intermittent catheterization, but only one patient has experienced unexpected permanent postoperative urinary retention (one patient had expected urinary retention). Of the 92 patients available for follow-up (range 1–10 mo), 63 (68.5%) are totally dry, 12 (13.0%) have persistent mild SUI, 4 (4.3%) have persistent urge incontinence, 9 ((9.8%) have had *de novo* urge incontinence, and 2 (2.2%) have mixed incontinence.

## *Urge Incontinence*

The true incidence of bladder overactivity in the general population has been estimated to be 10%. Diokno et al. urodynamically studied 169 randomly selected noninstitutionalized women, and found that 8% showed evidence of detrusor instability. In the absence of other pathology, such as urinary-tract infection, bladder tumors, or bladder stones, symptoms of urgency and urge incontinence may be caused by bladder overactivity. The term "detrusor instability" is used to describe the urodynamic findings of detrusor

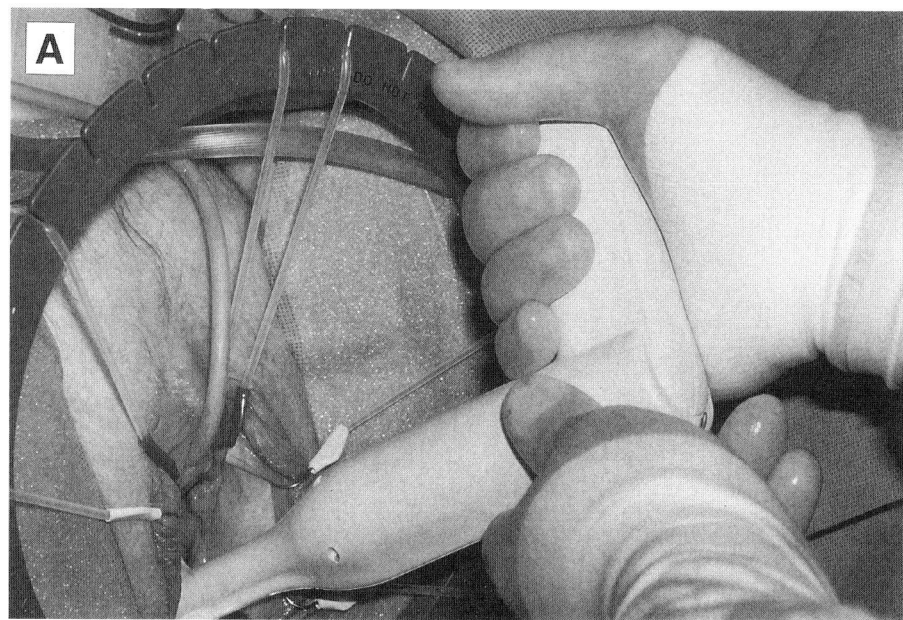

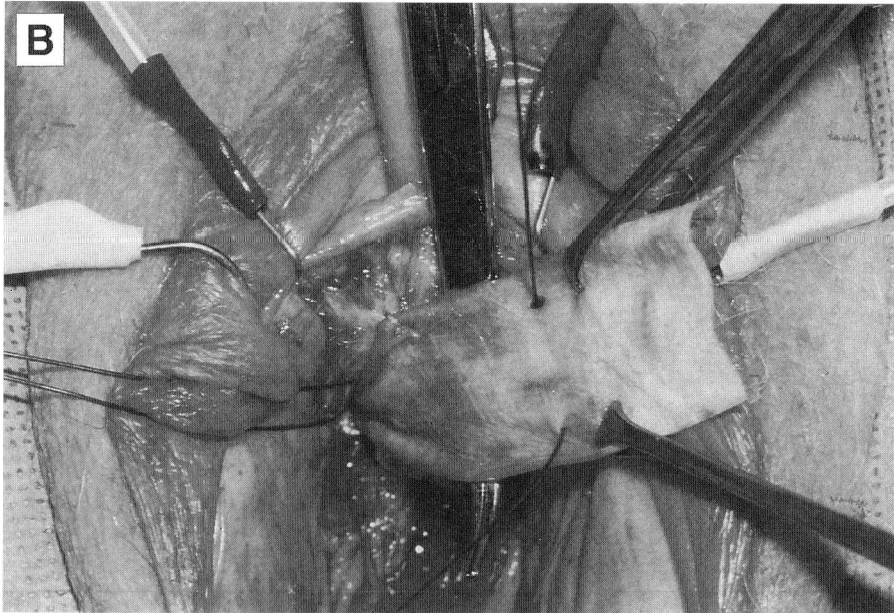

Fig. 3. **(A)** Placement of the transvaginal device used for placement of the bone anchors. **(B)** The cadaveric fascial strip is placed flat and snug on a right-angle clamp to ensure proper tension on the sling.

overactivity in patients with no neuropathology. Any rise in bladder pressure as the patient attempts to inhibit micturition falls into this definition (*see* Fig. 4). In those patients with neurologic disease, the same urodynamic findings are termed "detrusor hyperreflexia." In other words, the terminology describes the same condition, but indicates whether the patient has a neurologic cause for the unstable bladder.

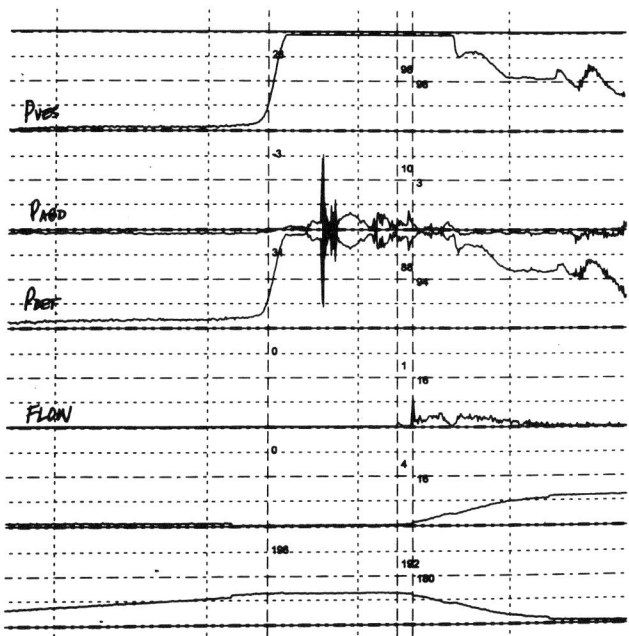

**Fig. 4.** Multichannel urodynamics study illustrates high detrusor pressures with concomitant low urinary flow rate as is seen in patients with bladder-outlet obstruction.

## Nonsurgical Options

Treatment of detrusor instability or hyperreflexia is optimally nonsurgical, with surgical therapy used only as a last resort.

**Medications.** Agents that inhibit bladder contractility can increase bladder capacity and may also decrease intravesical pressures. Also, sustained elevation of intravesical pressures above 40 cm $H_2O$—seen especially in those patients with myelodysplasia—puts the patient at risk for upper-tract damage. Patients who fall into this group should be evaluated with renal ultrasound to rule out the presence of hydronephrosis.

*Anticholinergics and Musculotropics.* Anticholinergic medications competitively inhibit acetylcholine at the postganglionic autonomic (muscarinic) receptors. Musculotropics act directly on smooth-muscle contractility through a papaverine-like action and also have varying anesthetic properties. Medications and their respective dosages are listed in Table 5. Probantheline is more selective than atropine for the lower urinary tract.

Adverse effects of this group of these medications vary with the systemic absorption and tend to be the most pronounced with oxybutynin (Ditropan®). Effects include dry mouth, constipation, blurred vision, tachycardia, drowsiness, precipitation of urinary retention, and confusion. Narrow-angle glaucoma is an absolute contraindication to the use of this group of medications. The adverse effects often result in poor compliance on the part of the patients. The hepatic metabolites of oxybutynin are responsible for the severity of its side effects. Patients who are unable to tolerate the adverse effects of oral oxybutynin, have failed other oral therapies, and are willing to undergo catheter-

Table 5
Anticholinergics and Musculotropics for Treatment of the Overactive Bladder

| Medication | Dosage |
|---|---|
| Anticholinergics | |
| Probantheline bromide (Pro-Banthine®) | 15–30 mg QID |
| Hyoscyamine sulfate (Levsin®, Levsinex®) | #1 BID (available in capsule, slow-release, elixir) |
| Musculotropics | |
| Oxybutynin (Ditropan®) | 2.5–5.0 mg QD to TID; May try intravesical instillation |
| Ditropan XL® | 5–10 mg QD |
| Dicyclomine hydrochloride (Bentyl®) | 20–30 mg TID |
| Flavoxate hydrochloride (Urispas®) | 100–300 mg TID |
| Belladonna/opium (B&O suppository®) | 1/3–1 per rectum TID |
| Tolterodene (Detrol®) | 2 mg BID |

ization are candidates for intravesical oxybutynin. Intravesical instillation of oxybutynin bypasses the liver, and therefore the tolerance of this route of administration is better. In this study, 42 patients with detrusor instability ($n = 19$), detrusor hyperreflexia ($n = 20$), or bowel/bladder overactivity following augmentation cystoplasty ($n = 3$) were placed on intravesical ditropan (5 mg/30 cm$^3$ saline bid-tid) with a mean follow-up of 18.4 mo. No patients had adverse effects, but 21% ($n = 9$) dropped out of the study secondary to difficulty tolerating the catheterization required for intravesical instillation. Of the remaining 33 patients, 55% ($n = 18$) showed a significant improvement in their symptoms.

Tolterodine (Detrol®) is a competitive muscarinic antagonist that was released for use in the United States in mid-1998. Detrol is administered at 2 mg twice a day. Because of its higher specificity for bladder muscarinic receptors (as compared to the salivary-gland muscarinic receptors), its systemic and central side effects are significantly decreased, and it is far better tolerated than Ditropan. Notably, one of the most common side effects leading to patient discontinuation of Ditropan is dry mouth, an effect that is significantly decreased with the use of Detrol. Once-a-day slow-release oxybutynin (Ditropan XL®) is now FDA-approved, and has just become available on the market. One study, which compared oxybutynin 5 mg BID to 10 mg QD showed no significant differences in the efficacy or adverse effects, affording only the advantage of once-a-day dosing. However, Brown found that although the efficacy of immediate-release (IR) oxybutynin was equivalent to that of Ditropan XL, the incidence of dry mouth was significantly lower for the latter (see Table 6). The incidence of other anticholinergic adverse effects was similar in both groups.

*Tricyclic Antidepressants.* TCAs have both anticholinergic and local anesthetic effects, which make them a good choice for treatment of detrusor instability. The increase in norepinephrine also increases alpha-stimulation at the bladder neck to

Table 6
Incidence of Dry Mouth with Oxy-IR (Immediate-Release) vs Ditropan XL

| Degree of dry mouth | Oxy-IR (n = 53) | Ditropan XL (n = 52) |
|---|---|---|
| Any | 86.5% | 67.9% |
| Moderate/severe | 46.2% | 24.5% |

increase bladder-outlet resistance, and may theoretically have some effect on the smooth-muscle receptors in the bladder body, resulting in smooth muscle relaxation. The authors use imipramine (Tofranil®) at a dose of 10–25 mg TID.

*DDAVP (1-Desaminocystine 8-D-Argininevasopressin).* Administration of such an agent as DDAVP—a synthetic analog of the antidiuretic hormone, vasopressin—decreases urine production. In this manner, the *problem* of the bladder instability may be eluded all together, although not *treated*. This drug is primarily used in patients with nocturnal enuresis and diabetes insipidis and is not routinely administered in the therapy of detrusor instability. Adverse effects of DDAVP are rare and usually occur within the first few weeks of therapy. The main risk includes water intoxication and hyponatremia, and therefore, the drug must be used with caution in the elderly—particularly in patients with a history of congestive heart failure.

**Behavioral Modification/Bladder Training/Biofeedback.** Fluid restriction to 30–40 oz/d with avoidance of caffeine and alcohol is imperative. This is particularly true in patients who experience urgency and urge incontinence at higher bladder volumes. Often, patients will increase fluid intake in response to the dry mouth they experience when on anticholinergic medications. Patients must be counseled strongly to avoid drinking more fluid. Helpful tips for the patients include candy, gum, artificial saliva, or small sips of fluid to overcome dry mouth. Additionally, the constipation also experienced by many patients on anticholinergics can be treated with Mitrolan, a wafer laxative that does not require the intake of the large amounts of fluid required by some fiber supplements.

Behavioral modification for treatment of urinary incontinence is based on the concept that instability is a result of frequent voiding. Patients are trained to postpone urination and void according to the clock rather than according to the urge to void. Using biofeedback, they are taught to inhibit or resist the sensation of urgency. Initially, the goal is set for urination every 1–2 h, then gradually increased to 3–4 h. For patients with instability only at high volumes, timed voiding every 2–3 h may be helpful in avoiding the uninhibited contractions that result in the symptoms of urgency.

Results vary according to the reporting source. Fantl et al. reviewed and reported on the literature available studying pelvic-floor rehabilitation (PFR) and bladder training for treatment of urge incontinence. Overall, approx 20% of patients became continent, and 75% improved by at least 50% in the number of incontinence episodes with PFR—as opposed to <15% cure, and approx 50% with at least 50% reduction in symptoms with bladder training. The range of follow-up was not specified. Burgio et al. studied 197 volunteer women with urge incontinence or mixed incontinence with urge as the predominant component. Patients were randomized to biofeedback (four sessions in 8 wk), drug therapy (oxybutynin 2.5–5.0 mg TID), or placebo. The biofeedback group had the greatest objective and perceived improvement (80.7 and 74.1%, respectively) as compared to the medication group (68.5 and 50.9%) and the placebo group (39.% and 26.9%). Follow-up continued over 6 yr. Clearly, patients must be compliant and willing to continue the behavioral changes they learn in the program indefinitely.

Detrusor hyperreflexia with impaired contractility (DHIC) is a condition that includes bladder overactivity and incomplete emptying, causing symptoms of urgency and urge incontinence concomitant with impaired contractility, such that the patient is unable to sustain a contraction sufficient for complete bladder emptying. Resnick et al. performed detailed urodynamics studies on 245 institutionalized patients (mean age 89 yr). Detrusor instability was the cause of incontinence in 61% of the patients, and DHIC was found to be the second most common cause (33%) of incontinence in that population. Anticholinergic medications and clean, intermittent catheterization are indicated in patients with DHIC. The anticholinergic agents may help control the symptoms of urgency related to the detrusor overactivity, and regular catheterization not only helps avoid the complication of urinary-tract infections that may be seen as a result of poor emptying, but also often alleviates the symptoms of urgency associated with higher vesical volumes.

**Electrical Stimulation.** Sacral nerve stimulation is currently increasing in usage in the United States. A temporary percutaneous stimulation device for stimulation of the third sacral nerve root is placed under fluoroscopic guidance. If the trial is successful in inhibition of bladder contractility, a permanent stimulator is implanted surgically. The postulated mechanism of action is through activation of spinal or beta-adrenergic nerves. Up to 60–70% success has been reported in the initial studies. Shaker and Hassouna placed a permanent sacral neurostimulator in 18 of 18 patients following a positive response after percutaneous nerve stimulation. Mean follow-up was 18.8 mo (range 3–83 mo), and all patients showed a marked reduction in urinary incontinence episodes from a mean of 6.49 to 1.98 episodes in 24 h. Twelve (66%) of patients were completely dry or had one or fewer incontinence episodes per day (44 and 22%, respectively).

**Intravesical Instillation.** As mentioned previously, intravesical oxybutynin instillation has shown promising results in the treatment of urinary urgency. The use of intravesical capsaicin, although not available in the United States, has been used widely in Europe with excellent results. The theory is that intravesical capsaicin renders the unmyelinated sensory afferent C-fibers in the bladder unresponsive to further stimulation, thereby decreasing detrusor instability and the associated pain.

Seventy-nine patients with urge incontinence—including 74 patients with multiple sclerosis and four neurologically normal patients—were treated with intravesical capsaicin instillation. Dosage was 1–2 mmol/L in 30% ethanol in saline. Complete continence was achieved in 44%, 36% improved, and 20% failed. In another series, 16 patients received 1 mmol of capsaicin intravescially. Decreased frequency was experienced by 14 of 16 patients, and 10 of the 14 achieved continence. There was a significant increase in the mean volume at first urge as well as the mean bladder capacity, with effects lasting up to 12 mo.

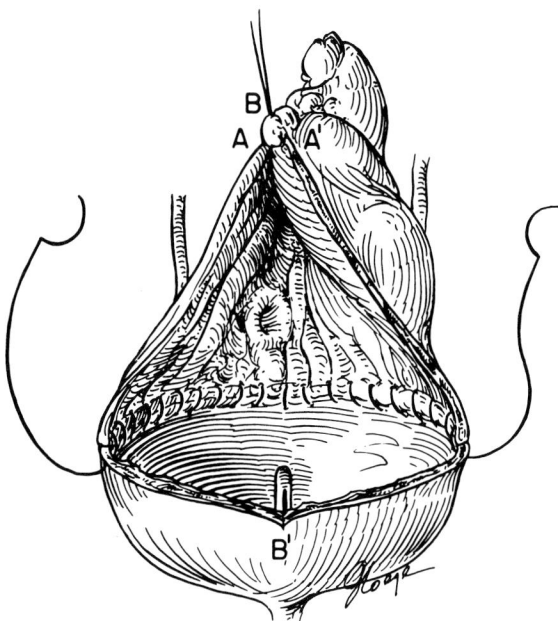

**Fig. 5.** A segment of bowel is resected, detubularized, and placed onto the bivalved bladder to augment its capacity and decrease intravesical pressures.

**Acupuncture.** Acupuncture is not widely used in the United States, and therefore the majority of the literature comes from abroad. Kitakoji performed an average of 7 (range 4–12) acupuncture treatments on 11 patients for treatment of an overactive bladder with undetermined follow-up. A needle was inserted bilaterally at a point designated as Zhongliao point BL-33. Nine patients had preprocedural urge incontinence and two had urgency. Urgency resolved in both patients. Five of nine patients with urge incontinence became dry, and two had subjective improvement.

## Surgical Options

Surgery is the last resort for treatment of urge incontinence. It may be offered to patients who have poor results with medications, biofeedback, or electrical stimulation, or who are unable to continue medications secondary to the adverse effects.

**Augmentation Cystoplasty.** A patch of ileum or colon may be used to augment the bladder to decrease intravesical pressure and instability and increase bladder capacity (*see* Fig. 5). The literature suggests that patients must be counseled on the 30–40% chance of requiring postoperative intermittent catheterization. The authors counsel their patients that lifelong intermittent catheterization may be expected in 100% of patients postoperatively. Success rates for augmentation cystoplasty have been reported to be in the 69–97% range. Risks include a possible increased risk of developing carcinoma in the bowel patch, gastrointestinal complications including diarrhea, constipation, or bowel obstruction, electrolyte disturbances (which vary depending on the bowel segment used), mucus production by the bowel patch, and the possibility of a minimally increased risk of infection. Patients are instructed on periodic irrigation of the mucus from the bladder to minimize the risk of infection or outlet obstruction secondary to a mucus plug. Periodic cystoscopy should be performed to ensure that no stones or large mucus plugs are within the augmented bladder.

**Urinary Diversion.** Urinary diversion or augmentation cystoplasty with creation of an abdominal stoma is a logical consideration for patients who may have difficulty accessing the urethra for catheterization.

### *Mixed Stress and Urge Incontinence*

Up to 56% of patients with urinary incontinence have components of both stress and urge incontinence. It is important to determine as best as possible the proportion of stress symptoms and urgency symptoms in each individual to help direct treatment options.

## Nonsurgical Options

**Medications.** Medications that increase the bladder-outlet resistance *and* decrease detrusor contractility are ideal. As discussed in previous sections, imipramine has properties that result in both an increase in outlet resistance and detrusor relaxation. It is therefore an optimal choice for treatment of mixed incontinence with mild to moderate symptoms of stress and/or urgency. Medications may also be tried in conjunction with other nonsurgical treatment options. In fact, nonsurgical therapy alone is typically unsuccessful if the type of SUI involved is ISD.

**Behavioral Therapy/Biofeedback.** Behavioral therapy and biofeedback involve fluid restriction, avoidance of caffeinated and alcoholic beverages, bladder training, conscious postponement of urination, and pelvic-floor exercises. This program can be combined with pharmacologic therapy, often with excellent results.

**Electrical Stimulation.** Electrical stimulation is discussed in the section covering urge incontinence.

## Surgical Options

If a patient's primary complaints consist of stress symptoms and there is urodynamically documented SUI, a pubovaginal sling may be considered. Detrusor instability is alleviated following antiincontinence surgery in up to 60% of patients with mixed incontinence.

In extreme cases in which nonsurgical therapy is not enough to control the patient's symptoms, augmentation cystoplasty with or without collagen injection therapy or pubovaginal sling may be considered. Patients must be counseled on the necessity for postoperative catheterization.

### *Overflow Incontinence*

Treatment of overflow incontinence is important, especially if the patient experiences recurrent urinary-tract infections or deterioration of renal function is apparent. The goal of treatment is complete emptying of the bladder. First, the patient's medication profile should be reviewed in consideration of the possibility of urinary retention secondary to anticholinergic side effects of medications. Any medications that could be contributing to the problem should be discontinued, if possible. In the case of persistent retention, or when discontinuation of contributing medications is not feasible, the patient should ideally be placed on intermittent catheterization.

**Nonsurgical Options**

**Medications.** In theory, medications that decrease bladder-outlet resistance or increase detrusor contractility should promote bladder emptying. However, no evidence supports the belief that the available medications accomplish this satisfactorily. Medications that have been used include bethanechol (Urecholine®), although this agent has not been shown to be efficacious.

**Clean-Intermittent Catheterization.** Clean, intermittent catheterization is the treatment of choice for overflow incontinence. However, this option requires compliant patients (or caretakers) with the mental capacity and manual dexterity to perform catheterization. In nursing homes, a sterile technique may be preferred, although not necessarily practical, for the sake of infection control.

**Indwelling Foley Catheter or Suprapubic Tube.** Because of the risks of long-term catheters, indwelling catheters are a last resort. Complications include urethral damage, infections, stones, and tumors. If a long-term indwelling catheter is needed despite these risks, a suprapubic cystostomy is preferred to avoid urethral damage. Catheters should be changed monthly.

**Surgical Options**

Surgical therapy for treatment of female overflow incontinence is rarely a viable option. However, in the case of bladder-outlet obstruction secondary to periurethral scarring or suture "kinking" the urethra—such as that seen following anti-incontinence surgery—urethrolysis with Martius fat-pad graft may be performed to relieve the obstruction. Bladder-outlet obstruction is confirmed by urodynamics studies, ideally with video imaging of the bladder, bladder neck, and urethra, and pressure-flow studies. The sine qua non of obstruction on a pressure-flow curve is high detrusor pressure, low urinary flow rate, and incomplete bladder emptying (*see* Fig. 6). Again, in patients who are unable to catheterize through the urethra, creation of a catheterizable abdominal stoma may be a consideration.

Controversy exists regarding urethral resuspension at the time of urethrolysis. We do not advocate this practice because if postoperative urinary retention occurs, it is difficult to determine whether it is secondary to persistent outlet obstruction or caused by the anti-incontinence procedure. Goldman et al. reviewed their results in 31 patients who underwent urethrolysis without resuspension to relieve obstruction following anti-incontinence surgery. Twenty-six (84%) patients voided well or had significant improvement following the surgery, and only six (19%) had recurrence of any degree of incontinence. Four of the patients with SUI (66%) became dry following collagen injection, and 16% remained obstructed after urethrolysis.

## CONCLUSIONS

Urinary incontinence is a prevalent and costly health-care problem affecting all sectors of the population. Regardless of the cause of incontinence, most of the cases can be treated successfully once they are recognized. Patient education regarding the

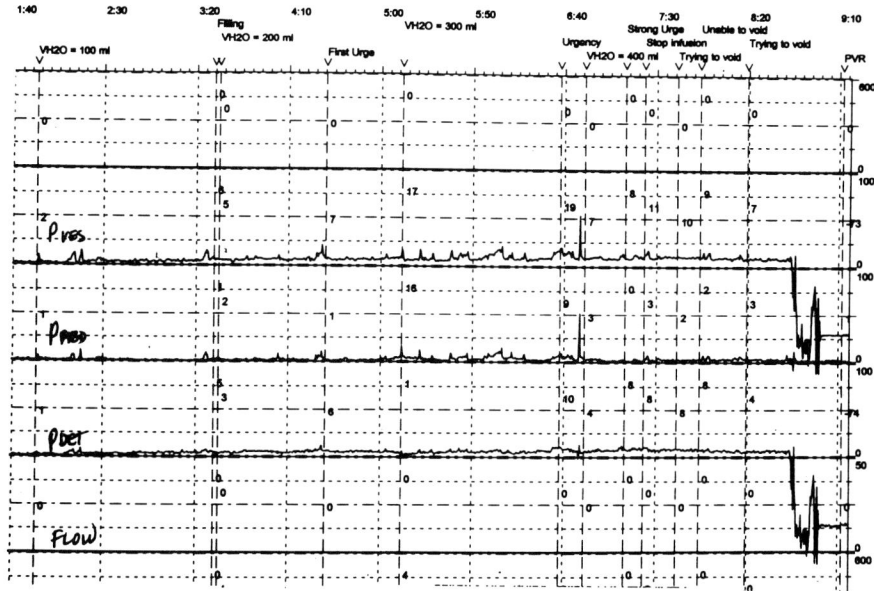

**Fig. 6.** Urodynamics during an attempted void demonstrating no evidence of detrusor contraction (no rise in detrusor pressure), as may be seen in patients with overflow incontinence.

prevalence of urinary incontinence and the availability of therapy and relief certainly reveals many patients who are ashamed to seek help for the problem secondary to the stigma attached to incontinence, or are simply unaware that incontinence is a treatable condition that they need not endure. Careful evaluation can result in successful treatment and an improvement in the quality of life for patients who suffer from urinary incontinence.

## SELECTED READING

Appell RA (1998) Surgery for the treatment of overactive bladder. *Urology* 51(Suppl 2A):27–29.

Abrams P (1998) Tolterodine. *Br J Urol.*

Blaivas JG, Jacobs BZ (1991) Pubovaginal fascial sling for the treatment of complicated stress urinary incontinence. *J Urol* 145(6):1214–1218.

Blaivas JG, Romanzi LJ, Heritz DM (1998) Urinary incontinence: pathophysiology, evaluation, treatment overview, and nonsurgical management. In: Walsh PC, Retik AB, Vaughan ED, Wein AJ, eds., *Campbell's Urology*, 7th edition. Philadelphia: WB Saunders Co., pp. 1007–10043.

Brown J (1998) Comparison of tolerability and efficacy of once-a-day vs immediate-release oxybutynin chloride in patients with urge urinary incontinence. Oxybutynin XL Study Group, University of California, San Francisco.

Burgio KL, Locher JL, Goode PS, Hardin JM, McDowell BJ, Dombrowski M, Candib D (1998) Behavioral vs drug treatment for urge urinary incontinence in older women: a randomized controlled trial. *JAMA* 280(23):1995–2000.

Buyse G, Waldeck K, Verpoorten C, Bjork H, Casaer P, Anderson KE (1998) Intravesical oxybutynin for neurogenic bladder dysfunction: less systemic side effects due to reduces first pass metabolism. *J Urol* 160:892–896.

Cammu H, Van Nylen M (1998) Pelvic floor exercises versus vaginal weight cones in genuine stress incontinence. *Eur J Obstet Gynecol Reprod Biol* 7(1):89–93.

Carr LK, Walsh PJ, Abraham VE, Webster GD (1997) Favorable outcome of pubovaginal slings for geriatric women with stress incontinence. *J Urol* 157(1):125–128.

Cervigni M (1996) Hormonal influences in the lower urinary tract. In: Raz S, ed., *Female Urology.* Philadelphia: WB Saunders Co.

Chaikin DC, Rosenthal J, Blaivas J (1998) Pubovaginal fascial sling for all types of stress urinary incontinence: long-term analysis. *J Urol* 160(4):1312–1316.

Clemmens JQ, Stern JA, Bushman WA, Schaeffer AJ (1998) Long-term results of the Stamey bladder neck suspension: Direct comparison with the Marshall Marchetti Krantz procedure. *J Urol* 160:372–376.

Constantinou CE (1985) Resting and stress urethral pressures as a clinical guide to the mechanism of continence in the female patient. *Urol Clin N Am* 12(2):247–258.

Cross CA, Cespedes RD, McGuire EJ (1998) Our experience with pubovaginal slings in patients with stress urinary incontinence. *J Urol* 159:1195–1198.

Cross CA, English SF, Cespedes RD, McGuire EJ (1998) A follow-up on transurethal collagen injection therapy for urinary incontinence. *J Urol* 159:106–108.

Cruz F, Guimaraes M, Silva C, Rio ME, Coimbra A, Reis M (1997) Desensitization of bladder sensory fibers by intravesical capsaicin has long lasting clinical and urodynamic effects in patients with hyperactive or hypersensitive bladder dysfunction. *J Urol* 157(2):585–589.

De Ridder D, Chandiramani V, Dasgaputa P, Van Poppel H, Baert L, Fowler CJ (1997) Intravesical capsaicin as a treatment for refractory detrusor hyperreflexia: a dual center study with long-term follow-up. *J Urol* 158(6):2087–2092.

Diokno AC, Brown MB, Brock BM (1988) Clinical and cystometric characteristics of continent and incontinent non-institutionalized elderly. *J Urol* 145:567.

Elkabir JJ, Mee AD (1998) Long-term evaluation of the Gittes procedure for urinary stress incontinence. *J Urol* 159:1203–1205.

Fantl JA, Wyman JF, McClish DK (1991) Efficacy of bladder training in older women with urinary incontinence. *JAMA* 265:609–613.

Fink RS, Collins WP, Papdaki L (1985) Vaginal oestriol: effective menopausal therapy not associated with endometrial hyperplasia. *J Gynaecol Endocrinol* 1–2:1.

Finkbeiner AE (1985) Is bethanecol chloride clinically effective in promoting bladder emptying? A literature review. *J Urol* 1134(3):443–449.

Fuertes EM, Casado SJ, Cuesta AJ, Cid GM, de Behtencourt RF, Briso HJ, Tamayo JC, Dehaini DA, Fernandez LR, Estevez RL, Chapado SM (1998) [Occlusive urethral systems: can they constitute an alternative in the management of female stress incontinence? (abstract)]. *Arch Esp Urol* 51(1):71–77.

Gilja I, Puskar D, Mazuran B, Radej M (1998) Comparative analysis of bladder neck suspension using Raz, Burch, and transvaginal Burch procedures. *Eur Urol* 33:298–302.

Gillberg PG, Sudnquist S (1998) Tolterodine. *Eur J Pharm* 349(2–3):285–292.

Goldman HB, Rackley RR, Appell RA (1999) The efficacy of urethrolysis without resuspension for iatrogenic urethral obstruction. *J Urol* 161:196–199.

Govier FE, Gibbons RP, Correa RJ, Weissman RM, Pritchett TR, Hefty TRL (1997) Pubovaginal sling using fascia lata for the treatment of instrinsic sphincter deficiency. *J Urol* 157(1):117–121.

Haab F, Zimmern PE, Leach GE (1997) Urinary stress incontinence due to intrinsic sphincteric deficiency: experience with fat and collagen periurethral injections. *J Urol* 157(4):1283–1286.

Herschorn S, Steele DJ, Radomski SB (1996) Followup of intraurethral collagen for female stress urinary incontinence. *J Urol* 156(4):1305–1309.

Kato K, Kondo A (1997) Clinical value of vaginal cones for the management of female stress incontinence. *Int Urogynecol J Pelvic Floor Dysfunct* 8(5):314–317.

Kitakoji H, Terasaki T, Honjo H, Odahara Y, Ukimura O, Kojima M, Watanabe H (1995) Effect of acupuncture on the overactive bladder (abstract). *Nippon Hinyokika Gakkai Zasshi* 86(10):1514–1519.

Kondo A, Kato K, Gotoh M, Narushima M, Saito M (1998) The Stamey and Gittes procedures: long-term followup in relation to incontinence and types and patient age. *J Urol* 160:756–768.

Leach GE (1998) Bone fixation technique for transvaginal needle suspension. *Urology* 31(5):388–390.

Leach GE, Dmochowski RR, Appell RA, Blaivas JG, Hadley HR, Luber KM, et al. (1997) Female SUI clinical guidelines panel summary report on surgical management of female stress urinary incontinence. The American Urological Association, *J Urol* 158:875–880.

Mark SD, Webster GD (1996) Detrusor hyperactivity. In: Raz S, ed., *Female Urology.* Philadelphia: WB Saunders Co.

Mattsson LA, Cullberg G (1983) A clinical evaluation of treatment with estriol vaginal cream versus suppository in postmenopausal women. *Acta Obstet Gynecol Scand* 62:397.

Nilsson CG, Lukkari E, Haarala M, Kivel A, Hakonen T, Kiiholma P (1997) Comparison of a 10-mg controlled release oxybutynin tablet with a 5-mg oxybutynin tablet in urge incontinent patients. *Neurourol Urodyn* 16(6):533–542.

Nielsen KK, Walter S, Maegaard E, Kromann-Andersen B (1993) The urethral plug II: an alternative treatment in women with genuine urinary stress incontinence. *Br J Urol* 72(4):428–432.

Payne CK (1998) Epidemiology, pathophysiology and evaluation of urinary incontinence and overactive bladder. *Urology* (2A Suppl):3–10.

Resnick NM, Yalla SV, Laurino E (1989) The pathophysiology of urinary incontinence among institutionalized elderly persons. *N Engl J Med* 320(1):1–7.

Shaker HS, Hassouna M (1998) Sacral nerve root neuromodulation: an effective treatment for refractory urge incontinence. *J Urol* 159(5):1516–1519.

Simonds RJ, Homberg SD, Hurwitz RL, Coleman TR, Bottenfield S, Conley LJ, Kohlenberg SH, Castro KG, Dahan BA, Schable CA (1992) Transmission of human immunodeficiency virus type 1 from a seronegative organ tissue donor. *N Engl J Med* 326(11):726–732.

Stein M, Discippio W, Davia M, Taub H (1995) Biofeedback for the treatment of stress and urge incontinence. *J Urol* 153:641–643.

Stothers L, Goldenberg SL (1998) Delayed hypersensitivity and systemic arthralgia following transurethral collagen injection for stress urinary incontinence. *J Urol* 159:1507–1509.

Sweat SD, Lightner DJ (1999) Complications of sterile abscess formation and pulmonary embolism following periurethral bulking agents. *J Urol* 161:93–96.

Trockman B, Leach GE, Hamilton J, Sakamoto M, Santiago L, Zimmern P (1995) Modified Pereyra bladder neck suspension: 10-year follow-up using outcomes analysis in 125 patients. *J Urol* 154:1481.

Vandersteen DR, Husmann DA (1998) Treatment of primary nocturnal enuresis persisting into adulthood. *J Urol* 161:90–92.

Wagner TH, Hu TW (1998) Economic costs of urinary incontinence in 1995. *Urology* 51:355–361.

Wein AJ (1995) Pharmacology of incontinence. *Urol Clin N Am* 22(3): 557–577.

Wein AJ (1998) Chillies: from antiquity to urology (comment). *J Urol* 160(3):965.

Weese D, Roskamp D, Leach GE, Zimmern PE (1993) Intravesical oxybutinin chloride: experience with 42 patients. *Urology* 41(6):527.

Wheatcroft SM, Vardy SJ, Tyers AG (1997) Complications of fascia lata harvesting for ptosis surgery. *Br J Ophthalmol* 82(3):333,334.

Wilson PD, Borland M (1990) Vaginal cones for the treatment of genuine stress urinary incontinence. *Aust NZ J Obstet Gynaecol* 30(2):157–160.

Wright EJ, Iselin CE, Carr LK, Webster GD (1998) Pubovaginal sling using cadaveric allograft fascia for the treatment of ISD. *J Urol* 160:759–762.

Zarazoga MR (1996) Expanded indications for the pubovaginal sling: treatment of type 2 or 3 stress incontinence. *J Urol* 156(5):1620–1622.

# 33 Managing Incontinence in the Geriatric Patient

*Patricia S. Goode, MD
and Kathryn L. Burgio, PhD*

**Contents**

EPIDEMIOLOGY OF INCONTINENCE IN OLDER ADULTS
PRESENTATION OF INCONTINENCE IN THE GERIATRIC PATIENT
EVALUATION OF THE GERIATRIC PATIENT WITH INCONTINENCE
TREATMENT OF PERSISTENT INCONTINENCE IN THE
    GERIATRIC PATIENT
SELECTED READING

## EPIDEMIOLOGY OF INCONTINENCE IN OLDER ADULTS

The highest prevalence of incontinence in adults occurs in the elderly. Among community-dwelling older men and women, the prevalence is approx 15 and 30% respectively. The prevalence is much higher among nursing-home residents—well over half of this population are incontinent. Half of home-bound older individuals are also incontinent. The costs of incontinence are enormous—estimated at $11.2 billion annually in the community and $5.2 billion in nursing homes.

The psychosocial burden of incontinence is significant, and the sequelae is insidious. At first, believing that incontinence is a normal aging change, an older individual may wear a pad and continue social activities. However, as the incontinence worsens, lifestyle changes result. A large and embarrassing urge accident on the golf course may end participation in this activity. Frequent trips to the bathroom and accidental urine loss during a bridge game or church service may make these activities seem too bothersome. As incontinence causes older individuals to leave their homes less and less frequently, the decrease in physical activity causes deconditioning. Ultimately, the ensuing frailty increases the incidence of falls and depression, increasing morbidity and mortality.

## PRESENTATION OF INCONTINENCE IN THE GERIATRIC PATIENT

### Stress Incontinence

Stress incontinence—the involuntary loss of urine during coughing, sneezing, or other physical activities that increase intravesical pressure to exceed outlet resistance—

From: *Current Clinical Urology: Office Urology: The Clinician's Guide*
Edited by: E. D. Kursh and J. C. Ulchaker © Humana Press Inc., Totowa, NJ

is quite common in older women. The older woman's pelvic floor provides less support because of age-associated atrophy as well as weight gain and chronic straining at stool in some women. In addition, urethral-closure pressures decrease with estrogen deficiency. Stress incontinence is rare in men except after urethral surgery. Surveys of men taken more than a year after radical prostatectomy reveal that well over one-half suffer from minor stress incontinence, with 24–56% wearing absorbent pads or other devices.

### *Urge Incontinence*

Urge incontinence—the involuntary loss of urine associated with a strong desire to void—becomes increasingly prevalent with age. Older persons have a higher prevalence of comorbidities associated with detrusor instability or decreased mobility, such as stroke and Parkinson's disease. Estrogen depletion is associated with urge incontinence as well as stress incontinence in women. Congestive heart failure and hypertension—common in the elderly—are often treated with diuretics, which can precipitate urgency and urge incontinence. Another common cause of increased urine output and urge incontinence is diabetes, which is poorly controlled in many older persons.

### *Overflow Incontinence*

Overflow incontinence—the involuntary loss of urine associated with insufficient bladder emptying and overdistension of the bladder—is also more prevalent in older persons. Urethral obstruction from prostatic hypertrophy or severe uterine or bladder prolapse may result in overflow incontinence. Diabetic neuropathy, or medications with anticholinergic side effects that are commonly prescribed for older persons, may impair bladder contractility and precipitate overflow incontinence. Overflow incontinence can present with a misleading clinical picture of urinary frequency, stress-induced leakage, or constant dribbling. For this reason, postvoid residual-urine volume determination is an essential part of the work-up of incontinence in the geriatric patient.

### *Functional Incontinence*

Functional incontinence is very common in elderly persons with physical or mental impairments that interfere with their ability to use the bathroom regularly. Dementia in the elderly approaches 50% of those persons 90 yr of age and older. Demented patients initially fail to respond appropriately to the urge to void. Later, they have difficulty finding the bathroom, or become so apraxic that they cannot remember what to do once they get to the bathroom. In the end stages of dementia, they are bed-bound and totally incontinent. It should be noted that incontinence in patients with mild dementia is seldom caused by their dementia. The incontinence can be cured or improved with diagnosis and treatment of the actual underlying cause or causes. Although prevalent, dementia is not a normal aging change, and patients suspected of being demented should be referred for a thorough evaluation for reversible causes.

### *Mixed and Other Types of Incontinence*

Mixed incontinence—most commonly urge and stress incontinence—is the most prevalent incontinence syndrome in elderly women. In postprostatectomy male patients, some urodynamic studies have shown mixed incontinence to be the most common, but clinically, stress incontinence is much more prevalent in this population. Unconscious or reflex incontinence, occurring without sensory awareness, is less common in older individuals. Usually, when geriatric patients state that they leak all the time, they have severe stress incontinence and have "tuned out" the multitude of small accidents. Similarly, nighttime urge incontinence is sometimes mistaken for nocturnal enuresis, but a careful history reveals that patients do not wake up wet, but have a precipitous urge and are incontinent before they can get out of bed.

## EVALUATION OF THE GERIATRIC PATIENT WITH INCONTINENCE

Evaluations of incontinence in men and women are well-described elsewhere in the text. In this chapter, the focus is on features that are unique for elderly individuals. One of the most difficult steps in the evaluation usually occurs before the patient presents to the urologist. Only one in three community-dwelling incontinent elderly persons has ever told their physician about their incontinence. Elderly persons may believe it to be a normal aging change. Also, they may be afraid that if their incontinence is discovered, they will be placed in a nursing home. The geriatric patient needs to be assured that incontinence, although common, is not a normal part of aging, and that it is very responsive to treatment. Many older patients can be cured of incontinence, and the remainder can improve enough to restore their lifestyle.

### *Geriatric Incontinence History*

**The History**

In geriatric patients, the history is often the most important component of the incontinence evaluation. An optimal history includes determining the symptoms that are bothering the patient the most. For example, a 78-yr-old woman who gives a history of mixed stress and urge incontinence, demonstrates stress leakage on examination, has no detrusor instability on urodynamic studies, and then undergoes endoscopic bladder suspension can be disappointed when she is not cured of the urge accidents that were the actual reason she sought urologic evaluation.

The majority of elderly patients can provide an extremely helpful history, if given sufficient time. However, the patient with dementia presents a special challenge. In the early stages, these patients are extremely skilled at covering up the degree of their impairment with social skills. Their history is vague, or the details vary from visit to visit as they confabulate to hide their memory impairment. Also, these patients often respond poorly to behavioral therapy or confuse their medication regimens. If surgical therapy is chosen, they are at extremely high risk of perioperative delirium. The best way to diagnose dementia is with a brief screening instrument, such as the Mini-Mental State Examination. Any elderly patient who presents with a confusing or vague history, or has an unusual therapeutic response, should have a brief mental status examination.

New geriatric patients often are accompanied by an apparent caregiver. When the interview begins, that person should be invited to step out to the waiting room. Even if the person accompanying the patient is the spouse, the patient may not want them present for the history. If the caregiver remains with the patient's permission, he or she should be asked to step out when it comes time for the physical examination. The patient can then be asked questions about issues such as sexuality that were not appropriate to ask with the caregiver present. For the demented patient, the caregiver is crucial to supplement the history, particularly to provide information useful to evaluate treatment response. However, the elderly patient's autonomy and dignity must be preserved. A supplemental history should be obtained only with the patient's permission.

**Hearing Impairment**

Elderly patients—particularly men—have a high rate of hearing impairment. However, it is inappropriate to speak loudly to all older persons, because the majority are not hearing impaired. If the patient is having a difficult time hearing, one can face them so they can use lip-reading cues, speak in a normal pitch, and slow the pace slightly. An important investment for any urology office is a hearing amplification device consisting of a headset and a clip-on amplifier. These cost <$35.00, are available at many stereo/electronic supply stores, and can facilitate an adequate history or an informed consent from a hearing-impaired individual.

## *Transient Causes of Incontinence—Presentation and Treatment*

A very important goal of the geriatric incontinence history is to uncover transient causes of incontinence (*see* Table 1).

**Medications**

Geriatric patients take an average of 3–5 prescription medications and even more over-the-counter medications. Table 1 provides a list of commonly prescribed drugs and the types of incontinence they may precipitate. For example, in reviewing the medication list of a patient with stress incontinence, one may discover an alpha-blocker, such as doxazosin or terazosin prescribed for hypertension, that may have precipitated the incontinence. After discontinuing or changing a drug, it is important to schedule the patient for a timely follow-up visit, because patients who are not cured may require additional treatment. If the visit is not scheduled, the elderly patient may assume that there is nothing more to be done for their incontinence.

Another example of drug-induced incontinence is the case of an elderly man with overflow incontinence. This patient may have his overflow incontinence relieved without surgery by discontinuing as many anticholinergic prescription medications as possible, changing from a low potency to a high-potency antipsychotic medication, and/or discontinuing self-prescribed anticholinergic medications for allergy and sleep. If the allergy medications also contain decongestants, the alpha-agonist properties may be increasing tone in the bladder neck and proximal urethra, contributing to the outlet obstruction. In addition to medication changes, 2–4 wk of indwelling catheter drainage may be necessary to allow the overdistended bladder to recover its contractile ability.

Nocturnal enuresis or troubling nocturia in an elderly patient with congestive heart failure can be caused by a bedtime diuretic dose that could be given just as effectively in the late afternoon, allowing the major diuresis to occur before bedtime. Other pharmacologic causes of nocturnal enuresis include excessive evening alcohol intake and oversedation for insomnia. The older person has a decreased lean body mass, resulting in a smaller volume of distribution for alcohol, causing intoxication with lesser amounts of alcohol than the patient may have tolerated quite well in his younger days. Nonpharmacologic measures for insomnia, such as a warm bath, a glass of warm milk, or relaxation techniques, are safer, often as effective as sleeping pills, and much less likely to precipitate nocturnal enuresis. Dietary changes—especially discon-

## Table 1
### Transient Causes of Incontinence[a]

| Cause | Type of Incontinence | Mechanism |
|---|---|---|
| **D**rugs | | |
| Alcohol | Functional | Altered sensory awareness |
| | Urge, nocturnal enuresis | Diuretic effect |
| Alpha-blockers | Stress in women | Decreased urethral-closure pressure |
| Anticholinergic agents | Overflow | Decreased detrusor contractility |
| | Functional | Confusion |
| Antipsychotics | Functional | Both potencies can decrease sensory awareness |
| High potency | Functional | Decreased mobility |
| Low potency | Overflow | Anticholinergic |
| Artificial sweeteners | Urge | Increased sensory urgency |
| Caffeine | Urge | Diuretic, increased sensory urgency |
| Diuretics | Urge, nocturnal enuresis | Increased urine production |
| Narcotics | Functional | Decreased sensory awareness, |
| | Overflow | Decreased detrusor contractility |
| | Urge | Fecal impaction |
| Sedatives | Functional | Altered sensory awareness |
| **I**nfection | Urge | Increased sensory urgency |
| **A**trophic urethritis | Stress | Urethral mucosa thinning |
| | Urge | Decreased alpha-adrenergic sensitivity, increased sensory urgency |
| **P**sychological | | |
| Depression | Functional | Decreased motivation to toilet and neglect of personal hygiene |
| Delirium | Functional | Altered sensory awareness |
| **E**ndocrine | | |
| Diabetes | Urge | Hyperglycemia induced osmotic diuresis—polyuria |
| Hypercalcemia | Urge | Polyuria |
| **R**estricted mobility | Functional | Impaired ability to toilet |
| **S**tool impaction | Urge | Stimulation of detrusor instability |
| | Overflow | Opioid receptor stimulation |

[a]Adapted from Resnick.

tinuing artificial sweeteners and tapering off caffeine—may benefit patients with urge incontinence.

## Infection

Asymptomatic bacteriuria is common in the elderly, is not associated with increased morbidity or mortality, and does not require treatment. However, elderly patients who present with incontinence and are found to have bacteriuria should be treated and the effect on the incontinence determined.

## Atrophic Urethritis

Atrophic urethritis is commonly associated with incontinence in postmenopausal women. The thinning of the urethral mucosa induces stress leakage, and the sensory urgency that accompanies estrogen deficiency in some women precipitates urge incontinence.

**Psychological Factors**

Depression and delirium are psychological factors commonly associated with incontinence. Depression rarely causes incontinence; however, the inattention to personal hygiene that often accompanies depression may bring previously undiagnosed incontinence to medical attention. It is essential to treat depression, because it can interfere with the effectiveness of any treatment.

Delirium is altered sensorium, characterized by acute onset, wandering attention, restlessness, confusion, disorientation, and frequently, incontinence. In the geriatric patient, it is usually associated with an underlying medical condition. The most common presentation in a urology practice would be the patient who is brought in for incontinence, but who has had an abrupt functional decline. The accompanying family member reports that the patient was managing the checkbook last week, and is now confused and incontinent. If the underlying occult infection, metabolic disturbance, or other underlying causes of delirium are not diagnosed and treated, the mortality rate can approach 50%. The hallmark of delirium is the history of a sudden onset of functional decline.

**Endocrine Causes**

Diabetes becomes more prevalent with age. Urge incontinence, frequency, and nocturia are exacerbated by the osmotic diuresis that accompanies poorly controlled diabetes. Explaining the interrelationship of the urologic problem and diabetic control can motivate the elderly patient to adhere to a diabetic diet, self-glucose monitoring, and other therapeutic modalities. Primary hyperparathyroidism is not rare in older patients, and should be considered in the differential diagnosis for any patient who has polyuria.

**Mobility Impairment**

Impaired mobility can be an important factor in urge incontinence. Geriatric patients have multiple causes of decreased mobility, and the most common are osteoarthritis, deconditioning, sequelae of stroke, and fear of falling. Referral for outpatient or home physical therapy can increase mobility and help reduce urge accidents. A bedside commode can also be useful if the bathroom is far from the bedroom.

**Constipation**

Constipation is extremely common in older patients, and fecal impaction is reported to precipitate incontinence. It may be that the bulk of the impaction provokes detrusor instability, or that stimulation of opioid receptors results in urinary retention and overflow incontinence. Disimpaction followed by establishment of a bowel program with bulk-forming agents, stool softeners, adequate fluid intake, increased mobility, and laxatives if necessary, is essential to prevent recurrence.

## *Bladder Diary*

A bladder diary (*see* Fig. 1), in which the patient or caregiver records the time of each void, the number and severity of accidents, and precipitating factors for each episode of leakage, is extremely important for diagnosis and treatment of incontinence. The bladder diary helps define the type of incontinence, makes the patient or caregiver

| Time urinated | Small Accident[a] | Large Accident[b] | Reason for accident |
|---|---|---|---|
| | | | |
| | | | |
| | | | |
| | | | |
| | | | |
| | | | |
| | | | |

[a] wet or dampen underclothes
[b] wet or dampen outer clothes

Number of pads used today: _____

Notes: _____

Fig. 1. Bladder diary. Used with permission from Burgio, 1989.

more aware of the circumstance of leakage, and serves as a baseline from which improvement can be measured. It is also an integral part of behavioral therapy.

## *Geriatric Physical Examination*

A high-low examination table is extremely helpful in a practice with a large number of elderly patients, because it permits transfers from a wheelchair and allows safe access with a walker or cane. In the geriatric physical examination, special attention should be given to mobility status. Any patient who has difficulty ambulating around the office or getting onto an examining table should be considered for a referral for a physical therapy assessment.

The urologic physical should include a pelvic examination in the older woman. Atrophic vaginitis, with thin, dry, pale, friable vaginal tissue, is diagnostic of atrophic vaginitis—a common condition in elderly women. Treatment of atrophic vaginitis optimizes the outcome of most treatments for incontinence. However, not all abnormal pelvic findings in the elderly woman require treatment. Pelvic-organ prolapse is a very common finding, but its presence does not necessarily relate to the urinary symptoms. Without treatment of the prolapse, elderly women with normal post void residual volumes respond quite well to behavioral treatment. Another common finding is perineal skin irritation from contact with urine or stool. Suggestions for a gentle perineal skin cleanser, treatment of candidiasis if present, and a moisture barrier ointment can greatly increase patient comfort. The rectal exam should include checking anal wink, resting sphincter tone, and ability to voluntarily contract the sphincter, as well as checking for fecal impaction.

## *Postvoid Residual Volume Determination*

Postvoid residual volume (PVR) tends to be higher in geriatric patients, but values consistently 200 or greater are indicative of inadequate bladder emptying. Caution is advised when interpreting the 50–199 mL postvoid residual volumes. Geriatric patients frequently visit the bathroom immediately after reaching the clinic; thus, they may not have had an urge to void before the PVR is measured. A repeated PVR on a subsequent visit after a "normal" void may be more accurate. Portable ultrasonic bladder scanners are quite accurate, less invasive than catheterization, and should be considered in any urology practice that evaluates a sufficient number of patients with incontinence.

### Laboratory Testing

Laboratory tests for evaluation of urinary incontinence in the older person include a urinalysis and a blood-urea nitrogen and creatinine. If polyuria is present, a serum glucose and calcium should be ordered. For diabetics, a glycosylated hemoglobin, which indicates the state of glucose control over the past 90 d, is a much better indicator of diabetic control than a random blood sugar.

### Urodynamic Testing

Elderly patients with stress and/or urge incontinence, normal PVR, and no complicating factors (eg, hematuria) do not require further urodynamic testing before undergoing initial treatment. Urodynamic findings often do not correlate well with the type of incontinence that is causing the most trouble for geriatric patients, and may even be misleading. For example, detrusor instability is extremely common in healthy older adults with no urologic symptoms at all. An elderly patient with a clear history of stress incontinence alone may demonstrate detrusor instability on cystometrogram, yet usually only requires treatment for stress incontinence. Patients with an uncertain diagnosis after initial evaluation (history, physical, urinalysis, and PVR) who demonstrate a consistently elevated PVR, or who fail to respond as expected to conservative therapies, may need urodynamic, endoscopic, or imaging studies before further therapy can be prescribed.

## TREATMENT OF PERSISTENT INCONTINENCE IN THE GERIATRIC PATIENT

Before treating persistent incontinence, all transient causes should be diagnosed and optimally treated (Table 1). If incontinence remains after treatment of transient causes, then therapy for persistent incontinence can be undertaken. As a general rule, the least invasive treatment should be tried first.

### Hormone Replacement Therapy

If a postmenopausal woman has genital atrophy, hormone replacement therapy should be initiated along with other treatments. Estrogen is helpful in the treatment of both urge and stress incontinence, because it can reduce sensory urgency and increases mucosal thickness, improving urethral coaptation. Estrogen has also been shown to have a protective effect against coronary artery disease, stroke, osteoporosis, and possibly Alzheimer's dementia. Most studies show a small increased risk of breast cancer, which is greatly outweighed by the benefit of cardiovascular risk reduction in large samples of women. Starting at half the replacement dose (0.3 mg conjugated estrogens or 0.5 mg estradiol daily) for the first 2–3 mo may improve long-term compliance by decreasing side effects, particularly breast tenderness. If the uterus is still present, combination estrogen and progestin therapy is recommended to protect against endometrial hyperplasia and ultimately, uterine cancer. Using 2.5 mg of progesterone daily, as opposed to cycled regimens, will decrease the chance of bleeding and increase compliance.

Some women already on full-dose hormone replacement therapy still show atrophy on examination or Pap smear, and can benefit from vaginal estrogen (0.5–1 g) 2–3 times/wk. Also, elderly women who decline oral hormone replacement therapy may consider vaginal estrogen, which is quite successful in reversing genital atrophy over a period of 4–6 wk. The dose is 0.5–1 g applied vaginally 2–3 times/wk at bedtime. Women who are reluctant to use a vaginal applicator can spread the labia and apply the cream externally at the vaginal introitus with equivalent results. Alternatively, the estradiol vaginal ring (Estring™), which can be placed in the vagina, releases 7.5 µg/24 h in a consistent, stable manner over 90 d. The serum estrogen levels are extremely low, and some practitioners have felt the ring is the safest alternative for patients with severe vaginal atrophy and a history of breast cancer or deep venous thrombosis.

## *Behavioral Treatments*

The effectiveness of a well-designed behavioral program is greatly underestimated by most physicians. These seemingly simple treatments, combined, can cure up to one-third of patients, and will improve the vast majority of patients with urge and or stress incontinence. Behavioral treatments are ideal for older patients because they are safe and have no side effects. The keys to success are clear directions to the patient, use of self-monitoring (bladder diary), and frequent brief follow-up visits to encourage treatment adherence. A nurse-practitioner trained in behavioral treatment of incontinence is a wonderful addition to a urology practice.

**Fluid Management**

It is rare to find an elderly patient who is drinking too much water. Usually, they have restricted fluid intake in an attempt to avoid incontinent episodes. Although timing of fluids can be helpful (eg, avoiding evening beverages to limit nocturia), general fluid restriction will simply produce more concentrated and odorous urine and increase the probability of urinary-tract infections. One fluid-management strategy that may be helpful is advising patients with urge incontinence to taper off caffeine and avoid artificially sweetened beverages. Both sugar substitutes and caffeine are bladder irritants, and tend to worsen urge incontinence.

**Voiding Schedules**

Older patients with urge incontinence often have reduced bladder capacity and/or detrusor instability accompanied by frequent urination. Bladder training has been quite successful for these patients, and has become more widely accepted as a first-line treatment. The intervention consists of placing the patient on a regular voiding schedule that they can tolerate. Gradually, over several weeks, the interval between voids is lengthened to an optimal 3–4-h schedule. To assist them in postponing urination and adhering to the schedule, patients are taught strategies such as distraction or pelvic-muscle contraction to cope with or decrease urgency.

In other patients, a different pattern occurs, reflecting infrequent voiding followed by large urge accidents on the way to the bathroom. Elderly patients who are sedentary, or hesitate to get up to go to the bathroom because of arthritic pain or dyspnea, and demented patients who fail to recognize and respond to urgency, may elicit a detrusor contraction from a full bladder when they get out of a chair. A regular voiding schedule can permit the bladder to empty before large, unmanageable volumes accumulate. Even patients with moderately advanced dementia should be placed on a prompted voiding schedule for 2–3 d, and many will respond. Two schedules have demonstrated success: every 2 h while awake, or first thing in the morning, before and after every meal, and at bedtime. A printed instruction sheet—explaining the rationale of a schedule of voiding before urgency occurs—and outlining the specific schedule will increase success.

**Pelvic Muscle Exercises**

Pelvic muscle exercises are helpful for both stress and urge incontinence, as well as for postvoid dribbling. A fundamental step in teaching the patient pelvic muscle exercises is helping the patient identify the proper muscles. Arnold Kegel, in 1948, used home biofeedback via vaginal manometry to successfully teach pelvic muscle exercises for stress incontinence. Burgio has shown that a single session of biofeedback followed by practice at home without biofeedback is successful in the majority of patients with urge and mixed urge and stress incontinence. Pelvic muscle exercises can also be taught during the physical examination by having the patient contract the perivaginal muscles or the external anal sphincter around the examining finger. During pelvic muscle exercises, the pubococcygeus and the levator ani contract in concert; therefore, anal palpation is effective in teaching pelvic muscle contraction.

When doing pelvic muscle exercises, elderly patients with weak pelvic muscles tend to recruit their abdominal muscles, contraction of which actually increases bladder pressure. They also may contract their buttocks, abduct their hips, and use a variety of other unproductive efforts. Instructing them do to a "medium" squeeze of the pelvic muscles helps prevent recruitment of undesirable muscles. Also, instructing them to place a hand on the abdomen or not to hold their breath during contractions helps prevent Valsalva maneuvering, which pushes urine out of the bladder.

Burgio and colleagues described a program of pelvic muscle exercises that is simple and effective. Each pelvic muscle exercise consists of contracting the pelvic muscles for 1–10 s, depending on the patient's ability, followed by an equal period of relaxation. As the patient gains strength, the duration of each squeeze is increased gradually up to 10 s. The home exercise regimen consists of 15 exercises, three times daily for a total of 45 exercises per day. Because pelvic muscle control needs to be used in a variety of positions, and a pelvic muscle contraction feels different in various positions, it is helpful for the patient to practice one session standing, one session lying, and one session sitting. Once established, the exercises are integrated into daily life by pairing them with routine activities to help increase treatment adherence. For example, a patient may do standing exercises before brushing his teeth each morning, sitting during a television commercial, and lying down immediately after retiring for the evening.

If not contraindicated, the patient is instructed to interrupt the urinary stream once each day by squeezing the pelvic muscles. If the patient cannot fully stop it, even slowing of the stream demonstrates that the patient is using the correct muscles. Interrupting the stream more often than once a day may lead to dysfunctional voiding with retained urine, and should be discouraged.

**Using the Pelvic Muscles—Strategies**

**Stress Incontinence Strategies.** The simple maneuver of squeezing the pelvic muscles just before and holding them tightly during any activity likely to precipitate stress leakage can reduce or cure stress incontinence. This is true of men with postprostatectomy stress leakage as well. A bladder diary can help patients to recognize activities, such as coughing, lifting a grandchild, or blowing one's nose, that precipitate stress leakage. Initially the strategy requires conscious effort, but with repetition, stress strategies usually become automatic.

**Postvoid Dribbling Strategies.** Many patients complain of urine leakage immediately after voiding. Squeezing the pelvic muscles once voiding is complete may express pooled urine from the urethra and increase urethral resistance to continued seepage of urine from the postvoid residual volume in the bladder.

**Urge Strategies.** The usual response to urgency is to rush to the bathroom—a counterproductive behavior that can precipitate detrusor contractions and interfere with the concentration needed to suppress the urge. Patients can learn to manage urgency and urge incontinence by changing their response to the sensation to void. Instead of rushing, they can use their pelvic muscles to occlude the urethra and abort premature detrusor contractions. Most patients can learn the skill through simple verbal instruction and home practice. Patients are told to squeeze their pelvic muscles tightly 3–4 times when they first feel an urge to void, sit or stand until the urge passes, and then proceed to the bathroom at a normal pace. If the urge returns on the way to the bathroom, the urge strategy is repeated until the urge is again suppressed. Urge strategies can be done in an anticipatory manner when the bladder is full before standing up from a chair or getting out of bed. With practice, this too can become automatic. Urinary frequency often improves dramatically as the patient gains skill in using urge strategies.

### *Pharmacotherapy of Incontinence in the Geriatric Patient*

Medications may be added if behavioral therapy alone is insufficient to control incontinence or if the patient declines behavioral therapy. For postmenopausal women, hormone replacement therapy is extremely helpful for both urge and stress incontinence.

**Pharmacotherapy of Stress Incontinence**

Stress incontinence is ideally treated with behavioral therapy, collagen injections, a pessary, or bladder suspension surgery rather than with medication. Some women do benefit from alpha-adrenergic agonists (*see* Table 2). Pseudoephedrine is recommended over phenylpropanolamine for older patients because of a higher incidence of blood-pressure elevation with the latter. Hypertension affects one-half of elderly patients, so caution is warranted with both of these medications. A drug-free interval at night is optimal to prevent insomnia, a common side effect of alpha-agonists. This can be accomplished using 12-h sustained release (60 mg) pseudoephedrine instead of the 24-h sustained-release preparation (120 mg). Imipramine is helpful for some patients, but usually causes too much drowsiness to be used for daytime stress incontinence in

Table 2
Pharmacotherapy of Incontinence in Geriatric Patients

| Indication | Drug | Dose |
|---|---|---|
| Stress incontinence | Pseudoephedrine (Sudafed) | 15–30 mg tid |
|  | Pseudoephedrine—sustained release | 60 mg QAM |
| Urge incontinence | Oxybutynin (Ditropan), | 2.5 mg daily–5.0 mg tid |
|  | oxybutynin—sustained release |  |
|  | (Ditropan XL) | 5–20 mg once daily |
|  | Tolterodine (Detrol) | 1–2 mg bid |
|  | Hyoscyamine (Levsin) 0.125 | 1–2 tablets Q 4 h prn |
|  | Hyoscyamine 0.374 | 1 tablet bid |
| Nocturnal enuresis, bothersome nocturia, or nighttime urge incontinence | Imipramine (Tofranil) | 10–50 mg Q h.s. |

geriatric patients. Imipramine can also cause postural hypotension and cardiac conduction disturbances, and should be avoided in the frail elderly.

**Pharmacotherapy of Urge Incontinence**

Urge incontinence responds well to pharmacotherapy. Because of frequent side effects—including dry mouth, constipation, blurred vision, urinary hesitancy, and incomplete bladder emptying—behavioral therapy should be tried first in geriatric patients. In severe incontinence, pharmacotherapy may be started along with the behavioral therapy, with the option of tapering the drug when the patient improves strength and control of the pelvic muscles. Specific drugs and dosage regimens are presented in Table 2. Side effects can be lessened by starting with very low dosages and prescribing the medication specifically when needed. For example, if the patient manages well at home and really needs medication just before going to church or going out to dine, single doses of oxybutynin or hyoscyamine are useful. If nocturia and nighttime accidents are the major problem, a single bedtime dose of oxybutynin may be quite effective. Imipramine is also very useful for nighttime problems, but in the frail elderly, postural hypotension may precipitate a fall during the night. Because Medicare and the supplemental health insurance held by most older patients do not cover medications, budget is often a factor in prescribing medications. Propantheline is inexpensive, but causes too many side effects in elderly patients. Generic oxybutynin may be the optimal choice in these cases.

### *Surgery and Collagen Injection for the Geriatric Patient*

For properly selected patients, periurethral collagen injections can be quite helpful and are well tolerated. Surgery should be considered for elderly women with stress incontinence who have not had adequate improvement from nonsurgical management, or in women with symptomatic pelvic prolapse. Surgery may also be indicated in elderly men in whom incontinence is associated with outflow obstruction. Age itself should not be a contraindication to surgery. The general health status of the patient rather than age should be considered when weighing the potential risks and benefits of surgery. A consultation with a geriatrician or internist can help minimize surgical risk.

## SELECTED READING

Burgio KL, Locher JL, Goode PS, Hardin JM, McDowell BJ, Candib D (1998) Behavioral vs. drug treatment for urge urinary incontinence in older women: a randomized clinical trial. *JAMA* 280:1995–2000.

Burgio KL, Pearce KL, Lucco AJ (1989) *Staying Dry: A Practical Guide to Bladder Control.* Baltimore: The Johns Hopkins University Press.

Fantl JA, Newman DK, Colling J, et al. (1996) *Urinary incontinence in adults: acute and chronic management. Clinical Practice Guideline,* No. 2, 1996 update. Rockville, MD: AHCPR Publication No. 96-0682, US Department of Health and Human Services, Public Health Service, Agency for Health Care Policy and Research.

Folstein MF, Folstein S, McHugh PR (1975) Mini-Mental State: a practical method for grading the cognitive state of patients for the clinician. *J Psychiatr Res* 12:189–198.

Resnick NM (1995) Urinary incontinence. *Lancet* 346:94–100.

# XI  OTHER PROBLEMS

# 34 Evaluation and Differential Diagnosis of Hematuria

*Dimitri Kuznetsov, MD
and Charles Brendler, MD*

**CONTENTS**
>   INTRODUCTION
>   OVERVIEW
>   HISTORY
>   PHYSICAL EXAMINATION
>   EVALUATION
>   CYTOLOGY
>   UNUSUAL UROLOGIC CAUSES OF HEMATURIA
>   NONUROLOGIC CAUSES OF HEMATURIA
>   COMMON RENAL CAUSES OF HEMATURIA
>   SUMMARY AND CONCLUSIONS
>   SELECTED READING

## INTRODUCTION

Hematuria is an extremely common condition, and almost always requires a complete urologic evaluation. The urologist must have a thorough knowledge of the urologic causes of hematuria as well as the nonurologic causes. In this chapter we provide an overview of hematuria and discuss important aspects of the history and physical examination. We then discuss the evaluation and differential diagnosis of hematuria, including unusual urologic causes and the more common nonurologic causes of hematuria.

## OVERVIEW

Significant hematuria is generally defined by gross hematuria, or by more than three red blood cells per high-powered field on microscopic examination. The urinary dipstick is a quick and inexpensive method to detect hematuria, with nearly 90% sensitivity. Proper collection and handling of a urinary specimen increases the accuracy of both the dipstick and microscopic analysis in detecting hematuria. Menstrual blood flow or preputial bleeding can render a urine sample falsely positive, whereas prolonged storage of a warm, dilute, alkaline urine will result in lysis of red blood cells, and, therefore will increase the likelihood of a false-negative result. It is important to emphasize that hematuria is often intermittent, and repeat urinalyses may be required to document its presence.

Other heme-containing pigments can produce a false-positive result, and therefore, microscopic analysis must always be performed to validate the dipstick result. The two pigments that can produce false-positive results are hemoglobin and myoglobin. Hemoglobinuria results from intravascular hemolysis, and myoglobinuria from massive muscle breakdown. Since a positive result on the dipstick results from oxidation of the chromogen reagent in the heme indicator portion of the dipstick, a specimen that lacks whole red blood cells containing only hemoglobin or myoglobin will yield a false-positive result. A centrifuged urinary specimen that contains intact red blood cells on microscopic examination establishes the diagnosis of hematuria.

It is also important to determine the urinary specific gravity before performing the microscopic examination. A highly concentrated urine sample can falsely elevate the number of red cells detected per high-powered field, resulting in an overestimation of the degree of hematuria. Conversely, a dilute urine sample will not only decrease the number of red blood cells detected, but will also predispose the red blood cells to hemolysis. Hemolysis results from passive transudation of hypotonic urine into the red blood cells, resulting in cell lysis and a falsely low number of red blood cells subsequently detected on microscopy.

Microscopy can confirm the diagnosis of hematuria, and can sometimes establish the anatomic origin of the bleeding. The presence of proteinuria or casts suggests a medical rather than a urologic cause for hematuria. Even with gross hematuria of urologic origin, it is unusual to find proteinuria >300 mg/d. This distinction may be complicated when a patient with chronic renal disease presents with new-onset hematuria. In this situation, the urologist must first exclude a urologic cause for the hematuria and then refer the patient for further medical evaluation. It is imperative not to overlook a common urologic problem, such as a tumor or stone, in patients who have comorbid conditions that may complicate a seemingly straightforward diagnosis.

## *Glomerular vs Nonglomerular Hematuria*

Hematuria secondary to an underlying urologic disorder usually produces little protein and no casts identified in the urine. The finding of proteinuria >300 mg/d or red blood-cell casts should raise suspicion of either a glomerular or nonglomerular renal cause of the hematuria. Glomerular hematuria implies bleeding that originates from the renal glomerulus. The finding of dysmorphic red blood cells, red blood-cell casts, and proteinuria is strongly suggestive of glomerular hematuria. Table 1 lists common disorders typically associated with glomerular hematuria and Fig. 1 demonstrates the general work-up for glomerular hematuria.

Nonglomerular hematuria can originate from the renal tubulointerstitium, have a renovascular cause, or be secondary to a systemic disorder. With nonglomerular hematuria, the urine usually contains normal-appearing, circular red blood cells, and no red blood-cell casts, although significant proteinuria is often present. The algorithm in Fig. 2 illustrates a guide to the evaluation of nonglomerular renal hematuria.

Table 1
Glomerular Disorders in Patients with Glomerular Hematuria[a]

| Disorder | Percentage of patients |
|---|---|
| IgA nephropathy (Berger's disease) | 30 |
| Mesangioproliferative GN | 14 |
| Focal segmental proliferative GN | 13 |
| Familial nephritis (e.g., Alport syndrome) | 11 |
| Membranous GN | 7 |
| Mesangiocapillary GN | 6 |
| Focal segmental sclerosis | 4 |
| Unclassifiable | 4 |
| Systemic lupus erythematosus | 3 |
| Postinfectious GN | 2 |
| Subacute bacterial endocarditis | 2 |
| Others | 4 |
| Total | 100 |

[a]Adapted from Fassett, RG, et al.: *Lancet*, 1:1432, 1982.

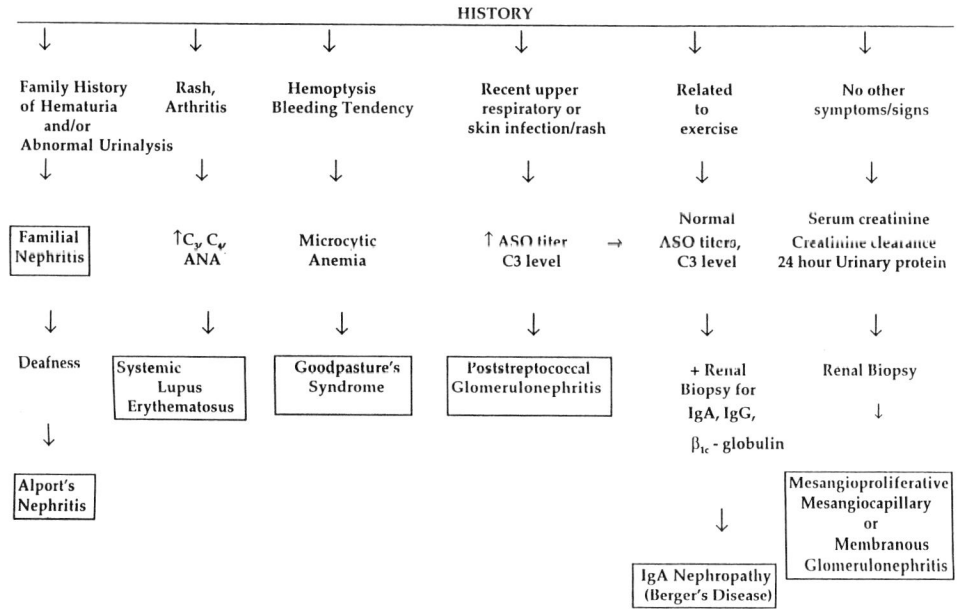

**Fig. 1.** Evaluation of glomerular hematuria (dysmorphic erythrocytes, erythrocyte casts, ± proteinuria).

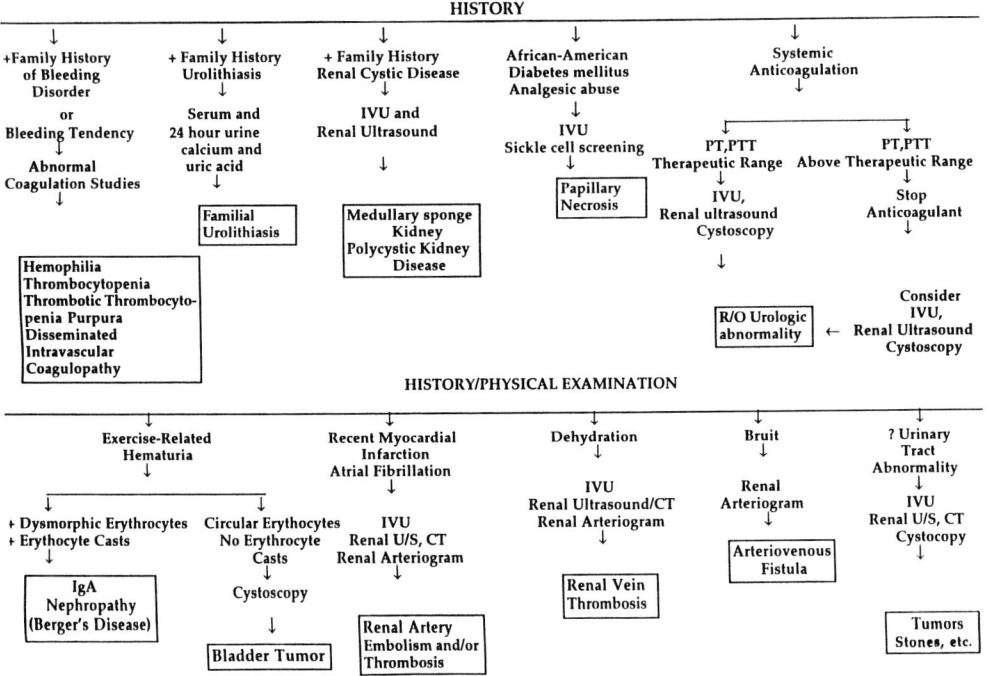

Fig. 2. Evaluation of nonglomerular renal hematuria (circular erythrocytes, no erythrocyte casts, ± proteinuria).

## *Pseudohematuria*

Pseudohematuria occurs when ingestion of pigment-forming substances results in red discoloration of the urine. Such medications as rifampin, pyridium, and various phenothiazines will result in red discoloration of the urine, mimicking hematuria. Other substances that may result in pseudohematuria are listed in Table 2. A finding of heme pigment on the dipstick in the presence of red blood cells on microscopic examination will establish the diagnosis of hematuria.

## HISTORY

### *Characteristics of Hematuria*

The specific characteristics of hematuria can help establish the etiology. The timing of hematuria is extremely important, and is usually classified as initial, total, or terminal. Hematuria that occurs at the start of urination commonly reflects urethral pathology, whereas terminal hematuria usually arises from the prostate or bladder neck. Total hematuria, which occurs most commonly, usually originates in the bladder or upper urinary tracts.

Hematuria is usually painless unless it is associated with infection or obstruction of the urinary tract. In regard to infection, it is important to remember that bladder tumors may become secondarily infected, and, therefore, result in both pyuria and hematuria. Thus, almost any adult who presents with gross hematuria, regardless of whether a urinary-tract infection is also present, should undergo a complete urologic evaluation.

Table 2
Common Causes of Abnormal Color

| | |
|---|---|
| Colorless | Very dilute urine |
| | Overhydration |
| Cloudy/Milky | Phosphaturia |
| | Pyuria |
| | Chyluria |
| Red | Hematuria |
| | Hemoglobinuria/myoglobinuria |
| | Anthrocyanin in beets and blackberries |
| | Chronic lead and mercury poisoning |
| | Phenolphthalein (in bowel evacuants) |
| | Phenothiazines (Compazine, and so forth) |
| | Rifampin |
| Orange | Dehydration |
| | Phenazopyridine (Pyridium) |
| | Sulfasalazine (Azulfadine) |
| Yellow | Normal |
| | Phenacetin |
| | Riboflavin |
| Green-Blue | Biliverdin |
| | Indicanuria (tryptophan indole metabolites) |
| | Amitriptyline (Elavil) |
| | Indigo carmine |
| | Methylene blue |
| | Phenois (IV cimetidine [Tagamet], IV promethazine [Phenergan], and others) |
| | Resorcinol |
| | Triampterene (Dyrenium) |
| Brown | Urobilinogen |
| | Porphyria |
| | Aloe, fava beans, and rhubarb |
| | Chloroquine and primaquine |
| | Furazolidone (Furoxone) |
| | Metronidazole (Flagyl) |
| | Nitrofurantoin (Furadantin) |
| Brown-Black | Alcaptonuria (homogentisic acid) |
| | Hemorrhage |
| | Melanin |
| | Tyrosinosis (hydroxyphenylpyruvic acid) |
| | Cascara, senna (laxatives) |
| | Methocarbamol (Robaxin) |
| | Methyldopa (Aldomet) |
| | Sorbitol |

The only exception to this rule is a young woman who presents with her first or second episode of hemorrhagic bacterial cystitis.

Finally, the presence or absence of clots and the shape of the clots will help establish the location of the hematuria. Clot formation usually correlates with heavier bleeding, and often reflects the amount of time that blood spends in the bladder. Therefore, it is

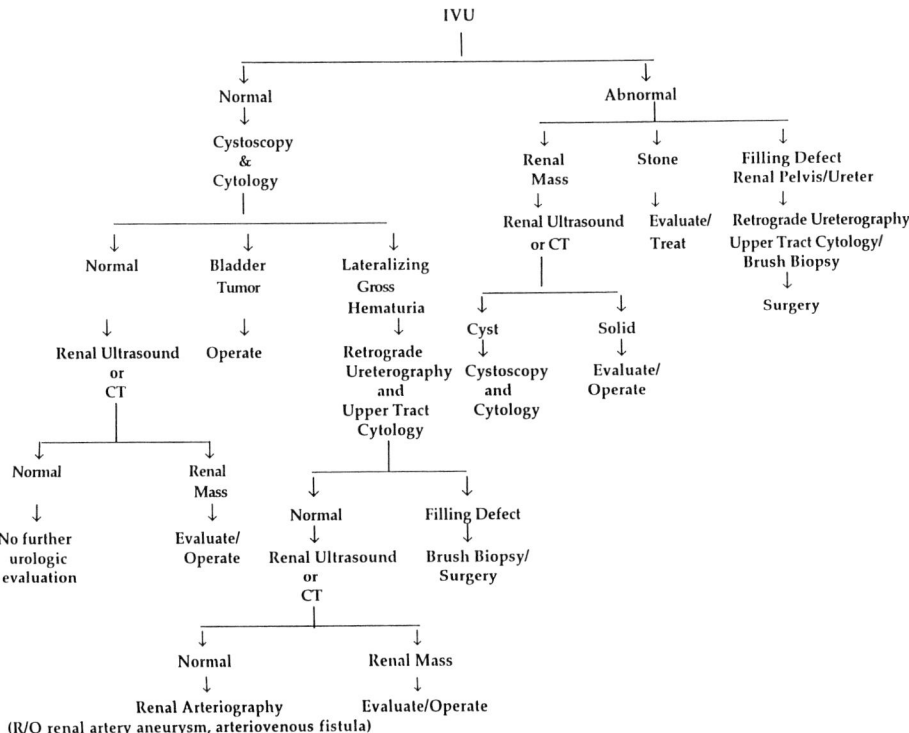

Fig. 3. Evaluation of essential hematuria (circular erythrocytes, no erythrocyte casts, no significant proteinuria).

unusual to see clot formation in a patient with urethral bleeding. Usually, clots are amorphous and of bladder origin, but, less commonly, clots may assume a vermiform or "worm-like" shape, indicating that the hematuria is of kidney or ureteral origin with clots having formed in the ureter.

The historical evaluation of hematuria of urologic origin is generally straightforward, and follows the algorithm shown in Fig. 3. The history is of greater significance in the evaluation of hematuria of nonurologic origin. A history of a bleeding disorder, anticoagulant therapy, sickle-cell or HIV disease, or strenuous exercise are all important issues that need to be ascertained. These conditions are discussed more fully later in the chapter under nonurologic causes of hematuria.

## PHYSICAL EXAMINATION

Except in cases of trauma, the physical examination is not particularly helpful in the evaluation of hematuria. However, physical examination is useful in the diagnosis of dermatologic causes of hematuria, such as inflammation of the prepuce or glans penis, and occasionally with squamous-cell cancer of the penis.

Trauma involving lower rib fractures, or a flank contusion associated with hematuria, signifies a possible renal injury. In patients with pelvic fractures, the finding of blood at the urethral meatus is pathognomonic of a urethral injury. A partial or complete disruption of the membranous urethra can present with this sign, and any associated perineal or genital swelling can signify either blood or urinary extravasation into the surrounding tissues. Classically, this is characterized by a perineal hematoma that is contained within Colles' fascia, which resembles a butterfly. Another sentinel finding noted with disruption of the membranous urethra is seen when the prostate cannot be palpated or is replaced by a pelvic hematoma during rectal examination.

## EVALUATION

The evaluation of hematuria requires a complete assessment of both the upper and lower urinary tracts. This point cannot be overemphasized, since the multifocal nature and diversity of genitourinary pathology can result in delayed or inappropriate treatment if the entire urothelium is not completely evaluated. The main modalities used for upper urinary-tract evaluation are intravenous urography, ultrasonography, and computerized tomography. Cystoscopy remains the gold standard in evaluating the bladder and urethra.

### *Intravenous Urography (IVU)*

IVU historically has been the procedure of choice in the evaluation of the upper urinary tracts, because it allows for assessment of both upper urinary-tract anatomy and function, and because urologists are very comfortable interpreting an IVU. It is now clear, however, that both ultrasonography and computerized tomography (CT) are superior to the IVU in the evaluation of the renal parenchyma. Furthermore, the potential complications of the IVU, including contrast-induced renal toxicity, allergic reactions to contrast, and the potential cardiovascular effects of a high osmotic load, have led to increased enthusiasm for both ultrasonography and noninfused CT. Nevertheless, the IVU continues to be the initial test of choice in evaluating the renal pelvis and ureter.

Traditionally, the IVU has been considered the basic test in the evaluation of urologic trauma. CT provides much more accurate information regarding the extent of renal trauma, and has to a great extent replaced IVU. Nevertheless, the IVU remains helpful in determining renal function and the presence of a contralateral kidney. It is particularly useful when the patient has already been taken to the operating room, at which time a single-shot IVP can provide critical information.

In summary, the IVU remains a useful screening test in the initial evaluation of hematuria, but the benefits of this procedure must be weighed against the potential complications, particularly when alternative tests that provide more comprehensive information are available.

### *Ultrasonography*

Ultrasonography is noninvasive, relatively inexpensive, and avoids the risks of intravenous contrast and radiation exposure. Spencer and colleagues concluded that ultrasonography in combination with a plain radiograph is the preferred initial modality in the evaluation of hematuria. Ultrasonography was noted to be superior to the IVU in detecting and defining small renal parenchymal lesions, and was reasonably accurate in evaluating renal obstruction and renal pelvic pathology. Nonetheless, IVU is still regarded as a better test for the evaluation of the renal pelvis and ureter, because ultrasonography may miss a renal pelvic lesion, ureteral calculus, or tumor. For this reason, if one suspects a soft-tissue urothelial lesion in the renal pelvis or ureter, either an IVU or retrograde pyelogram should be obtained.

## Computerized Tomography (CT)

CT is extremely helpful in the evaluation of hematuria because of its accuracy in identifying renal and retroperitoneal pathology that may be associated with hematuria. Furthermore, a noninfused spiral CT is now regarded by many as the test of choice in the evaluation of the patient with a suspected ureteral calculus. Several studies have demonstrated that a noninfused spiral CT is rapid, cost-effective, and highly accurate in the evaluation of stone disease.

In patients with asymptomatic hematuria, an infused CT scan can be obtained if the etiology of hematuria has not been established with an IVU and cystoscopy, and if further evaluation of the renal parenchyma and retroperitoneum is required. In an attempt to devise a cost-effective approach in the evaluation of hematuria, Perlman combined a limited CT evaluation within 2 h after obtaining an IVU. This combination, known as CT-urography, was concluded to be cost-effective and time-saving, and minimized the amount of intravenous contrast needed to provide a thorough evaluation of both the urothelium and the renal parenchyma.

## Retrograde Pyelography (RP)

RP is extremely valuable in the evaluation of the renal pelvis and ureter when the IVU is inconclusive. RP can be performed at the time of cystoscopy when the IVU is contraindicated or does not adequately define the upper urinary tracts. Subsequently, filling defects can be approached ureteroscopically or managed in an antegrade fashion through a nephroscope. Both antegrade and retrograde methods allow for visualization, biopsy, and minimally invasive treatment of urologic pathology.

# CYTOLOGY

Urinary cytology is an important adjunct in the evaluation of hematuria. Cytologic specimens can be obtained from voided urine, but a greater number of cells can be obtained by saline barbotage of the bladder. The specimen should be examined within 2 h or refrigerated, because urinary stasis can result in cell degeneration that diminishes the accuracy of the cytologic specimen.

The finding of either severe atypia or malignant cells in the cytologic specimen often signifies transitional-cell carcinoma. Severe atypia or malignant cells without grossly visible lesions on cystoscopy should prompt random biopsies of the bladder and prostate, which may detect carcinoma *in situ*. If the bladder and prostate are excluded as the sites of pathology, retrograde pyelography with ureteral cytologic washings should be obtained to assess the upper urinary tracts, particularly if intravenous pyelography is inconclusive in the evaluation of the renal pelvis and ureter.

The sensitivity of urinary cytology is 70%, and the specificity 90–95% in detecting carcinoma *in situ*. These poorly differentiated high-grade lesions are much more likely to be detected with cytology than well- or moderately differentiated tumors, since they are more prone to slough into the urine than less abnormal cells. High-grade lesions are more likely to have abnormal intercellular adhesion molecules, which makes these cells more loosely attached to the surrounding tissues. Occasionally, false-positives will occur as a result of other processes, including inflammation, infection, previous radiation, or intravesical chemotherapy. In summary, cytology is easily performed as part of the evaluation of hematuria and is particularly useful in diagnosing transitional-cell carcinoma *in situ* of the urinary bladder and upper urinary tracts in cases in which the radiologic and endoscopic findings may be normal.

## UNUSUAL UROLOGIC CAUSES OF HEMATURIA

Although the etiology of urologic hematuria is usually readily identifiable, certain rare urologic conditions may need to be included in the differential diagnosis. These include: chronic unilateral hematuria, autosomal dominant polycystic kidney disease, and hematuria secondary to recurrent urothelial carcinoma following cystectomy or nephrectomy.

### *Chronic Unilateral Hematuria*

Chronic unilateral hematuria—also known as either benign essential hematuria or lateralizing hematuria—results from a vascular malformation of the renal urothelium. The hematuria is typically painless and intermittent but recurrent, and eventually may result in low-grade anemia or renal colic from clot formation with ureteral obstruction. This condition is rarely life-threatening, but occasionally, the hematuria may be severe enough to necessitate surgery. The diagnosis is difficult to establish radiographically, but can readily be made ureteroscopically. Patients are usually young people who have previously undergone an extensive nondiagnostic evaluation. The sentinel clue to the diagnosis is the finding of unilateral hematuria on cystoscopy during an episode of active bleeding. Subsequent ureteroscopy will demonstrate angiomatous, slightly elevated, and well-demarcated erythematous lesions located on the renal papilla. Endoscopic fulguration of these lesions will usually cure the patient of this troubling condition.

### *Autosomal Dominant Polycystic Kidney Disease (ADPKD)*

Except in patients with autosomal dominant polycystic kidney disease (ADPKD), benign renal-cyst rupture is rarely a cause of hematuria. In ADPKD, however, gross hematuria resulting from cyst rupture occurs in over one-third of cases. Furthermore, gross hematuria resulting from cyst rupture is often the first clinical symptom of this disease. The hematuria is frequently associated with a concomitant episode of pyelonephritis that predisposes to renal cystic-pressure elevation with subsequent rupture and communication with the pyelocalyceal system.

### *Recurrent Urothelial Carcinoma Following Cystectomy or Nephrectomy*

Recurrent urothelial carcinoma following cystectomy frequently results in hematuria. The incidence of urethral carcinoma following cystectomy is about 5%, and ureteral carcinoma, about 3%. Urethral washing cytology is the best means to evaluate the urethra following cystectomy, and should be done annually. Patients with glandular or stromal involvement of the prostate are at particularly high risk for urethral recurrence, and, if the urethra has not been removed primarily, these patients should be followed particularly closely. The cardinal sign of recurrent transitional-cell carcinoma of the urethra is a bloody urethral discharge, which should immediately prompt further evaluation.

Patients with positive distal ureteral margins at the time of cystectomy are at an increased risk for subsequent recurrent disease in the ureters. Every effort should be made to obtain negative distal ureteral margins on frozen section at the time of cystectomy, and patients should be followed with an intravenous pyelogram at regular intervals.

Although rare, transitional-cell carcinoma involving the ureteral stump following nephrectomy can result in hematuria. The diagnosis may not be readily apparent, because routine upper-tract imaging will fail to demonstrate the ureter in the absence of the kidney. Indeed, Dr. Alfred Blalock, the renowned cardiac surgeon from Johns Hopkins, died of transitional-cell carcinoma of the ureter, which developed many years after he underwent a simple nephrectomy for tuberculosis. In cases of unexplained hematuria following a nephrectomy, a retrograde ureterogram of the remaining ureteral stump should be obtained.

## NONUROLOGIC CAUSES OF HEMATURIA

### Bleeding Disorders

Hemophilia and von Willebrand's disease are the two most common disorders of hemostasis that result in hematuria. Usually these disorders have been identified previously. If not, a careful history can reveal distinctive symptoms, such as frequent epistaxis and easy bruisability, and a physical examination may reveal important findings, such as petechiae.

With these disorders, severe bleeding may result and present with either renal colic from ureteral obstruction, or anemia from more severe blood loss. Usually, the hematuria results from the primary hematologic disorder, but a full urologic evaluation is indicated to rule out unrelated urologic pathology.

Disorders of platelet function are detected by an elevated bleeding time. In von Willebrand's disease, the interaction of von Willebrand's factor with platelets is effected, resulting in a prolonged bleeding time.

### Anticoagulation Therapy

Patients who are receiving anticoagulant medications and whose clotting parameters are in the normal therapeutic range must undergo a complete urologic evaluation for hematuria. Such patients are frequently found to have underlying urologic pathology, with the most common etiologies being cancer, calculi, infection, renal infarction, and benign prostatic hyperplasia. It is estimated that as many as 70% of the pathology identified in such patients is clinically significant and requires treatment.

### Sickle-Cell Disease

African-Americans or individuals who have a family history of sickle-cell disease, sickle-cell trait, or hemoglobin SC disease frequently present with gross hematuria as a result of these inherited disorders. In these patients, hematuria is thought to arise from the capillary bed of the renal medulla and the relatively hypoxic, hypertonic, and acidic environment of the capillary bed is thought to predispose the red blood cells to sickle, resulting in hematuria. Furthermore, individuals with sickle-cell disease are predisposed to papillary necrosis and cortical infarction, which often results in gross hematuria. With an appropriate level of suspicion, the various hemoglobin abnormalities can easily be identified using hemoglobin electrophoresis to detect sickle-cell disease or its variants as the cause of hematuria.

### Human Immunodeficiency Virus (HIV)

Hematuria occurs in about 20–25% of patients infected with HIV. Possible etiologies include viral renal infection, glomerulonephritis, urinary-tract infections, sexually transmitted urethritis, subclinical Kaposi's sarcoma, and thrombocytopenia. A recent study concluded that in young, asymptomatic, HIV-infected patients, a urologic evaluation can safely be omitted in the presence of normal renal function and absence of significant urologic history. On the other hand, no data exist regarding the need for a urologic evaluation in older HIV-infected patients who are more susceptible to other urologic diseases. As the natural history of HIV disease is further established, its impact on the urologic system and guidelines regarding the need for evaluation and treatment will become better defined.

One newly discovered entity that may result in hematuria in HIV patients involves the use of indinivir sulfate, a protease inhibitor used to treat HIV infection. Renal stones develop in 8–15% of patients who receive indinivir. These calculi are frequently radiolucent and difficult to diagnose on plain radiographs, and also on computerized tomography.

### *Arteriovenous Fistula*

About 5–10% of individuals who undergo a needle biopsy of the kidney experience transient hematuria that is severe enough to warrant a blood transfusion in 1–3% of patients. About 15–18% of patients who undergo a renal biopsy or placement of a percutaneous nephrostomy subsequently develop an arteriovenous fistula or renal arterial aneurysm. Most of these arteriovenous fistulae are clinically silent, and resolve spontaneously within 2 yr. Less commonly, treatment is required when hematuria persists or if hypertension or congestive heart failure develops. Initially, minimally invasive treatment should be attempted using interventional radiology techniques, but with persistent bleeding, a partial or even total nephrectomy may be required.

### *Exercise and Hematuria*

It is well-recognized that strenuous exercise may result in hematuria, which may stem from two different causes. First, glomerular trauma may result in red blood-cell excretion following intense exercise. Second, repetitive trauma resulting from the dome of the bladder striking the trigone in long-distance runners can result in either microscopic of even gross hematuria. Both of these conditions are benign and transient, neither lasting longer then 48 h after completion of exercise. A complete urologic evaluation should be performed, but in general, patients can be reassured regarding the benign nature of these conditions.

## COMMON RENAL CAUSES OF HEMATURIA

IgA nephropathy (Berger's disease) and thin basement membrane disease, also known as benign hematuria, are two common renal diseases that may present with hematuria. These two conditions are the most common nonurologic causes of hematuria, and IgA nephropathy is the most common glomerulopathy worldwide.

### *IgA Nephropathy (Berger's Disease)*

The pathogenesis of Berger's disease is unknown, but is thought to result from immune dysregulation. The most common clinical presentation is that of painless hematuria, which develops 48–72 h after an acute upper-respiratory infection or gastrointestinal illness. A finding of proteinuria in the range of 2 g of protein/24 h is seen in

50% of patients. On renal biopsy, deposits of IgA, IgG, and C3 are found in the mesangial region of the renal glomeruli, which confirms the diagnosis. This syndrome usually resolves without treatment, but chronic hypertension develops in 20–30% and nephrotic syndrome in about 10% of cases. Cases that do not resolve rapidly can become chronic and last decades, with intermittent episodes of hematuria, eventually leading to end-stage renal disease in 20–50% of such cases. Risk factors for progression include renal insufficiency prior to onset, hypertension, and significant proteinuria at the time of diagnosis. Although no single therapy exists to treat this disease, the cornerstone of treatment is effective control of blood pressure, which has been shown to slow progression.

### *Thin Basement Membrane Disease (Benign Hematuria)*

The pathophysiology of this disorder is related to decreased thickness of the glomerular basement membrane that is readily identified through electron microscopy. This is a common autosomal, dominant, inherited disorder that manifests itself in childhood with persistent asymptomatic hematuria. As the name implies, the condition is benign and not associated with an alteration in renal function. If the serum creatinine is elevated or proteinuria is identified, another diagnosis should be considered.

## SUMMARY AND CONCLUSIONS

In summary, hematuria is an extremely common finding—one that an office urologist encounters on an almost daily basis. The diverse nature of pathology resulting in hematuria requires the urologist to have a thorough understanding of urologic and nonurologic causes of hematuria. Often, insight into the patient's past medical history and current comorbid conditions will be instrumental in the diagnosis and subsequent treatment. A systematic approach to the evaluation of hematuria, using algorithms such as those included in the chapter, will usually enable the urologist to establish the correct diagnosis.

## SELECTED READING

Abarbanel J, Benet AE, Lask D, Kimche D (1990) Sports hematuria. *J Urol* 143:887–890.
Brendler CB (1998) Evaluation of the urologic patient. In: Walsh PC, Retik AB, Vaughan ED, Wein AJ, eds., *Campbell's Urology* (7th ed.), Philadelphia: WB Saunders Co., pp. 146.
Brendler CB (1998) Evaluation of the urologic patient. In: Walsh PC, Retik AB, Vaughan ED, Wein AJ, eds., *Campbell's Urology* (7th ed.), Philadelphia: WB Saunders Co., pp. 148.
D'Amico G (1987) The commonest glomerulonephritis in the world: IgA Nephropathy. *Q J Med* 245:709–727.
Fielding JR, Steele G, Fox LA, Heller H, Loughlin KR (1997) Spiral computerized tomography in the evaluation of acute flank pain: a replacement for excretory urography. *J Urol* 157:2071–2073.
Freeman JA, Esrig D, Stein JP, Skinner DG (1994) Management of the patient with bladder cancer. Urethral recurrence. *Urol Clin N Am* 21:645.
Gabow PA, Duley I, Johnson AM (1992) Clinical profiles of gross hematuria in autosomal dominant polycystic kidney disease. *Am J Kidney Dis* 20:140–143.
Hernandez-Graulau JM (1997) Indication for percutaneous nephrostomy in non-calculous disease. In: Sosa RE, et al. *Textbook of Endourology*. Philadelphia: WB Saunders Co., pp. 152, 153.
Kasiske BL, Keane WF (1996) Laboratory Assessment of Renal Disease: Clearance, Urinalysis, and Renal Biopsy. In: Brenner BM, *The Kidney* (5th ed.), Philadelphia: WB Saunders Co., pp. 1164–1165.
Kenworthy P, Tanguay S, Dinney CP (1996) The risk of upper tract recurrence following cystectomy in patients with transitional cell carcinoma involving the distal ureter. *J Urol* 155:501–503.

Lakkis FG, Campbell OC, Badr KF (1996) Microvascular diseases of the kidney. In: Brenner BM, ed., *The Kidney* (5th ed.) Philadelphia: WB Saunders Co., pp. 1723–1724.

Libertino JA (1998) Renovascular Surgery. In: Walsh PC, Retik AB, Vaughan ED, Wein AJ, eds., *Campbell's Urology* (7th ed.), Philadelphia: WB Saunders Co., pp. 462.

Morey AF, McAninch JW, Tiller BK, Duckett CP, Carroll PR (1999) Single shot intraoperative excretory urography for the immediate evaluation of renal trauma. *J Urol* 161:1088–1092.

Perlman ES, Rosenfield AT, Wexler JS, Glickman MG (1996) CT urography in the evaluation of urinary tract disease. *J Comput Assist Tomogr* 20:620–626.

Peterson JC, Adler S, Burkart JM, Greene T, Hebert I, Hunsicker I, et al. (1995) Blood pressure control, proteinuria, and the progression of renal disease. *Am Int Med* 123:754–762.

Pettersson E (1997) IgA nephropathy: 30 years on. *J Intern Med* 242:349–353.

Schuster GA, Lewis GA (1987) Clinical significance of hematuria in patients on anticoagulant therapy. *J Urol* 137:923–925.

Schwartz BF, Schenkman N, Armenakas NA, Stoller ML (1999) Imaging Characteristics of Indinavir Calculi. *J Urol* 161:1085–1087.

Shaw ST, Pan SY, Wong ET (1956) Routine urinalysis: is the dipstick enough? *JAMA* 253.

Siegel AJ, Hennkens CH, Solomon HS, Van Boeckel B (1979) Exercise-related hematuria. Findings in a group of marathon runners. *JAMA* 241:391–392.

Spencer J, Lindsell D, Mastorakou I (1990) Ultrasonography compared with intravenous urography in the investigation of adults with hematuria. *Br Med Bull* 301:1074–1076.

Sundaram PC, Saltzman B (1998) Utility of CT in the evaluation of patients with Indinavir Urolithiasis. *J Urol* (Supplement), 159:324.

# 35 Evaluation and Management of Recurrent Stone Disease

*Stephen J. Savage, MD*
*and Stevan B. Streem, MD*

**CONTENTS**
> INTRODUCTION
> RECURRENT CALCIUM STONES
> URIC ACID STONES
> CYSTINE STONES
> INFECTION-RELATED (STRUVITE) CALCULI
> REFERENCES

## INTRODUCTION

It has been estimated that in the United States, stone disease affects 3–5% of the population, with the higher incidence occurring in men. Once a patient has developed even a single stone, the probability of a recurrence has been estimated at 50–90% within 5–10 yr. Therefore, a primary concern for most patients is prevention of another episode. Although the decision to undertake an evaluation to determine the etiology of the stone disease is itself often a difficult one, our general approach is to offer investigation to those patients for whom we would be willing to prescribe long-term medication. In general, patients with their first stone episode or recurrent episodes many years apart are treated with general dietary advice. In contrast, those patients with recurrent stones within a few years, multiple stones at the time of presentation, or stones that present at a particularly young age—especially in women—will be more likely to undergo investigation and be treated with long-term specific therapy.

In general, stones form when the urine is supersaturated with any of these crystals or salts. As such, an evaluation of the pathogenesis of the stone disease begins with determination of 24-h urinary constituents that make the patient prone to stone formation. At the same time, serum studies are obtained, which often act to exclude systemic disease as well as specific renal tubular problems. Finally, whenever a stone is available, chemical or crystallographic analysis should be obtained.

Table 1 summarizes our current basic metabolic evaluation in terms of serum and 24-h urinary studies.

From: *Current Clinical Urology: Office Urology: The Clinician's Guide*
Edited by: E. D. Kursh and J. C. Ulchaker © Humana Press Inc., Totowa, NJ

Table 1
Metabolic Evaluation

| Blood analysis | 24° Urine analysis | Stone analysis |
|---|---|---|
| Calcium | Volume | Calcium ox/po4 |
| Phosphate | Creatinine | Uric acid |
| Uric acid | Calcium | Struvite |
| Creatinine | Oxalate | Cystine |
| $CO_2$ | Uric acid | |
| Potassium | Citrate | |
| Sodium | Sodium | |
| Chloride | Cystine if: | |
| PTH if: |   Cystine stone | |
|   Elevated serum Ca |   Family history | |
|   Decreased serum $PO_4$ | | |

Table 2
Calcium Nephrolithiasis Risk Factors[a]

Idiopathic hypercalciuria: 60%
Hypocitraturia: 39%
Hyperuricosuria: 35%
Hyperoxaluria: 8%
1° HPTH: 3%
RTA: 2%
MSK

[a]From Levy et al. (1995) *Am J Med* 98:50.

## RECURRENT CALCIUM STONES

Calcium stones develop when the urine is supersaturated with calcium, oxalate, or phosphate. The major risk factors for this are hypercalciuria, hyperoxaluria, hyperuricosuria, and hypocitraturia. As summarized in Table 2, these risk factors may be present alone or in combination such that in general, hypercalciuria is present in 60% of recurrent calcium stone-formers, hypocitraturia in 40%, hyperuricosuria in 35%, and hyperoxaluria in 8%. Primary hyperparathyroidism has been found in as many as 3% of recurrent calcium stone-formers, and Renal Tubular Acidosis (RTA) is the cause in 2%. Medullary Sponge Kidney is another important risk factor for calcium nephrolithiasis, although the metabolic evaluation in those patients diagnosed radiographically will mirror that of a general population of recurrent calcium stone-formers.

### *Idiopathic Hypercalciuria*

Idiopathic hypercalciuria may be defined as daily urinary calcium excretion in excess of 300 mg in men or 250 mg in women, although perhaps a better definition is excretion of calcium in excess of 4 mg/kg/d. The hypercalciuria is termed "idiopathic" only in the absence of hypercalcemia or other known causes of hypercalciuria.

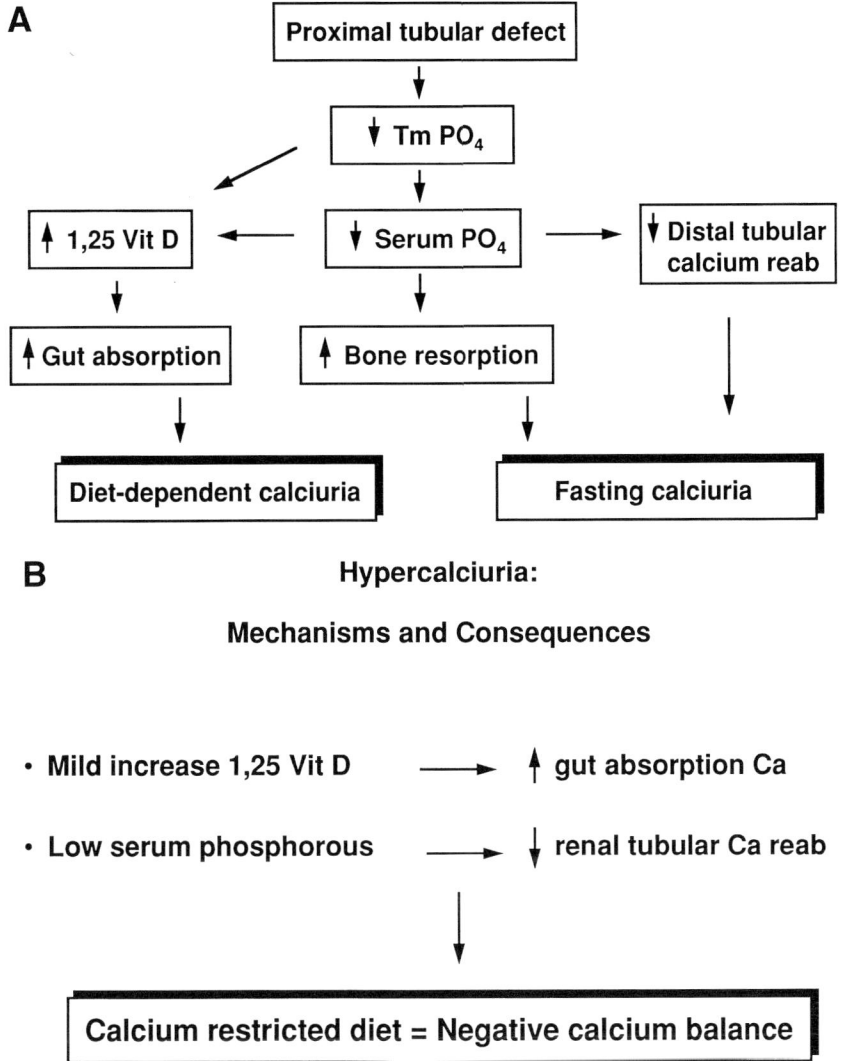

Fig. 1. Schematic demonstrating the effects of a diminished $T_{max}$ for phosphate that lead to hypocalciuria.

Idiopathic hypercalciuria is characterized by a higher incidence in men than women, at a ratio as high as 3:1. In general, affected patients exhibit a low to low-normal serum phosphate, and if tested, exhibit hyperabsorption of calcium from the gut. Idiopathic hypercalciuria may also be characterized by disordered regulation of $1,25(OH_2)$ Vit $D_3$. Finally, dietary calcium restriction in these patients is associated with a negative calcium balance—that is, bone resorption.

One accepted explanation for the hypercalciuria in these patients is that the problem is primarily characterized by a proximal tubular defect that leads to a diminished $T_{max}$ for phosphate. The result is a low serum phosphate and an elevated 1,25 vitamin D. As summarized in Fig. 1, the result is increased gut absorption, increased bone resorption, and diminished distal tubular calcium reabsorption. Clinically this can appear as either diet-dependent calciuria or fasting calciuria. Although some centers try to differentiate these, we believe that for the vast majority of patients, a low-calcium diet will result in a negative calcium balance and bone resorption. As such, we no longer differentiate hyperabsorption from "renal leak." Rather, we treat the whole patient by increasing the tubular calcium reabsorption. In several long-term studies of dietary calcium and supplemental calcium as a risk factor for stones, there appears to be no increased risk of calcium stone formation with either form. In fact, the long-term age adjusted risk for stones may be diminished for those with increased dietary calcium.

Although the role of dietary calcium restriction in most of these patients is at best controversial, it does seem clear that there is a role for dietary sodium restriction, because a high sodium intake increases urinary calcium, especially in hypercalciuric patients. Once the diagnosis of idiopathic hypercalciuria has been made in a patient with recurrent stones, a conservative dietary approach would include oral fluids >2 L/d, no added salt (< 4 g NaCl/d), a normal calcium intake, and moderate oxalate restriction. A high-fiber, low-fat, and modest protein-restricted diet may also be beneficial.

For those patients who fail dietary therapy alone—or who either present with multiple stones or have rapidly recurrent stones—medication is clearly indicated. Our preference is hydrochlorothiazide, 25–50 mg daily, which will increase tubular reasorption of calcium, thereby negating the adverse effects of long-term negative calcium balance and bone resorption. Hydrochlorothiazide may be associated with adverse side effects, many of which are the result of potassium depletion. For these patients, amiloride (5 mg daily) is an excellent alternative.

## *Hypocitraturia*

Hypocitraturia is present alone or with other risk factors in approx 40% of patients with recurrent stones. Although laboratories differ, a reasonable definition is excretion <320 mg/d.

There are several risk factors for hypocitraturia, although the most frequent is a metabolic acidosis. This can result from renal tubular acidosis, inflammatory bowel disease that leads to alkaline intestinal losses, thiazide-induced hypokalemia, or a diet high in animal protein. Hypocitraturia may also be present in the case of intestinal citrate malabsorption or decreased urinary magnesium. Other causes to consider include strenuous physical exercise, high sodium intake, and active urinary infection.

The diagnosis is established by 24-h urinary citrate excretion of <320 mg/d in the absence of active infection. Serum electrolytes are necessary to exclude renal tubular acidosis. Suggestive serum studies would include a hyperchloremic, hypokalemic acidosis. Patients with RTA generally also exhibit hypercalciuria.

Treatment should include citrate supplementation with potassium citrate or balanced citrates that are available as a syrup or crystal packet forms. For patients who cannot tolerate citrates, sodium bicarbonate—which is inexpensive and is generally well-tolerated—may be given as an alternative. This will treat the metabolic acidosis and increase the urinary citrate levels as well. However, the sodium load may increase urinary calcium. When sodium bicarbonate is used to treat RTA, potassium supplementation is generally also required.

When thiazide therapy results in hypokalemia with or without hypocitraturia, potassium citrate is an excellent supplement. However, it should not be given concurrently with potassium-sparing diuretics.

### *Hyperuricosuria*

Hyperuricosuria is a risk factor found in approx 35% of recurrent calcium stone-formers. In our laboratory, this is defined as daily uric-acid excretion exceeding 750 mg. In the setting of a supersaturated urine, the uric acid may act as a nidus for calcium crystallization through "epitaxy." Lowering the urinary uric acid decreases this relative risk for crystallization. In a prospective, double-blind randomized study, allopurinol (300 mg daily) significantly reduced recurrent stone events. For patients with recurrent calcium stones and hyperuricosuria, allopurinol is an important therapeutic option.

### *Hyperoxaluria*

Hyperoxaluria is a risk factor found in approx 8% of patients with recurrent calcium stones. Oxalate is a metabolic end product of glyoxalate. Glyoxalate can be either transaminated—that is, detoxified—to glycine, or oxidized to oxalate. Oxalate forms an insoluble complex with calcium, whether in the gut or the urine. The normal urinary excretion of oxalate is <50 mg daily, and greater amounts would be classified as hyperoxaluria.

Hyperoxaluria can result from endogenous or exogenous sources. Endogenous hyperoxaluria is a result of increased production. The most severe forms are congenital, and these are termed primary hyperoxaluria. At least two enzyme deficiencies have been associated with this condition, and both result in a decreased transamination (detoxification) to glycine, and an increased oxidation to oxalate. The diagnosis is made by liver biopsy to assay the deficient enzyme.

Endogenous hyperoxaluria may also result from increased hepatic conversion resulting from methoxyflurane anesthesia or ethylene glycol ingestion. Pyridoxine deficiency and ingestion of Vitamin C at >2 g/d can also be associated with hyperoxaluria. Pyridoxine is a coenzyme required for the transamination of glycine, whereas oxalate results from the metabolism of ascorbic acid in Vitamin C. Although generally not as severe, exogenous or acquired hyperoxaluria is the most frequent variety. This generally results from dietary excess of foods high in oxalates or enteric hyperabsorption. In that instance, jejunoileal bypass and inflammatory bowel disease are the most frequently associated conditions. In those cases, the dietary calcium has been saponified in association with rapid intestinal transport. As such, oxalate in the gut is not bound to the calcium, and is thus available for absorption. Dietary calcium restriction may also result in hyperoxaluria, again because of the lack of calcium available to bind with the oxalate.

The treatment of hyperoxaluria depends on the primary problem. For congenital hyperoxaluria, standard treatment is hydration and pyridoxine, 200–400 mg daily. Again, pyridoxine is a cofactor in the transamination of glyoxlate to glycine. In refractory, end-stage cases, a liver/kidney transplant is curative.

For exogenous (acquired) hyperoxaluria, the best treatment is hydration, dietary oxalate restriction, and pyridoxine. For patients with rapid intestinal transport from any cause, calcium supplementation and oral citrates may prove helpful. In those patients with a jejunoileal bypass, reversal should be strongly considered when the stone disease cannot otherwise be controlled.

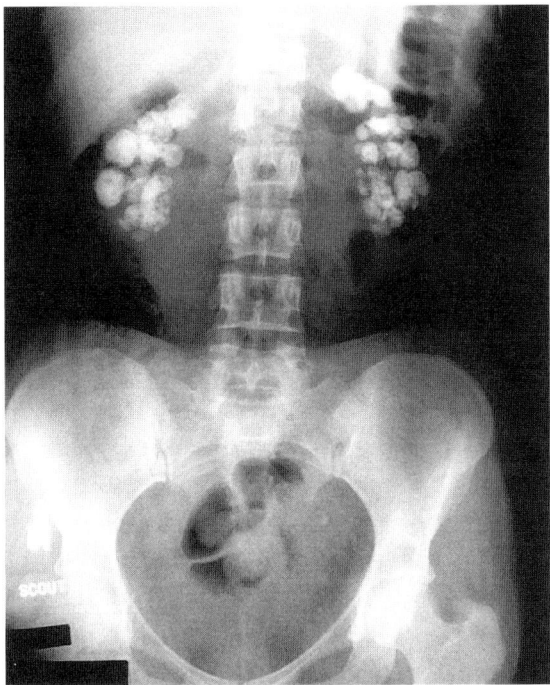

**Fig. 2.** Plain abdominal radiograph of patient with Type I (distal) renal tubular acidosis demonstrating nephrocalcinosis.

## *Primary Hyperparathyroidism*

Primary hyperparathyroidism may be present in up to 3% of patients who present with recurrent calcium stones. The diagnosis is made by the finding of an elevated serum calcium and a decreased serum phosphate. Determination of parathyroid hormone levels should be diagnostic, especially when other causes of hypercalcemia have been excluded. A parathyroidectomy is curative.

## *Renal Tubular Acidosis (RTA)*

Calcium stones occur in association with Type I (distal) renal tubular acidosis. The primary problem is a deficiency of distal tubular excretion of hydrogen ions. This leads to an increase in urinary potassium, sodium, and calcium, which subsequently results in decreased serum potassium, chloride, and $CO_2$. Ultimately, the result is an alkaline, calciuric, hypocitraturic urine.

Clues to the diagnosis of renal tubular acidosis include radiographic evidence of nephrocalcinosis (*see* Fig. 2), which may be present, and a urinary pH that is fixed at >5.5, even on fasting morning specimens. It is more common in young women than in men, and should also be considered whenever the stone composition has a preponderance of calcium phosphate, although this is not a prerequisite. Serum electrolytes consistent with hyperchloremic, hypokalemic acidosis are highly suggestive, as is a 24-h urine with profound hypocitraturia and hypercalciuria. Appropriate treatment is citrate supplementation with potassium citrate or balanced citrates at a dose sufficient to normalize the metabolic acidosis. This should also resolve the hypocitraturia and hypercalciuria.

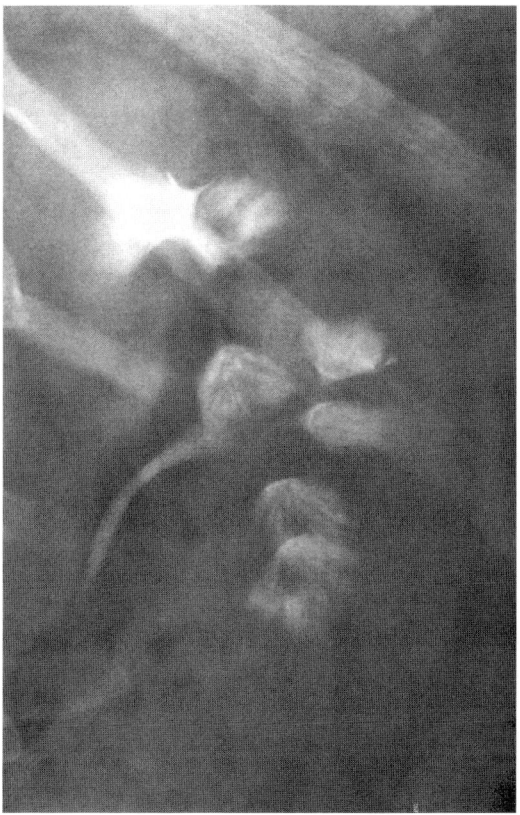

**Fig. 3.** Intravenous pyelogram illustrating the classic "paintbrush" appearance of the calyceal tips in a patient with medullary sponge kidney.

## *Medullary Sponge Kidney (MSK)*

MSK represents a congenital dilatation of the collecting ducts. This process generally presents in the second or third decade of life. The clinical manifestations include stones as well as pyelonephritis, especially in women who are otherwise more prone to bacteruria. The diagnosis is made on radiographic contrast studies, such as an IVP or CT, which reveal intracavitary/parenchymal calcifications associated with tubular ectasia or a "paintbrush" appearance to the calyceal tips (*see* Fig. 3). The calcifications in MSK are often asymmetric between the kidneys and segmental within any involved renal unit. Although the etiology of stone formation in affected patients is somewhat controversial, a standard metabolic evaluation should be performed, because the results will be similar to those for the general stone-forming population. Treatment depends on the specific abnormality found, and includes appropriate dietary restriction and supplementation, antibiotic suppression for patients with recurrent infection, and treatment of any primary metabolic disorder discovered. When a specific metabolic abnormality cannot be discerned, empiric therapy with citrates or thiazides is generally appropriate.

## *Idiopathic Calcium Nephrolithiasis*

At times, despite a thorough metabolic evaluation in the setting of recurrent calcium stones, a specific metabolic abnormality cannot be found. Such patients are deemed to

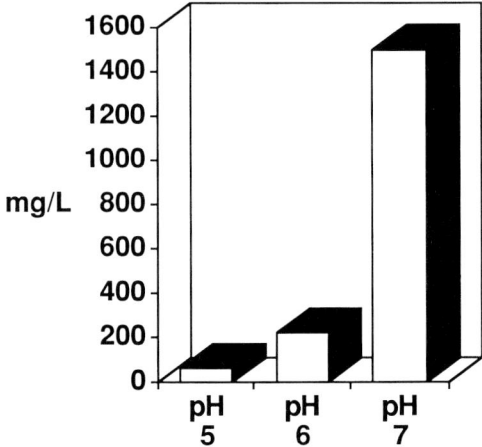

**Fig. 4.** Solubility of uric acid at varying acidity.

have "idiopathic calcium nephrolithiasis." Reasonable treatment options for these patients include appropriate dietary advice—hydration, oxalate and salt restriction, low fat, high fiber, and moderate protein restriction. When a dietary regimen alone is not successful, "empiric" therapy may be initiated with citrates or thiazides. The role of allopurinol in this setting is unproven.

## URIC ACID STONES

Uric acid stones account for 8–12% of calculi. Unlike most mammals, humans are prone to uric acid stones because they lack uricase, an enzyme that normally allows the conversion of uric acid to the freely soluble allantoin. As such, human uric acid levels are ten times those of other mammals. Despite relatively high urate levels, most people do not suffer from uric acid stones because of the normal range of urinary pH throughout the day. The pKa of uric acid is 5.75. The pH at which one-half of the uric acid in solution will be in the free form, and one-half will exist as the urate salt. Free uric acid is relatively insoluble, whereas urate salts are relatively soluble. In fact, at a urinary pH of 5.0, the urine is saturated with uric acid at only 60 mg/L, whereas at a urinary pH of 6.0, the solubility is increased almost fourfold to 220 mg/L (*see* Fig. 4).

Most patients affected with uric acid stones have prolonged periods of urinary acidity when the urinary pH is <6.0, and often fixed at 5.0. These patients lack the usual postprandial "alkaline tide," and therefore, more uric acid is in the free, or less soluble, form. A disturbance in ammonium regulation has been theorized.

The medical evaluation of patients with uric acid stones is straightforward. The urologist should check for a history of gout or GI disorder, including an intestinal diversion. Gout results in hyperuricemia and hyperuricosuria, and any condition associated with a chronic diarrheal state results in chronic dehydration, as well as an acid urine secondary to alkaline GI losses. Chemotherapy—especially for blood dyscrasias—can result in hyperuricemia and hyperuricosuria secondary to rapid cellular breakdown. Yet, most affected patients will have a fixed-acid urine. Completion of the metabolic evaluation of uric acid stone formers requires only measurement of serum uric acid and 24-h urinary uric-acid excretion. The patient should also be instructed to record serial urine pH.

The diagnosis of urate calculi should also be considered from the radiographic appearance of the stones. Uric acid stones are relatively radiolucent, although very large uric acid stones, even when pure, can be lightly opaque. Plain tomograms may help in this situation. Uric acid stones are highly echogenic, with acoustic shadowing on ultrasound, and exhibit high Hounsfield units on CT scanning without intravenous contrast. On such studies, they are indistinguishable from any other stone.

Treatment of uric acid stones can involve both dissolution and prevention. Dissolution is accomplished by reducing urinary uric acid concentration and increasing urinary uric acid solubility. During dissolution, oral fluids should be increased to allow urinary output of 2–3 L daily. Allopurinol can be considered to reduce urinary uric acid excretion, although this alone will not allow dissolution of active stones. That can only be accomplished by increasing urinary uric-acid solubility through urinary alkalization. Medication is given to keep the urinary pH between 6.0 and 6.5. Higher levels of pH do not increase uric acid solubility further, and may allow precipitation of calcium phosphate which is pH-dependent.

The best agents to accomplish urinary alkalization are potassium citrate or balanced citrates. Doses in the range of 60–120 mEq citrate per day in 3–4 divided doses will often accomplish the desired urinary pH range. Sodium bicarbonate is a useful alternative, although theoretically the sodium load will increase urinary calcium excretion. However, sodium bicarbonate does have the advantage of being inexpensive and generally well-tolerated.

Once the active stones are dissolved or passed, preventive therapy is important, because untreated uric acid stones are almost always recurrent. Dietary modification includes increased oral fluids and moderate purine restriction, especially if the patient is hyperuricosuric. Sodium restriction will also be valuable in preventing associated calciuria. The most pathophysiologically appropriate approach to the hyperuricosemic and hyperuricosuric patient is allopurinol. A dose of 300 mg daily is generally appropriate. Allopurinol inhibits uric acid production as a competitive inhibitor of xanthine oxidase. When the primary problem is a persistently acid urine rather than hyperuricosuria, urinary alkalization once or twice daily at a dose of 20–30 mEq citrate should be adequate.

For patients who are intolerant of allopurinol or failed allopurinol for prevention, alkalization may be used instead. Similarly, for alkalization failures or intolerance, allopurinol should be considered.

## CYSTINE STONES

Cystine stones account for 1–2% of calculi in the United States. The etiology is always an inherited enzymatic deficiency in the renal and intestinal tubular reabsorption of four dibasic amino acids. These include cystine, ornithine lysine, and arginine. The only clinically important aspect of this genetic disorder is the propensity for urinary calculi. The disease is inherited in a complex autosomal recessive pattern, and the recessive gene frequency has been estimated at 1:200, whereas the disease frequency is between 1:20,000 and 1:100,000. Normals excrete <100 mg of cystine daily, and heterozygotes excrete between 100 and 400 mg but are affected by cystine stones only

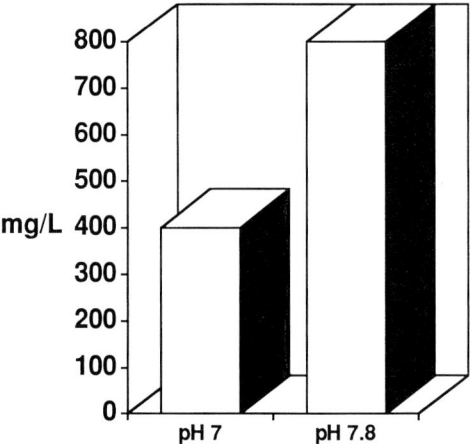

**Fig. 5.** Twofold increase in solubility of cystine at pH 7.8 vs 7.0.

rarely. Homozygotes excrete more than 400 mg daily, which puts them at significant risk for stones.

Cystine biochemistry is important in pathophysiology and treatment. Cystine contains a disulfide bond, which has therapeutic significance. Its solubility in urine is pH-dependent, which is therapeutically important. Cystine is the least soluble of the four dibasic amino acids, and is therefore the only one that precipitates in urine to form stones. As noted in Fig. 5, although the solubility of cystine is pH-dependent, it is not nearly as pH-dependent as uric acid, although the solubility is doubled at a pH of 7.8 compared to a pH of 7.0.

The patient evaluation includes determining whether there is a family history of stones, especially in siblings—as heterozygotes are rarely affected. Cystinuria should be considered whenever the stone disease presents in the pediatric age group, although cystine stones can first develop in the geriatric age group as well. Radiographically, they have a homogenous, "ground glass" (lightly opaque) appearance. The diagnosis can be suggested by cyanide nitroprusside urine screening, but a 24-h chromatographic quantitative analysis will be diagnostic. A urinalysis revealing characteristic hexagonal crystals is also diagnostic, because only cystinuria is associated with this finding. In some cases, the diagnosis will be made unexpectedly at the time of stone analysis.

Treatment of recurrent cystine stones is intended to reduce urinary cystine concentration and increase urinary cystine solubility. Dietary modification to reduce urinary cystine concentration includes forced hydration to >3–4 L per day. Sodium intake should be restricted, because sodium increases urinary cystine excretion. Methionine is a precursor of cystine, and theoretically, a methionine-restricted diet might be useful. In practice, however, it is unpalatable, and has little effect on cystine excretion. Reasonable advice might be to avoid methionine-rich foods.

Urinary alkalization is a mainstay of treatment along with forced hydration, because it increases urinary solubility. Sodium bicarbonate is inexpensive and well-tolerated. However, the sodium load will—at least theoretically—increase urinary cystine and calcium, and this should be avoided. The best alternatives are potassium citrate or balanced citrates. A dose of 90–120 mEq/d in three or four divided doses is generally required to keep the urinary pH at approx 7.5–8.0. When citrates are not tolerated, sodium bicarbonate is a reasonable alternative.

When hydration and alkalization alone fail to prevent or dissolve active cystine stones, urinary cystine concentration is reduced with the use of thiol derivatives. D-penicillamine (D-pcn) had been a mainstay of treatment at 1–2 g/d in four divided doses, with the goal of keeping the urinary cystine excretion below 400 mg/d. D-pcn acts through a thiol-disulfide exchange that converts cystine to cysteine, which is much more soluble than cystine. However, D-pcn use is limited by a relatively high incidence of significant side effects. In its place, alpha-mercaptopropionylglycine (alpha-MPG)—which acts through thiol-disulfide exchange—is being increasingly used. A dose of 800–1200 mg/d in four divided doses is generally sufficient. Although the spectrum of side effects is similar to that with D-pcn, the incidence and severity are significantly lower, and this is currently the thiol of choice for cystinuria.

Captopril, an ACE inhibitor, also has a free sulfhydryl group, and allows thiol-disulfide exchange. At a dose of 50 mg three times daily, captopril has been shown to significantly reduce urinary cystine excretion in at least some affected patients. It is reasonable to add captopril to the regimen for any cystinuric who otherwise requires antihypertensive medication, or who has failed hydration, alkalization, and standard thiol treatment.

## INFECTION-RELATED (STRUVITE) CALCULI

Infection-related calculi account for approx 10% of stones in the United States. They do however, account for the majority of opaque "staghorn," or branched calculi. They are the only type of stone that affects women more frequently than men.

Infection-related stones are composed primarily of magnesium-ammonium phosphate (struvite). However, in almost all instances calcium phosphate is admixed, and at time these have been referred to as "triple phosphate." Carbonate-apatite is another infection-related stone with a similar pathophysiology.

As summarized in Fig. 6, the basic abnormality is a persistently alkaline urine, with a pH >7.2. This is always associated with a urease-producing bacterial infection. In that setting, urea is hydrolyzed through the action of bacterial urease to ammonia and carbon dioxide. The ammonia is further hydrolyzed to ammonium, resulting in an alkaline urine. An alkaline, ammoniac urine is supersaturated with struvite.

As mentioned previously, women are affected more frequently than men. Affected patients may present with febrile urinary-tract infection or flank pain, or alternatively, they may be asymptomatic and the diagnosis may be found when chronic bacteriuria is evaluated. Women especially may present with recurrent cystitis without upper-tract symptoms. Patients at an increased risk for these stones are those at increased risk for urinary infection: all patients with neurogenic bladders, indwelling catheters, or a urinary diversion. Although the patient evaluation should include a search for anatomic or functional abnormalities, a metabolic evaluation is important, because 30–50% of patients affected with infection-related calculi will be found to have an underlying metabolic abnormality.

Treatment of these patients involves complete removal of the stone. In contemporary practice, this generally involves percutaneous techniques with or without supplemental shock wave lithotripsy, especially when the stone is large and extensively branched.

## Pathophysiology

**Basic abnormality = persistently alkaline urine (pH > 7.2)**
**Always a/w urease - producing bacterial infection:**

$$NH_2 - CO - NH_2 + H_2O \underset{}{\overset{urease}{\longleftrightarrow}} 2NH_3 + CO_2$$
(Urea) (ammonia)

$$NH_3 + H_2O \longleftrightarrow NH_4^+ + OH^- \text{ (alkaline urine)}$$
(ammonium)

**Alkaline urine + ammonuria = supersaturation c̄ struvite**

**Fig. 6.** Pathophysiology of the formation of infection-related stones. Urease-producing bacteria infection leads to alkaline urine and ammonia, allowing supersaturation of struvite.

When the stone is removed, long-term antibiotic suppression or prophylaxis plays a role. Urease inhibitors (acetohydramic acid) are indicated whenever a bacterial infection cannot be successfully suppressed in a patient with a history of struvite stones. However, the use of these agents has been limited by a fairly high incidence of significant side effects. When an underlying metabolic abnormality has been revealed, it should be treated specifically.

## SELECTED READING

Chow GK, Streem SB (1996) Medical management of cystinuria: results of contemporary clinical practice. *J Urol* 156:1576.
Cole F (1984) Treatment of hypercalciuria. *N Engl J Med* 311:116.
Curhan GC, Willett WC, Rimm EB, Stampfer MJ (1993) A prospective study of dietary calcium and other nutrients and risk of symptomatic kidney stones. *N Engl J Med* 328 (12):833.
Dretler SP (1998) The Physiologic approach to the medical management of stone disease. *Urol Clin N Am* 25(4):613.
Ettinger B, Tang A, Citron JT, Livermore B, Williams T (1986) Randomized trial of allopurinol in the prevention of calcium oxalate calculi. *N Engl J Med* 315:1386.
Levy FL, Adams-Huet B, Pack CYC (1998) Ambulatory evaluation of nephrolithiasis: an update of a 1980 protocol. *Am J Med* 50:1995.
National Institutes of Health Consensus Development Conferences on Prevention and Treatment of Kidney Stones (1989) *J Urol* 141 (3, Part II).
Pak CYC, Fuller C, Sakhaee K, Preminger GM, Britton F (1985) Long-term treatment of calcium nepholithiasis with potassium citrate. *J Urol* 134:11.
Parivar F, Low RK, Stoller ML (1996) The influence of diet on uninary stone disease. *J Urol* 155:432.
Pholman T, Hruska KA, Menon M (1998) Renal tubular acidosis. *J Urol* 132:431.
Smith LH, Fromm H, Hofmann AF (1972) Acquired hyperoxaluria, nephrolithiasis and intestinal disease. *N Engl J Med* 286 (26):1371.

# 36 Common Pediatric Problems

*Jonathan H. Ross,* MD *and Robert Kay,* MD

**CONTENTS**
> UNDESCENDED TESTICLES
> SCROTAL SWELLING
> PENIS PROBLEMS
> VOIDING DYSFUNCTION
> URINARY-TRACT INFECTIONS
> HEMATURIA IN CHILDREN
> SELECTED READING

## UNDESCENDED TESTICLES

Undescended testis is one of the most common congenital genitourinary anomalies. The incidence of undescended testis is 3% in term infants and 30% in premature infants. Many undescended testes will descend spontaneously in the first months of life, and the incidence at 1 yr of age is 0.8%.

Men with a history of an undescended testis are at risk for infertility and testicular tumors. The incidence of infertility is only slightly increased in cases of unilateral cryptorchidism, but is 40–70% in men with a history of bilateral undescended testis. Circumstantial evidence suggests that early orchidopexy (at 1 yr as opposed to school-age) may improve ultimate fertility.

The risk of testicular cancer in men with a history of cryptorchidism is 5–10 times that of the general population. This increased risk is greater for intra-abdominal than inguinal testes. Carcinoma *in situ* occurs in 2–3% of men with a history of cryptorchidism, and 20% of testis tumors in these men occur in the normally descended contralateral testis. There is no direct evidence that orchidopexy reduces tumor risk, but it puts the testicle in a location where tumors are more easily palpated and therefore detected earlier. All men with a history of undescended testis should perform routine testicular self-exams after puberty.

An undescended testis is defined as a testis that has become arrested in its descent through the normal pathway. This is distinguished from the rarer ectopic testis, which is a testis that has deviated from the normal pathway of descent. The most common location for undescended testes is the inguinal canal. Other sites include the high scrotum, pubic tubercle, superficial inguinal pouch, and the abdomen. Ectopic testicles may be found in the femoral canal, perineum, prepubic space, or the contralateral scrotum.

Because most undescended testes are located in the inguinal canal, they can be evaluated during a clinical exam. Impalpable testes present a more challenging problem, and require a more extensive evaluation.

## *History and Physical*

In a child with an undescended testicle, as with any congenital anomaly, a thorough history of the pregnancy and infancy is important. The parents should also be questioned regarding whether anyone has ever felt the testis. Was the undescended testis noted at birth? This is particularly important in older children who may have retractile testes. A history of the testis having been in a normal location at one time—either on examination by the primary care physician, or as noted by the parents—suggests that the testis is retractile. Obviously, any history of previous inguinal surgery is important as a possible cause of secondary testicular ascent or atrophy. Although clinical hernias are rare in children with an undescended testis, most have a patent processus vaginalis, and it is important to determine a history of hernia.

The physical examination of the child with an undescended testis is the most important part of the evaluation. It is essential that the child be relaxed and warm during the examination. A cold room or a nervous child will exaggerate retractile testes. Before touching the child, the genitalia and inguinal region should be visually examined. Because the first touch may stimulate a cremasteric reflex, the best opportunity to see the testis in the scrotum is on initial inspection. A true undescended testis is often associated with a poorly developed hemiscrotum on the ipsilateral side. Placing the child in the frog-leg position and gently milking from the inguinal canal to the scrotum will often bring a high retractile testis down. If the testis can be brought down in this way, and remains in the hemiscrotum without tension, the diagnosis of a retractile testis is made. Applying a small dab of liquid soap to the examining hand can reduce friction and improve sensitivity in detecting an inguinal testis. Ectopic sites should also be palpated if no testis is felt in the inguinal region or scrotum.

## *Palpable Undescended Testes*

The physical examination will allow for a distinction among an impalpable testis, a palpable undescended testis, and a retractile testis. In equivocal cases, reexamination at a later date will often clarify the diagnosis. When serial examinations leave the question of a retractile testis vs an undescended testis uncertain, an HCG stimulation test may be administered. A variety of regimens may be used. We administer 500–2000 IU (depending on body size) every other day for a total of five doses. It is generally agreed that a retractile testis will "descend" in response to HCG stimulation. Some truly undescended testes may also descend in response to HCG, although the actual success rate is controversial. Reported success rates range from 6 to 70%. Patients with retractile testes may be reassured that no further evaluation is necessary.

In the case of a palpable undescended testis, no further evaluation is necessary unless there are other associated genital anomalies. The most important is hypospadias, which occurs in 5–10% of boys with an undescended testicle. Hypospadias in association with even one undescended testicle raises the possibility of intersex. Patients with a unilateral undescended testis and hypospadias may have mixed gonadal dysgenesis. These patients generally have a mosaic kayotype of 45XO/46XY. Therefore, patients with an undescended testis and hypospadias should undergo a karyotype. In the newborn,

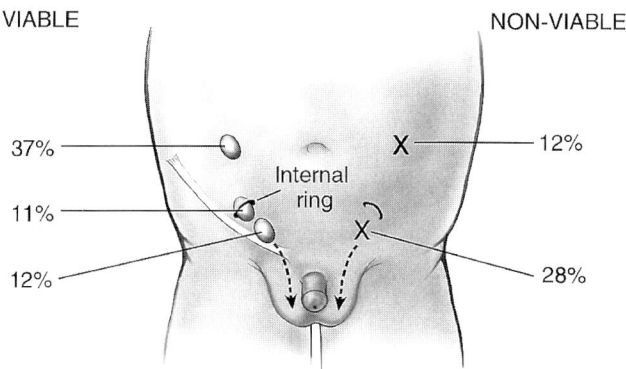

Fig. 1. The location of impalpable testes determined at laparoscopy (based on data from Cisek, 1998).

if both testes are undescended—particularly if they are impalpable—then congenital adrenal hyperplasia or other less common forms of intersex should also be considered.

## *Impalpable Testes*

In a boy with bilateral impalpable testes, the question arises regarding whether the testes are intra-abdominal or are absent (*see* Fig. 1). Bilateral anorchia can be diagnosed biochemically with an HCG stimulation test. This is accomplished by administering three doses of 1500 U of HCG on alternate days. If there is no rise in serum testosterone, and baseline gonadotropin levels are elevated, then the child has anorchia and no further evaluation is necessary. If there is a rise in testosterone after the administration of HCG, then the child has at least one functioning testis—presumably intra-abdominal. Occasionally, boys with low testosterone levels and normal gonadotropin levels will have testicles present; hence the dual requirement of a negative HCG stimulation test and elevated baseline gonadotropins.

In the boy with a unilateral impalpable testis, an HCG stimulation test is obviously of no value. In these boys, and in boys with bilateral impalpable testes and a positive HCG stimulation test, further evaluation is indicated. Several radiologic tests are available to identify an intra-abdominal testis. Ultrasound, computerized tomography, and magnetic resonance imaging have all been used. The overall accuracy of these testes in localizing an undescended testis is 80–90%. However, the majority of testes in reported series are inguinal. The accuracy of these imaging studies for localizing an intra-abdominal testis is <25%. Gonadal venography is more accurate, and able to locate or confirm the absence of an intra-abdominal testis in 75% of cases. However, this modality requires heavy sedation or anesthesia in children, is invasive, and is technically difficult in patients <6 yr old.

Since the readily available tests are not sensitive for detecting an intra-abdominal testis, they are of little benefit. In the minority of cases when a radiologic study identifies an intra-abdominal testis, an operation to bring the testicle down will be required. However, the failure of any of these tests to identify a testis does not mean the testis is absent—each test has a significant false-negative rate. Therefore, a negative study also mandates an operation to locate an intra-abdominal testis, or prove definitively that it is absent. Because the results of radiologic tests will not alter management, there is little value in performing them. A possible exception is the child whose body habitus makes physical examination of the inguinal region difficult. If ultrasound can identify an inguinal testis in such a child, then the child will be spared laparoscopy.

### *Surgical Evaluation of Impalpable Testes*

Approximately 50% of boys with a unilateral impalpable testis will in fact have an absent testis on that side. Because of the inability of radiologic studies to reliably identify an intra-abdominal testis, an operation is required to determine the presence or absence of an impalpable testis. Historically, this has been approached through an inguinal incision, which could be extended into the abdomen if necessary. Although open exploration is still an accepted approach, the addition of laparoscopy to the operative armamentarium can reduce the morbidity of these explorations. Prior to a formal operative incision, laparoscopy is performed through a supra- or infraumbilical incision. If an intra-abdominal testis is identified, then an orchidopexy is performed. This can usually be accomplished laparoscopically with the addition of two working ports. For high intra-abdominal testes, a first-stage Fowler-Stephens may be performed laparoscopically.

If blind-ending vessels are identified in the abdomen, the procedure is terminated. If vessels are seen entering the inguinal canal, then an inguinal exploration is undertaken. This allows removal of any testicular "nubbin," which may contain some seminiferous tubules at risk for malignant degeneration. In some cases, the inguinal exploration will reveal a viable testis that was missed on physical exam.

## SCROTAL SWELLING

### *Acute Scrotal Swelling*

The differential diagnosis of acute scrotal swelling in children includes spermatic-cord torsion (testicular torsion), torsion of the appendix testis, epididymo-orchitis, hernia, hydrocele, and testis tumor. The last three do not usually present acutely, but may on occasion. The evaluation and management of the acute scrotum are discussed in Chapter 26.

### *Hydrocele/Hernia*

Hydroceles and hernias may present as an acute scrotal mass, but usually present as intermittent scrotal swelling. Hydroceles are non tender and transilluminate. A normal testis should be palpable. In equivocal cases, an ultrasound is diagnostic. Most infant hydroceles resolve by 1 yr of age. Persistent hydroceles should be repaired to prevent the development of a hernia. Contralateral exploration is not routinely performed. Hernias do not transilluminate, and can usually be palpated up to the inguinal ring. Bowel sounds may be auscultated. Again, ultrasound is helpful in equivocal cases. Hernias that cannot be reduced should be repaired immediately. If reducible, they may be repaired electively, but as soon as possible.

### *Neonatal Scrotal Masses*

Testicular torsions can occur in the neonatal period, and should be considered in a neonate with a unilateral hard scrotal mass. Although the mechanism is different in

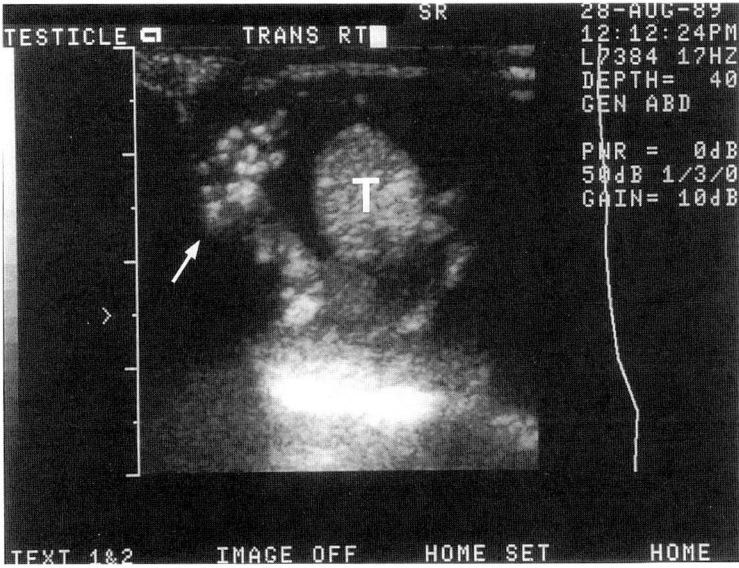

Fig. 2. Scrotal ultrasound of newborn with meconium peritonitis presenting with a hard scrotal mass. Note the peripheral calcifications (arrow) and normal testis (T).

neonates than in older children, orchiectomy and contralateral orchidopexy are indicated, because metachronous contralateral torsions have been described. If present at birth, the testis is invariably necrotic, and the operation may be delayed until 24–48 h of life to allow for a thorough preoperative evaluation of the newborn. Frequent scrotal exams should be performed so that an early contralateral torsion is not missed.

A bilateral hard scrotum may be caused by dystrophic calcification in a child with meconium peritonitis. Because the processus vaginalis is patent in the fetus, meconium can migrate into the scrotum and cause calcifications analogous to those seen in the abdomen. An ultrasound reveals peripheral scrotal calcifications with a normal testis (see Fig. 2). A plain film of the abdomen confirms the diagnosis. No specific treatment of the scrotal calcifications is required.

Testicular tumors are extremely rare in the neonate. However, they must be considered in the differential diagnosis of a neonatal scrotal mass. An ultrasound may be helpful in differentiating torsion from a tumor. However, if any doubt exists, then the patient should undergo an inguinal exploration, rather than the scrotal approach more commonly used for presumed testicular torsion.

### *Adolescent Varicocele*

The incidence of varicoceles in adolescent boys is 15%—the same as in adult men. Epidemiologic evidence suggests that approx 20% of these boys will have significant fertility problems. Given the high incidence of incidental varicocele in boys, the indications for repair are controversial. The most widely accepted indication is a consistently smaller testicle on the affected side. Studies have clearly shown that varicocele repair in these patients results in catch-up growth of the testis and ultimately, a better spermiogram. However, the impact on fertility is yet to be determined. Since roughly half of boys with a varicocele have ipsilateral testicular hypotrophy, even this indication would result in 5–10% of all boys undergoing a repair—and most of them would probably be fertile in adulthood, with or without a repair at that time. If a repair is undertaken, the approach is the same as in adults.

## PENIS PROBLEMS

Uncircumcised boys may develop phimosis, balanoposthitis, or paraphimosis. Phimosis is a progressive scarring of the prepuce usually caused by recurrent inflammation. The normal attachment of the foreskin to the glans penis, and the normal inability to retract the foreskin in young children, should not be confused with pathologic phimosis. Evolution of the potential space between the glans and prepuce is a developmental phenomenon that occurs slowly after birth. Although the foreskin is rarely retractable in the newborn, by 1 yr of age, 50% are retractable, and by 5 yr of age at least 90% are retractable. Virtually all foreskins become retractable in puberty. Thus, "phimosis" is not a pathologic condition in young children unless it is associated with balanitis or, rarely, urinary retention. Failure of physicians and parents to appreciate this normal process has led to an overdiagnosis of phimosis.

Balanoposthitis refers to inflammation of the prepuce and glans penis. It generally resolves with warm baths and topical or enteral antibiotics.

In children, paraphimosis is often iatrogenic. It may be mistaken as balanitis by emergency and primary care physicians who assume the child is circumcised. Management is the same as in adults, although heavy sedation or a brief general anesthetic are usually required.

Many penile problems may be avoided in uncircumcised boys if parents are properly educated in the care of the uncircumcised penis. The penis should be washed like any other part of the body, and the foreskin should not be retracted in a way that causes pain or preputial bleeding. Forceful retraction is painful, and may result in secondary phimosis. Desquamated skin (keratin pearls) that collects under the prepuce is harmless and does not need to be removed from under the unretractable foreskin. Indeed, this is part of the natural mechanism by which the foreskin eventually separates from the glans. In older boys, the foreskin is easily retracted, and the entire glans and preputial skin may be washed daily.

The most common complication of circumcision is meatitis, which may result in meatal stenosis. Many boys have small urethral meati. A small meatus is not necessarily a stenotic meatus. The diagnosis of meatal stenosis should only be made if the meatus is obviously scarred, or if the observed urinary stream is thin or deflected. Meatal stenosis is easily treated with an office meatotomy using a lidocaine/prilocaine emulsion (EMLA cream). The cream is applied to the glans, with an attempt to allow some to enter the meatus. It is secured with plastic wrap or the finger of a glove and tape. After ½ h, the penis is checked and additional cream is added as needed. After the cream has been on for 1 h, it is removed with a damp cloth. A painless clamp and cut meatotomy can then be performed. If the boy experiences discomfort as the procedure is initiated, cream is reapplied for an additional 30 min. Distraction with a video or video game is extremely helpful.

Hypospadias occurs in fewer than 1% of newborn boys. It should be repaired between 6 and 12 mo of age. Older children have significant genital awareness, leading to much greater psychological stress. Nearly all hypospadias repairs can be accomplished as an outpatient in a single operation.

## VOIDING DYSFUNCTION

### Bladder Instability

The most frequent cause of incontinence in children is bladder instability. These children present with urge incontinence and squatting behavior, or "potty dancing." Most have been wet since toilet training, although a dry period of several months after toilet training is not uncommon. Bladder instability represents a normal stage in the development of bladder control. As infants, a normal coordinated bladder contraction occurs with bladder filling. When toilet-trained, most children initially prevent wetting by activation of the external sphincter when a bladder contraction is reflexively initiated with bladder filling. Most children quickly progress to direct central inhibition of bladder contractions with filling, until an appropriate opportunity to void presents itself. A delay in this ability to centrally inhibit bladder contractions leads to the typical symptoms of bladder instability. These symptoms will resolve spontaneously, but may persist for many years in some children.

Indications to treat the problem include associated urinary-tract infections or vesicoureteral reflux. In the absence of these indications, treatment is initiated if the problem is causing enough psychosocial stress that the parents and/or child desire therapy. Conservative measures include timed voiding and treating any constipation that may be present because constipation is a common cause of bladder instability. If conservative measures fail, then medical management is initiated. Oxybutinin chloride is prescribed at 0.5 mg/kg/d divided TID. Parents should be warned about the possible side effects of a dry mouth, facial flushing, heat intolerance, and constipation. Patients with associated recurrent UTIs are also placed on antibiotic prophylaxis with trimethoprim/sulfamethoxazole 0.25–0.5 cm$^3$/kg once daily, or nitrofurantoin 1–2 mg/kg once daily. Medical therapy is discontinued every 6–12 mo to determine if it is still required. Urethral dilation is an unproven and inappropriate therapy for pediatric voiding dysfunction.

Young children with typical bladder instability do not require radiographic evaluation. Boys with severe symptoms or any child with symptoms that are not improving should undergo a screening ultrasound of the kidneys and bladder. A VCUG is obtained in any child with evidence of bladder-wall thickening or hydronephrosis (to rule out reflux, a neurogenic bladder, and posterior urethral valves). Urodynamics are unnecessary in children with typical bladder instability, because they will predictably reveal normal bladder compliance with uninhibited bladder contractions. An MRI of the spine should be considered in children with atypical symptoms, and particularly those who were initially dry and later develop urge incontinence.

### Urinary Frequency Syndrome

The "urinary frequency syndrome" refers to the acute onset of urinary frequency in school-age children with normal baseline voiding patterns. These children may urinate as often as every 15 min. However, incontinence is rare, even when a toilet is unavailable. This sensory urgency is distinct from the more common bladder instability. Children with urinary frequency syndrome rarely wake at night to void. When the typical symptoms are present and the physical exam and urinalysis are normal, no further evaluation is necessary. However, an ultrasound may be obtained to rule out a serious underlying abnormality. Behavioral and viral etiologies have been suggested, but the syndrome remains idiopathic. There is no effective therapy for the syndrome, which resolves spontaneously in a matter of weeks or months.

## *Nocturnal Enuresis*

The vast majority of children with bed-wetting have primary nocturnal enuresis. These are children who have wet the bed all their life (although a dry interval of several months following toilet-training is not unusual). The diagnosis is made in the absence of any daytime symptoms or history of urinary-tract infections. The physical exam and urinalysis should be normal. A positive family history supports the diagnosis. In older children, a screening renal and bladder ultrasound may be obtained, but this is generally unnecessary. Virtually all bed-wetting will resolve spontaneously at some point prior to adulthood. No treatment is necessary unless the problem is distressing to the child. Treatment is discouraged in children under 6 yr of age.

The safest, most effective, and least expensive treatment is a bed-wetting alarm. This should be the first treatment used. It requires a commitment from the child and family to use the alarm for several weeks before results are obtained. Medications are reserved for those who fail an alarm.

Two medical treatments are widely used. Nasal desmopressin acetate is an extremely expensive, but relatively safe form of therapy. Treatment should be initiated with four puffs at bedtime. If this fails, then treatment is abandoned. If it is successful, then the dose is lowered by one puff every week or so, until the lowest effective dose is determined. Treatment should be discontinued every 6 mo to see if it is still required. An oral form of desmopressin has recently become available and may be more convenient for some patients.

Imipramine is an older medical treatment that is effective in many patients. Treatment is initiated at 25 mg QHS. The dose may be increased to 50 mg—and in older children, to 75 mg—as needed. It takes several weeks to achieve an optimal effect. Side effects include anticholinergic effects, alteration in sleep patterns, and behavioral changes. Parents should be warned about the risk of accidental death by overdose in younger siblings.

## URINARY-TRACT INFECTIONS

Urinary-tract infections in children are a significant source of morbidity, particularly when associated with anatomic abnormalities. Vesicoureteral reflux is the most commonly associated abnormality. Reflux allows the ascent of lower urinary-tract infections, initiating pyelonephritis. This can lead to renal scarring. Renal scarring is associated with hypertension in 10–20% of patients, and reflux nephropathy is a significant cause of end-stage renal disease in children and adolescents. However, when reflux is recognized early, and managed appropriately, renal insufficiency is exceedingly rare. Children with significant reflux may present with a single UTI. Other infections leading to severe bilateral scarring may be subclinical, or mistaken for other entities, such as otitis. Therefore, even a single documented infection in a child must be taken seriously.

## Diagnosis

Children with UTIs do not always present with the classic symptoms of irritative voiding or flank pain. Infants often present with fever and irritability. Even older children may have nonspecific symptoms, such as abdominal pain or an unexplained fever. When a UTI is suspected, a urinalysis and urine culture should be obtained. Because a documented infection warrants thorough radiographic evaluation, empiric treatment on the basis of symptoms or a positive urinalysis alone should be avoided.

Although the most accurate means of obtaining a urine culture is by suprapubic aspiration, the procedure can be anxiety-provoking for the child, parent, and physician. Urine specimens are therefore most often obtained by placing a plastic bag over the perineum of infants, and by obtaining a voided specimen in older children. Because "bag" and voided specimens may be contaminated, they must be analyzed in conjunction with the urinalysis and clinical setting. In patients with complicated histories, when the uncertainty of contamination must be avoided, a catheterized specimen can be obtained.

Although the presence or absence of a true UTI is occasionally difficult to determine, the distinction between cystitis and pyelonephritis is even more problematic. No clinical findings (such as fever or flank pain) and no laboratory studies (such as erythrocyte sedimentation rate or white blood-cell count) provide an accurate means of distinguishing pyelonephritis from cystitis. Fortunately, this distinction is rarely crucial. The management of the child is dictated by the clinical severity of the illness rather than the specific site of infection in the urinary tract. Furthermore, since the risk of reflux is similar in all patients with a UTI, the distinction between cystitis and pyelonephritis is not important in guiding the radiographic evaluation.

In rare circumstances, when it is critical to distinguish the diagnosis of pyelonephritis from some other infection, a $^{99m}$technetium dimercaptosuccinic acid (DMSA) renal flow scan is the best study to obtain. Patients with a normal scan during an acute infection do not have pyelonephritis and will not develop scarring. On the other hand, an area of photopenia on a DMSA scan identifies a region of pyelonephritis that is at risk for eventual scar formation. Because this test is invasive, expensive, exposes the child to radiation, and is unlikely to alter the child's management, it is not used in the routine evaluation of children with a UTI.

## Treatment

Because UTIs are usually caused by gram-negative rods, particularly *Escherichia coli*, any oral antibiotic with good gram-negative coverage is a reasonable choice for treatment. Trimethoprim/sulfamethoxazole offers good coverage and is inexpensive. It is given in suspension form at 4 mg trimethoprim per kg twice daily. Other commonly used antibiotics include amoxicillin (10 mg/kg three times daily) and nitrofurantoin (2.5 mg/kg, three times daily). Cephalosporins may be indicated if infection with a more resistant organism is suspected.

Children who require hospitalization should be placed on broad-spectrum intravenous antibiotics pending the results of a urine culture. Because most community acquired UTIs are caused by gram-negative bacilli, coverage should include an aminoglycoside, cephalosporin, or broad-spectrum penicillin derivative. Coverage may need to be broader in children with recent hospitalization, recent instrumentation, or recurrent infections, since they may be infected with gram-positive organisms, such as enterococcus or coagulase negative staphylococcus. A urine gram-stain may be helpful in the initial selection of antibiotics.

## *Radiographic Evaluation*

The most significant anomaly associated with UTIs in children is vesicoureteral reflux, which occurs in 30–50% of these patients. Despite the high rate of association, no randomized prospective studies demonstrate the benefit of screening these patients for anomalies. However, there is no doubt that vesicoureteral reflux is associated with scarring because it allows lower-tract infections to ascend, resulting in pyelonephritis. Since antibiotic prophylaxis can prevent recurrent UTIs, it seems prudent to screen children with UTIs who are at risk for renal scarring. This would certainly include children with recurrent UTIs. Since children are at greatest risk for renal scarring in the first few years of life, reflux screening is also recommended for any child with a single UTI prior to toilet-training. Older children with consistent pediatric care (so that a pattern of recurrent UTIs will not be missed) may not be screened after a single infection. A renal ultrasound may be reassuring in these patients. Although ultrasound is a poor screening test for reflux, it could be argued that missed reflux is of little concern in an older child with a single infection and normal kidneys sonographically.

Children should be screened for reflux with a cystogram. A cystogram performed by an experienced pediatric radiologist is well-tolerated by most children. A few doses of antibiotics may be given around the time of the cystogram to prevent an iatrogenic infection. Although renal ultrasounds are less invasive, they are normal in 50–75% of patients with reflux, and therefore ineffective for screening. A DMSA renal scan is the best study for detecting renal scarring, and therefore might identify patients at particular risk for reflux. Unfortunately, a renal scan cannot detect children with reflux who have not yet developed a scar—the very ones who might benefit most from antibiotic prophylaxis.

When a child presents with a UTI, a cystogram should be delayed for at least 48 h after initiating antibiotic therapy so bacteremia is not induced in a bacteruric patient by instrumenting the urinary tract. There is no need to delay the cystogram beyond that point. Concern that obtaining a cystogram too soon after a UTI may result in a false-positive study is ill-founded. Even children who only reflux when they have cystitis have significant reflux, since reflux causes scarring by allowing cystitis to ascend.

A renal ultrasound is obtained in children with a UTI to rule out obstructive uropathy. An ultrasound can also detect gross renal scarring or marked asymmetry of renal size in patients with vesicoureteral reflux. When accurate detection of renal scarring is important, a DMSA renal flow scan is the best study.

Two types of cystogram are currently available. A nuclear cystogram may be obtained by instilling a radionuclide into the bladder and imaging with a gamma camera. Nuclear cystography is at least as sensitive for the detection of reflux as a standard voiding cystourethrogram (VCUG) and exposes the child to less radiation. However, grading of reflux is less precise, and associated bladder abnormalities cannot be detected with nuclear cystography. Therefore, a VCUG is preferred as the initial study in the evaluation of a child with a urinary-tract infection. Nuclear cystography is used in follow-up of patients with vesicoureteral reflux who are on the observation protocol. Vesicoureteral reflux is present in one-third of siblings of refluxers, and in two-thirds of the children of refluxers. Nuclear cystography may be employed for screening these children as well.

## *Management of Vesicoureteral Reflux*

Reflux will resolve spontaneously in some patients. It is more likely to resolve if it is low-grade, unilateral, and not associated with other anomalies. The grade of reflux is the most important factor. Over several years of observation reflux will resolve in approx 80% of patients with grade 1 or 2 reflux, 50% of patients with grade 3 reflux, and 25% of patients with grade 4 reflux. Because of this tendency to resolve, most patients with reflux are initially treated on an observation protocol. The mainstay of medical management is antibiotic prophylaxis. Because scarring usually occurs only with the reflux of infected urine, prevention of UTIs is essential. The most frequently used agents are nitrofurantoin (1–2 mg/kg) and trimethoprim/sulfamethoxazole liquid (0.25–0.5 cm$^3$/kg) in a once-daily dose. Cystograms are obtained annually, and chemoprophylaxis is discontinued when reflux resolves. Upper tract studies are obtained periodically as dictated by the patient's clinical course. Findings suggestive of detrusor instability should be sought and, if present, treatment with anticholinergic agents is initiated. Constipation should also be treated.

Any patient on observation who develops a breakthrough urinary tract infection or new renal scarring should undergo surgical correction of his/her reflux. Surgery is also appropriate in patients who cannot comply with close follow-up and long-term antibiotic prophylaxis. This would include patients who wish to avoid repeated cystograms and office visits. Patients with high-grade reflux may be considered for immediate surgical intervention.

Surgical treatment is usually done by ureteral reimplantation. Subtrigonal collagen injection therapy is an alternative for patients who require surgical intervention. Subtrigonal injection is an outpatient procedure in which collagen is injected endoscopically under the bladder mucosa at the ureteral orifice. Subtrigonal collagen injection corrects reflux in 60–70% of cases, although more than one injection is occasionally required.

Regardless of management, patients with renal scarring require life-long follow-up for the detection of hypertension, proteinuria, and deteriorating renal function (reflux nephropathy). In cases of unilateral reflux nephropathy with hypertension and a very poorly functioning kidney on the affected side, simple nephrectomy may be appropriate.

## *Recurrent UTIs*

Some children with no discernable anatomic anomaly develop recurrent UTIs. Many of these children present after toilet training, when normal reflex voiding is interfered with by social constraints. The risk of renal scarring in these patients is low, but not absent. Some of these children will have symptoms of bladder instability, such as urge incontinence or squatting behavior, in the absence of an infection. These voiding symptoms often respond to anticholinergic agents, such as oxybutynin chloride. Even when the symptoms are subtle, and not in themselves troublesome, recurrent infections can be prevented—or reduced in frequency—by anticholinergic therapy in conjunction with antibiotic prophylaxis. Constipation can predispose to bladder instability and recurrent UTIs, and therefore should be aggressively managed.

Even an anatomically and functionally normal urinary tract may be predisposed to recurrent infections. Certain host factors may play a role, such as antigen expression on the bladder epithelium. However, there is no specific therapy for these host factors, so children with frequent infections are managed with antibiotic prophylaxis administered in the same fashion as for patients with vesicoureteral reflux. However, in the absence of reflux, upper-tract monitoring and routine urine cultures are rarely indicated, as treatment of asymptomatic bacteriuria in this setting is unnecessary.

### *The Foreskin and Urinary-Tract Infections*

Routine neonatal circumcision has become more popular in the last decade because of recently described associations between an intact foreskin and infant UTI. This was best illustrated by a series of systematic studies by Wiswell and colleagues at US Army hospitals. In several large epidemiologic studies, they found that the incidence of significant UTIs in uncircumcised male infants <6 mo of age was 1–2%. The incidence in circumcised infants was only 0.1–0.2%.

Because of the data demonstrating an increased risk of UTI in uncircumcised infants, routine circumcision has been advocated by some authors, who point out that there is significant mortality and renal scarring associated with UTIs occurring in early infancy. However, circumcision is a permanent solution to a problem that only affects males in the first 6 mo of life. There may be alternative nonsurgical means for preventing these infections, and whether all boys should be circumcised to prevent infection in 1–2% remains debatable. It is also unclear whether circumcision would augment the benefit of antibiotic prophylaxis in boys with reflux or other urologic anomalies.

## HEMATURIA IN CHILDREN

Hematuria in children is usually more alarming for parents than it is significant for the child. Life-threatening causes of hematuria in children are rare, and are easily excluded with noninvasive studies. The differential diagnosis of hematuria in children is very different from that in adults, and the typical adult evaluation of an intravenous pyelogram and cystoscopy is rarely appropriate for children (*see* Fig. 3).

The initial step in evaluating hematuria in children is a careful history and physical examination. If signs or symptoms suggest a specific diagnosis, such as a urinary-tract infection, the appropriate confirmatory studies are obtained. However, in the absence of specific signs or symptoms, the first distinction to be made is between medical renal disease, such as glomerulonephritis, and "urologic" diseases. Patients suspected to have the former should be referred early to a pediatric nephrologist (before extensive urologic evaluation). Patients with "urologic" hematuria can be divided into those with microscopic (or mild gross) hematuria and those with troublesome gross hematuria.

Several nephrologic causes of hematuria are benign or untreatable, and several uncommon urologic causes require treatment only if they lead to significant bleeding. Therefore, patients with asymptomatic microscopic hematuria need only be evaluated for disorders that are treatable and pose a threat to their health. Once those disorders are excluded, no further evaluation is indicated, although a specific diagnosis may not have been reached. Patients with gross hematuria, for whom the amount of blood loss

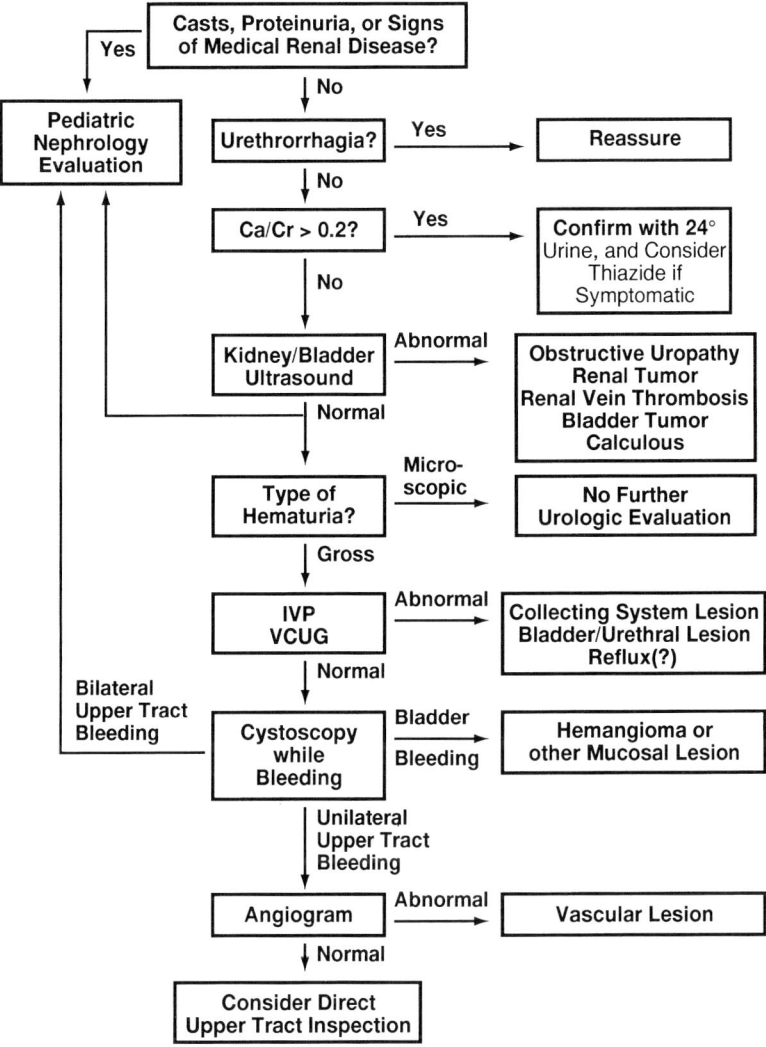

Fig. 3. Algorithm for evaluating hematuria in children.

is significant, may require invasive testing before a cause is found. This type of evaluation is justified in these patients only if the bleeding itself requires treatment.

### "Nephrologic" vs "Urologic" Hematuria

Most hematuria in children is "nephrologic." The distinction between "nephrologic" and "urologic" causes of hematuria is usually made at the initial clinical evaluation. A history of recent Streptococcal infection or systemic illness, a family history of hematuria, or a history of hemoglobinopathy suggest a nephrologic cause. Physical findings of edema (suggesting nephrotic syndrome) or a rash consistent with Henoch-Schöenlein purpura also indicate a nephrologic cause. The most important part of the initial evaluation is the urinalysis. The presence of significant proteinuria or red blood-cell casts mandates an evaluation by a pediatric nephrologist. In children with hematuria, it is essential to look at many microscopic fields of the urinalysis so that casts will be detected if present, and the patient will be spared an unnecessary urologic evaluation.

## *Causes That Can Be Detected by Noninvasive Means*

It is important to rule out serious disorders in children with hematuria. This can almost always be accomplished with a thorough physical examination (including a rectal exam), a urinalysis, and an ultrasound of the urinary tract. It is essential that the ultrasound include imaging of the kidneys, ureters, and bladder.

A "pink diaper" is a form of pseudohematuria, most often caused by precipitation of urates in acid urine as it cools to room temperature. A pink diaper may also be caused by production of red pigment by *Serratia marcescens*, the predominant bacterium in the intestinal tract of newborns. A urinalysis will confirm that the infant does not have true hematuria.

Urethrorrhagia is a benign idiopathic condition seen most often in peripubertal boys. The most frequent complaint is of blood-staining in the underwear. The bleeding is urethral, which can be confirmed by demonstrating significantly more blood in an initial-stream specimen than in a midstream specimen. If the remainder of the history and physical (including a rectal exam) is normal, then the family should be reassured. The disorder is self-limited, but may take months to resolve and is occasionally recurrent. The temptation to perform cystoscopy should be avoided, because the incidence of urethral stricture in these patients following instrumentation is high.

Hypercalcuria is a relatively common cause of hematuria in asymptomatic children without a urinary-tract infection or proteinuria. It may cause dysuria, suprapubic pain, or flank pain, but is often asymptomatic. It is more common in patients with a family history of stone disease. Hypercalcuria may be diagnosed by checking a spot urine for calcium/creatinine ratio (normal <0.2). Definitive diagnosis is made by demonstrating a urine calcium excretion rate of >4 mg/kg/24 h. Thiazide diuretics are prescribed for children with significant symptoms. Making the diagnosis in an asymptomatic patient reassures the family of a benign etiology for the hematuria, and identifies the patient as being at risk for developing renal calculi. Despite this risk of stone formation, routine treatment of asymptomatic patients with thiazides is not indicated. Conservative measures, including dietary modifications and increasing fluid intake, may be reasonable.

Patients with obstructive uropathy may present with hematuria, sometimes following unnoticed minor trauma. Patients with obstructive uropathy will have an abnormal ultrasound that suggests the diagnosis. Patients with posterior urethral valves may also have hematuria, although they usually have other symptoms that suggest the disorder. Most patients with valves will have an abnormal ultrasound with hydronephrosis, bladder-wall thickening, and/or a dilated posterior urethra.

Renal-vein thrombosis is a common cause of neonatal hematuria. It occurs in a setting of dehydration and/or polycythemia. In older children it may be associated with the nephrotic syndrome. Ultrasound will show an enlarged kidney, and a clot may be visualized in the renal vein.

Renal malignancies are rare in children. The most common is Wilms' tumor, although some cases of renal-cell carcinoma have been reported. Angiomyolipomas occur in the setting of tuberous sclerosis and may cause significant gross hematuria. All of these tumors may be diagnosed by ultrasound.

Malignant bladder tumors are extremely rare in children. Rhabdomyosarcoma of the bladder or prostate occurs most commonly in children under 5 yr of age. The tumors are often palpable on bimanual exam and are evaluated initially with ultrasound. The diagnosis is confirmed by biopsy. Transitional-cell carcinoma has been reported in approx 120 patients under the age of 20 (most in their teens). More than 90% have hematuria, and these tumors can usually be seen on ultrasound, because they are almost universally low-grade, low-stage, papillary tumors. Leiomyosarcoma occurs in the wall of the bladder and gives an abnormal appearance on ultrasound. Benign bladder tumors, such as neurofibroma and pheochromocytoma can also be detected by ultrasound and usually occur in typical clinical settings.

Stone disease is uncommon in childhood. It occurs more frequently in neonates in the ICU, patients with a positive family history, and children with hypercalcuria. Although ultrasound is a good screening test for calculous disease, an intravenous pyelogram may be indicated in patients at high-risk for stones. Metabolic stone disease is more common in children than adults, but calcium stones are still the most common stones found in children.

### *Causes Requiring Invasive Methods for Detection*

Virtually all serious causes of hematuria in children can be detected by noninvasive means. The only indication to perform invasive studies is when gross hematuria is, in itself, a problem. This is a somewhat subjective determination. However, if a patient has frequent bright-red bleeding with clots, or if enough blood is being lost to cause anemia, then a definitive diagnosis must be reached. All of these patients require a nephrologic evaluation before invasive testing is initiated. Furthermore, although ultrasound in children is an excellent modality, an IVP and VCUG should be obtained prior to invasive studies. An IVP displays the anatomy of the collecting system better than an ultrasound, and may demonstrate subtle abnormalities to guide the invasive evaluation.

The treatable lesions to be considered include urothelial lesions, such as hemangiomas, and vascular lesions, such as arteriovenous malformations. If all noninvasive studies—including an IVP—are normal, then the next step is to perform cystoscopy during an episode of acute bleeding. This allows the source of the bleeding to be localized to the bladder or one of the upper tracts. If blood is seen coming from both orifices, a systemic or nephrologic cause should be reconsidered. Bladder lesions can usually be managed endoscopically. Bladder hemangiomas are well-managed with laser.

If blood is seen coming from a ureteral orifice, then the next step is an arteriogram of the affected kidney. This should rule out any vascular lesions, and, if one is found, it may be possible to manage it percutaneously. If angiography is normal, and significant bleeding persists, then visualization of the ureteral, renal pelvic, and calyceal urothelium may be indicated. How this is accomplished will depend, in part, on the experience and preference of the urologist. The options are ureteropyeloscopy from below, or percutaneous nephroscopy. In some patients, both procedures may be required before a lesion is found.

## SELECTED READING

### *Undescended Testicle*

Cendron M, Huff D, Keating MA, Snyder HM III, Duckett JW (1993) Anatomical, morphological and volumetric analysis: a review of 759 cases of testicular maldescent. *J Urol* 149:570–573.

Cisek LJ, Peters CA, Atala A, Bauer SB, Diamond DA, Retik AB (1998) Current findings in diagnostic laparoscopic evaluation of the nonpalpable testis. *J Urol* 160:1145–1149.

Hrebinko RL, Bellinger MF (1993) The Limited role of imaging techniques in managing children with undescended testes. *J Urol* 150:458–460.

Moore RG, Peters CA, Bauer SB, Mandell J, Retik AB (1994) Laparoscopic evaluation of the nonpalpable testis: a prospective assessment of accuracy. *J Urol* 151:728–731.

Rajfer J, Handelsman DJ, Swerdloff RS, Hurwitz R, Kaplan H, Vandergast T, Ehrlich RM (1986) Hormonal therapy of cryptorchidism. *N Engl J Med* 314:466–470.

Turek PJ, Ewalt DH, Snyder HM III, Stampfers D, Blyth B, Huff DS, Duckett JW (1994) The absent cryptorchid testis: surgical findings and their implications for diagnosis and etiology. *J Urol* 151:718–721.

## Scrotal Swelling

Kass EJ, Belman AB (1987) Reversal of testicular growth failure by varicocele ligation. *J Urol* 137:475, 476.

Kass EJ, Marcon B (1992) Results of varicocele surgery in adolescents: a comparison of techniques. *J Urol* 148:694–696.

Kemmotsu H, Oshima Y, Joe K, Mouri T (1998) The features of contralateral manifestations after the repair of unilateral inguinal hernia. *J Pediatr Surg* 33:1099–1103.

Podesta ML, Gottlieb S, Medel R, Jr, Ropelato G, Bergada C, Quesada EM (1994) Hormonal parameters and testicular volume in children and adolescents with unilateral varicocele: preoperative and postoperative findings. *J Urol* 152:794–797.

Skoog SJ, Conlin MJ (1995) Pediatric hernia and hydroceles. The urologist's perspective. *Urol Clin N Amer* 22:119–130.

## Penis Problems

Herzog IW, Alvarez SR (1986) The treatment of foreskin problems in uncircumcised children. *Am J Dis Child* 140:254–256.

Kaplan GW (1983) Complications of circumcision. *Urol Clin N Am* 10:543–549.

Ross J, Kay R (1997) Use of a deepithelialized skin flap in hypospadias repairs accomplished by tubularization of the incised urethral plate. *Urology* 50:110–112.

## Voiding Dysfunction

Koff SA, Byard M (1998) The daytime urinary frequency syndrome of childhood. *J Urol* 140:1280, 1281.

Loening-Baucke V (1997) Urinary incontinence and urinary tract infection and their resolution with treatment of chronic constipation of childhood. *Pediatr*, 100:228–232.

Monda JM, Husmann DA (1995) Primary nocturnal enuresis: a comparison among observation, imipramine, desmopressin acetate and bed-wetting alarm systems. *J Urol* 154:745–748.

O'Regan S, Yazbeck S, Schick E (1985) Constipation, bladder instability, urinary tract infection syndrome. *Clin Nephrol* 23:152–154.

## Urinary-Tract Infections

Blane CE, ct al. (1993) Renal sonography is not a reliable screening examination for vesicoureteral reflux. *J Urol* 150:752.

Koff S (1992) Relationship between dysfunctional voiding and reflux. *J Urol* 148:1703.

Lebowitz RL (1992) The detection and characterization of vesicoureteral reflux in the child. *J Urol* 148:1640.

Rushton H, et al. (1992) Dimercaptosuccinic acid renal scintigraphy for the evaluation of pyelonephritis and scarring: a review of experimental and clinical studies. *J Urol* 148:1726.

Weiss R, et al. (1992) Results of a randomized clinical trial of medical versus surgical management of infants and children with grades III and IV primary vesicoureteral reflux (US). *J Urol* 148:1667.

Wiswell TE, Hatchey WE (1993) Urinary tract infections and the uncircumcised state: an update. *Clin Pediatr* 32:130–134.

## Hematuria in Children

Baumgardner DJ (1990) The infant with a reddish diaper. *Postgrad Med* 88:199–202.

Kaplan GW, Brock WA (1982) Idiopathic urethrorrhagia in boys. *J Urol* 128:1001.

Leonard MP, Neckel JC, Morales A (1988) Cavernous hemangiomas of the bladder in the pediatric age group. *J Urol* 140:1503, 1504.

Lieu TA, Grasmeder HM III, Kaplan BS (1991) An approach to the evaluation and treatment of microscopic hematuria. *Pediatr Clin N Am* 38:579–592.

Stapleton FB (1990) Idiopathic hypercalcuria: association with isolated hematuria and risk for urolithiasis in children. *Kidney Int* 37:807–811.

# INDEX

**A**

Abdomen, examination of, 83
Abdominal ultrasound probe, 97f
Abscess, 329
Access, 11
   patient expectations, 10
Accounting software, 50
ACD, 311–313, 312f–313f
ACE inhibitors, 170
Acetohydramic acid, 494
Acupuncture, female urge incontinence and, 447
Acute bacterial prostatitis, 115t
Acute scrotum, 355–367
   differential diagnosis, 359–367
   laboratory evaluation, 357
   medical history, 355–356
   physical examination, 356–357
   radiologic evaluation, 357
   ultrasound, 357–358
Acyclovir, HSV and, 123
Adjunctive hormonal therapy, prostate cancer and, 297–298
Adolescents, varioceles in, 499–500
ADPKD, 477
Adrenal antiandrogens, prostate cancer and, 298
Adriamycin, toxicity of, 186
Advanced information systems, 45–53
   accounting software, 50
   appointment scheduling, 51
   benchmarking, 52
   benefits, 50–52
   billing, 49
   clinical protocols, 52
   competing, 46–47
   consensus, 52
   consultants, 53
   electronic time clock, 50
   e-mail, 49
   EMRs, 49
   future, 47–50
   imaging software, 49
   implementation, 52–53
   network-based fax, 49
   operating system, 48
   reporting capabilities, 51–52
AIP, 117t
Albarran bridge, 89–90, 90f
Alcohol
   IC, 135
   male infertility, 383
Alcohol abuse, ED and, 347
Allergic contact dermatitis (ACD), 311–313
Alpha-adrenergic agonists
   female SUI, 433, 433t
   geriatric stress incontinence, 463
Alpha-adrenergic blockers
   BPH, 228–231, 233–234
   ED, 349–350
   genital pain, 373
5-alpha-reductase inhibitors, BPH and, 231–233
Alprostadil, ED and, 350
Ambulatory surgical centers, safe harbor and, 61
American Urological Association Index
   BPH, 227f
   LUTS, 218
Anabolic steroids, male infertility and, 383
Androgen blockade, intermittent, prostate cancer and, 297
Androgens, 292
Anesthesia, local, elective sterilization and, 397
Anesthetic blocks, local, genital pain and, 374
Angioedema, 318
Angiography
   RCC, 157f
   renal mass, 149–150
Angiokeratoma corporis diffusum, 308
Angiokeratomas of Fordyce, 308, 309f
Angiomyolipomas, 508
Angiotensin-converting enzyme (ACE) inhibitors, 170
Anorchia, 497
Antiandrogens, prostate cancer and, 298
Anticholinergics, female urge incontinence and, 443–444, 444t
Anticoagulants, 478
Antidepressants, IC and, 136–137
Aphthous ulcers, 323

Apocrine hydrocystomas, 308
Apomorphine, ED and, 349–350
Appointment scheduling, advanced information systems for, 51
Arteriovenous fistula, 479
Associations, public speaking and, 20
Asymptomatic inflammatory prostatitis (AIP), 117t
Atrophic urethritis, geriatric incontinence and, 457–458
Audience for public speaking, 20–22
Augmentation cytoplasty, female urge incontinence and, 447–448, 447f
Autologous fat, 435
Autologous slings, female SUI and, 439–441
Autosomal dominant polycystic kidney disease (ADPKD), 477
Azithromycin
    chancroid, 125
    chlamydia trachomatis, 123
    gonorrhea, 125
    mollicutes, 127

## B

Bacillus Calmette-Guerin (BCG)
    bladder cancer progression, 197
    CIS, 197
    dose reduction trials, 199t
    failures, options for, 200–201
    IC, 138
    optimization, 197–198
    prophylaxis, for bladder cancer, 194
    toxicity, 186, 198–199
    tumor recurrence, 196t
    urothelial cancer, 179–180
Bacterial vaginosis, 127–128
Bactrim, fixed drug eruptions and, 318f
Balanitis circinata, 314
Balanitis circumscripta plasmacellularis, 317
Balanitis xerotica obliterans, 309–310
Balanoposthitis, 311, 312f, 328–329
    children, 500
Balantitis, 311
Basal-cell carcinoma (BCC), 336–337
BCC, 336–337
BCG. *See* Bacillus Calmette-Guerin
BCGosis, 198–200
Behavioral modification, female urge incontinence and, 445–446
Behavioral therapy, female SUI and, 434–435
Behcet's disease, 323–324, 324f
Benchmarking, advanced information systems for, 52

Benefits, 5
Benign familial pemphigus, 322–323
Benign hematuria, 480
Benign prostatic hyperplasia (BPH), 215, 416
    alpha-blockers, 228–231, 233–234
    5-alpha-reductase inhibitors, 231–233
    high-intensity focused ultrasound, 249
    ILC, 244–247
    medical therapy
        efficacy vs. effectiveness, 226–228
        monitoring, 225–226
    minimally invasive therapy, 239
    phytotherapy, 234
    prostatic urethral stents, 249–251
    thermal damage, 238–239
    transurethral balloon dilation, 251
    transurethral needle ablation, 247–248
    TUMT, 239–244
Benzthiazide penicillin-G, syphilis and, 124
Berger's disease, 479–480
Bethanechol, overflow incontinence and, 449
Bilateral orchiectomy, prostate cancer and, 293
Billing. *See also* Coding
    advanced information systems, 49
    fraud and abuse, 43–44
    methodology, 34
    third-party payers, 42–43
Bill stuffers, 23
Biofeedback
    female SUI, 435
    female urge incontinence, 445–446
    office-based unit, 100f
    urinary stress incontinence, 99–100
Biopsy
    needle, prostate cancer and, 260–261
    percutaneous, renal mass and, 160–161
    prostatic needle, 99
    transrectal needle, prostate and, 99
    TRUS, efficacy of, 269–270
    urothelial cancer, 177–178
Bladder
    examination, 83
    instability, and children, 501
    ultrasound, 94f, 95
Bladder cancer
    chemotherapy, 205–206
    intravesical therapy. *See* Intravesical therapy
    radiation therapy, 205–206
    radical cystectomy, 204
    risk assessment, 186, 187t
Bladder compliance, 412–413

Bladder diary, 410
  geriatric incontinence, 458–459, 459f
Bladder-neck obstruction, 416
Bladder-outlet obstruction, uroflowmetry and, 100, 101f
Bladder training, female urge incontinence and, 445–446
Bleeding disorders, 478
Bonuses, 5
Bosniak classification of cystic renal masses, 150, 151f–152f
Bougies, 92, 93f
Bowenoid papulosis, 336, 337f
BPH. *See* Benign prostatic hyperplasia
Brown bag presentations, 22
Bullous pemphigoid, 321
Bundling
  procedural coding, 41–42
  third-party payers, 43
Buschke-Lowenstein tumor, 335–336, 336f
Business process, associated costs of, 47

## C

CAB, prostate cancer and, 296
Cadaveric fascia lata, female SUI and, 441
Caffeine, IC and, 135
Calcium-channel blockers, male infertility and, 383
Calcium glycerophosphate, IC and, 135
Calcium nephrolithiasis
  idiopathic, 489–490
  risk factors, 484t
Calcium oxalate crystals, urinalysis for, 87
Calcium stones, recurrent, 484–490
Calculi. *See* Stones
CAM, 419
*Candida albicans*, 128
*Candida intertrigo*, 326, 326f
Capillary hemangiomas, 331–332, 332f
Captopril, 493
Carbonate-apatite, 493
Carcinoma *in situ* (CIS)
  BCG, 197
  radical cystectomy, 204–205
  voiding symptoms, 176
Casts, urinalysis and, 86
Catheters, 93–95, 94f
  Foley, 93, 449
  intravesical therapy, 189
  nonretention, 93, 94f
Cautery unit, self-contained, 98f
CAVD, 386

CBAVD, 386
Cefixime, gonorrhea and, 125
Ceftriaxone
  chancroid, 125
  gonorrhea, 125
  syphilis, 124
Cellulitis, 327
Cephalosporin, gonorrhea and, 125
Cerebrovascular accident, 415
Chancroid, 125
Children
  bladder instability, 501
  hematuria, 506–509, 507f
  nocturnal enuresis, 501–502
  penis problems, 500–501
  scrotal swelling, 498–500
  undescended testicles, 495–498
  urinary frequency syndrome, 501–502
  UTIs, 502–506
  voiding dysfunction, 501–502
*Chlamydia trachomatis*, 121, 123, 124
Chlorpactin, IC and, 138
Chronic bacterial prostatitis, 116t
Chronic pain syndrome, 376
Chronic pelvic pain syndrome
  inflammatory, 116t
  noninflammatory, 116t
Chronic unilateral hematuria, 477
Cicatricial pemphigoid, 321, 321f
Ciprofloxacin
  chancroid, 125
  gonorrhea, 125
Circumcision, complications from, 500
CIS
  BCG, 197
  radical cystectomy, 204–205
  voiding symptoms, 176
Clean-intermittent catheterization, overflow incontinence and, 449
Clindamycin, bacterial vaginosis and, 128
Clinical decision making, EMRs and, 47–48
Clinical laboratory services, fraud alerts and, 62
Clinically advanced prostate cancer, hormone ablation therapy for, 286–287
Clinically localized prostate cancer
  cryotherapy, 286
  external-beam radiation therapy, 282–285
  interstitial radioactive seed implants, 285–286
  observation, 278–280
  radical prostatectomy, 280–282
Clinical protocols
  advanced information systems, 52
  EMRs, 47–48

Coagulation necrosis, BPH and, 238
Coding, materials, 34. *See also* E/M coding
Coding system, 34–35
Colectomy, total, male infertility and, 384
Collagen, 428–429, 435, 464–465
Color-coded prescription pads, 267
Color Doppler ultrasound, acute scrotum and, 357–358
Combined androgen blockade (CAB) prostate cancer, 296
Communication
  referrals, 28–30
  staff, 12
Computed tomography (CT)
  hematuria, 476
  RCC, 156f, 158
  renal mass, 149
Computers. *See* Advanced information systems
Conduits, 208
*Condylomata acuminata*, 126
Confidentiality, 11
Confirmatory consults, E/M coding and, 36
Conflict, ED and, 346
Congenital absence of the vas deferens (CAVD), 386
Congenital bilateral absence of the vas deferens (CBAVD), 386
Consensus, advanced information systems and, 52
Constipation, geriatric incontinence and, 458
Consultants, advanced information systems and, 53
Consults
  CPT criteria, 35
  E/M coding, 35–36
  exception, E/M coding and, 36
  Medicare criteria, 35
  third-party payers, 43
Continent cutaneous urinary diversion, 209
Continuous ambulatory monitoring (CAM), 419
Conversion factor, third-party payers and, 42–43
Cooperative hospital organizations, safe harbor and, 61
Corporate practice of medicine, 55
*Corynebacterium minutissimum*, 328
*Corynebacterium tenuis*, 328
Costs
  business process, 47
  fixed, 45
  patient expectations, 10
  reduction, 50

Coumarin, skin necrosis and, 318
Counseling, elective sterilization and, 396
CPT
  consults, 35
  E/M global, 40
Crab louse, 330–331, 331f
Crohn's disease, 325
Cryoglobulinemia, 325
Cryotherapy
  clinically localized prostate cancer, 286
  genital warts, 126–127
Cryptorchidism, male infertility and, 383–384
CT
  hematuria, 476
  RCC, 156f, 158
  renal mass, 149
Current Procedural Terminology (CPT)
  consults, 35
  E/M global, 40
Cystectomy
  elderly, 208
  evaluation, 206–207
  indications, 204–205
  nonsurgical alternatives, 205–206
  preoperative assessment, 207–208
  preoperative education, 210–211
  radical, 204–205
  surgical clearance, 207–208
Cystectomy patient, laboratory evaluation of, 206–207
Cystic renal masses, 150
Cystine, solubility of, 492f
Cystine crystals, urinalysis and, 87
Cystine stones, 491–493
Cystitis, 106
Cystogram, nuclear, 504–505
Cystometry, 100, 411–416
  IC, 134
  methods, 413–415
  terminology, 411–412, 412t
Cystoscopes, 89–90, 90f
Cysts, 308
Cytoplasty, augmentation of, female urge incontinence and, 447–448, 447f

# D

DDAVP (1-Desaminocystine 8-D-Argininevasopressin), female urge incontinence and, 445
De minimis compensation, Self-Referral statute and, 71
Depression, ED and, 346

Dermatitis, penis and, 311
1-Desaminocystine 8-D-Argininevasopressin (DDAVP), female urge incontinence and, 445
Desmopressin acetate, 502
Detrol, female urge incontinence and, 444
Detrusor hyperreflexia, 418–419, 446
Detrusor instability (DI), 221
Diabetic neurogenic bladder, 416
Diet, modification of, and IC, 135, 135t
Digital rectal examination (DRE), LUTS and, 216–217
Dimethyl sulfoxide (DMSO), IC and, 137
Discipline, of employees, 10
Discounts, safe harbor and, 60
Ditropan, adverse effects of, 443–444
DMSO, IC and, 137
Document templates, 47
Doxazosin, BPH and, 228–230
Doxorubicin, toxicity of, 186
Doxycycline
    lymphogranuloma venereum, 124
    mollicutes, 127
D-pcn, 493
D-penicillamine (D-pcn), 493
DRE, LUTS and, 216–217
Drug eruptions, fixed, 317–318, 318f
Drug-induced geriatric incontinence, 456–457
Drug instillation, intravesical therapy and, 189
Drug reactions, 317–318
Drug representatives, referrals from, 30–31

**E**

EB, 322–323
ED. *See* Erectile dysfunction
Editing, of lay articles, 18
Education, referrals and, 30
Educational materials, practice efficiency of, 27
Elderly, cystectomy and, 208
Elective sterilization, 395–402
    complications, 401–402
    counseling, 396
    evaluation, 396
    local anesthesia, 397
    patient selection, 395
    postoperative care, 400–401
    vas delivery and occlusions, 397–400
Electrical stimulation, female urge incontinence and, 446
Electronic medical records (EMRs), 49
    accuracy, 50–51
    clinical decision making, 47–48
    clinical protocols, 47–48

Electronic order forms, 51
Elmiron, IC and, 136
EM, 320
E-mail, 49
E/M coding, 35–42
    category, 35–36
        consults, 35–36
    E/M global, 39–40
    established patients, 37–38
    level, 36–39
        history, 37–39
        medical decision-making, 38–39
        physical examination, 38
        time vs. components, 39
    methodology, 36
    new patients, 37–38
    procedural, 41–42
E/M global, 39–40
    CPT, 40
    Medicare, 40
    modifiers, 40
EMLA cream, 500
EM major, 320
Employees
    discipline, 10
    hiring, 7–8
    hospital, referrals and, 30
    interviewing, 7–8
    orientation, 8–10
    performance appraisal, 9–10
    productivity, 45–46
    recognition, 13
    recruiting, 7
    salaries, safe harbor and, 59
    supervision, 9–10
    termination, 5, 10
    training, 8–10
Employment policies, 5
EMRs, 49
    accuracy, 50–51
    clinical decision making, 47–48
    clinical protocols, 47–48
Endocrine therapy, prostate cancer and, 291–299
Enterostomal therapy (ET) nurse, 211
Enuresis, nocturnal, 501–502
Environment, 11
    patient expectations, 10
Epidermal inclusion cysts, 308
    scrotum, 308f
Epidermolysis bullosa (EB), 322–323
Epididymectomy, 374
Epididymitis, 361–362

Equipment rental, Self-Referral statute and, 68
Erectile dysfunction (ED), 343–351
  associated disorders, 346–348
  laboratory studies, 346
  medical history, 345
  physical examination, 345–346
  psychogenic, 347–348
  radical prostatectomy, 282
  sexual history, 345
  treatment, 348–351, 349f, 349t
  urological history, 81, 83t
  vascular surgery, 351
Erysipelas, 327
Erythema multiforme (EM), 320
Erythema multiforme (EM) major, 320
Erythrasma, 328, 328f
Erythrocytes, urinalysis and, 86
Erythromycin
  chancroid, 125
  chlamydia trachomatis, 123
  lymphogranuloma venereum, 124
  mollicutes, 127
Erythroplasia of Queryrat, 333–334, 334f–335f
ESPRC, 256
Established patients
  E/M coding
    history, 37–38
    physical examination, 38
Estrogen, 292
  female SUI, 434
  prostate cancer, 293–294
ET nurse, 211
European Randomized Study of Prostate Cancer (ESPRC), 256
Exercise, hematuria and, 479
Existing patients
  marketing, 22–25
    educating, 22–23
    networking, 24–25
    newsletters, 23–24
    value-added services, 23
External-beam radiation therapy
  BCG failures, 201
  clinically localized prostate cancer, 282–285
Extramammary Paget's disease, 337–339, 338f
Extravaginal torsion, 359

# F

Fabry's disease, 308
Factitial ulcers, 325
Fair market value, 68, 71
Fax, 49

Federal Anti-Kickback Statute, 58–63
  advisory opinions, 62–63
  fraud alerts, 61–62
  Safe Harbor regulations, 59–61
Federal discrimination laws, and interviewing, 7–8
Federal Physician "Self-Referral" Statute, 63–73
  advisory opinions, 71
  compliance, 72–73
  legislative history, 63
  penalties and sanctions, 71–72
  reporting requirements, 71
  statutory exceptions, 65–71
Female genitals, examination of, 84–85
Female incontinence, 417–429
  assessment, 420–422, 421f
  motor-urge incontinence, 420
  stress incontinence, 422–427
  surgery, 427–429
  symptoms, 418
  urge incontinence, 418–419
Female mixed stress and urge incontinence, 448
Female overflow incontinence, 448–449
Female "self cath" catheters, 94f
Female urge incontinence, treatment of, 441–448
Female urinary incontinence, 431–450
  treatment, 432–448
    mixed stress and urge incontinence, 448
    overflow incontinence, 448–449
    SUI, 432–441
    urge incontinence, 441–449
Filiform, 92, 93f
Filling cystometry, LUTS and, 221
Finasteride
  BPH, 231–234
  side effects, 232–233
Fixed costs, 45
Fixed drug eruptions, 317–318, 318f
Flags, 50–51
Flexible cystoscopy, 118
Flexible fiberoptic cystoscopes, 90, 91f
Flexible foreign-body forceps, 90, 91f
Fluconazole, vulvovaginal candidiasis and, 129
Fluid management, geriatric incontinence and, 461
Fluoroquinolones, UTIs and, 110
5-fluorouracil (5-FU), genital warts and, 126–127
Fluoxetine hydrochloride, IC and, 137
Foley catheters, 93, 449
Follicle stimulating hormone (FSH), 388

# Index

Follicular occlusion triad, 329–330
Folliculitis, 329
Followers, 92, 93f
Followup consults, E/M coding and, 36
Foods, avoidance of, IC and, 135, 135t
Foreskin, and UTIs in children, 506
Foscarnet, adverse effects of, 318
Fournier's gangrene, 327–328, 367
Fraud alerts, 61–62
Fraud and abuse, billing and, 43–44
FSH, 388
5-FU, genital warts and, 126–127
Furuncle, 329

## G

Genital pain, 369–379
    causes, 370
    defined, 371
    evaluation, 372–373
    local anesthetic blocks, 374
    medical therapy, 373–374
    multidisciplinary approach, 377–379
    neuromuscular pelvic-floor dysfunction, 376–377
    psychological factors, 375–376
    scrotum innervation, 371–372
    stress, 376t
    surgery, 374–375
    testicular innervation, 371–372
Genitals, examination of, 84–85
Genital ulcer disease, 128t
Genital warts, 126–127
Genitourinary system
    segmental innervation, 409t
Geriatric functional incontinence, 454
Geriatric incontinence, 453–465
    behavioral therapy, 461–463
    bladder diary, 458–459, 459f
    drug-induced, 456–457
    endocrine causes, 458
    epidemiology, 453
    evaluation, 455–460
    laboratory testing, 460
    medical history, 455–456
    physical examination, 459
    presentation, 453–455
    psychological factors, 458
    PVR, 459–460
    transient causes, 456–458, 457t
    treatment, 460–465
    urodynamic testing, 460
Geriatric mixed incontinence, 454–455
Geriatric overflow incontinence, 454
Geriatric stress incontinence, 453–454
Geriatric urge incontinence, 454
Glans, tattoo on, 319, 319f
Global, procedural coding and, 41
Glomerular hematuria
    evaluation, 471f
    glomerular disorders, 471t
Glucocorticoids, prostate cancer and, 298
Glucosuria, 86
GnRH, 388
Gonadal venography, 497
Gonadotoxins, male infertility and, 382–384, 383t
Gonadotropin-releasing hormone (GnRH), 388
Gonorrhea, 124–125
Group practice investments, safe harbor and, 61
Group purchasing organizations, safe harbor and, 60

## H

*Haemophilus ducreyi*, 125
Hailey-Hailey disease, 322–323, 323f
HCFA compliance plan, billing and, 44
HCG stimulation test, 497
Health benefits, 5
Health-care regulatory compliance, 58–73
    Federal Anti-Kickback Statute, 58–63
    Federal Physician "Self-Referral" Statute, 63–73
*Health Exchange*, 24
Health Professionals Shortage Area, 60
Hematoma, 401
Hematospermia, urological history and, 78
Hematuria, 175–176, 469–481
    causes, 473t, 477–480
    characteristics, 472–474
    children, 506–509, 507f
        nephrologic vs. urologic, 507–508
    cytology, 476–477
    evaluation, 475–476
    glomerular, evaluation of, 471f
    glomerular disorders, 471t
    glomerular vs. nonglomerular, 469
    nonglomerular, evaluation of, 472f
    physical examination, 474–475
    urological history, 78, 78t
Hemophilia, 478
Henoch-Schonlein purpura, 366–367
Heparin, IC and, 138
Hernia, in children, 498
Hernia repair, male infertility and, 384

Herpes simplex virus (HSV)
  diagnosis, 122–123
  incidence, 121
  treatment, 123
Hidradenitis suppurativa, 329–330, 329f
HIFU, BPH and, 249
High-intensity focused ultrasound (HIFU), BPH and, 249
Hiring, of employees, 7–8
History, E/M coding and, 37–38
HIV, 478
Home health services, fraud alerts and, 62
Hormonal therapy, adjunctive, prostate cancer and, 297–298
Hormone ablation therapy, clinically advanced prostate cancer and, 286–287
Hormone replacement therapy, geriatric incontinence and, 460–461
Hospital-based physicians, fraud alerts and, 61
Hospital coinsurance waivers, safe harbor and, 60
Hospital employees, referrals for, 30
Hospital incentives, fraud alerts and, 62
HSV
  diagnosis, 122–123
  incidence, 121
  treatment, 123
Human immunodeficiency virus (HIV), 478
Hyaline casts, urinalysis and, 86
Hydrocele, 363–364
  children, 498
Hydrochlorothiazide, idiopathic hypercalciuria and, 486
Hydroxyzine, IC and, 137
Hyoscyamine, geriatric urge incontinence and, 464
Hypercalciuria, 508
  idiopathic, 484–486
Hyperoxaluria, 487
Hyperparathyroidism, 488
Hyperprolactinemia, ED and, 347
Hyperthermia, BPH and, 238
Hyperuricosuria, 487
Hypocalciuria, 485f
Hypocitraturia, 486–487
Hypogonadism, ED and, 346–347
Hypospadias, 500–501

I

IC. *See* Interstitial cystitis
ICD-9, Medicare and, 40
Idiopathic calcium nephrolithiasis, 489–490
Idiopathic hypercalciuria, 484–486

IgA nephropathy, 479–480
ILC. *See* Interstitial laser coagulation
Illicit drug use, ED and, 347
Imaging software, 49
Imipramine
  geriatric stress incontinence, 463–464
  geriatric urge incontinence, 464
  nocturnal enuresis, 502
In-111 capromab pendetide, 262
Incontinence
  female. *See* Female incontinence
  geriatric. *See* Geriatric incontinence
  prostatectomy, 416
  stress. *See* Stress incontinence
  urinary. *See* Urinary incontinence
Indigo 830e Diode Laser System, 245
Indwelling Foley catheter, overflow incontinence and, 449
Infection, geriatric incontinence and, 457
Infection-related stones, pathophysiology of, 493f
Infection-related (struvite) calculi, 493–494
Infertility, male. *See* Male infertility
Infestations, 330–331
Inflammatory chronic pelvic pain syndrome, 116t
Inflammatory renal masses, 160
Inguinal hernia, 363–364
Injection therapy, female SUI and, 435
Inpatient consults, E/M coding and, 36
Interferon-alpha
  bladder cancer, 194
  toxicity, 186
Intermittent androgen blockade, prostate cancer and, 297
International Prostate Symptom Score (IPPS), 218, 219t, 239
Interstitial Cystitis Association, 135
Interstitial cystitis (IC), 131–140
  behavioral therapy, 136
  diagnosis, 132–135
  dietary modification, 135, 135t
  fluid management, 136
  intravesical agents, 137–138
  NIDDK research criteria, 132, 132t
  oral pharmacotherapy, 136–137
  pain management, 138–139
  physical therapy, 136
  surgery, 139–140
Interstitial laser coagulation (ILC)
  BPH, 239, 244–247
    adverse events, 247
    anesthesia, 246
    preoperative assessment, 244–246

results, 247
technique, 246
Interstitial radioactive seed implants, clinically localized prostate cancer and, 285–286
Interviews
employees, 7–8
radio, 19
television, 19
Intraurethral pharmacotherapy, ED and, 350
Intravaginal torsion, 359–361
Intravascular papillary endothelial hyperplasia, 332
Intravenous pyelography (IVP), urothelial cancer and, 176–177
Intravenous urography (IVU)
hematuria, 475
renal mass, 148–149, 155f
Intravesical therapy
bladder cancer, 185–201
BCG, 194–201
BCG prophylaxis, 194
chemotherapy crossover, 194
CIS, 193–194
efficacy, 190
financial aspects, 187–189, 189t
interferon-alpha, 194
optimization, 189–190
residual disease, 193, 197
toxicity, 186, 188t
tumor prophylaxis, 190–193, 192t
female urge incontinence, 446
toxicity, 186, 188t
Investigational agents, ED and, 349–350
Investments, safe harbor and, 59
Iowa needle trumpet, 99, 99f
IPPS, 218, 219t, 239
Irritant dermatitis, 313–314, 314f
IVP, urothelial cancer and, 176–177
IVU
hematuria, 475
renal mass, 148–149, 155f

## J

Job descriptions, 5–6
receptionist, sample, 5–6
Jock itch, 327
Joint ventures, fraud alerts and, 61

## K

Kaposi's sarcoma, 337, 338f
KCl instillation test, IC and, 134–135
Kidney, examination of, 83

## L

Lay articles, 16–19
editing, 18
query letters, 17–18
topic selection, 17
writing, 18
Leadership, 12–13
Lease agreements, safe harbor and, 59
Legal entity, medical practice as, 55–57
Lentigines, 319
Leukocytes, urinalysis and, 86
Leukocytospermia, 392
LH, 388
LHRH, prostate cancer and, 294–295, 296t
Lichen nitidus, 316–317, 316f
Lichen planus, 315–316, 316f
Lichen sclerosis, 309–310, 310f
Lichen sclerosis et atrophicus (LSA), 309–310, 310f–311f
Lidocaine/prilocaine emulsion (EMLA cream), 500
Limited liability company (LLC), 57
Lindane, scabies and, 127
LLC, 57
Local anesthesia, elective sterilization and, 397
Local anesthetic blocks, genital pain and, 374
Localized renal-cell carcinoma (RCC)
nephron-sparing surgery, 166–171, 166t
partial nephrectomy, 169t
radical nephrectomy, 165–166
Loops, 208
Lower urinary-tract localization studies, 117–118, 117t
Lower urinary-tract symptoms (LUTS)
causes, 216t
evaluation, 215–222
filling cystometry, 221
medical history, 216
physical examination, 216–217
postvoid residual urine, 221
pressure-flow study, 220–221
surgical indications, 220
symptoms, 218–220, 219t
upper urinary tract imaging, 221
urethrocystoscopy, 221
urodynamics, 220
uroflowmetry, 220
urological history, 79–80, 80t
LSA, 309–310, 310f–311f
Luteinizing hormone (LH), 388
Luteinizing hormone-releasing hormone agonists (LHRH), prostate cancer and, 294–295, 296t

LUTS. *See* Lower urinary-tract symptoms
Lymphangioma circumscriptum, 332, 333f
Lymphogranuloma venereum, 124

## M

Male genitals, examination of, 84
Male infertility, 381–394
    chemotherapy, 383
    gonadotoxins, 382–384, 383t
    medical history, 382
    physical examination, 384–385
    semen analysis, 386–388
    sperm function tests, 392–393, 393t
    systems review, 384
    varicocele, 385
    vas deferens absence, 385–386
Malpractice, 11
Malpractice insurance, obstetrical, subsidies for, 60–61
Managed care
    marketing, 31
    safe harbor, 60
Management contracts, safe harbor and, 59
Marijuana, male infertility and, 382–383
Marketing, 15–32
    benefits, 16
    effectiveness, 31–32
    existing patients, 22–25
    managed care, 31
    new patients, 16–22
    practice efficiency, 25–28
    referrals, 28–31
Masden Symptom Score, 239
Massachusetts male aging study (MMAS), 343
Masson's tumor, 332
Mearees/Stamey Four-Glass Test, 117t
Meatitis, 500
Median raphe cyst, 308
Medical decision-making, E/M coding and, 38–39
Medical practice, as a legal entity, 55–57
Medicare
    consults, 35
    E/M global, 40
    fraud and abuse, billing and, 43–44
    ICD-9, 40
Medullary sponge kidney (MSK), 389, 484
Melanocytic nevi, 319
Melanoma, 337
Melanotic macules, 318–319
Men. *See* Male
Metrogel, bacterial vaginosis and, 128

Metronidazole
    bacterial vaginosis, 128
    trichomoniasis, 126
Mitomycin
    BCG failures, 201
    CIS, 193
    urothelial cancer, 178–179
Mixed stress and urge incontinence, female, 448
MMAS, 343
Mobility impariment geriatric incontinence and, 458
Modifiers
    E/M global, 40
    third-party payers, 43
Moles, 319
Mollicutes, 127
Morphine, IC and, 139
Motor-urge incontinence, female, 420
MSK, 389, 484
Multiple procedural reductions, third-party payers and, 43
Multiple sclerosis, 416
Muscularis mucosae, 180–181
Musculotropics, female urge incontinence and, 443–444, 444t
MUSE, 350
Mutual funds, Self-Referral statute and, 67
*Mycoplasma genitalium*, 127
*Mycoplasma hominis*, 127

## N

Narcotics
    acetaminophen levels, 139t
    IC, 138–139
National Institute of Arthritis, Diabetes, Digestive and Kidney Diseases (NIDDK) research criteria, IC and, 132, 132t
National Institutes of Health Interstitial Cystitis Database Study, 132–133
Nd:YAG laser, BPH and, 244
Needle biopsy
    prostate cancer, 260–261
    transrectal, prostate and, 99
Needle suspension, female SUI and, 438
Neodymium yttrium-aluminum-garnet (Nd:YAG) laser, BPH and, 244
Neonatal scrotal masses, 498–500, 499f
Nephrectomy, RCC and, 165–171
Nephron-sparing surgery (NSS)
    RCC, 166–168, 166t
        follow-up, 168–171
        VHLD, 168

Network-based fax, 49
Networked information systems, 48, 53
Networking, with existing patients, 24–25
Neurogenic bladder, diabetic, 416
Neuromuscular pelvic-floor dysfunction, 376–377
New patients, 11
  attraction, 16–22
    lay articles, 16–19
    public speaking, 19–22
  E/M coding
    history, 37
    physical examination, 38
Newsletters, 23–24
  referrals, 30
NIDDK research criteria, IC and, 132, 132t
Nitrofurantoin
  bladder instability, 501
  male infertility, 383
  UTIs, 110, 503
Nocturnal enuresis, 501–502
Noncontinent urinary diversion, 208
Nonglomerular hematuria, evaluation of, 472f
Noninflammatory chronic pelvic pain syndrome, 116t
Nonrentention catheters, 93, 94f
"No-scalpel" instruments, 98f
NSS
  RCC, 166–168, 166t
    follow-up, 168–171
  VHLD, 168
Nuclear cystogram, 504–505
Nuclear orchiogram, acute scrotum and, 358–359
Nurses, referrals for, 30

## O

Observation, of clinically localized prostate cancer, 278–280
Obstetrical malpractice insurance, subsidies for, safe harbor and, 60–61
Office management, 3–13
  employee hiring, 7–8
  employee training, 8–10
  leadership, 12–13
  patient satisfaction, 10–12
  practice organization, 4–7
Office rental, Self-Referral statute and, 68
Office urodynamics, 407–416
  bladder diary, 410
  clinical assessment, 409
  cystometry, 411–416
    laboratory, 408
    physical examination, 409–410
    tests, 410–411
Ofloxacin
  chlamydia trachomatis, 123
  gonorrhea, 125
  mollicutes, 127
Oligospermia, semen analysis for, 390–391
Operating system, 48
Orchialgia, diagnosis of, 373t
Orchiectomy, 293, 375
Orchiogram, nuclear, acute scrotum and, 358–359
Orchitis, 361–362
Order forms, electronic, 51
Organizational chart, 5, 5f
Organizations, public speaking and, 20
Orientation, of employees, 8–10
Orthotopic neobladder, 209–210
Outpatient consults, E/M coding and, 35–36
Overflow incontinence, female, 448–449
Oxybutynin
  adverse effects, 443–444
  bladder instability, 501
  geriatric urge incontinence, 464
Oxycodone, IC and, 139
Oxycontin, IC and, 139

## P

Pain
  genital. See Genital pain
  IC, 138–139
  urological history, 78–79, 79t
Paraneoplastic pemphigus, 322, 322f
Paraphimosis, in children, 500
Parkinson's disease, 415
Partial nephrectomy, and RCC, postoperative surveillance of, 169t
Patient compliance, 11
Patient education
  bill stuffers, 23
  cystectomy, 210–211
  practitioner expertise, 22–23
  videos, do-it-yourself, 25–26
Patient expectations, 10
Patient networking, 24–25
Patient reception, standards for, 5
Patients
  established, 37–38
  follow-up, 12
  new. See New patients
  position, intravesical therapy and, 189–190
  referrals. See Referrals

Patient satisfaction, 10–12
  telephones, 11–12
Pearly penile papules, 307–308, 307f
Pediculosis pubis, 330–331
Pelvic examination, and the incontinent woman, 420–422, 421f
Pelvic-floor rehabilitation (PFR), 445–446
Pelvic muscle exercises, geriatric incontinence and, 462–463
Pemphigus, 321–323
Pemphigus foliaceus, 322
Pemphigus vegetans, 322
Pemphigus vulgaris, 321–322
Penile arterial revascularization, 351
Penile prosthesis implantation, 350
Penis
  bacterial infections, 327–330
  benign tumors, 331–332
  blistering disorders, 320–323
  children, 500–501
  cysts, 209
  dermatological conditions, 306t
  examination, 84
  hypopigmentation, 319–320
  inflammatory dermatoses, 311–313
  metastatic tumors, 339, 339f
  mycoticinfections, 326–327
  pigmented lesions, 318–320
  postinflammatory pigment changes, 319–320
  SCC, 332–334, 334f–333f
  ulcerative conditions, 323–325
  viral infections, 325–326
Pentosan polysulfate sodium (PPS), IC and, 136
Percutaneous biopsy, renal mass and, 160–161
Performance appraisals, 5, 9–10
Permethrin cream, scabies and, 127
Personal anecdotes, in speeches, 22
Personal service arrangements, Self-Referral statute and, 69
Personal service contracts, safe harbor and, 59
Personnel policies, 5
PFR, 445–446
Pharmaceutical representatives, referrals from, 30–31
Pharmacists, referrals from, 30
Phentolamine, ED and, 349–350
Phimosis, inchildren, 500
*Phthirus pubis*, 330–331, 331f
Physical examination, 82–85
  abdomen, 83
  cystectomy patient, 206
  E/M coding, 38
  genitals, 83–84
  IC, 133–134
  LUTS, 216–217
  prostate cancer, 257
  renal mass, 147–148
Physical therapy evaluation, genital pain and, 378
Physicians
  hospital-based, fraud alerts and, 61
  patient expectations, 10
Physician services, Self-Referral statute and, 65
Phytotherapy, BPH and, 234
Pink diaper, 508
PIVOT, 278
PKMB, 336
Plasma-cell balanitis, 317, 317f
PLCO screening trial, 256
PLESS, 228, 233
Pneumatruia, urological history and, 81
Podofilox, genital warts and, 126–127
Policy and procedure manual, 4
Position descriptions, 5–6
  receptionist, sample, 5–6
Posthitis, 311
Postvoid residual urine (PVR)
  geriatric incontinence, 459–460
  LUTS, 221
Potassium chloride (KCl) instillation test, IC and, 134–135
Potassium citrate
  hypocitraturia, 486
  RTA, 488
  uric acid stones, 491
PPMT, 117t
PPS, IC and, 136
Practice efficiency, 25–28
  color-coded prescription pads, 27
  educational materials, 27
  patient education videos, 26
Practice organization, 4–7
  job descriptions, 5–6
  organizational chart, 5, 5f
  personnel policies, 5
  policy and procedure manual, 4
  standards, 4–5
Practitioners, recruitment of
  safe harbor, 60
  Self-Referral statute, 70
Prazosin, BPH and, 230
Pre- and Post-massage Test (PPMT), 117t
PREDICT trial, 233
Preoperative education, for cystectomy, 210–211
Prepaid health plans, Self-Referral statute and, 67

Prescription medications, for ED, 347
Pressure-flow studies, 118
    LUTS, 220–221
Primary urethritis, 106
Privacy, 11
Probe
    abdominal ultrasound, 97f
    rectal, 96f
Probentheline, female urge incontinence and, 443–444
Procedural coding, 41–42
    bundling, 41–42
    global, 41
    specificity, 41
    third-party payers, 43
Proctitis, 122
Professional corporation, 56–57
Prolapse, 423–426, 424f–426f
Propantheline, geriatric urge incontinence and, 464
Props, for public speaking, 19
Proscar, BPH and, 231–233
Proscar Long-Term Efficacy and Safety Study (PLESS), 228, 233
Prostasoft 2.0 software, 242–243
Prostate
    biopsies, regions of, 270f
    needle biopsy, 99
    normal, ultrasonographic characteristics of, 266–268, 267f–268f
    ultrasound, 95, 95f–96f
    urethral stents, BPH and, 249–251
Prostate, Lung, Colorectal, Ovarian (PLCO) screening trial, 256
Prostate cancer
    adjunctive hormonal therapy, 297–298
    bilateral orchiectomy, 293
    CAB, 296
    clinically advanced, hormone ablation therapy and, 286–287
    clinically localized. See Clinically localized prostate cancer
    clinical staging, 261–262
    diagnosis, 256–262
    endocrine therapy, 291–299
        early vs. delayed, 297
    endocrinology, 291–292
    estrogens, 293–294
    hormone therapy, second line, 298
    intermittent androgen blockade, 297
    LHRH, 294–295, 296t
    management algorithm, 299t
    medical history, 256–257
    needle biopsy, 260–261
    physical examination, 257
    PSA testing, 257
    PSA velocity, 257–258
    RIS, 262
    screening, 255–256, 258f
    TRUS, 260–261
Prostate Cancer Intervention Versus Observation Trial (PIVOT), 278
Prostatectomy, adjunctive hormonal therapy and, 297
Prostatectomy incontinence, 416
Prostate gland, examination of, 84
Prostatic-specific antigen (PSA)
    age-specific range, 258
    density, 258
    free, 258–259
    LUTS, 217
    screening, 255–256
    testing, 257
    velocity, 257–258
Prostatitis, 113–120
    classification, 114–115, 115t
    diagnosis, 114–117
        clinical, 115–117
    etiology, 113–114
    lower urinary-tract localization studies, 117–118, 117t
    pathogenesis, 113–114
    prevalence, 113
    treatment, 118–120
Prostatodynia, 373
Prostatron, 240
Protocols, clinical, advanced information systems and, 52
Providers, patient expectations of, 10
Prozac, IC and, 137
PSA. See Prostatic-specific antigen
Pseudoephedrine, geriatric stress incontinence and, 463
Pseudoepitheliomatous keratotic and micaceous balanitis (PKMB), 336
Pseudohematuria, 472
*Pseudomonas aeruginosa*, 328
Psoriasis, 314–315, 315f
Psychological evaluation, genital pain and, 378
Public speaking, 19–22
    audience
        knowing, 20–21
        selection, 20
    preparation, 21–22
    props, 19

Pubovaginal sling
    female mixed stress and urge incontinence, 448
    female SUI, 438–439
PVR
    geriatric incontinence, 459–460
    LUTS, 221
Pyelonephritis, 106
Pyoderma gangrenosum, 324–325, 324f
Pyridoxine, hyperoxaluria and, 487

## Q

Quality of care, 10
Query letters
    lay articles, 17–18
    public speaking, 20

## R

RA, 484, 488, 488f
Radiation therapy
    bladder cancer, 205–206
    external-beam
        BCG failures, 201
        clinically localized prostate cancer, 282–285
Radical cystectomy
    bladder cancer, 204
    CIS, 204–205
    indications, 204–205, 205t
Radical nephrectomy, RCC and, 165–166
    follow-up, 168–171
    postoperative surveillance, 170t
Radical prostatectomy, clinically localized prostate cancer and, 280–282
Radio interviews, 19
Radioimmunoscintigraphy (RIS), prostate cancer and, 262
Radiotherapy, adjunctive hormonal therapy and, 297–298
RCC. See Renal-cell carcinoma
Receptionist
    job description, sample, 5–6
    telephone, 11
Recognition of employees, 13
Recruiting employees, 7
Rectal probe, 96f
Rectum, male, examination of, 84
Recurrent calcium stones, 484–490
Recurrent stone disease, 483
    metabolic evaluation, 484t
Recurrent urinary-tract infections (UTIs), 105–111
    evaluation, 108–109
    treatment, 109–110
Referrals
    communication, 28–30
    education, 30
    marketing, 28–31
    newsletters, 30
    nontraditional, 30–31
    safe harbor, 60, 61
Reiter's syndrome, 314
Relative values, third-party payers and, 42–43
Renal angiomyolipoma, 152–153, 153f
    vs. RCC, 153
Renal-cell carcinoma (RCC), 154–155
    angiography, 157f
    CT, 156f, 158
        vs. MRI, 158
    familial forms, 147
    localized, 165–168
    metastatic evaluation, 158–159
    MRI, 159f
    nephron-sparing surgery, 166–168, 166t
        follow-up, 168–171
    partial nephrectomy, postoperative surveillance of, 169t
    radical nephrectomy, 165–166
        follow-up, 168–171
        postoperative surveillance, 170t
    retroperitoneal lymph node, 157f
    signs and symptoms, 147t
    staging evaluation, 155, 158–159, 158t
Renal hyperfiltration
    dietary intervention, 170
    pharmacologic intervention, 170
Renal mass
    clinical evaluation, 146–148
    differential diagnosis, 145–146, 146t
    inflammatory, 160
    laboratory testing, 148
    MRI, 149, 158
    percutaneous biopsy, 160–161
    physical examination, 147–148
    radiographic evaluation, 148–150
    sonographic features, 156f
Renal oncocytoma, 154, 171
Renal tubular acidosis (RA), 484, 488, 488f
Renal ultrasound, 504
Renal-vein thrombosis, 508
Reports, advanced information systems and, 51–52
Resignation, 5
Retrograde pyelography, hematuria and, 476

Retropubic suspension, female SUI and, 438
Rhabdomyosarcoma, 509
Rigid cystoscopes, 89–90, 90f
RIS, prostate cancer and, 262
Robinson catheters, nonrentention of, 93, 94f

## S

Safe Harbor regulations, 59–61
Salaries, 5
    safe harbor, 59
*Sarcoptes scabiei*, 127, 330
Saw palmetto plant, 234
Scabies, 127, 330, 331f
SCC
    penis, 332–335, 334f–335f
    scrotum, 335
Scheduling
    staff, 12
    standards, 5
Sclerosing lymphangitis, 308, 309f
S corporations, 57
Scrotum
    acute. *See* Acute scrotum
    epidermal inclusion cysts, 308f
    examination, 84
    innervation, 371–372
    masses, neonatal, 498–500, 499f
    metastatic tumors, 339, 340
    SCC, 335
    swelling, in children, 498–500
Sebaceous hyperplasia, 332
Seborrheic keratoses, 332
Securities, Self-Referral statute and, 67
"Self cath" catheters, female, 94f
Semen
    analysis, 386–392
        concentration, 388
        hormonal evaluation, 388–390
        leukocytospermia, 392
        motility, 391–392
        oligospermia, 390–391
        teratozoospermia, 392
        volume, 386–388
    normal, 386t
Seminal-vesicle biopsies, 270
*Serenoa repens*, 234
Serotonin uptake inhibitors, IC and, 137
*Serratia marcescens*, 508
Sertraline hydrochloride, IC and, 137
Serum creatine, LUTS and, 217
Sextant biopsies, 270
Sex therapy, 347–348

Sexual intercourse, UTIs and, 107
Sexually transmitted disease, 121–129
    incidence, 121–122
Shingles, 325, 325f
Shock wave lithotripsy, 494
Sickle-cell disease, 478
Sildenafil citrate, ED and, 348–349
Silver nitrate, IC and, 138
Sleep disorders, ED and, 347
Slings, 438–441, 448
Smoking, ED and, 347
Sodium bicarbonate
    cystine stones, 492–493
    uric acid stones, 491
Sodium oxychlorosene, IC and, 138
Software, 49–50, 242–243
Sole proprietorship
    advantages, 56
    disadvantages, 55–56
Sonography, urothelial cancer and, 176
Sounds, 90–92, 92f
Specific gravity, of urine, 85
Spectinomycin, gonorrhea and, 125
Speeches. *See also* Public speaking
    celebrities, 22
    goals, 21
    historical figures, 22
    personal anecdotes, 22
    point of view, 21
    preparation, 21–22
Sperm
    function tests, 392–393, 393t
    granulomas, 401
    motility, 391–392
Spermatic cords, laparoscopic resection of, 374
Spermatocele, 364–365
Spinal cord injury, 415
Spring-loaded biopsy needle, 99, 99f
Squamous cell carcinoma (SCC)
    penis, 332–335, 334f–335f
    scrotum, 335
Squamous epithelial cells, urinalysis and, 86
Staff
    clerical vs. clinical, 12
    communication, 12
    productivity, 45–46
    scheduling, 12
Staff meetings, 4, 12–13
Staff retreats, 12
*Staphylococcus aureus*, 327
Stark law. *See* Federal Physician "Self-Referral" statute

Stat Operative Note, 29
Stents, urethral, BPH and, 249–251
Sterilization, elective. *See* Elective sterilization
Steroids, anabolic, male infertility and, 383
Stevens-Johnson syndrome, 320
Stones
    cystine, 491–493
    infection-related, 493–494
    recurrent, 483
        metabolic evaluation, 484t
    recurrent calcium, 484–490
    uric acid, 490–491
Stress incontinence, 416
    cystoceles, 426–427, 427f
    prolapse, 423–426, 424f–426f
    surgery, 427–428
    urodynamics, 419–420
    woman, 422–427
Stress urinary incontinence (SUI), 431–432
    female, treatment of, 432–441
Structured notes, 51
Struvite calculi, 493–494
SUI, 431–432
    female, treatment of, 432–441
Sulfasalazine, male infertility and, 383
Sulfisoxazole, lymphogranuloma venereum and, 124
Supervision, of employees, 9–10
Supplies, third-party payers and, 43
Support groups, 23
Swollen scrotum. *See* Acute scrotum
Synthetic slings, female SUI and, 439, 439t–440t
Syphilis, 124
    incidence, 121

**T**

Tamsulosin, BPH and, 230
Targis, 240–241, 243
Tattoo, on the glans, 319, 319f
TCA
    female SUI, 433–434
    female urge incontinence, 444–445
    IC, 136–137
Team work, 4
Telephone receptionist, 11
Telephones
    patient satisfaction, 11–12
    standards, 4–5
Television interviews, 19
TEN, 320–321
Teratozoospermia, 392
Terazosin, BPH and, 228–230
Termination of employees, 5, 10

Testicles
    appendages, torsion of, 362–363
    denervation, 374
    innervation, 371–372
    torsion, 359–367
    tumor, 366
    ultrasound, 96
Testosterone replacement therapy, 346–347
Thermotherapy, BPH and, 238–239
Thiazide, hypocitraturia and, 487
Thin basement membrane disease, 480
Thiotepa
    CIS, 193
    toxicity, 186
    urothelial cancer, 178–179
Third-party payers
    billing, 42–43
    conversion factor, 42–43
    relative values, 42–43
Time, reduction of, advanced information systems and, 50
Time management, 13
Time-off, 5
*Tinea cruris*, 327, 328
Titan Intraprostatic ASI Stent, 249–250
TMP/sulfa, UTIs and, 109–110, 503
Tobacco, male infertility and, 382–383
Tolterodine, female urge incontinence and, 444
Total colectomy, male infertility and, 384
Toxic Epidermal Necrolysis (TEN), 320–321
Training of employees, 8–10
Transabdominal ultrasound, 95, 97f
Transitional-cell cancer, 159–160, 509
    urinary bladder, incidence of, 175
Transitional cells, urinalysis and, 86
Transition-zone biopsy, 270
Transrectal needle biopsy, prostate and, 99
Transrectal ultrasound (TRUS)
    efficacy, 268
    LUTS, 216–217
    prostate cancer, 260–261
Transrectal ultrasound (TRUS)-guided biopsies
    complications, 272–274
    efficacy, 269–270
    patient preparation, 271
    procedure, 271–272
    repeat, 274
Transurethral balloon dilation, BPH and, 251
Transurethral laser-induced prostatectomy (TULIP), 244–245
Transurethral microwave thermotherapy (TUMT), BPH and, 239–244
    adverse effects, 243–244

anesthesia, 241–242
  patient selection, 241
  results, 242–243
Transurethral needle ablation (TUNA), BPH and, 239, 247–248
Transurethral resection of the bladder tumor (TURB), 190
  tumor recurrence, 195t
Transurethral resection (TUR), urothelial cancer and, 178
Trauma, 364–365
*Treponema pallidum*, 124
Triage, 12
*Trichomonas vaginalis*, 125
Trichomoniasis, 125–126
Trichomycosis, 328
*Trichophyton rubrum*, 327
Tricyclic antidepressants (TCA)
  female SUI, 433–434
  female urge incontinence, 444–445
  IC, 136–137
Trimethoprim/sulfamethoxazole (TMP/sulfa), UTIs and, 109–110, 503
TRUS, efficacy of, 268
TRUS-guided biopsies. See Transrectal ultrasound (TRUS)-guided biopsies
TULIP (transurethral laser-induced prostatectomy), 244–245
TUMT. *See* Transurethral microwave thermotherapy
TUNA, BPH and, 239, 247–248
TUR, urothelial cancer and, 178
TURB, 190
  tumor recurrence, 195t

## U

Ultrasonic bladder scanner, portable, 94f
Ultrasound, 94f–95f, 95–96
  acute scrotum, 357–358
  bladder, 94f, 95
  color Doppler, acute scrotum and, 357–358
  hematuria, 475
  high-intensity focused, BPH and, 249
  physics, 265–266
  prostate, 95, 95f–96f
  renal, 504
  renal mass, 149
  testicular, 96
  transabdominal, 95, 97f
  transrectal, LUTS and, 216–217
Ultrasound unit, office-based, 95f
Undescended testicles, 495–498
  impalpable, 497–498, 497f, 498

  medical history, 496
  palpable, 496–497
  physical examination, 496
Unix operating system, 48
Upper urinary tract imaging, LUTS and, 221
*Ureaplasma urealyticum*, 127
Ureter
  examination, 83
  reimplantation, 505
Urethra
  anesthesia, 97–99, 97f
  male, examination of, 84
  plugs, female SUI and, 436–437
  stents, for prostate, BPH and, 249–251
Urethral
  catheters, 93, 95
  discharge, urological history of, 81
Urethritis
  atrophic, geriatric incontinence and, 457–458
  primary, 106
Urethrocystoscopy, LUTS and, 221
Urethrolysis, overflow incontinence and, 449
Urethrorrhagia, 508
Urge incontinence
  female, treatment for, 441–448
  incontinent woman, 418–419
Uric acid, solubility of, 490f
Uric acid stones, 490–491
Urinalysis, 85–87
  chemical testing, 85–86
  LUTS, 217
  microscopic examination, 86–87
Urinary bladder, and transitional-cell cancer, incidence of, 175
Urinary crystals, urinalysis and, 87
Urinary diversion
  female urge incontinence, 448
  noncontinent, 208
  patient selection, 208–210
Urinary frequency syndrome, in children, 501–502
Urinary incontinence
  defined, 431
  female. See Female urinary incontinence
  radical prostatectomy, 282
  types, 431–432, 432t
  urological history, 81, 82t
Urinary stress incontinence, biofeedback and, 99–100
Urinary-tract infections (UTIs)
  children, 502–506
    diagnosis, 503
    foreskin, 506

radiographic evaluation, 504–505
   recurrent, 505–506
   treatment, 503–504
   vesicoureteral reflux, 505
classification, 106
diagnosis, 107
epidemiology, 105–106
incidence, 105
pathogenesis, 107–108
recurrent, 105–111
   evaluation, 108–109
   treatment, 109–110
sexual intercourse, 107
Urine
   culture, 177
   cytology, 177
   microscopic examination, 86
   specific gravity, 85
Urodynamic instrumentation, 100
Urodynamics
   laboratory, 408
   LUTS, 220
   terminology, 407–408, 408t
Uroflowmetry, 413–415, 414t–415t
   bladder-outlet obstruction, 100, 101f
   LUTS, 220
Urological history, 77–82
   erectile dysfunction, 81, 83t
   hematospermia, 78
   hematuria, 78, 78t
   lower urinary-tract symptoms, 79–80, 80t
   pain, 78–79, 79t
   past medical history, 81–82
   pneumatruria, 81
   urethral discharge, 81
   urinary incontinence, 81, 82t
UroLume Wallstent, 249–250
Urothelial cancer
   clinical presentation, 175–176
   office evaluation, 176–181
   tumor recurrence, 178
Urothelial carcinoma, recurrent, 477–478
UTI. *See* Urinary-tract infections

## V

Vacum constriction devices (VCDs), ED and, 350
Valacyclovir, HSV and, 123
Valrubicin
   BCG failures, 201
   toxicity, 186
Value-added services, 23

Van Buren sounds, 90–92, 92f
Variable costs, 45–46
Varicella zoster virus, 325–326, 325f
Varicocele, 365–366
   adolescents, 499–500
   male infertility, 385
Varicose veins, 332
Vas, delivery and occlusions, elective sterilization and, 397–400, 397f–399f
Vasectomy, instrumentation of, 99
Vasectomy tray, 98f
VCDs, ED and, 350
Verruciform xanthoma, 332
Verrucous carcinoma, 335–336, 336f
Vesicoureteral reflux, in children, 505
Veterans Administrative Cooperative Research Group trial, 297
VHLD, nephron-sparing surgery and, 168
Videos, as patient education, 25–26
Vitiligo, 320
Voiding
   dysfunction
      children, 501–502
      classification, 408t
   schedules, geriatric incontinence and, 461–462
   symptoms, 80t
Von Hippel-Lindau disease (VHLD), and nephron-sparing surgery, 168
Von Willebrand's disease, 478
Vulvovaginal candidiasis, 128–129
Vytone Cream, 311

## W

Wages, 5
Waiting time
   patient expectations, 10
   standards, 5
Walther sounds, 92, 92f
Warranties, safe harbor and, 60
Welcome Package, 11
Wilms' tumor, 508
Windows NT-based operating system, 48
Women. *See* Female
Writing lay articles, 16–19

## Y

YV-plasty, male infertility and, 384

## Z

Zoloft, IC and, 137
Zoon's balanitis, 317, 317f